D0443299

NORMAL FAMILY PROCESSES

Third Edition

NORMAL FAMILY PROCESSES

Growing Diversity and Complexity

THIRD EDITION

EDITED BY

Froma Walsh

THE GUILFORD PRESS
New York/London

ABOUT THE EDITOR

Froma Walsh, MSW, PhD, is a Professor in the School of Social Service Administration and the Department of Psychiatry, Pritzker School of Medicine, and Co-Director of the Center for Family Health at the University of Chicago. She is on the Board of Directors of *Family Process,* a past editor of the *Journal of Marital and Family Therapy,* a past president of the American Family Therapy Academy, and a recipient of numerous awards for her distinguished contributions to the field of mental health. She is the author of *Strengthening Family Resilience,* editor of *Spiritual Resources in Family Therapy* and the first and second editions of *Normal Family Processes,* and coeditor of *Living beyond Loss, Women in Families,* and *Chronic Disorders and the Family.*

CONTRIBUTORS

Carol M. Anderson, MSW, PhD, Department of Psychiatry, University of Pittsburgh, Pittsburgh, PA

Edward R. Anderson, PhD, Department of Human Ecology, The University of Texas at Austin, Austin, TX

W. Robert Beavers, MD, Department of Psychiatry, University of Texas Southwestern Medical Center, and President, Family Studies Center, Dallas, TX

Duane S. Bishop, MD, Department of Psychiatry and Human Behavior, Brown University, Providence, RI

Nancy Boyd-Franklin, PhD, Graduate School of Applied and Professional Psychology, Rutgers University, Busch Campus, Piscataway, NJ

Betty Carter, MSW, Founder and Director Emerita, Family Institute of Westchester, Harrison, NY

Carolyn Pape Cowan, PhD, Department of Psychology and the Institute of Human Development, University of California at Berkeley, Berkeley, CA

Philip A. Cowan, PhD, Department of Psychology and the Institute of Human Development, University of California at Berkeley, Berkeley, CA

David S. DeGarmo, PhD, Oregon Social Learning Center, Eugene, OR

Janice Driver, PhD candidate, Department of Psychology, University of Washington, Seattle, WA

Marina Eovaldi, PhD, The Family Institute, Northwestern University, Evanston, IL

Nathan E. Epstein, MD, Department of Psychiatry and Human Behavior, Brown University, Providence, RI

Celia Jaes Falicov, PhD, Department of Psychiatry, University of California at San Diego, San Diego, CA

Marion S. Forgatch, PhD, Oregon Social Learning Center, Eugene, OR

Peter Fraenkel, PhD, Doctoral Subprogram in Clinical Psychology, The City University of New York; Director, Center for Time, Work, and the Family, Ackerman Institute for the Family, New York, NY

Dean M. Gorall, PhD, Family Social Science, University of Minnesota, Minneapolis, MN

John M. Gottman, PhD, Department of Psychology, University of Washington, Seattle, WA

Shannon M. Greene, PhD, Department of Human Ecology, The University of Texas at Austin, Austin, TX

Shelley A. Haddock, PhD, Human Development and Family Studies Department, Colorado State University, Fort Collins, CO

Robert B. Hampson, PhD, Department of Psychology, Southern Methodist University, Dallas, TX

Ann Hartman, DSW, Smith College School for Social Work, Northampton, MA

E. Mavis Hetherington, PhD, Department of Psychology, University of Virginia, Charlottesville, VA

Gabor I. Keitner, MD, Department of Psychiatry and Human Behavior, Brown University, Providence, RI

Joan Laird, MS, Smith College School for Social Work, Northampton, MA

Kevin P. Lyness, PhD, Human Development and Family Studies Department, Colorado State University, Fort Collins, CO

Cassandra Ma, PsyD, The Family Institute, Northwestern University, Evanston, IL

Monica McGoldrick, MSW, The Multicultural Family Institute, Highland Park, NJ

Ivan W. Miller, PhD, Department of Psychiatry and Human Behavior, Brown University, Providence, RI

Eun Young Nahm, PhD candidate, Department of Psychology, University of Washington, Seattle, WA

David H. Olson, PhD, Life Innovations, Minneapolis, MN

Kay Pasley, EdD, Human Development and Family Studies, University of North Carolina at Greensboro, Greensboro, NC

Julia Pryce, MSW, School of Social Service Administration, University of Chicago, Chicago, IL

Cheryl Rampage, PhD, The Family Institute, Northwestern University, Evanston, IL

David Reiss, MD, Department of Psychiatry, George Washington University Medical Center, Washington, DC

John S. Rolland, MD, Department of Psychiatry and Center for Family Health, University of Chicago, Chicago, IL

Christine E. Ryan, PhD, Department of Psychiatry and Human Behavior, Brown University, Providence, RI

Alyson Shapiro, PhD candidate, Department of Psychology, University of Washington, Seattle, WA

Erica Spotts, PhD, Department of Medical Epidemiology, Karolinska Institutet, Stockholm, Sweden

Amber Tabares, PhD candidate, Department of Psychology, University of Washington, Seattle, WA

Hilary Towers, PhD, Center for Family Research, George Washington University Medical Center, Washington, DC

Emily B. Visher, PhD (deceased), California School of Professional Psychology, Alameda, CA

John S. Visher, MD, Department of Psychiatry, Stanford University, Stanford, CA

Froma Walsh, PhD, School of Social Service Administration, Department of Psychiatry, and Center for Family Health, University of Chicago, Chicago, IL

Catherine Weigel-Foy, MSW, The Family Institute, Northwestern University, Evanston, IL

Toni Schindler Zimmerman, PhD, Human Development and Family Studies Department, Colorado State University, Fort Collins, CO

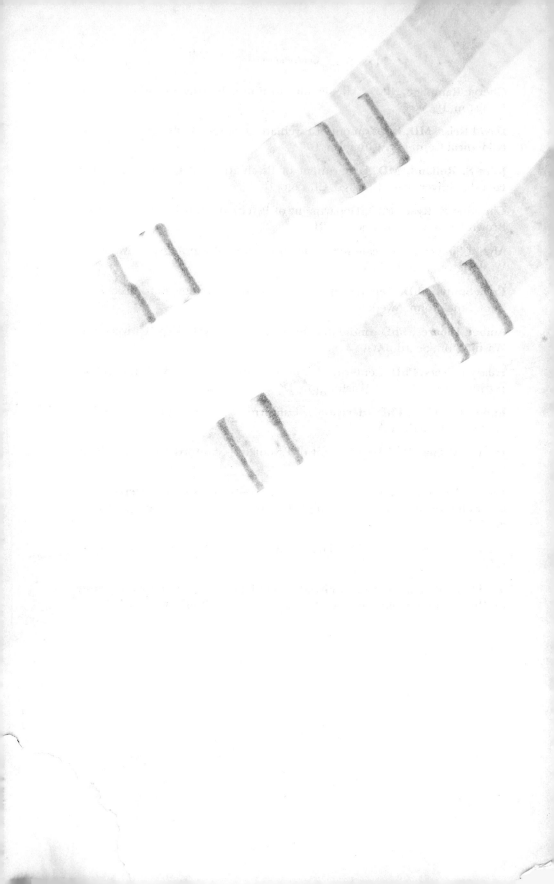

PREFACE

What is a normal family in the 21st century? With the growing diversity and complexity of families in our rapidly changing world, no single model of normality and health fits most families; a pluralistic view is required. Drawing on the latest research, this volume illuminates our understanding of the strengths and challenges in the broad spectrum of normal families in our times.

The first edition of *Normal Family Processes*, published in 1982, was hailed as a landmark volume in the clinical literature. With traditional mental health training and practice focused on family deficits and blind to family strengths, I remarked then, only half-jokingly, that a normal family might be defined as one that had not yet been clinically assessed! This groundbreaking text was the first to examine normality from a family systems orientation, presenting pioneering research and conceptualization of family normality and health. Offering a fresh perspective on "nonclinical" families, the book proved to be widely influential in rebalancing the skewed clinical focus that had tended to pathologize families. In the following decade, the field of family therapy shifted attention to greater recognition and fostering of family strengths. The second edition of *Normal Family Processes*, in 1993, presented advances made by leading researchers and clinical scholars in the conceptualization and assessment of family functioning and gave greater attention to the increasing diversity of families as well.

This third edition updates and expands our knowledge and perspectives on well-functioning families as family life and societies worldwide have become more diverse and complex. Most scholars and clinicians have moved a healthy distance beyond the simplistic quest to discover—or recover—a universal blueprint for healthy family functioning and to mold families to fit that standard. Additionally, postmodern theory has heightened awareness that views of normality are socially constructed, influenced by cultural and professional values and biases. Nevertheless, it is imperative to examine notions of normality because they still profoundly influence family assessment, intervention, social policy, and the popular media. Families still tend to be pathologized and stigmatized when they don't conform to the reified standard of "the normal family"—a mythical ideal of the so-called "traditional" middle-class, intact, nuclear family of the 1950s, headed by a breadwinner-father and supported by a full-time homemaker-mother. Clinicians, and families themselves, too often set unrealistic or inappropriate goals to meet this standard, reinforcing a sense of failure and deficiency. Chapters in this volume are attuned to the changing landscape of families today, whose cultural and personal beliefs, structural arrangements, socioeconomic conditions, gender roles, sexual orientation, and life-cycle patterns are so varied. Based on a growing body of research, the authors reveal that healthy functioning can be found—and fostered by clinicians—in a variety of family forms; what matters most are family processes that nurture and sustain caring, secure, and committed relationships.

The authors in this new edition are at the forefront of research, knowledge building, and clinical training. They present the latest data, identify trends, and offer useful frameworks to guide intervention and prevention efforts to reduce family vulnerabilities and build family strengths. As in the earlier editions, contributors have been selected because of their significant contributions to clinically relevant theory and research. In Part I, I present a conceptual overview, grounding the volume in a systemic framework, with ecological and developmental perspectives on family processes and healthy functioning. Emerging trends in contemporary family life are highlighted and considered in sociohistorical and cross-cultural contexts. Clinical views of normal and healthy family functioning are examined as they relate to formulations of dysfunction and influence therapeutic goals. Recommendations for clinical practice, training, and research are offered. Recent developments in strengths-based approaches to family therapy are noted, and the advantages of a family resilience framework for intervention and prevention are suggested.

Parts II, III, and IV address the diversity and complexity of patterns of family functioning relevant to varying structural forms, sociocultural contexts, and developmental challenges. Family risk, coping, adaptation, and resilience are considered in relation to intrafamilial and environmental stressors. As the chapters demonstrate, some family patterns and adaptive strategies may be more functional than others in mastering a particular set of challenges—be it stepfamily integration, immigration, or conditions of poverty and racism. Drawing on research and clinical experience, two questions frame the discussion: (1) What are the "normal"—that is, expectable, typical—challenges and responses associated with various conditions? (2) Can we identify key family processes that promote coping and mastery of life challenges (e.g., in successful single-parent families, in optimal functioning and well-being with serious illness or disability)?

In Part II, Varying Family Forms and Challenges, topics include navigating work and family challenges in two-parent families, by Peter

Fraenkel; risk and resilience after divorce, by Mavis Hetherington's research team; single-parent households, by Carol Anderson; remarriage and stepparenting, by Emily B. and John S. Visher and Kay Pasley; lesbian and gay families, by Joan Laird; and adoptive families, by Cheryl Rampage and her colleagues. In Part III, Cultural Dimensions in Family Functioning, the topics are culture and normality, by Monica McGoldrick; race, class, and poverty, by Nancy Boyd-Franklin; immigrant families, by Celia Jaes Falicov; changing gender norms, by Shelley Haddock and her colleagues; and the spiritual dimension of family life, by Froma Walsh and Julia Pryce. In Part IV, Developmental Perspectives on Family Functioning, topics include the family life cycle, by Monica McGoldrick and Betty Carter; family resilience, by Froma Walsh; normal family transitions and healthy child development, by Philip A. and Carolyn Pape Cowan; and family challenges with illness and disability, by John S. Rolland.

In Part V, pioneering family systems investigators present and update their research findings, offer assessment tools, and identify key processes that distinguish well-functioning couples and families. Chapter subjects include interactional patterns in marital success or failure, by John M. Gottman's research team; David H. Olson's Circumplex Model for couple and family assessment; the Beavers Systems Model; Nathan B. Epstein and his colleagues' McMaster Model of Family Functioning; and the groundbreaking research by David Reiss and his colleagues on the complex intertwining of genetic and environmental influences on family relationships. In Part VI, Ann Hartman's chapter examines societal constructions of family normality, their influence on recent family policy developments, and the opportunities and challenges ahead if we are to support families in their efforts to thrive.

This volume is designed to serve as a basic textbook in clinical training for social workers, marriage and family therapists, psychologists, counselors, and psychiatrists; as a sourcebook for practitioners in a wide range of mental health, healthcare, and human service professions; for scholars and students in the social sciences; and for those formulating family policy in public and private arenas. It is intended as a resource for all who strive to improve the quality of family life and the well-being of all members, from the newborn to the eldest. It provides up-to-date, essential knowledge and perspectives for all who want to gain an understanding of contemporary families, their strengths, and their challenges. The valuable contributions in this volume, all by distinguished authors at the forefront of the field, can inform and enrich intervention and prevention efforts, family research, social policy, and program planning, shifting focus from how families fail to how they can succeed.

In the aftermath of the terrorist attacks of September 11, 2001, our very conception of normality has been fundamentally altered. We question assumptions and reaffirm values, we reexamine our identity and connections to others in our shared world, and we try to adapt to a more uncertain and insecure future. Mastering these challenges will require great wisdom and humanity in the years ahead. Notably, one finding has stood out among the widespread responses: a heightened appreciation of the significance of family bonds—in their diversity and complexity—as mattering above all else in people's lives. In these troubled times, more than ever, I share with all the authors an appreciation of the families we have been privileged to know and learn from, who do their best to love well as they face life's adversities, forging their own adaptive pathways.

ACKNOWLEDGMENTS

On behalf of all the authors, I would like to express our gratitude to the many ordinary and extraordinary families who have informed our research and enriched our teaching and practice. We are also indebted to our own families, who have grounded us in the reality of the myriad challenges we all must navigate to sustain loving relationships. I am grateful to Allison Werner-Lin, my research assistant, for her keen eye and mind in surveying emerging census data and literature. I want to thank the staff at The Guilford Press for their support in the production of this volume and for their conviction that a third edition is, indeed, timely and needed. I have most appreciated the wise counsel and thoughtful feedback offered by Jim Nageotte and the stunning cover designed by Paul Gordon, who captured the essence of the diversity, centrality, and enduring value of families in our lives.

We were saddened by the death, last fall, of our highly esteemed colleague Emily B. Visher, who was a valued contributor to all three editions of this volume. She and her husband, John, were early pioneers in the study of stepfamilies and founders of the Stepfamily Association of America. Ahead of her times, she was a woman of uncommon wisdom, courage, and grace. This book is dedicated to her memory.

CONTENTS

PART I

Overview

CHAPTER 1

CHANGING FAMILIES IN A CHANGING WORLD
Reconstructing Family Normality

Froma Walsh

> All happy families are alike; every unhappy family is
> unhappy in its own way.
> —TOLSTOY

> All happy families are more or less dissimilar; all unhappy
> ones are more or less alike.
> —NABOKOV

The first edition of this volume (Walsh, 1982) posed the question, "What is a normal family?" Many believed that Tolstoy was right: that families must conform to one model to be happy and raise their children well. The second edition (Walsh, 1993) grappled with the dilemmas in defining family normality, with their growing diversity and the recognition that "normality" is socially constructed. Over the past two decades, families have become increasingly varied and complex. Despite the dire predictions of family demise by single model advocates, it appears that Nabokov got it right: Research attests to the potential for healthy functioning in a variety of family arrangements. In the turmoil of our rapidly changing world, families in their rich diversity are more important than ever. As Maya Angelou put it, "The ache for home lives in all of us; the safe place where we can go. . . ." Yet families today face unprecedented challenges that need to be understood and addressed.

This overview chapter seeks to advance our knowledge of the diversity and complexity of contemporary families. First, we consider the social construction of family normality and clarify four major perspectives from the clinical field and the social sciences. The value of a systems orientation is highlighted, to understand "normal" family processes in terms of typical and optimal family functioning. Next, we survey the emerging trends and challenges for families, examining the myths of idealized family models and actual family patterns from sociohistorical and multicultural perspectives. Chapter 2 examines the implications for clinical practice, family research, and social policy.

WHAT IS A NORMAL FAMILY?

The Social Construction of Normality

Clinicians and family scholars have become increasingly aware that definitions of normality are socially constructed, influenced by subjective worldviews and by the larger culture (Gergen, 1991; Hoffman, 1990). Family therapists have become wary of the term "normal," taking to heart Foucault's (1980) criticism that too often in history, theories of normality have been constructed by dominant groups, reified by religion or science, and used to pathologize or oppress others who do not fit ideal standards.

The very concept of the family has been undergoing redefinition as tumultuous social and economic changes of recent decades have altered the landscape of family life (Coontz, 1997). Societies worldwide are experiencing rapid transformation and uncertainties about the future. Amid the turmoil, couples and families have been forging new and varied arrangements as they strive to build caring and committed relationships. These efforts are made more difficult by questions about their normality. Therefore, our current conceptualizations of normal family processes— both typical and optimal—must take into account the changing views of changing families in a changing world.

Although some might argue that the subjectivity of any constructions of normality, along with the growing complexity and diversity of families, make it impossible or unwise to address the topic at all, this very subjectivity makes it all the more imperative. Notions of normality sanction and privilege certain family arrangements while stigmatizing and marginalizing others. They powerfully influence all clinical theory, practice, research, and policy. It is crucial to be aware of the explicit and implicit assumptions about normal families that are embedded in our cultural, professional, and personal belief systems.

Perspectives on Family Normality

The definition of family normality is also problematic in that the term "normal" is used to refer to quite different concepts, from varying frames of reference, influenced by the subjective position of the observer and the surrounding culture. The label may hold quite different meanings to a clinician, a researcher, or a family concerned about its own normality. Our language confounds understanding when such terms as "healthy," "typical," and "functional" are used interchangeably with the label "normal." In an overview of concepts of mental health in the clinical and social science literature, Offer and Sabshin (1974) were struck by the varied definitions of a "normal" person. Building on their synthesis of views of individual normality, four perspectives can be usefully distinguished to clarify conceptions of a normal family (Walsh, 1982, 1993): (1) normal as asymptomatic; (2) normal as typical, average; (3) normal as ideal; and (4) normal in relation to systemic transactional processes.

Normal Families as Asymptomatic

From this clinical perspective grounded in the medical/psychiatric model, the judgment of normality is based on a negative criterion: the absence of pathology. Therefore, a family is regarded as normal—and healthy—if there are no symptoms of disorder in any member. This perspective is limited by its deficit-based skew and inattention to positive attributes of family well-being. Healthy family functioning involves more than the absence of problems and can be found in the midst of problems, as in family resilience (Walsh, 1998; see also Chapter 15, this volume). As Minuchin (1974) has emphasized, no families are problem-free. Thus, the presence of distress is not necessarily an indication of family pathology. Similarly, freedom from symptoms is rare: Kleinman (1988) reported that, at any given time, 75% of all people are "symptomatic," experiencing physical or psychological distress. Most do not seek treatment but instead define it as part of normal life.

Another problem lies in the common assumption that an individual disorder is invariably a symptom of family dysfunction. It is erroneous to presume that all individual problems are necessarily symptomatic of—and caused by—a dysfunctional family. Conversely, it cannot be assumed that a healthy person is the product of a healthy family. Studies of resilience find many healthy individuals who successfully overcome the adversities of growing up in seriously troubled families (see Walsh, 1996).

Further problems arise when therapy is used as the marker for family health or dysfunction, such as when researchers compare clinical and nonclinical families as disturbed and normal samples. Simply because no family member is in treatment, we cannot presume that a family is healthy. "Nonclinical" families are a heterogeneous group spanning the entire range of functioning. What is defined as a problem and whether help is sought vary with different family and cultural norms; worrisome conflict in one family might be considered a healthy airing of differences in another. A troubled family may not seek therapy or may attempt to handle problems in other ways, such as through kin support or religion. Conversely, as mental health professionals are the first to avow, seeking help can be a sign of health.

Normal Families as Typical, Average

From this perspective, a family is viewed as normal if it fits patterns that are common or expectable in ordinary families. This approach has been widely used by social scientists, with statistical measures of frequency or central tendency. In the normal distribution (or bell-shaped curve), the middle range on a continuum is taken as normal and both extremes as deviant. Thus, by definition, families deviating from the norm are "abnormal." Unfortunately, the negative connotations of deviance lead to the pathologizing of difference. Note also that from this perspective, an optimally functioning family would be abnormal (i.e., atypical). This approach disengages the concept of normality from health and absence of symptoms. Family patterns that are common are not necessarily healthy and may even be destructive, as in violence. Moreover, because average families have occasional problems, this would not in itself signal family abnormality/pathology.

Normal Families as Ideal, Healthy

This perspective on normality defines a *healthy* family in terms of ideal traits for optimal functioning. A well-functioning family is seen as successful in accomplishing family tasks and promoting the growth and well-being of individual members. We must be cautious about standards of healthy families derived from clinical theory based on inference from disturbed cases. The pervasiveness of cultural ideals must also be considered. Social norms of the ideal family are culturally constructed values that prescribe how families ought to be. A certain range of conduct and particular family form and roles are considered desirable, or even essential, according to prevailing standards in the dominant society. Yet ideals may vary with particular ethnic or religious values. Moreover, unconventional family arrangements may be optimal for the functioning of a particular family in its context.

It is crucial not to conflate concepts of normal as typical and normal as ideal. Talcott Parsons's influential studies of "the normal family" in the 1950s made a theoretical leap from description of a sample of typical white, middle-class, suburban, nuclear families to the prescription of those patterns, such as rigid gender roles, as universal and essential for the healthy development of offspring (Parsons & Bales, 1955). Psychiatrists then extrapolated from that model to hold that deviation from those patterns is inherently pathogenic for children, even contributing to schizophrenia (Lidz, 1963; Lidz, Fleck, & Cornelison, 1965). Such pathologizing of differences from the norm—either typical or ideal—stigmatizes families that do not conform to the standard, such as single-parent and gay and lesbian families (see Part II, this volume).

Normal Family Processes

This perspective, grounded in systems theory, considers both typical and optimal functioning in terms of basic processes in human systems, dependent on an interaction of biopsychosocial variables (Bertalanffy, 1968; Grinker, 1967). Viewing functioning in developmental and cultural contexts, this approach allows for unique coping styles and multiple adaptational pathways. This transactional view attends to ongoing processes *over time* (Wynne, 1988). In contrast, others have generally sought to identify fixed traits of a so-called normal family—thought of as a static, timeless entity or viewed cross-sectionally at a single point in time.

Normal functioning is conceptualized in terms of basic patterns of interaction (Bateson, 1979; Watzlawick, Beavin, & Jackson, 1967). Such processes support the integration and maintenance of the family unit and its ability to carry out essential tasks for the growth and well-being of its members, such as the nurturance and protection of children, elders, and other vulnerable members. Families develop their own internal norms, expressed through explicit and unspoken relationship rules (Jackson, 1965). Conveyed in family stories and ongoing transactions, a relatively small set of patterned and predictable rules regulate family processes and provide expectations about roles, actions, and consequences. Family belief systems are shared values and assumptions that provide meaning and organize experience in the social world and guide family life (Hess & Handel, 1959; Reiss, 1981). Cultural and religious values strongly influence family norms (Spiegel, 1971; McGoldrick, Giordano, & Pearce, 1996; see McGoldrick, Chapter 9, Walsh and Pryce, Chapter 13, this volume, and Walsh, 1999b).

A *biopsychosocial systems orientation* takes into account the multiple, recursive influences in individual and family functioning. Thus, there is no simple 1:1 correlation between individual and family health or dysfunction. A disturbed child is not necessarily the product of a dysfunctional family; genetic/biological vulnerabilities and larger social influences must be assessed (Reiss, Hetherington, Plomin, & Neiderhiser, 2000; see Towers et al., Chapter 22, this volume). From an ecosystemic perspective (Bronfenbrenner, 1979; Keeney & Sprenkle, 1982), each family's capabilities and coping style are considered in relation to the needs of individual members and to the larger social systems in which the family is embedded. Successful family functioning is dependent on the *fit,* or compatibility, between the family, its individual members, and other social systems. Family distress is viewed in context: It may be generated by internal stressors, such as the strain of coping with an illness, and complicated by external influences, such as inadequate health care (see Rolland, Chapter 17, this volume).

A *family life-cycle framework* considers processes in the multigenerational system as it moves forward over time (Carter & McGoldrick, 1999; see McGoldrick & Carter, Chapter 14, this volume). Normal family development is conceptualized in terms of adaptational processes that involve mastery of life-stage tasks and transitional stress (Duvall, 1977). The concept of normal as typical is useful systemically to describe expectable strains and transactional patterns over the course of the family life cycle. Optimal family processes vary with different developmental demands and structural configurations. For example, high cohesion is optimal in rearing small children but shifts in adolescence toward more autonomy (see Olson & Gorall, Chapter 19, this volume).

Normative stressors are those that are common and predictable (Boss, 2001). It is normal, and not necessarily indicative of family pathology, for disruption to be experienced with major transitions, such as the birth of the first child (see Cowan & Cowan, Chapter 16, this volume). Non-normative stressors, which are uncommon, unexpected, or "off-time" in the life cycle (Neugarten, 1976), tend to be more traumatic for families, as in the untimely death of a child. Family distress at such times is to be expected (i.e., normal, typical). Strains may be worsened by a pileup of stressors, or barriers of poverty and racism (see Boyd-Franklin, Chapter 10, this volume). How the family responds as a functional unit is critical for recovery (Harway, 1996; Walsh & McGoldrick, 1991). Many adaptational pathways are possible, with healthier families thought to use a larger variety of coping techniques, more effective problem-solving strategies, and more flexibility in dealing with internal and external life events. More recent work has sought to understand better the key elements in family resilience (McCubbin, McCubbin, McCubbin, & Futrell, 1998; McCubbin, McCubbin, Thompson, & Fromer, 1998; Walsh, 1998; see Walsh, Chapter 15, this volume).

In summary, the integration of systemic and developmental perspectives forms an overarching framework for considering normality. The definition of average and optimal family processes is contingent on both social and developmental contexts. What is normal—either typical or optimal— varies with different internal and external demands posing challenges for both continuity and change over the course of the family life cycle (Falicov, 1988). This developmental systems paradigm provides a common foundation for family therapy and family process research, and for the conceptual models by contributors to the present volume.

It is important also to clarify the terms "functional" and "dysfunctional," which have commonly replaced more value-laden labels of "normal" and "pathological." Functional essentially means workable. It refers to the utility of family patterns in achieving family goals, including instrumental tasks, such as problem solving, and the socioemotional well-being of family members. Whether processes are functional is contingent on each family's aims—involving family members' beliefs about normality and health, as well as situational and life-stage demands, resources, and sociocultural influences. Thus, the goodness of fit is crucial.

Dysfunctional, in a purely descriptive sense, simply refers to family patterns that are not working and associated with symptoms of distress—regardless of a problem's source. However, the term "dysfunctional" has come to connote serious disturbance and causal attributions that tend to pathologize families and blame them for individual and social problems. Popular self-help and recovery movements abound for "survivors" of dysfunctional families (Kaminer, 1992). Because individual problems are not invariably caused by family pathology, caution is urged in labeling families, distinguishing those with serious disturbance, abuse, and neglect from most families that are struggling with ordinary problems in living. It is preferable, and less stigmatizing, to identify particular family patterns, or processes, as dysfunctional rather than to label the family.

When a family pattern is deemed functional, we need to consider what is meant: functional to what end and for whom? A pattern may be functional at one systems level but dysfunctional at another. As a classic example, interactional rules that stabilize a fragile couple relationship (e.g., conflict avoidance) may have dysfunctional consequences for a child who becomes the go-between. Furthermore, assessment of family functioning must not be limited to the interior of the family but must also evaluate available resources and the impact of other systems. For instance, workplace policies deemed necessary for productivity are too often detrimental for families (see Fraenkel, Chapter 3, this volume). Dual-earner and single-parent households experience tremendous role strain with the pressures of multiple, conflicting demands and inadequate resources. Many parents manage to keep their families intact and their children functional only at a high cost to couple relationships and personal well-being.

BEYOND THE MYTHS OF THE NORMAL FAMILY: THE CHANGING LANDSCAPE OF FAMILY LIFE

In a cultural climate of uncertainty about the future of the family, anxiety has focused on supposed deficits in families that deviate from idealized normal family images of the past. The family has been regarded as the linchpin of the social order (Hareven, 2000). Yet controversy and change have surrounded the definition of the family throughout our history, especially in times of transition (Skolnick, 1991). Other generations, too, have worried about the breakdown of the "traditional family," a popular image at the time of what families were supposed to be like, but by no means a correct recollection of the past. Fears of the demise of the family have escalated in periods of social turbulence, as in our times, fueling nostalgia for return to families of the past.

As societies have been changing dramatically, cherished myths of the traditional family have persisted, lagging behind emerging social realities, yet exerting a powerful influence. In the United States, two eras have become idealized in our "normal family" folklore: the extended family of the preindustrial past and the modern nuclear family of the 1950s. Just as storytelling has served in every age and culture to transmit family norms, since the mid-20th century, television—now beamed by satellite to the most remote parts of the world—has become the prime medium for transmitting family folklore, both shaping and reflecting the values and beliefs of the dominant culture. Series such as "Little House on the Prairie" transported viewers back to the distant past, to a simpler time of large families, homespun values, and multigenerational connectedness. Family life portrayed in such shows as "Ozzie and Harriet" and "Leave it to Beaver" exemplified the more recent "tradition" of the middle-class nuclear family, headed by the breadwinner father and supported by the homemaker mother. The lasting popularity of such images expresses longing for not only a romanticized notion of the family but also simpler, happier, and more secure times (Coontz, 1993). A sociohistorical lens offers a valuable perspective on the challenges and future directions of families in the 21st century.

Changing Families in a Changing World

Our understanding of family functioning and our approaches to strengthen families must be relevant to our times and viewed in sociohistorical context. The norms and structures of societies worldwide are in transformation. As our world grows increasingly complex and unpredictable, families face unprecedented challenges. With profound social and economic upheavals over recent decades, families and the world around them are changing at an accelerated pace (Teachman, Tedrow, & Crowder, 2000). At the forefront of emerging trends are the following:

- Varied family forms
- Changing gender roles
- Cultural diversity and socioeconomic disparity
- Varying and expanded family life-cycle course

Varied Family Forms

The idealized image of intact, multigenerational family households of the preindustrial past distorts their actual instability and diversity (Hareven, 2000). Family patterns were no more orderly and stable than today's complex and varied family structures and roles. In fact, family transitions were more unpredictable due to many life uncertainties, particularly unplanned pregnancies and untimely death. The risk of not growing up in an intact family was high. Family units were commonly disrupted by early parental death, which led to remarriage and stepfamilies, or to child placements with extended family, foster care, or orphanages. Most families now have greater control over options and timing of marriage and parenting, largely due to birth control and medical advances that have increased life expectancy.

Family households in the past were quite diverse and complex, as continues to be true in most parts of the world. Their flexibility enabled resilience in weathering instabilities. Households commonly included nonkin boarders, providing surrogate families for individuals on their own and facilitating adaptation of new immigrants, as well as income and companionship for widows and the elderly (Aries, 1962). In many cultures, it is still expected that a brother will marry the widow of a deceased husband, making their future children both cousins and half-siblings of his own children by another marriage. Actually, the current proliferation of diverse family arrangements and informal support networks, although termed "nontraditional family forms," continues this tradition. For instance, when two single parents combine households and resources, they strengthen their family functioning.

The nuclear family structure arose with the industrial era and peaked in the 1950s. The household comprised an intact, two-parent family unit headed by a male breadwinner and supported by his full-time homemaker wife, who devoted herself to household management, raising children, and elder care. Many mistake this model for an essential, and now endangered, institution, when it was actually peculiar to its times (Skolnick & Skolnick, 1992). Following the Great Depression and World War II, prosperity was fueled by a strong postwar economy and government benefits that provided for education, jobs, and home ownership, enabling most families to live comfortably on one income. After a steady decline in the birth rate, couples married younger and in greater numbers, producing the "baby boom."

In earlier eras, the family fulfilled a broad array of economic, educational, social, and religious functions intertwined with the larger community. Relationships were valued for a variety of contributions to the collective family unit. The modern nuclear family household, fitting the resurgent ethos of the rugged individual, was expected to be self-reliant within the borders of its white picket fence. It became a rigid, closed system, isolated from extended kin and community connections that had been sources of adaptability. It also lost the flexibility and diversity that had enabled households to reconfigure according to need. Marital disillusionment also resulted from unrealistically high expectations for spouses to fulfill all needs for romantic love, support, and companionship. Yet nostalgia for the stability, security, and prosperity of those times is understandable.

Today, the idealized 1950s model of the white, middle-class, intact nuclear family, headed by a breadwinner father and supported by a homemaker mother, is only a narrow band on the broad spectrum of normal families (Teachman et al., 2000). In its place, a diverse reshaping of contemporary family life, termed the "postmodern family" (Stacey, 1990), is a hodgepodge of multiple, evolving family cultures and structures: working mothers and two-earner households; divorced, single-parent, remarried, and adoptive families; and domestic partners, both gay and straight.

Dual-earner families now comprise over two-thirds of all two-parent households (Barnett & Rivers, 1996; see Fraenkel, Chapter 3, this volume). Two paychecks have become essential for most families to maintain a modest standard of living. Traditional gender role divisions are no longer typical, as women's career aspirations, divorce, and economic pressures have brought over 70% of all mothers into the workforce. By choice, and even more, by necessity, most mothers (married and single-parent) are currently in the workforce—nearly three-fourths of mothers of school-age children; over two-thirds of mothers of preschool children. Flexible work schedules and affordable, quality child care are still difficult to obtain, in contrast to most European societies, which provide generous benefits and services to support families of working parents.

More people are living on their own as the number of single adults has nearly doubled over the past two decades. At the same time, more young adults live with their parents, delaying launching or returning home for financial reasons. Marriage and childbearing are being postponed. The average age at marriage is 27 for men and 25 for women, up from ages 22 and 20, respectively, in 1960. The number of unmarried couples living together has risen dramatically to nearly 9% of all unions. Nearly half of all adults live in a cohabiting relationship without marriage at some time in their lives. Although many go on to marry, others break up within 3 years. When there are children, instability in such relationships increases the risk of adjustment problems.

Single-parent households—including families headed by unmarried and divorced parents—have become increasingly common. Nearly half of all children—and over 60% of poor minority children—are expected to live at least part of their childhood in a single-parent household (Bumpass & Raley, 1995; see Anderson, Chapter 5, this volume). Single mothers head 25% of all households (up from 5% in 1960) and over half of African American families (Cherlin, 1998). Growing numbers of older, more financially secure single adults, both straight and gay, have been choosing single parenthood through adoption and a variety of reproductive strategies (Seltzer, 2000). Unwed teen pregnancy, a growing concern a decade ago, has declined. At the same time, it has become increasingly common for grandparents, especially grandmothers, to assume primary caregiver roles for their grandchildren when parents are unable to provide such care (Minkler & Roe, 1993).

Adoptive families have also been on the rise for single parents as well as couples (see Rampage et al., Chapter 8, this volume). Most adoptions are now open, based on findings that children benefit psychologically and developmentally if they know who their birth families are, have the option for contact, and especially in biracial and international adoptions, are encouraged to connect with cultural traditions (Pertman, 2000). In foster care, permanency in placement is seen as optimal, keeping siblings together and with extended kin wherever possible, and avoiding the instability and losses in multiple placements (Ehrle & Geen, 2002).

Postdivorce and remarriage families have become typical. Divorce rates, after climbing rapidly in the 1970s and 1980s, have leveled off at just under 50% for first marriages (Bramlett & Mosher, 2001; Goldstein, 1999). The vast majority of divorced individuals go on to remarry, making stepfamilies increasingly common (Ganong & Coleman, 1999; see Visher et al., Chapter 6, this volume). Yet the complexity of stepfamily integration contributes to a divorce rate of nearly 60% of remarriages. Claims that divorce inevitably damages all children, based on small, nonrepresentative clinical samples (e.g., Wallerstein, Lewis, & Blakeslee, 2000) have not been substantiated in large-scale, carefully controlled research (Amato, 2000; Booth & Amato, 2001; Furstenberg & Cherlin, 1991; Hetherington & Kelly, 2002; see Greene et al., Chapter 4, this volume). Although some studies have found more problems in children of divorced families than those in intact families (23% compared to 12%), Hetherington and colleagues have found that the vast majority of children—over 75%—do reasonably well after divorce, and many do very well. They have tracked family patterns associated with successful adaptation versus dysfunction in the predivorce climate, through divorce processes, subsequent reorganization, and later stepfamily integration. In high-conflict families, children tend to do better in cases of divorce than those in families that remain intact. Moreover, other factors, such as economic strain and a noncustodial parent's cutoff, are critical variables that can make a difference. Most studies conclude that children's healthy development depends most on the quality of relationships with and between parents.

Although family structures are changing dramatically, people still view a loving, committed relationship as one of the most important sources of life happiness (Waite & Gallagher, 2000), and nearly 90% legally marry at least once by the age of 50. Growing numbers will marry more than once in their lifetime or form committed partnerships without legal remarriage, often in later life (see Greene et al., Chapter 4, this volume). The social movement for gay and lesbian rights has brought increasing visibility and advocacy for the normalization and legalization of same-sex domestic partners (see Laird, Chapter 7, this volume). Most people want to share their lives with a partner and seek an intimate relationship that provides comfort, intimacy, and long-term companionship.

Yet our language and preconceptions about "the normal family" can pathologize relationship patterns that do not conform to the model. Despite the growing involvement of fathers and the active contributions to family life by grandparents and other caregivers, it is still widely assumed that they stand in for a working or absent mother, whose influence is seen as primary for the well-being of children. The label "latchkey child" implies *maternal* neglect when parents must work. The term "single-parent family" can blind us to the involvement or potential contribution of a non-custodial parent. A stepparent or adoptive parent relationship is viewed as inherently deficient when framed as not the "real" or "natural" parent. One judge denied a parental rights request by a lesbian woman, who shared parenting for her partner's biological child, on the grounds that it would be too confusing for a child to have two mothers. Similar preconceptions also disenfranchise stepparents and adoptive parents. However, gains are being made in broadening conceptions of the family. In one landmark court decision supporting gay parental rights, the judge concluded: "It is the totality of the relationship, as evidenced by the dedication, caring, and self-sacrifice of the parties which should, in the final analysis, control the definition of family" (cited in Stacey, 1990, p. 4). In another landmark decision in 2002, the American Pediatric Association endorsed the rights of gay and lesbian parents to adopt children, citing the large body of research finding that children in these families fare as well psychologically and socially as those raised by heterosexual parents.

As Sussman, Steinmetz, and Peterson (1999) conclude, it no longer makes sense to use the nuclear family as the standard against which various forms of the family are measured. We need to be mindful that families in the distant past and in most cultures worldwide have had multiple, varied structures. It is unfortunate when discourse is framed as "profamily" versus "antifamily" positions, attacking those who hold a pluralistic view of viable relationship options (Ahrons, 1994). A growing body of research finds that healthy family processes for caring, committed relationships matter more than family form for effective functioning and the well-being of children (Demo & Acock, 1996; Lansford, Ceballo, Abby, & Stewart, 2001; Stacey & Biblarz, 2001).

Changing Gender Roles and Rules

In viewing recent structural changes in the family as part of a historical continuum, the changing status of women emerges as the major ongoing dynamic from the end of the Victorian era to the present (Risman, 1999). Over the centuries (and still today in many cultures), marriage was viewed in functional terms: Matches were made by families on the basis of economic and social position, with wives and children the property of their husbands and fathers. The family patriarch held authority over the women and children, controlling all major decisions and resources. For the husband to be certain of his (male) heirs, the honor of the family required the absolute fidelity of the wife and the chastity of marriageable daughters. This value has been enforced in many Arab societies, for instance, through the veiling and cloistering of women in the household, and in some African cultures, through rites of genital mutilation of young girls, so that sex will never be a pleasurable temptation. In many patriarchal societies, polygamy has been considered the normal family arrangement. The husband, his co-wives, and their many children often live together in one household, and a man's social status is enhanced with each wife, whose status, as well, increases with the birth of each son.

Although families had many more children in the past, women invested relatively less parenting time, contributing to the shared family economy in varied ways, from weaving to bookkeeping. Fathers, older children, extended kin, and neighbors all participated actively in child rearing. The integration of family and work life allowed for intensive sharing of labor between husbands and wives, and parents and children. Industrialization and urbanization brought a redefinition of gender roles and functions. Family work and "productive" paid work became segregated into separate gendered spheres of home and workplace (Bernard, 1982). Domesticity became glorified, assigning to women exclusively the roles of custodian of the hearth, nurturer of the young, and caretaker of the old. Particularly in North American and British societies, the maternal role came to be reified to such an extent that mothers have been regarded as the primary, essential, and irreplaceable caregivers, responsible for the healthy development of children and blamed for any and all child and family problems (Braverman, 1989). Yet women's unpaid domestic work was devalued and rendered invisible, with their total dependency on the financial support of male breadwinners. When necessity brought women into the workforce, their wages and job status were lower than men's, and working women remained bound to their primary family obligations—a dual disparity that widely persists. The belief that women's full-time homemaking/parenting role was essential for the well-being of all family members furthered the myth that any outside work was harmful, undermining their husbands' esteem as breadwinners and endangering their children's healthy development.

The breadwinner/homemaker model was highly adaptive to the demands of the industrial economy of the times. However, the rigid gender roles, subordination of wives to their husbands, and most fathers' peripheral position due to workplace demands was not healthy for either the functioning of the family or the well-being of its members. The loss of community further isolated men and women from companionship and support. Role expectations for women to keep the family functional came at great personal cost, with a disproportionate burden in caring for others while denying their own needs and identities (McGoldrick, Anderson, & Walsh, 1989). For men, the work ethic and job schedules diminished involvement with their families. One critic wrote: "Each suburban family is somehow a broken home, consisting of a father who appears as an overnight guest, [and] a put-upon housewife with too much to do" (Skolnick, 1991, p. 60).

The belief that "proper gender roles" are essential for healthy family functioning and child development dominated sociological conceptualization of the normal American family, supported by Talcott Parsons's observations of white, middle-class suburban families in the 1950s (Parsons & Bales, 1955). In his view, the nuclear family structure provided for a healthy complementarity in the division of roles into male "instrumental" leadership and female "socioemotional" support. The fields of psychiatry and child development adhered to this family model and its corollary that the failure of a family to uphold proper gender roles would invariably damage children (Lidz, 1963).

The first wave of feminism came in reaction to the exploititive and stultifying effects of the modern family model, with its separate and unequal spheres for men and women. With reproductive choice and family planning, women turned to the work sphere, seeking the personal growth and status valued by society. The "Superwoman syndrome" soon emerged as women sought to "have it all," combining jobs and child rearing, but found they were adding on a "second shift" (Hochschild, 1989), since most men did not make reciprocal changes toward equal sharing of family responsibilities. Accordingly, the second wave of the Women's Movement focused on family politics, in efforts to redefine and rebalance gendered role relations, so that both men and women could seek personal fulfillment, be gainfully employed, and share in the responsibilities and joys of family life (McGoldrick et al., 1989). Still, numerous studies have found that employed women continue to carry upwards of 80% of household and child care obligations. Although many men are doing substantially more than their own fathers did, it remains far less than most wives' share of the burden (Lamb, 1997, 1999). More recent men's movements have sought greater involvement in parenting by fathers and a reconnection with the fathers they barely knew (Kimmel, 1996). Although some advocate a return to the traditional patriarchal model, most men share with women the desire for a full and equal partnership in family life. Living out this aim is still a work in progress (Pleck, 1997; see Haddock et al., Chapter 12, this volume).

Cultural Diversity and Socioeconomic Disparity

One of the most striking features of North American families today is their increasing cultural diversity (Fine, Demo, & Allen, 2000). In the United States, the foreign-born population has tripled since 1970, with most coming from Latin America and Asia. In 2000, one in five persons was either foreign-born or a first-generation resident. Through immigration and earlier, higher birth rates in Hispanic, Asian, and African American families, the proportion of people of color in the U.S. has risen to nearly half of the population and is expected to increase further in coming decades. Hispanics now nearly equal blacks in number and are rapidly becoming the largest minority group. Non-Hispanic whites are now proportionally the minority (43.8%) in the 100 largest cities (U.S. Bureau of the Census, 2000).

The 2000 Census was the first to allow the option of checking more than one race. Five percent of blacks, 6% of Hispanics, 14% of Asians, and 2.5% of whites identified themselves as bi- or multiracial. Interracial and interfaith unions are increasingly common and more accepted, blending diversity within families and for offspring. There is also greater identification, especially by young blacks, with their many ancestors. Contrary to the myth of the melting pot, American families, with a long tradition of immigration, have always been ethnically diverse (see Falicov, Chapter 11, this volume). Cultural pluralism can be seen as a source of strength that vitalizes a society. Unfortunately, recent economic insecurity and fears of terrorism have aggravated racial discrimination and intolerance toward non-European immigrants and minorities, complicating their adaptive challenges.

Social scientists have too often generalized to all families on the basis of white, middle-class values and experience. Taking the intact, self-sufficient nuclear family as the norm, there has been insufficient appreciation of the strong extended family bonds that have fostered resilience in African American and immigrant families to survive conditions of poverty and discrimination (Boyd-Franklin, 1989; McAdoo, 1996; see Boyd-Franklin, Chapter 10, this volume). Over recent decades, due to structural changes in the economy, the broad middle class has been shrinking (Ehrenreich, 1989), and the gap of inequality has widened between the rich and poor (U.S. Bureau of the Census, 2000). The financial prospects of most young families today are lower than those of their parents, with a decline in median income and more families living in poverty. Even full-time employment doesn't sustain some families above the poverty line: Most require two incomes to support even a modest standard of living and their children's education. Many are struggling anxiously through uncertain times as businesses downsize and workers are let go despite loyal service. As the economy has shifted from the industrial sector to services and computer-based technology, the impact has hit hardest for working-class and poor families, with limited education, job skills, and employment opportunities.

Declining economic conditions and job dislocation can have a devastating impact on family stability and well-being, fueling substance abuse, family conflict and violence, marital dissolution, homelessness, and an increase in poor, single-parent households. Social and economic disempowerment have also contributed to the high rate of unwed teenage parenting. Studies find that young inner-city fathers are less likely to marry and assume financial responsibility for their children when they lack job opportunities and face bleak earning prospects, reinforced by racism (Johnson, 2000; Wilson, 1996).

Harry Aponte (1994) stresses that emotional and relational problems of poor minority families require understanding within the fabric of their socioeconomic and political contexts: They are dependent on and vulnerable to the overreaching power of society and cannot insulate themselves from society's ills. Aponte notes, "They cannot buy their children private schooling when their public school fails [or] buy into an upscale neighborhood when their housing project becomes too dangerous. When society stumbles, its poorest citizens are tossed about and often crushed" (p. 8).

The economic and social conditions of women and children have worsened disproportionately. Gender inequities persist in the workplace. The earnings gap between men and women, although slightly improved over the past decade—due in part to a drop in male earnings—still leaves women currently earning 73 cents to each dollar earned by men (U.S. Bureau of the Census, 2000). The glass ceiling has barely shown a crack as women in management positions have lost ground in comparable earnings over the past decade. The number of children in poverty has increased over 40% since 1970. Life chances are worsened by persistent conditions of discrimination, neighborhood decay, poor schools, crime, violence, and lack of opportunity to rise above those obstacles.

The Index of Social Health, developed by Fordham University social scientists, compiles a number of indicators of social well-being in the U.S. each year, including statistics on the number of jobless, affordable housing, number of children and families in poverty, teen suicide, and high school completion. On a scale of 1 to 100, the nation's social health was rated at 77 in 1973; it plummeted to 38 in 1995. Such an index, if published annually like the stock market's economic indicators, could heighten public awareness of the urgent need to address our nation's social well-being. Such immense structural disparities perpetuate a vast chasm between the rich and the poor, increasing the vulnerability of growing numbers of families living on the fault line (Rubin, 1994). Despite public rhetoric promoting strong families, insufficient support is given for families to thrive (Stacy, 1996; See Hartman, Chapter 23, this volume).

Varying and Extended Family Life-Cycle Course

Families and societies worldwide are rapidly aging. Currently, the median age in the U.S. is 35 years old, and over 13% of the population is over 65 (up from 8% in 1950). By 2020, aging baby-boomers will swell the over-65 age group to exceed 20%. Increased life expectancy, now at 75 years (79 for women and 73 for men), has made possible—and more challenging—long-lasting couple and intergenerational relations. Four- and five-generation families are increasingly common (Bengston, 2001; Walsh, 1999a). Sibling relations assume growing significance for most people as they age (Bank, 1997; Cicirelli, 1995).

Yet serious and chronic illnesses pose increasing family caregiving challenges (Institute for Health & Aging, 1996). With medical advances, more people are living longer with chronic health conditions. Adults over age 85 are the fastest growing and most vulnerable segment of society; half are likely to be affected by dementia. With women still shouldering the preponderance of caregiving responsibilities, those at midlife have been dubbed "the sandwich generation," also in the workforce and carrying responsibilities for adolescent and college-age children. With fewer young people in families to support the growing number of elders, threats to Social Security and health care benefits will likely fuel growing insecurity and intergenerational tensions.

In part, the current high divorce rate is due to the expectation that, unlike the past, couples have another 20–40 years after launching children. It's difficult for one relationship to meet the changing developmental needs and priorities of both partners over so many years. As Margaret Mead (1972) noted, in youth, romance and passion stand out in choosing a partner. In rearing children, relationship satisfaction is linked more to sharing family joys and responsibilities. In later life, needs for companionship and mutual caregiving come to the fore. In view of these shifts, Mead envisioned time-limited, renegotiable contracts, suggesting that perhaps serial monogamy best fits the challenges over a lengthened life course. Although many would see her prescription as undermining the family, today's families are increasingly living out this pattern. Despite the high divorce rate, most people remain optimistic: They long for a romantic, committed relationship and, if their attempt fails, they try again, with hope overcoming disappointment. Two or three commited relationships in a (long) lifetime, along with periods of cohabitation and single living, are likely to become increasingly common. Thus, most adults and their children will move in and out of a variety of family structures as they separate and recombine. We will need to learn how to buffer transitions and live successfully in complex arrangements.

Our view of the family must also be expanded to the varied course of the life cycle, to a wider range of normative (typical) developmental phases and transitions fitting the diverse preferences and challenges that make each family unique. Some become first-time parents at the age when others become grandparents. Others start second families at midlife. Adults who remain single (Anderson & Stewart, 1995), or couples who are unmarried or without children, forge a variety of intimate relationships and significant kin and friendship bonds, such as the close-knit networks of gay men and lesbians termed "families of choice" (Weston, 1991). New technologies enabling conception and others prolonging life and the dying process pose unprecedented opportunities and dilemmas for families (see Rolland, Chapter 17, this volume). Yet, in impoverished communities, the lack of adequate health care and early death through violence, substance abuse, and AIDS drastically foreshorten the life cycle for many (Burton, 1990).

Families Facing the Future

Periods of major social and economic turmoil are tremendously disruptive of family life. We are in the midst of a stressful transformation to a postindustrial, technologically based global economy. Family patterns have been altered by a host of interconnected factors (Amato & Booth, 1997), most notably, growing cultural diversity, economic restructuring, a widening gap between rich and poor, aging of societies, declining birth rates, and movements for equality and social justice for women, gay men and lesbians, and people of color. Families are facing the future with growing diversity and complexity in structure, gender, culture, class, and life-cycle patterns.

Many of the strains challenging families are not of their own making, but are generated by larger forces in the world around them. Over recent decades, families have experienced multiple dislocations. Job security, health care coverage, and retirement benefits are increasingly uncertain. Conflicting work and family demands create time binds, pressuring lives at an accelerated pace as family members seek elusive "quality time" (Hochschild, 1997). Children are exposed to a toxic social environment (Garbarino, 1997). Besieged parents are unsure how to raise their children well in a hazardous world, and how to counter pressures of the internet and pop culture that saturate homes and minds with alluring and destructive images of beauty, wealth, sex, and violence (Pipher, 1997). The American ethos of the "rugged individual," along with geographic mobility, has contributed to the breakdown of communities and the fraying of our social fabric (Bellah, Madsen, Sullivan, Swidler, & Tipton, 1983; Booth, 2001; Galbraith, 1996). Social policies fail to provide safety nets for vulnerable families or to create programs and services to help struggling families succeed. Seen in context, it is more understandable that family stability has become so precarious—and all the more remarkable that over half of all marriages remain intact. Yearnings for "family," "home," and "community" are stronger than ever, heightened by the continuing threat of terrorism.

Life was never more secure in earlier times or distant places, yet in the relativism of the postmodernism era, many are alarmed by a seeming collapse of universal family values (Doherty, 1996; Stacey, 1996). Families today do have strong values, yet they are in unfamiliar territory, lacking a map to guide their passage. Debates about the future of the family have touched a vulnerable core of anxiety and uncertainty about contemporary life. The many discontinuities and unknowns generate an uncomfortable tension. Myths of the ideal family compound the sense of deficiency and failure for families in transition even when they don't fit emerging needs and challenges. A widespread sense of confusion about family relationships leads people to question what is normal (i.e., typical, expectable) in family life and how to construct healthy (i.e., optimally functioning) families. The chapters in this volume offer useful maps for navigating new terrain.

Kenneth Gergen (1991) observes that when we become aware of the multiplicity in diverse human experience, we begin to see that each ethnic community, political group, and economic class has its own limited, partial perspective and frames the world in its own terms. Although we may lose safe and sure claims to truth, objectivity, or authority and the idea of self as the center of meaning, we may gain the reality, the centrality, and the fundamental necessity of relatedness.

In today's world marked by breathtaking change and fragmentation, our lives do seem unpredictable, with few absolutes. Yet rather than becoming alarmed and collapsing under these pressures and threats, Robert Lifton (1993) contends that humans are surprisingly resilient. He compares our predicament and response to that of the Greek god Proteus, who was able to change shape in response to crisis, just as we create new psychological, social, and family configurations, exploring new options and transforming our lives many times over. Many families do show remarkable resilience, making the best of their situations and inventing new models of human connectedness. These "brave new families," as sociologist Judith Stacey (1990) termed them, are creatively reworking family life in a variety of household and kinship arrangements. As Stacey found in her ethnographic study of working-class families, people today are drawing on a wide array of resources and fashioning them into new gender and relationship strategies to cope with new challenges. Men and women are increasingly sharing household work and child care; unmarried working women and men, both straight and gay, are choosing to raise children on their own; longtime close friends are claiming kinship; and extended family connections are being sustained across serial marriages. Stacy was particularly impressed by creative initiatives to reshape the experience of divorce from a painful, bitter schism and loss of resources into a viable kin network, involving new partners and former mates, multiple sets of children, stepkin, and friends in households and support systems collaborating to survive and flourish. It is ironic that such families are termed "nontraditional." Their flexibility, diversity, and community show the resiliencies found in the varied households and loosely knit clans of the past and still today in many cultures.

Mary Catherine Bateson (1994) believes that adaptation comes out of encounters with novelty that may seem chaotic. An intense multiplicity of vision, enhancing insight and creativity, is needed by families today. Although we can never be fully prepared for the demands of the moment, Bateson argues that we can be strengthened to meet uncertainty:

> The quality of improvisation characterizes more and more lives today, lived in uncertainty, full of the inklings of alternatives. In a rapidly changing and interdependent world, single models are less likely to be

> viable and plans more likely to go awry. The effort to combine multiple models risks the disasters of conflict and runaway misunderstanding, but the effort to adhere blindly to some traditional model for a life risks disaster not only for the person who follows it but for the entire system in which he or she is embedded, indeed for all other living systems with which that life is linked. (p. 8)

If we knew the future of particular families, we might prepare them with the necessary skills and attitudes. But it is doubtful that such stability or certainty ever existed. Today's families are constantly adapting to meet emerging demands of a dynamic society and a changing global environment (Sussman et al., 1999). As Bateson observes, ambiguity is the warp of life, and cannot be eliminated. Thus, we must help families to find *coherence within complexity*. In Bateson's apt metaphor, "We are called to join in a dance whose steps must be learned along the way. Even in uncertainty we are responsible for our steps" (p. 10).

Amid the swirling confusions and upheavals, Bateson (1994) urges us to encourage families to carry on the process of learning throughout the life cycle in all they do, ". . . like a mother balancing her child on her hip as she goes about her work with the other hand and uses it to open the doors of the unknown" (p. 9). The ability to combine multiple roles and adapt to new challenges can be learned. Encouraging such vision and skills is a core element of strengths-based approaches to family therapy.

REFERENCES

Ahrons, C. (1994). *The good divorce: Keeping your family together when your marriage comes apart.* New York: HarperCollins.

Amato, P. R. (2000). The consequences of divorce for adults and children. *Journal of Marriage and the Family, 62,* 1269–1287.

Amato, P. R., & Booth, A. (1997). *A generation at risk: Growing up in an era of family upheaval.* Cambridge, MA: Harvard University Press.

Anderson, C., & Stewart, S. (1995). *Flying solo: Single women at midlife.* New York: Norton.

Aponte, H. (1994). *Bread and spirit: Therapy with the new poor.* New York: Norton.

Aries, P. (1962). *Centuries of childhood: A social history of family life.* New York: Knopf.

Bank, S. (1997). *The sibling bond* (rev. ed.). New York: Basic Books.

Barnett, R. C., & Rivers, C. (1996). *She works/he works: How two-income families are happier, healthier, and better off.* San Francisco: Harper.

Bateson, G. (1979). *Mind and nature: A necessary unity.* New York: Dutton.

Bateson, M.C. (1994). *Peripheral visions.* New York: HarperCollins.

Bellah, R., Madsen, R., Sullivàn, W., Swidler, A., & Tipton, S. (1985). *Habits of the heart: Individualism and commitment in American life.* Berkeley: University of California Press.

Bengston, V. G. (2001). Beyond the nuclear family: The increasing importance of multigenerational bonds. *Journal of Marriage and the Family, 63,* 1–16.

Bernard, J. (1982). *The future of marriage.* New Haven, CT: Yale University Press.

Bertalanffy, L. (1968). *General system theory and psychiatry: Foundation, developments, applications.* New York: Braziller.

Booth, A. (2001). *Does it take a village?: Community effects on children, adolescents, and families.* Mahwah, NJ: Erlbaum.

Booth, A., & Amato, P. R. (2001). Parental divorce relations and offspring post-divorce well-being. *Journal of Marriage and the Family, 63,* 197–212.

Boss, P. (2001). *Family stress management: A contextual approach.* Thousand Oaks, CA: Sage.

Boyd-Franklin, N. (1989). *Black families in family therapy: A multi-systems approach.* New York: Guilford Press.

Bramlett, M. D., & Mosher, W. D. (2001). First marriage dissolution, divorce, and remarriage in the United States. In *Advance data from vital and health statistics.* Washington, DC: National Center for Health Statistics.

Braverman, L. (1989). The myths of motherhood. In M. McGoldrick, C. Anderson, & F. Walsh (Eds.), *Women in families: Framework for family therapy* (pp. 227–243). New York: Norton.

Bronfenbrenner, U. (1979). *The ecology of human development.* Cambridge, MA: Harvard University Press.

Bumpass, L. L., & Raley, R. K. (1995). Redefining single-parent families: Cohabitation and changing family reality. *Demography, 32,* 97–109.

Burton, L. (1990). Teenage childbearing as an alternative life-course strategy in multigeneration black families. *Human Nature, 1,* 123–143.

Carter, B., & McGoldrick, M. (1999). *The expanded family life cycle: Individual, family, and social perspectives* (3rd ed.). Needham Heights, MA: Allyn & Bacon.

Cherlin, A. J. (1998). Marriage and dissolution among black Americans. *Journal of Comparative Family Studies, 29,* 147–159.

Cicirelli, V. G. (1995). *Sibling relationships across the life span.* New York: Plenum Press.

Coontz, S. (1993). *The way we never were: The American family and the nostalgia trip.* New York: Basic Books.

Coontz, S. (1997). *The way we really are: Coming to terms with America's changing families.* New York: Basic Books.

Demo, J., & Acock, A. C. (1996). Family structure, family process, and adolescent well-being. *Journal of Research on Adolescence, 6,* 457–488.

Doherty, W. (1996). *The intentional family.* Reading, MA: Addison-Wesley.

Duvall, E. (1977). *Marriage and family development.* (15th ed.). Philadelphia: Lippincott.

Ehrenreich, B. (1989). *Fear of falling: The inner life of the middle class.* New York: Pantheon.

Ehrle, J. & Geen, R. (2002). *Children cared for by relatives: Identifying service needs.* Washington, DC: Urban Institute, National Survey of America's Families.

Falicov, C. (Ed.). (1988). *Family transitions: Continuity and change over the life cycle.* New York: Guilford Press.

Fine, M.A., Demo, D.H., & Allen, K.A. (2000). Family diversity in the twenty-first century. In D.H. Demo, K.A. Allen, & M.A. Fine (Eds.), *Handbook of family diversity* (pp. 440–448). New York: Oxford University Press.

Foucault, M. (1980). *Power/knowledge: Selected interviews and other writings.* New York: Pantheon.

Furstenberg, F., & Cherlin, A. (1991). *Divided families: What happens to children when parents part.* Cambridge, MA: Harvard University Press.

Galbraith, J. K. (1996). *The good society: The humane agenda.* New York: Houghton Mifflin.

Ganong, L., & Coleman, M. (1999). *Changing families, changing responsibilities: Family obligations following divorce and remarriage.* Thousand Oaks, CA: Sage.

Garbarino, J. (1997). *Raising children in a socially toxic environment.* San Francisco: Jossey-Bass.

Gergen, K. (1991). *The saturated self.* New York: Basic Books.

Goldstein, J. R. (1999). The leveling of divorce in the United States. *Demography, 36(6),* 409–414.

Grinker, R. R. (1967). Normality viewed as a system. *Archives of General Psychiatry, 17,* 320–324.

Hareven, T. (2000). *Families, history, and social change: Life course and cross-cultural perspectives.* New York: Westview.

Harway, M. (1996). *Treating the changing family: Handling normative and unusual events.* New York: Wiley.

Hess, G., & Handel, G. (1959). *Family worlds: A psychological approach to family life.* Chicago: University of Chicago Press.

Hetherington, E. M., & Kelly, J. (2002). *For better or for worse: Divorce reconsidered.* New York: Norton.

Hochschild, A. (1989). *The second shift: Working parents and the revolution at home.* New York: Viking Penguin.

Hochschild, A. (1997). *Time bind: When work becomes home and home becomes work.* New York: Holt.

Hoffman, L. (1990). Constructing realities: An art of lenses. *Family Process, 29,* 1–12.

Institute for Health and Aging. (1996). *Chronic care in America: A 21st century challenge.* Princeton, NJ: Robert Wood Johnson Foundation.

Jackson, D. D. (1965). The study of the family. *Family Process, 4,* 1–20.

Johnson, W. (2000). Work preparation and labor market experiences among urban, poor, nonresident fathers. In S. Danziger & A. Lin (Eds.), *Coping with poverty: The social contexts of neighborhood, work, and family in the African-American community.* Ann Arbor: University of Michigan Press.

Kaminer, W. (1992). *I'm dysfunctional, you're dysfunctional.* Redding, MA: Addison-Wesley.

Keeney, B., & Sprenkle, D. (1982). Ecosystemic epistemology: Critical implications for the aesthetics and pragmatics of family therapy. *Family Process, 21,* 1–19.

Kimmel, M. S. (1996). *Manhood in America: A cultural history.* New York: Free Press.

Kleinman, A. (1988). *Suffering, healing, and the human condition.* New York: Basic Books.

Lamb, M. (1997). *The role of the father in child development* (3rd ed.). New York: Wiley.

Lamb, M. (Ed.). (1999). *Parenting and child development in "non-traditional" families.* Mahwah, NJ: Erlbaum.

Lansford, J. E., Ceballo, R., Abby, A., & Stewart, A. J. (2001). Does family structure matter? A comparison of adoptive, two-parent biological, single-mother, stepfather, and stepmother households. *Journal of Marriage and the Family, 63,* 840–851.

Lidz, T. (1963). *The family and human adaptation.* New York: International Universities Press.

Lidz, T., Fleck, S., & Cornelison, A. (1965). *Schizophrenia and the family.* New York: International Universities Press.

Lifton, R. (1993). *The Protean self: Human resilience in an age of fragmentation.* New York: Basic Books.

McAdoo, H. (Ed.). (1996). *Black families* (3rd. ed.). Thousand Oaks, CA: Sage.

McCubbin, H., McCubbin, M., McCubbin, A., & Futrell, J. (Eds.). (1998). *Resiliency in ethnic minority families: Vol. II. African-American families.* Thousand Oaks, CA: Sage.

McCubbin, H., McCubbin, M., Thompson, E., & Fromer, J. (Eds.). (1998). *Resiliency in ethnic minority families: Vol. 1. Native and immigrant families.* Thousand Oaks, CA: Sage.

McGoldrick, M., Anderson, C., & Walsh, F. (Eds.). (1989). *Women in families: A framework for family therapy.* New York: Norton.

McGoldrick, M., Giordano, J., & Pearce, J. (Eds.). (1996). *Ethnicity and family therapy* (2nd ed.). New York: Guilford Press.

Mead, M. (1972). *Blackberry winter.* New York: William Morrow.

Minkler, M., & Roe, J. (1993). *Grandparents as caregivers.* Newbury Park, CA: Sage.

Minuchin, S. (1974). *Families and family therapy.* Cambridge, MA: Harvard University Press.

Nabokov, V. (1969). *Ada.* New York: McGraw-Hill.

Neugarten, B. (1976). Adaptation and the life cycle. *Counseling Psychologist, 6,* 16–20.

Offer, D., & Sabshin, M. (1974). *Normality: Theoretical and clinical concepts of mental health* (2nd ed.). New York: Basic Books.

Parsons, T., & Bales, R. F. (1955). *Family, socialization, and interaction processes.* Glencoe, IL: Free Press.

Pertman, A. (2000). *Adoption nation: How the adoption revolution is transforming America.* New York: Basic Books.

Pipher, M. (1997). *The shelter of each other: Rebuilding our families.* New York: Ballantine.

Pleck, J. (1997). Paternal involvement: Levels, sources, and consequences. In M. Lamb (Ed.), *The role of the father in child development.* New York: Wiley.

Reiss, D. (1981). *The family's construction of reality.* Cambridge, MA: Harvard University Press.

Reiss, D., Hetherington, E. M., Plomin, R., & Neiderhiser, J. (2000). *The relationship code: Deciphering genetic and social influences on adolescent development.* ambridge, MA: Harvard University Press.

Risman, B. (1999). *Gender vertigo: American families in transition.* New Haven, CT: Yale University Press.

Rubin, L. B. (1994). *Families on the faultline.* New York: HarperCollins.

Seltzer, J. A. (2000). Families formed outside of marriage. *Journal of Marriage and the Family, 62,* 1247–1268.

Skolnick, A. (1991). *Embattled paradise: The American family in an age of uncertainty.* New York: Basic Books.

Skolnick, A., & Skolnick, J. (1992). *Family in transition* (8th ed.). New York: HarperCollins.

Spiegel, J. (1971). *Transactions: The interplay between individual, family, and society.* New York: Science House.

Stacey, J. (1990). *Brave new families: Stories of domestic upheaval in late twentieth century America.* New York: Basic Books.

Stacey, J. (1996). *In the name of the family: Rethinking family values in the postmodern age.* Boston: Beacon.

Stacey, J., & Biblarz, T. J. (2001). How does the sexual orientation of parents matter? *American Sociological Review, 66*(2), 159–183.

Sussman, M. B., Steinmetz, S. K., & Peterson, G. W. (Eds.). (1999). *Handbook of marriage and the family* (2nd ed.) New York: Plenum Press.

Teachman, J. D., Tedrow, L. M., & Crowder, K. D. (2000). The changing demography of America's families. *Journal of Marriage and the Family, 62,* 1234–1246.

Tolstoy, L. (1946). *Anna Karenina.* New York: World.

U.S. Bureau of the Census. (2000). Retreived from American Factfinder: *http://factfinder.census.gov*

Waite, L. J., & Gallagher, M. (2000). *The case for marriage: Why married people are happier, healthier, and better off financially.* Cambridge, MA: Harvard University Press.

Wallerstein, J. S., Lewis, J. M., & Blakeslee, S. (2000). *The unexpected legacy of divorce: A 25 year longitudinal study.* New York: Hyperion.

Walsh, F. (1982). Conceptualizations of normal family functioning. In F. Walsh (Ed.), *Normal family processes* (pp. 3–42). New York: Guilford Press.

Walsh, F. (1983). Normal family ideologies: Myths and realities. In C. Falicov (Ed.), *Cultural dimensions in family therapy.* Rockville, MD: Aspen.

Walsh, F. (Ed.). (1993). *Normal family processes* (2nd ed.). New York: Guilford Press.

Walsh, F. (1996). The concept of family resilience: Crisis and challenge. *Family Process, 35,* 261–281.

Walsh, F. (1998). *Strengthening family resilience.* New York: Guilford Press.

Walsh, F. (1999a). Families in later life: Challenges and opportunities. In B. Carter & M. McGoldrick (Eds.), *The expanded family life cycle* (3rd ed., pp. 307–326). Needham Heights, MA: Allyn & Bacon.

Walsh, F. (Ed.).(1999b). *Spiritual resources in family therapy.* New York: Guilford Press.

Walsh, F., & McGoldrick, M. (1991). Loss and the family: A systemic perspective. In F. Walsh & M. McGoldrick (Eds.), *Living beyond loss: Death in the family* (pp. 1–29). New York: Norton.

Watzlawick, P., Beavin, J., & Jackson, D. (1967). *Pragmatics of human communication.* New York: Norton.

Weston, K. (1991). Families we choose: *Lesbians, gays, and kinship.* New York: Columbia University Press.

Wilson, W. J. (1996). *When work disappears: The world of the urban poor.* New York: Random House.

Wynne, L. (1988). An epigenetic model of family process. In C. Falicov (Ed.), *Family transitions: Continuity and change over the life cycle* (pp. 81–106). New York: Guilford Press.

CHAPTER 2

CLINICAL VIEWS OF FAMILY NORMALITY, HEALTH, AND DYSFUNCTION

From Deficit to Strengths Perspective

Froma Walsh

Constructions of family normality, health, and dysfunction, which are embedded in our cultural and professional belief systems, underlie all clinical theory and practice. These assumptions exert a powerful and largely unexamined influence in every family assessment and intervention.

THROUGH A DARK AND NARROW LENS

The field of mental *health* has long neglected the study and promotion of *health*. In the concentration on mental *illness*, family normality became equated with the absence of symptoms, a situation rarely, if ever, seen in the clinical setting. Assumptions about healthy families were largely speculative and utopian, extrapolated from experience with disturbed clinical cases. Typical family patterns received scant attention.

Grounded in medical and psychoanalytic paradigms, clinical practice and research became focused on the understanding and treatment of psychopathology, viewing the family darkly in terms of damaging influences in the etiology of individual disorders. Indeed, throughout much of the clinical literature, families have been portrayed as noxious and destructive influences. Focused narrowly on a dyadic view of early childhood, "parenting" has been equated with "mothering," with the terms used interchangeably. Parents—especially mothers—have been viewed harshly and blamed for all problems, as in the following family case analysis in a leading psychiatric journal:

> In this paper, it has been possible to examine minutely a specific family situation. The facts speak rather boldly for themselves. The mother and wife is a domineering, aggressive, and sadistic person with no redeeming good qualities. She crushes individual initiative and independent thinking in her husband, and prevents their inception in her children. (Gralnick, 1943, p. 323)

Such mother-blaming indictments have persisted, often formed without any direct contact with the family but deduced from theories of family pathogenesis. "Parent-ectomies" have frequently been recommended, keeping families at bay, without "intrusion" in treatment, offering a corrective influence (Walsh & Anderson, 1988). Family assessment, skewed toward identification of deficits and conflicts, has tended to be blind to family strengths and resources to such an extent that—only half jokingly—a normal family might be defined as one that has not yet been clinically assessed.

MODELS OF FAMILY THERAPY

The family systems perspective advanced conceptualization of the family from a linear, dyadic view of causality to the recognition of multiple, recursive influences within and beyond the family that shape individual and family functioning. Yet early family therapy theory and practice remained pathology-oriented, attending to dysfunctional family processes implicated in the ongoing *maintenance* of individual symptoms, if not their origins. In recent decades, there has been a welcome shift in therapeutic focus and aims toward greater recognition and enhancement of family strengths. It is important to examine the views of family normality, health, and dysfunction embedded in major approaches to family therapy because of their critical influence in clinical practice. The second edition of this volume (Walsh, 1993) surveyed the most influential founding models and more recent developments in the field, considering the four perspectives on family normality outlined in Chapter 1. Although generalizations in an evolving field must be made with caution, some basic premises about family normality, health, and dysfunction can be identified in the various approaches. Two questions frame discussion:

1. *Family processes:* What are the explicit and implicit assumptions about normal—typical and optimal—family functioning and views of dysfunction?
2. *Therapeutic goals and change processes:* How do these beliefs influence therapeutic objectives and intervention processes?

As can be seen in the brief summary and update that follows, various aspects of family and couple functioning receive selective attention as they fit different views of problem formation, therapeutic goals, and change processes (see Table 2.1, p. 42)

Brief Problem-Solving Approaches

Structural Model

The structural model of family therapy (Minuchin, 1974), emphasized the importance of organizational processes for family functioning and the well-being of members. Therapy focuses on the patterning of transactions in which symptoms are embedded, viewing problems as an indication of imbalance or rigidity in the family's organization.

Minuchin (1974) directly challenged the myth of "placid" normality—the idealized view of the normal family as nonstressful, living in constant harmony and cooperation. Such an image crumbles, he argued, when looking at any family with ordinary problems. Through interviews with effectively functioning families from different cultures, Minuchin illustrated normal (i.e., typical) difficulties of family life transcending cultural differences. In an ordinary family, the couple has many problems in relating, bringing up children, dealing with in-laws, and coping with the outside world. He noted, "Like all normal families, they are constantly struggling with these problems and negotiating the compromises that make a life in common possible" (p. 16).

Therefore, Minuchin cautioned therapists not to base judgments of family normality or abnormality on the presence or absence of problems. Instead, he proposed a conceptual schema of family functioning to guide family assessment and therapy. This structural model views the family as a social system in transformation, operating within specific social contexts and developing over time, with each stage requiring reorganization. Each system maintains preferred patterns, yet a functional family must be able to adapt to new circumstances, balancing continuity and change to further the psychosocial growth of members (see also Falicov, 1988). Symptoms are most commonly a sign of a maladaptive reaction to changing environmental or developmental demands. Normal (i.e., common, expectable) transitional strains may be misjudged or mislabeled as pathological. Minuchin advised:

> With this orientation, many more families who enter therapy would be seen and treated as average families in transitional situations, suffering the pains of accommodation to new circumstances. The label of pathology would be reserved for families who in the face of stress increase the rigidity of their transactional patterns and boundaries, and avoid or resist any exploration of alternatives. (1974, p. 60)

These distinctions led to different therapeutic strategies: In average families, the therapist relies more on the motivation of family resources as a pathway to transformation. With greater dysfunction, the therapist becomes more active in order to realign the system.

Patterns of closeness and separateness were likewise viewed as transactional styles or preferences and not as qualitative differences between functional and dysfunctional families, although extremes of enmeshment or disengagement were considered dysfunctional. Structural family therapists have recognized that cultural norms vary widely (Falicov, 1995), and patterns must shift to meet different requisites at various life-cycle stages, from rearing young children, through adolescence, to launching (Combrinck-Graham, 1985).

Structural family therapists have emphasized the importance of generational hierarchy and the clarity of family rules and boundaries to protect the differentiation of the system and parental authority (Wood, 1985). Stressed parents, especially single parents, often need to delegate some responsibilities to an older child or a grandparent; this can function well so long as lines of authority are clearly drawn and a child is not required to sacrifice his or her own needs. A strong parental subsystem—two-parent or single-parent—is required for child-rearing tasks. The unquestioned authority of the traditional patriarchal model has more recently been replaced by a concept of flexible, authoritative parenting (Avenoli, Sessa, & Steinberg, 1999). Minuchin (1974) notes that although the ideal family is often described as a democracy, this does not mean that a family is leaderless or a society of peers. Rather, effective family functioning requires the power to carry out essential functions. Thus, a primary structural objective in family therapy is to strengthen the parental subsystem.

In healthier families, spouses are seen to support their partners' better characteristics. At times, average couples may undermine partners in attempts to improve or rescue them, yet such patterns don't necessarily imply malevolent motivation or serious pathology. Minuchin noted that the spousal subsystem requires complementarity and mutual accommodation. Yet, in practice, early structural family therapists supported the gender-based hierarchy in power and status rooted in patriarchal cultural values (Goldner, 1988; Walsh & Scheinkman, 1989). Therapy was commonly directed to "rebalance" the family by diminishing the mother's influence, while enhancing the father's position of authority.

Structural family therapists have shown particular sensitivity to the barrage of external pressures and constraints on poor inner-city families that contribute to problems in family organization (Aponte, 1994; Falicov, 1998; Minuchin, Montalvo, Gurney, Rosman, & Schumer, 1967). In recent years, Minuchin and his colleagues have directed efforts to change in larger systems, such as court and foster care policies and practices that "dismember" poor families and undermine functioning (Minuchin, Colapinto, & Minuchin, 1998).

In summary, from a structural perspective, no family style is inherently normal or abnormal. Each family develops its own structure and preferences. Whether those organizational patterns are functional or dysfunctional depends largely on their *fit* with the family's developmental and social demands. Any style is potentially workable and may meet ordinary demands. For optimal functioning, a strong generational hierarchy and clear lines of parental authority are considered essential. The strength of the system requires clear yet flexible boundaries and subsystems for the ability to shift organizational patterns to accommodate needed change.

Strategic/Systemic Approaches

The strategic approach of the Mental Research Institute (MRI) in Palo Alto, the problem-solving model of Haley and Madanes, and the Milan systemic approach were more concerned with developing a theory of therapeutic change than a model of family functioning. Haley (1976) made a careful distinction between the two, believing that clinicians have been hampered by theory that attempts to explain pathology but does not lead to problem solution.

Symptoms are seen as a communicative act, appearing when an individual is locked into an interactional pattern and can't see a way to change it. Assuming that all families confront problems, the MRI model (Weakland, Fisch, Watzlawick, & Bodin, 1974) focuses on how families attempt to handle or resolve normal problems in living. Families may *maintain* a problem by the misguided means they are using to handle it. An attempted solution may worsen the problem, or may itself become a problem requiring change. Therapy focuses on problem resolution by altering feedback loops that maintain symptoms. The therapeutic task is to reformulate, or recast, the problem in solvable terms. The therapist's responsibility is limited to initiating change that will get a family "unstuck" from unworkable interactional patterns.

Strategic and systemic therapists view healthy families as highly flexible; the families draw on a large repertoire of behaviors to cope with problems in contrast to the rigidity and a paucity of alternatives in a dysfunctional family. Beyond this generalization, they deliberately avoid definitions of normality (Jackson, 1977), with a tolerance for differences and ideosyncracies of families (Madanes, 1991), and believe that each family must define what is normal or healthy for itself in its situation.

Haley (1976) saw descriptions of family interaction as a way of thinking for purposes of therapy where there is a disturbed child but stressed that it would be an error to deduce from that a model for what normal families *should* be like. In observations of over 200 normal—average—families, Haley found patterns so diverse that to talk about a "normal" family seemed to him naive:

How to raise children properly, as a normal family should, remains a mystery that awaits observational longitudinal studies with large samples. Thinking about the organization of a family to plan therapy is another issue. As an analogy, if a child breaks a leg, one can set it straight and put it in a plaster cast. But one should not conclude from such therapy that the way to bring about the normal development of children's legs is to place them in plaster casts. (p. 108)

Haley selectively focused on key family variables involving power and organization that he considered relevant to therapeutic change. Like Minuchin, he thought a variety of arrangements could be functional if the family deals with hierarchical issues (i.e., authority, nurturance, and discipline) and establishes clear rules to govern the power and status differential.

Implicitly, strategic and systemic therapists assumed an asymptomatic perspective on family normality, equating the absence of symptoms with normality and health, and limiting therapeutic responsibility to symptom reduction, freeing a family from unworkable patterns to define its own functional alternatives. They contend that most families do what they do because family members believe it is the right or best way to approach a problem, or because it is the only way they know. The therapeutic task is to interrupt ways of handling the problem that do not work, that is, patterns that are dysfunctional. The Milan team (Selvini, Palazzoli, Boscolo, Cecchin, & Prata, 1980) emphasized that this requires learning the language and beliefs of each family to see the problem through its members' eyes, taking into account their values and expectations that influence their approach to handling a problem and their inability to change.

Through techniques such as relabeling and reframing, a problem situation is strategically redefined to cast it in a new light and to shift a family's rigid view, to alter a destructive process. Similarly, circular questioning, positive connotation, and respectful curiosity (Boscolo, Cecchin, Hoffman, & Penn, 1986; Cecchin, 1987) are used to contextualize symptoms, attribute benign intentions, and generate hope. Problems are also depathologized by viewing them as normative life-cycle complications, considering their adaptive functions for the family, and suggesting the helpful, albeit misguided, intentions of caring members trying to help one another. In such reformulations, new solutions can become apparent.

Postmodern Approaches

Growing out of strategic/systemic models, solution-focused and narrative approaches are based in constructivist and social constructionist views of reality (Hoffman, 2002). They shift therapeutic focus from problems and the patterns that maintain them to solutions that have worked in the past or might work now, emphasizing future possibilities. As in the MRI model, they believe that people are constrained by narrow, pessimistic views of problems, limiting the range of alternatives for solution. However, they reject the earlier assumption that problems serve ulterior functions for families and are oriented toward recognizing and amplifying clients' positive strengths and potential resources (deShazer, 1988; Berg, 1997).

Postmodern therapists don't believe there is any single "correct" or "valid" way to live one's life (O'Hanlon & Weiner-Davis, 1989). What is unacceptable for some may be desirable or necessary for others. Thus, therapists shouldn't impose on clients what they think is normal. Rather than search for structural or psychic flaws in distressed families, they focus on the ways people describe themselves, their problems, and their aims.

Narrative therapists' avoidance of generalizations about what is normal or abnormal is grounded in Foucault's (1980) observations about the abusive power of dominant discourses. Nichols and Schwartz (2001) describe this concern:

> Too often in human history, judgments made by people in power have been imposed on those who have no voice. Families were judged to be healthy or unhealthy depending on their fit with ideal normative standards. With their bias hidden behind a cloak of science or religion, these conceptions became reified and internalized. One-size-fits-all standards have pathologized differences due to gender, cultural and ethnic background, sexual orientation, and socioeconomic status. (p. 294)

Postmodern therapists have been especially wary of claims of objectivity, which they regard as unobtainable. They eschew psychiatric diagnostic categories, as well as family typologies and evaluation schemas, as reductionistic, dehumanizing, and marginalizing differences from norms (Laird, 1998). Narrative therapists "situate" themselves with clients, and assume a nonexpert, collaborative stance (Freedman & Combs, 1996). Clients are encouraged to educate their therapists about their predicaments and to correct therapists' faulty assumptions that don't fit their experience (Anderson, 1997; Anderson & Goolishian, 1988). Because clinicians and families are both steeped in the larger cultural discourses, Michael White (1995) challenges therapists to be transparent: to disclose beliefs that inform their therapy and fully own their ideas as their subjective perspective, biased by race, culture, gender, and class. In short, therapists try not to make assumptions or judge clients in ways that objectify them, so as to honor their unique stories and cultural heritage.

Narrative therapy is guided by a few basic assumptions: that people have good intentions and neither want nor need problems; and that they can develop empowering stories when separated from their problems and constraining cultural beliefs. Problems aren't thought to be caused by family interaction or psychodynamics; instead, therapeutic focus shifts away from pathology within people or families and toward an appreciation of the toxic effects of many dominant discourses in the social world. For instance, anorexia nervosa can be viewed not as having a disease, a personality disorder, or a dysfunctional family, but rather as a product of internalization of cultural obsession with thinness and beauty for women. The technique of externalization (White & Epston, 1990) separates clients from their problems, so that they can unite in overcoming them. In contrast to a stance of neutrality, therapists are encouraged to challenge culturally based injustices, such as men over women, rich over poor, and whites over people of color.

Thus, therapeutic goals extend beyond problem solving to a collaborative effort to help people reauthor their life stories and rewrite their futures. Through language and perspective, problem situations are reframed toward more empowering constructions that enable problem resolution. Respectful inquiry and conversations aim to free clients from oppressive personal and cultural assumptions, enlarge and enrich their stories, and encourage them to take active charge of their own lives.

Cognitive-Behavioral Approaches

Behavioral approaches to family and couple therapy arose from behavior modification and social learning traditions in psychology and have increasingly incorporated a cognitive framework (Baucom, Epstein, & LaTaillade, 2002; Dimidjian, Christensen, & Martel, 2002; Epstein & Schlesinger, 1996). They emphasize the importance of family rules and communication processes. Therapy attends straightforwardly to the ongoing interactions and conditions under which social behavior is learned, influenced, and changed. Despite little direct attention to the question of family normality, behavioral approaches view a healthy family in terms of its adaptive, functional relationship properties (Alexander & Parsons, 1982).

Families are viewed as critical learning contexts created and responded to by members. In well-functioning families, the exchange of benefits far outweighs costs. Gottman (1994; see Driver et al., Chapter 18, this volume) found that happy couple relationships have five positive interactional exchanges for every negative exchange. Because relationships involve transactions over a wide range of possibilities, there are many opportunities for rewarding exchanges likely to sustain the relationship. In well-functioning families, adaptive behavior is rewarded through attention, acknowledgment, and approval, whereas maladaptive behavior is not reinforced. Relationship failure is explained by deficient reward exchanges, with reliance on coercive control and punishment (Patterson, Reid, Jones, & Conger, 1975). Families may be helped to change the interpersonal consequences of behavior (contingencies of reinforcement) for more positive acknowledgment and approval of desired behavior.

Behaviorally-oriented researchers have identified specific interactional processes that predict the longterm success or failure of marital relationships (Gottman, 1994; see Driver et al., Chapter 18, this volume). All emphasize flexibility in response to varied situations and adaptability as partners evolve together and cope with the many challenges and external forces in their lives. Also important is long-term reciprocity and trust that the give-and-take will be balanced out over time. In contrast, dysfunctional relationships are more rigid and skewed, lack mutual accommodation, and are restricted by short-term tit-for-tat exchanges (Patterson et al., 1975). There is increasing recognition of gender differences in interactional patterns, for example, in women's greater valuing of closeness for relationship satisfaction and the tendency for men to withdraw or "stonewall," to resist influence, or to become explosive in disputes (Gottman, 1994; see Driver et al., Chapter 18, this volume).

Communication skills—particularly clear, direct expression of feelings, affection, and opinions; negotiation; and problem solving—are considered key to functional couple and family processes and can be learned. Relationship success is predicted not by the absence of conflict, but by acceptance of differences (Jacobson & Christensen, 1996) and conflict management (Markman, Renick, Floyd, Stanley, & Clements, 1993). For effective problem solving, difficult issues are controlled, escalating conflicts slowed down, and arguments kept constructive. Therapists specify problems and goals in concrete, observable behavioral terms, guiding family members to learn more effective ways to deal with one another and to enhance pleasurable interaction.

Psychoeducational Approaches

The psychoeducational model was developed for family intervention with schizophrenia and other persistent mental illnesses (Anderson, Reiss, & Hogarty, 1986). This approach corrects the pathologizing tendency in traditional treatments to blame a "schizophrenogenic mother" or a "toxic" family for causing mental illness (Lefley, 1996). Based on over two decades of research, mental disorders are seen as the product of the interaction of a core biological vulnerability and environmental stresses. Families are viewed as struggling the best they know how in managing severe cognitive, emotional, and behavioral symptoms. Families are engaged as valued and essential collaborators in treatment, with respect for their caregiving challenges, serving as vital resources for their family member's long-term functioning in the community. Multifamily group interventions (McFarlane, 2002) are designed to reduce family stress and provide support, through practical information and management guidelines for predictably stressful periods that can be anticipated in the course of a chronic mental illness. Families are helped to develop coping skills and to plan how to handle future stress and crises. The group format provides social support, sharing of problem-solving experiences, and reduction of stigma and isolation of families.

Psychoeducational multifamily group approaches are finding application in a wide range of problem situations faced by normal (i.e., average) families, such as family psychosocial demands of chronic physical illness (Steinglass, 1998; Rolland, 1994; see Rolland, Chapter 17, this volume), and stressful family transitions, such as divorce, remarriage, or job loss (Walsh, 2002). By identifying common challenges associated with stressful situations, family distress is normalized and contextualized, and therapy is focused on mastering adaptational challenges.

INTERGENERATIONAL GROWTH-ORIENTED APPROACHES

Psychodynamically Oriented Approaches

Several intergenerational approaches to family therapy have bridged psychodynamic and family systems theories. Their construction of normal versus pathological family processes has broadened focus from maternal influences in early childhood to the dynamic processes in the whole family, across the generations and over the life cycle. Parents, individually and through couple and parental relationships, promote attachment, separation, and individuation processes considered essential for healthy development. An optimally functioning family provides a secure base for members, a context of security, trust, and nurturance to support both attachment and individual maturation (Bowlby, 1988; Byng-Hall, 1995).

Family interaction is conceptualized in terms of object relations, related internalizations, and processes of introjection and projection. The capacity to function as a spouse and a parent is seen as largely determined by family-of-origin experiences. A healthy marriage is viewed as a committed relationship, capable of intimacy, relatively well-differentiated and unambivalent, with partners projecting few irrational expectations, motives, and fantasies onto each other, and with acceptance of one's self and partner as "good enough" despite flaws and disappointments (Scharff & Scharff, 1987). A shared projection process, based on complementarity of needs, influences mate choice as well as couple and parent–child relationship patterns. In a healthy family, partners/parents take responsibility for their own (pathological) projections and can contain or modify projections by others. Parents are aware and free enough from their intrapsychic conflicts and unfulfilled needs to invest in parenting and be responsive to their children's developmental priorities. Over time, family interactions modify the images of spouses, parents, and siblings, so that perceptions can mature without becoming frozen or distorted.

In dysfunctional families, unresolved conflict or loss interferes with realistic appraisal of and response to other family members. Framo (1970) viewed symptoms as resulting primarily from unconscious attempts by spouses/parents to reenact, externalize, or master through current relationships their issues from the family of origin. A symptomatic member may serve as a scapegoat (Ackerman, 1958), or express an irrational role assignment or a projective transference distortion, reinforced by family myths and structural patterns. A significant loss may disrupt the entire family system, with emotional upheaval and unresolved grief expressed in symptoms by a family member or distress in other relationships (Paul & Paul, 1975). Adolescent separation problems may result from intense family pressures to either bind or expel members (Stierlin, 1974).

Assessment and treatment therefore explore the connection of multigenerational family dynamics to resulting disturbances in current functioning and relationships. The therapist facilitates awareness of covert emotional processes and encourages members to deal directly with one another to work through unresolved conflicts and losses, and to test out, update, and alter negative introjects from the past (Framo, 1992). The conjoint process serves to build mutual empathy in couple and family bonds.

The contextual approach of Boszormenyi-Nagy (1987) emphasizes the ethical dimension of family relationships in multigenerational legacies of accountability and loyalty that guide members across the life cycle. In well-functioning families, members are not bound by a real or imagined "ledger" of unpaid debts. Families are strengthened by actions toward trustworthiness and relational equitability, considering all members' interests for growth, autonomy, and relatedness. Flexibility, fairness, and reciprocity over time are seen as crucial. Ideally, family members openly negotiate transitions and changing loyalty commitments. Covert but powerful unresolved loyalty issues fuel dysfunction. Therapy aims toward reconciliation of current extended family relationships by resolving grievances.

In summary, from a psychodynamic perspective, family processes and psychopathology are conceptualized in terms of the interlocking of parental individual dynamics, multigenerational loyalties, conflicts, and losses, and transferences or unconscious role assignments from the past. These approaches hold a model of ideal functioning toward which therapeutic growth is encouraged, yet they focus on the reduction of pathological family dynamics through insight, facilitation of direct communication, and efforts toward relational repair. Assumptions about healthy family processes have been extrapolated from clinical theory based on dysfunctional cases. Little is said about average families, extrafamilial influences, or family and cultural diversity. The pathological bent is strong: Consideration of intergenerational dynamics focuses on negative influences to be contained or resolved, with scant attention to positive experiences and relationships in the family of origin that might contribute to healthy family processes.

Bowen Model

Bowen (1978) developed both a theory of the family emotional system and a method of therapy from observation of a wide range of families, viewing them on a continuum from the most impaired, to normal (i.e., average), to optimally functioning. In his view, psychiatry never adequately defined normality simply in terms of freedom from emotional symptoms or behavior in the normal range. Instead, he accounted for the variability in functioning by the degree of anxiety and differentiation in a family. When anxiety is low, most relationship systems appear normal, or symptom-free. When anxiety increases, tensions develop in the system, blocking differentiation and producing symptoms. Well-differentiated people can be stressed into dysfunction but use a variety of adaptive coping mechanisms to recover rapidly. At the low extreme, fusion, lives are dominated by automatic emotional processes and reactivity, which impair functioning and relationships. Most people function in the moderate range, with variable cognitive and emotional balance, and some reactivity to others out of needs for closeness and approval. Human problems and neurotic-level symptoms are thought to erupt when the emotional system is unbalanced.

In his profile of "moderate to good differentiation of self," Bowen (1978) described marital partners as able to enjoy a full range of emotional intimacy without losing their autonomy. Parents can permit their children to differentiate without undue anxiety or attempts to mold them in their own images. Family members take responsibility for themselves and don't blame others. As situations require, they can function well alone and together. Their lives are more orderly, and they can cope with a broad range of situations.

Bowen related individual and family dysfunction to several processes: (1) high *emotional reactivity* and *poor differentiation* in the family emotional system; (2) *triangles* formed when two members (e.g., parents), overloaded and anxious under stress, embroil a vulnerable third person (e.g., a child); (3) *family projection process* focusing parental anxiety on a child; and (4) *emotional cutoff* of highly charged relationships by distancing or denying their importance. Stresses on the family system, especially by death, lower differentiation and heighten reactivity, commonly resulting in triangulation or cutoffs. Underfunctioning may be reinforced by overfunctioning in other parts of the system in a compensatory cycle.

Bowen has been criticized for an implicit gender bias in valuing traditional masculine attributes as criteria for healthy functioning—autonomous, being-for-self, intellectual, and goal-directed, while pathologizing traditional feminine traits—dependent, seeking love and approval, and being-for-others (Luepnitz, 2002). For Carter and McGoldrick (2001), the main objective in Bowen therapy is the differentiation of self *in relation to others* to achieve richer, deeper relationships, not blocked by emotional reactivity, fusion, or distancing.

The Bowen model values exploration and change beyond symptom reduction. The therapist, as coach, guides client efforts to gather information, gain new perspectives on key family members and patterns, and redevelop relationships by repairing cutoffs, detriangling from conflicts, and changing one's own part in vicious cycles. Carter and McGoldrick (1999; 2001) and colleagues (McGoldrick, 1998; McGoldrick, Giordano, & Pearce, 1996; McGoldrick, Gerson, & Shellenberger, 1998) have expanded the therapeutic lens beyond the family of origin to include cultural influences of ethnicity, social class, gender, and such forms of discrimination as racism and the effects of slavery across the generations (See McGoldrick, Chapter 9, and McGoldrick & Carter, Chapter 14, this volume).

Experiential Approaches

Growth-oriented experiential approaches were developed by Virginia Satir and Carl Whitaker. While highly intuitive and relatively atheoretical, both held strong views on essential elements of healthy family functioning. Satir (1988) blended a communications approach with a humanistic orientation. She observed a consistent pattern in her experience with optimally functioning families—defined as untroubled, vital, and nurturing. Family members have high self-worth. Communication is direct, clear, specific, and honest. Family rules are flexible, human, and appropriate. Family links to society are open and hopeful. By contrast, in troubled families, self-worth is low; communication is indirect, vague, and dishonest; rules are rigid and non-negotiable; and social interactions are fearful, placating, and blaming. Regardless of the specific problem that brought a family to therapy, Satir believed that changing those key processes relieves family pain and enhances family vitality. She regarded those four aspects of family life as the basic forces operating in all families, whether an intact, one-parent, blended, or institutional family, and even more important, within the growing variety and complexity of families. She was ahead of her time in attending to the spiritual dimension of healing and growth.

Whitaker believed that all families are essentially normal but can become abnormal in the process of pain caused by trying to be normal! He distinguished healthy families by attributes similar to those noted by other early systems therapists (Napier & Whitaker, 1978; Whitaker & Keith, 1981). He emphasized the value of humor to diffuse tensions, and playfulness for creative fantasy and experimental problem solving. Whitaker also saw healthy families as having an evolutionary sense of time and becoming: a continual process of growth and change across the life cycle and the generations, facilitated by family rituals and a guiding mythology, or belief system.

Experiential approaches view symptoms as resulting from old pains that, regardless of intent, are aroused in current interaction. To change behavior, key elements in family process are addressed; all are believed to be modifiable. Therapists foster awareness and mutual appreciation through an intense, shared affective experience, with open communication of feelings and differences. In a phenomenological approach to assessment and change, therapists follow and reflect the immediate experience, and catalyze exploration and spontaneity to stimulate genuine and nondefensive relating. Marital enrichment approaches have drawn on these ideas and methods (Guerney, 1991).

SUMMARY OF CLINICAL MODELS

This brief survey of family therapy models reveals varied, yet in many respects overlapping, perspectives on family normality, health, and dysfunction. Table 2.1 summarizes these views and related therapeutic goals. All approaches, grounded in a systemic orientation, view normality in terms of ongoing transactional processes. Their differences reflect more a selective emphasis on particular aspects of functioning: structural patterns, communication and problem-solving processes, relational dynamics, or meaning systems (Sluzki, 1983). Components of family functioning posited in one domain have correlates in other domains. For example, differentiation supports and is supported by firm boundaries and clear communication. All models view flexibility as essential to healthy family functioning.

Problem-solving approaches (structural, strategic–systemic, postmodern, cognitive-behavioral, and psychoeducational models) tend to view normality in functional terms: processes that work for a family to handle its problems. These approaches tend to be immediate in focus on altering current unworkable patterns in the most proximate interactional context. Structural and narrative therapists tend to give more attention to broader sociocultural influences in health and dysfunction. The psychoeducational model attends to the interaction of biological and environmental influences in serious disorders. The growing field of family support (Kagan & Weissbourd, 1994) has much in common with these strengths-based approaches.

Growth-oriented intergenerational approaches (psychodynamic, Bowen, and experiential models) hold more explicit views of family normality in terms of relational dynamics and optimal processes for family/couple functioning and healthy development. They attend to historical influences in dysfunction, yet focus intervention on change in current family transactions. Although there is tacit recognition that ideal relationships are unattainable in most families, therapeutic goals aim beyond symptom reduction toward optimal functioning. In recent years, family therapists have increasingly been integrating elements of various approaches (Imber-Black & Roberts, 1992; Lebow, 1997; Pinsof, 1995), as in emotionally focused therapy (Johnson, 1996), which combines attachment theory and behavioral approaches to foster secure relationships.

Brief therapy approaches that focus too narrowly on problem solving may miss broader contextual variables; for instance, conflict between a daughter and stepmother may involve interlocking triangles from unresolved issues in the parents' divorce. A son's school dropout may be precipitated by his father's job loss. Or with the pressures of managed care for a quick fix, clinicians may err in presuming that family members, once unblocked from a dysfunctional pattern, will be able on their own to construct and sustain healthier modes. At the other extreme, growth-oriented approaches risk pushing families toward unrealistic ideals of functioning. Therapy can become an endless quest for vaguely defined, value-laden visions of family health reflecting the clinician's or societal ideals. As a consultant observing a couple's therapy session, I was struck that after a year of therapy, their objectives seemed obscure and the partners stuck in seeing themselves and their relationship as deficient. I suggested that they look back to the start of therapy and rate, from 1 to 10, how satisfied they had felt about their relationship at that time. They both replied "3 or 4." Asked for their current assessment, the wife rated it an 8 and the husband 9. She looked at him, astonished, saying, "I had no idea you're that satisfied! I gave it only 8 because I thought I wasn't meeting your needs enough. Just out of curiosity, what would make it a perfect 10 for you? The husband replied, "Just if you liked to go fishing." They both laughed, agreeing that they hadn't realized how far they had come. An animated conversation ensued about their unspoken assumptions that they still weren't "measuring up" to some fantasy of marital bliss.

CHALLENGES AND OPPORTUNITIES FOR CLINICAL PRACTICE AND RESEARCH

Clinicians' Views of Family Normality and Health

Perspectives from constructivism and social constructionism (Hoffman, 2002) have heightened awareness that clinicians—as well as researchers—co-construct the dysfunctional patterns they "discover" in families, as well as therapeutic goals tied to beliefs about family health. Therapists cannot avoid normative thinking at some level. Noticing what they are trained to see, they may be blind to strengths and too readily ascribe pathology. Clinical sensitivity to normative (typical) family challenges and judgments about optimal family functioning reflect therapists' values and beliefs rooted in cultural, professional, and personal orientations. It is important for clinical training programs to examine social constructions of family normality and explore how such basic premises influence family assessment and intervention (Walsh, 1987).

TABLE 2.1. Major Models of Family Therapy: Normality, Dysfunction, and Therapeutic Goals

Model of family therapy	View of normal/healthy family functioning	View of dysfunction/symptoms	Goals of therapy
		Problem-solving approaches	
Structural	Generational hierarchy; strong parental authority Clear boundaries, subsystems Flexibility: Continuity and change to fit developmental and environmental demands	Family structural imbalance: Malfunctioning generational hierarchy, boundaries Enmeshed or disengaged Maladaptive reaction to changing demands	Reorganize family structure: • Strengthen parental authority • Reinforce clear, flexible boundaries • Mobilize more adaptive alternative patterns
Strategic/Systemic	Flexibility Large behavioral repertoire for: • Problem solving • Life-cycle passage	Symptom is communicative act • Maintained by misguided problem-solving attempts • Rigidity; lack of alternatives • Serving function for family	Resolve presenting problem; specific pragmatic objective Interrupt rigid feedback cycle: symptom-maintaining sequence Shift perspective
Postmodern Solution-focused Narrative	Normality is socially constructed Many options; flexibility	Problem-saturated narratives constrain options Dominant discourse stigmatizes differences from "norm"	Search for exceptions to problem Envision new possibilities Reauthor life stories Empower clients
Cognitive-behavioral	Adaptive behavior is rewarded; More positive exchanges than negative (costs); reciprocity Good communication, problem-solving, conflict management Flexibility	Maladaptive, symptomatic behavior reinforced by: • Family attention and reward • Deficient exchanges (e.g., coercive, skewed) • Communication deficits	Concrete behavior goals: • Reward adaptive, not maladaptive, behavior • More benefits than costs • Communication, problem-solving skills
Psychoeducational	Successful coping and mastery of psychosocial challenges: • Chronic illness demands • Stressful events, transitions	Stress–diathesis in biologically based disorders Normative and non-normative stresses	Information, coping skills, and social support to: • Manage demands, master challenges • ↓ Stress and stigma

Psychodynamic	Relationships based on current realities, not past projections Provide secure base Trust, nurturance for bonding and individuation	Shared projection process Unresolved conflicts, losses, loyalty issues in family of origin • Scapegoating • Unconscious role assignment	Insight, resolution of family of origin conflicts and losses ↓ Projection processes Relationship reconstruction Mutual empathy
Bowen model	Differentiation of self in relation to others Intellectual/emotional balance	Functioning impaired by family of origin relationships: • Poor differentiation (fusion) • Anxiety (reactivity) • Triangulation • Emotional cutoff	Differentiation ↑ Cognitive functioning ↓ Emotional reactivity Change self in relationships: • Repair conflicts, cutoffs
Experiential	High self-worth Clear, honest communication Flexible rules and roles Open, hopeful social links Evolutionary growth, change Playful interaction, humor	Symptoms are nonverbal messages elicited by current communication dysfunction. Old pains are reactivated.	Direct, clear communication in immediate experience. Genuine relating. Catalyze exploration, experimentation, spontaneity.

In a survey of family therapists (Walsh, 1993), judgments of criteria for healthy family functioning varied widely, related to a clinician's favored practice model. Psychodynamically oriented therapists valued such qualities as empathy and absence of distorting projection processes; Bowen therapists emphasized differentiation; structural family therapists cited strong parental leadership and generational boundaries; behaviorally oriented therapists stressed communication skills. Notably, flexibility was a consistent value across models.

Beliefs about family normality from clinicians' own cultural backgrounds and life experiences also influence family evaluation and intervention goals. Of the clinicians surveyed, nearly half viewed their own family of origin as not having been "normal." Yet being "abnormal" held quite different meanings. Some saw their own families as very dysfunctional, or pathological. Others saw theirs as *atypical,* not conforming to average families in their community. Many felt their families failed to live up to the *ideal* normal family in the dominant society, as portrayed in television images popular when they were growing up. Family differences from either average or ideal norms were often experienced as stigmatized deviance (deficient, shame-laden, or harmful). Clinicians' perceptions were also influenced by their own experience in therapy. Those who had received traditional psychodynamically oriented individual therapy tended to view their own families as more pathological—especially mothers—and were more pessimistic about changing family patterns than those who had been in systems-oriented therapies, who were less blaming and more hopeful about change. It is essential for clinicians to reflect on their own perspectives on normality and how they influence their views of families in therapy, the goals they set, and the possibilities for change.

Training Experience with "Nonclinical" Families

The training of therapists benefits immeasurably from interviews with ordinary families who aren't in therapy. The format might include (1) family life narrative interviews (separate and conjoint) to gather different family members' perspectives on their family identity, history, current relationships, and future hopes and dreams; (2) reflection on a problem or crisis faced and the resources and strategies used for coping and resilience; (3) direct observation of family interaction on a brief structured task, such as planning a special trip together. A family functioning assessment scale, such as those presented in Chapters 19–21 of this volume, or the family resilience framework in Chapter 15, can also be useful to identify strengths and vulnerabilities in family functioning.

Interviews with nonclinical families attune students to the diversity of family perspectives and salient issues relative to their life-cycle phase, family form, gender, cultural/religious values, and socioeconomic influences

(Walsh, 1993). Discussion of the wide range of "normal" families encountered provides an opportunity to deconstruct stereotypes, myths, and faulty assumptions. Pathologizing tendencies inherent in the problem focus of clinical training are called into question. Guided to assess strengths and resources, as well as vulnerabilities, students gain awareness of family competencies and potential. It also becomes apparent that all families are challenged in one way or another over their life course, and all have some problematic areas of functioning alongside strengths. Multiple observer perspectives are afforded by having students team up to conduct the interview and later discuss their observations and assessments, noting similarities and differences related to their own gender, ethnic/religious background, and current developmental stage. Awareness is heightened that each clinician is part of every evaluation and influences what is observed, emerging information, and functional or dysfunctional judgments ascribed to individuals and relational patterns. In expanding perspectives on normality, the experience more importantly depathologizes views of clinical families in distress and humanizes the process of therapy.

Normalizing Family Distress

Ordinary families in our society worry a good deal about their own normality. In a culture that readily pathologizes families for any problem and touts the virtue in self-reliance, family members are likely to approach therapy feeling at fault for having a problem and deficient for being unable to solve it on their own. Feelings of inadequacy are compounded by the overwhelming and confusing changes in contemporary family life, along with a lack of resources and relevant models for effective functioning. Furthermore, referrals for family therapy are often based on the faulty presumption that if an individual, especially a child, is symptomatic, the family must be the "real" problem and cause, or must need the symptoms to serve a function. Much of what is label as family "resistance" in therapy stems from fears of being judged abnormal or deficient and blamed for their problems. This "resistance" is too often taken as further evidence of their pathology.

It is crucial to appreciate the shaming and stigmatizing experience of families who have felt prejudged and blamed in contacts with mental health professionals, schools, or courts. Such families are likely to expect a therapist to judge them negatively and may mistake a silent, neutral stance as confirmation of this view. Clinicians should explore families' beliefs and concerns about their own normality or deficiency, and the models and myths they hold as ideal. It's crucial to disengage assumptions of pathology from participation in therapy. Rather than presenting—or implying—family causality as the rationale for family therapy, we need to respect every family's challenges, affirm its members' best efforts, and involve them as valued collaborators in problem resolution.

The aim of normalizing family members' distress is to *depathologize* and *contextualize* their feelings and experience. It is not intended to reduce all problems and families to a common denominator and should not trivialize any individual suffering or family plight. Care is needed not to oversimplify the complexity of contemporary family life or to err in normalizing truly destructive family patterns.

Errors in Pathologizing Normal Processes

In practice, two types of errors can be made in regard to questions of normality. The first is to overpathologize families by mistakenly identifying a normal pattern as dysfunctional or misconstruing difference (deviance) as abnormal (pathological). Certain family patterns may be typical and expectable under stressful conditions. For instance, family distress generated by the strains associated with a member's chronic illness can be misdiagnosed as family pathology and presumed to have played a causal role in the development of the disorder. The family response may be quite typical of families *in that situation,* and members may be coping as well as could be reasonably expected in the face of such challenges (Rolland, 1994; see Rolland, Chapter 17, this volume).

Clinicians may also err in confounding family style variance with pathology when personal preferences and cultural differences aren't taken into account. A pattern that differs from dominant North American norms is not necessarily dysfunctional. For instance, the overused label "enmeshment" may pathologize families in which high cohesion is culturally normative, such as Latino and other immigrant families (Falicov, 1998; see Falicov, Chapter 11, this volume). In many cases, high connectedness and caretaking may be both functional and desirable, without being intrusive (Green & Werner, 1996). One study found that Lesbian couples, often labeled pathologically as "fused," scored at the "enmeshed" extreme on the cohesion scale of the Circumplex Model, yet both partners reported satisfaction with their high closeness (Zacks, Green, & Marrow, 1988). Viewed in context, it might also reflect the high relational orientation in female socialization and may serve to buffer strains in a homophobic social environment (see Laird, Chapter 7, this volume).

Clinicians should also be careful not to label a family by a single trait or stylistic feature, reducing the richness of family interaction to a one-dimensional label (e.g., "This is a chaotic family"). As Lewis, Beavers, Gosset, and Phillips (1974) observed in their pioneering study, "no single thread" distinguishes healthy from dysfunctional families. Rather, many strands are intertwined in family functioning (see Beavers & Hampson, Chapter 20; Epstein et al., Chapter 21; and Olson and Gorall, Chapter 19, this volume).

Errors in Normalizing Dysfunction

The second type of error is to fail to recognize and deal with a dysfunctional family pattern by assuming it to be normal. Here, too, clinicians should be aware of their own value-laden assumptions and the research on family and couple functioning. For example, the myth that healthy families are problem-free (Walsh, 1983) may lead to unquestioning acceptance of a couple's claims of perfect harmony. Conflict avoidance tends to be dysfunctional over time, heightening the risk for later marital dissatisfaction and divorce (Gottman, 1994; see Driver et al., Chapter 18, this volume). Violence or abuse should never be normalized, despite its all too common occurrence in families and our society, or its rationalization as sanctioned by cultural or religious beliefs. Acceptance of diversity is not the same as "anything goes," when family practices harm any member. Perhaps the most important dialogue in our field involves debunking the myth of therapeutic neutrality to examine ethical issues (Doherty, 1995).

Family Diversity and Complexity: Meeting the Challenges

A decade ago, the cultural ideal of the white, middle-class, intact nuclear family remained an implicit standard in most clinical practice, training, research, and social policy, lagging behind the changing family structures and challenges of most Americans. The generation of family therapists who have come to the fore have increased the attention to family diversity and greater recognition of the impact of larger systems and sociocultural influences on family well-being and dysfunction (e.g., Boyd-Franklin, 1989; Boyd-Franklin & Bry, 2000; Breunlin, Schwartz, & MacKune-Karrer, 1992; Falicov, 1995; Hardy & Laszloffy, 1995; Imber-Black, 1988; McGoldrick, 1998).

Varied Family Forms

A burgeoning clinical literature has addressed common adaptive challenges associated with different family forms (e.g., Laird & Green, 1996, with gay and lesbian families; Visher & Visher, 1996, with stepfamilies). Research with nonclinical families, especially longitudinal studies, can inform clinical efforts to identify predictable strains and encourage effective family processes. For instance, Hetherington's studies of significant variables in postdivorce and stepfamily adaptation (see Greene et al., Chapter 4, this volume) illuminate key processes that clinicians and family life educators can target to help families buffer stresses and facilitate optimal adjustment for children and their parents.

We must move beyond the myth of the self-reliant nuclear family household to expand attention to the multiple relationships and powerful connections among extended and informal kin living separately and even at great distance. Genograms and time lines (McGoldrick, Gerson, & Shellenberger, 1998) are valuable tools to diagram complex family structures and note the concurrence of stressful events with symptoms of distress. Postdivorce, stepfamily, and adoptive families may need assistance in dealing with normal challenges (i.e., common and expectable in their situation), balancing needs for a cohesive family unit with children's needs to maintain vital connections with noncustodial parents and extended family. "Families of choice" in gay communities provide strong bonds in the face of social stigma or family-of-origin cutoff. Close friendships, social networks, faith congregations, and community supports are invaluable resources, and new technologies, from cellphones to the Internet, offer unimagined opportunities for connection and information, as families navigate a myriad of challenges in today's complex world.

Gender and Sexism

Feminist scholars and family therapists have stimulated growing awareness of traditional, culturally based gender norms, stereotypes, and biases, as well as power imbalances in family roles and relationships (Goldner, 1988; Hare-Mustin, 1986; Jordan, Kaplan, Miller, Stiver, & Surrey, 1991; McGoldrick, Anderson, & Walsh, 1989). More recent attention to men's issues has focused on fathering but hasn't sufficiently addressed the gendered power dynamics and inequities that persist in couple and family relationships (see Haddock et al., Chapter 12, this volume). The widely accepted principle of therapist neutrality was first challenged in feminist critique for tacitly reinforcing the status quo of culturally sanctioned gender biases (Hare-Mustin, 1986). A neutral stance, combined with assumptions of circular causality, fails to address abuses of power or hold accountable perpetrators of violence.

Culture, Race, Class, and Spirituality

Family therapists are becoming more responsive to cultural diversity and more cautious not to pathologize differences that may be valued and functional—or even necessary for survival. Yet the effects of social class and racism are often confused with ethnic differences (see McGoldrick, Chapter 9, and Boyd-Franklin, Chapter 10, this volume). The debilitating impact of poverty and discrimination demands far more attention in practice strategies. Multisystemic, community-based approaches with vulnerable children and families are a significant development in the field (e.g., Henggeler, Schoenwald, Borduin, Rowland, & Cunningham, 1998).

   Our field is coming to recognize that spirituality is a vital dimension of family life and, like other aspects of culture, should not be ignored in clinical practice. While being cautious not to impose our beliefs, we need to understand our clients' spiritual sources of distress and resources in healing and growth (Griffith & Griffith, 2002; Walsh, 1999b; see Walsh & Pryce, Chapter 13, this volume).

Varied Life Cycle Challenges

Family therapy training and family process research have tended to focus on young, married, heterosexual couples rearing children and adolescents. With growing diversity in developmental pathways, greater attention is needed to address the full and varied course of individual and family life cycles (see McGoldrick & Carter, Chapter 14, this volume) and the relational and generative options of those who remain single or without children, whose lives are often stigmatized as incomplete. With the aging of societies, we need to attend to the graying of families and the opportunities for change and growth that accompany challenges (Walsh, 1999a).

Interactive Effects

Consideration of family diversity needs to be better integrated into clinical training and research designs, and not marginalized as "special issues." Falicov (1995) offers a useful multidimensional framework, viewing each family as occupying a complex ecological niche, sharing borders and common ground with other families, as well as differing positions (e.g., gender, social class, life stage, rural vs. urban). A holistic assessment includes the varied contexts a family inhabits, aiming to understand values, constraints, and resources.

   Greater attention should be given to the interactions of sexism, racism, heterosexism, ageism, classism, disabling conditions, and institutionalized forms of discrimination. Goldner (1985) cautioned that an emphasis of pragmatic therapy approaches on "what works is best" can blind therapists to harmful social and cultural influences. Systems-oriented therapists are increasingly assuming an affirmative responsibility to advocate for social justice and for changes in larger systems—workplace, education, health care, child- and elder care—to support strong families and the well-being of all members (see Hartman, Chapter 23, this volume).

Progress and Priorities in Family Research

Family research and funding priorities must be rebalanced from psychopathology to health and prevention if we are to move beyond the rhetoric of "family values" and "family strengths" to clearer understanding of key processes and social supports for healthy family functioning. Over the past three decades, a number of family systems theorists and researchers proposed a variety of systems-based conceptual schemas for mapping components of healthy family functioning (Fleck, 1980; Kantor & Lehr, 1975; Moos & Moos, 1976; Schumm, 1985; Skinner, Santa Barbara, & Steinhauer, 1983; Stinnett & DeFrain, 1985). In delineating variables thought to be crucial, all researchers, like clinicians, bring their own selective focus. The empirically based, multidimensional Beavers Systems Model (Beavers & Hampson, 1990), Olson's Circumplex Model and relational inventories (Olson, Russell, & Sprenkle, 1989), and the McMaster Model developed by Epstein, Bishop, and Levin (1978) have found wide application in family assessment. Originally normed primarily on white, middle-class, intact families, these research teams have expanded their database to a broader diversity of families (see Chapters 19–21, this volume). Gottman's laboratory studies have informed our understanding of couple interaction processes that strengthen marriages or lead to divorce (see Driver et al., Chapter 18, this volume). The theory development and research on family stress, adaptation, and resilience offer valuable frameworks for understanding key family processes in overcoming adversity (Boss, 2001; see Cowan & Cowan, Chapter 16, this volume; Walsh, 1996, 1998; see Walsh, Chapter 15, this volume).

The contributions of both quantitative and qualitative research are increasingly valued. Quantitative research has tended to focus on organizational and communication patterns that can be readily measured through direct observation, rating scales, and self-report questionnaires. Qualitative methods, such as narrative interviews, hold potential for exploring meanings and belief systems, perceptions, and other subjectivities of family experience (Doherty, Boss, LaRossa, Schumm, & Steinmetz, 1993; Gilgun, Daly, & Handel, 1993). Computerized genogram programs (McGoldrick et al., 1998) hold untapped potential for tracking patterns in multigenerational family research.

Multidisciplinary dialogue and collaboration should be more strongly encouraged in conferences, journals, and research projects. The chasm between clinicians and researchers needs to be bridged through mutual exchange of perspectives: We have much to offer one another toward our common aim to understand and promote healthy family functioning. In future research and theory construction, our challenge is to become more knowledgeable about family functioning *in its diversity*. First, we need to better understand the typical, expectable strains and patterns in families of varying forms, social contexts, and life challenges. Second, we need to identify key processes and mediating variables that foster effective family functioning, adaptation, and the well-being of members. We have much to learn from families who succeed—to inform clinical practice with families in distress and prevention efforts with those at risk.

FROM DEFICIT TO STRENGTHS PERSPECTIVE: ADVANTAGES OF A FAMILY RESILIENCE FRAMEWORK

Over the past decade, family therapists have rebalanced the skewed perspective that long dominated the clinical field. In the many, varied approaches, focus has shifted from deficits, limitations, and pathology to a competency-based, health-oriented paradigm, recognizing and amplifying family strengths and resources (Nichols & Schwartz, 2001; Walsh & Crosser, 2000). This positive, future-oriented stance shifts the emphasis of therapy from how families have failed to how they can succeed—envisioning positive goals and options that fit each family's values and situation, and are reachable through collaborative efforts.

Family therapy approaches have become more respectful in the awareness that the very language of therapy can pathologize the family. We have become more sensitive to the blame, shame, and guilt implicit in pejorative labels with attributions of family causality (Anderson, 1986). We have turned away from earlier models emphasizing a hierarchical therapist-as-expert stance and adversarial strategies to reduce family pathology. The therapeutic relationship has become more collaborative and empowering of clients, recognizing that effective interventions depend more on drawing out family resources than on therapist change techniques (Karpel, 1986). Interventions aim to reduce stress, enhance positive interactions, support coping efforts, and mobilize kin and community resources to foster loving relationships and effective family functioning.

The concept of family resilience is valuable as a metaframework that can be applied with various strength-based practice approaches (Walsh, 1996; 1998; 2002; see Walsh, Chapter 15, this volume). It holds several advantages.

1. Unlike unrealistic problem-free, ideal models of family health, by definition, resilience focuses on strengths forged under stress, in the context of adversity. Most families who seek help are struggling in the midst of crisis. A family resilience framework is useful in identifying and facilitating family processes and other mediating variables (e.g., community resources) that reduce risk and foster effective coping and adaptation.

2. Unlike a static, singular family model, or set of traits, resilience involves processes over time, which may vary depending on adverse conditions and available resources. In clinical practice, a family resilience framework has wide applicability: in recovery from crisis, trauma, or loss; in weathering persistent illness or other adversity; or in overcoming barriers of poverty or discrimination.

3. The framework can be helpful to target intervention and prevention efforts on key processes, yet it is flexible in relation to diverse family values, structures, and resources.

4. Although some families are more vulnerable or face more hardships than others, all are seen to have potential for greater resilience in mastering their life challenges. By strengthening family resilience as presenting problems are resolved, the family becomes more resourceful in facing future challenges.

5. A resilience-based approach goes beyond coping, adaptation, or

competence in managing difficulties to recognize and seize the opportunities for transformation and growth that can emerge out of crisis.

CONCLUSION

The societal upheavals of recent decades have heightened wariness about defining *any* family pattern as normal—either typical or optimal—for families to emulate, or for therapies and social policies to promote. The growing diversity and complexity of families make it imperative to examine the social constructions of normality that powerfully influence all clinical theory and practice, family research, and social policy. Just as therapeutic neutrality is impossible, because we can never be value-free, it is naive—and ethically questionable—to adopt a neutral position toward normality, dismissing it from consideration and maintaining a stance of "anything goes" or a "one size fits all" model of intervention. A well-intentioned silence on questions of normality may be mistaken as judgment of families as abnormal or deficient for having problems or failing to fit a cultural ideal of the normal family. Silence may be taken as tacit support of norms and practices that harm members or disenfranchise families who don't meet standards. We must challenge the stigmatizing of differences as pathological and work toward more inclusive policies and attitudes.

We need to be aware of the implicit assumptions about normality we bring to our work with families from our own worldviews, including cultural standards, clinical/research paradigms, and personal/family experience. Finally, many families in their growing diversity and complexity are confused and concerned about how to build and sustain strong, loving relationships and raise children well. It is important to explore each family's constraining views of normality and family members' values and preferences for healthy family functioning, if we are to be attuned and responsive to the broad spectrum of families in our times. Family systems therapists may differ in specific ways, yet all strengths-based approaches share a deep conviction in every family's potential for health and growth.

REFERENCES

Ackerman, N. W. (1958). *The psychodynamics of family life.* New York: Basic Books.
Alexander, J. F., & Parsons, B. V. (1982). *Functional family therapy.* Pacific Grove, CA: Brooks/Cole.
Anderson, C. M. (1986). The all-too-short trip from positive to negative connotation. *Journal of Marital and Family Therapy, 12,* 351–354.
Anderson, C. M., Reiss, D., & Hogarty, G. (1986). *Schizophrenia and the family.* New York: Guilford Press.

Anderson, H. (1997). *Conversation, language, and possibilities: A postmodern approach to therapy.* New York: Basic Books.

Anderson, H., & Goolishian, H. (1988). Human systems as linguistic systems: Preliminary and evolving ideas about the implications for clinical theory. *Family Process, 27,* 371–393.

Aponte, H. (1994). *Bread and spirit: Therapy with the new poor.* New York: Norton.

Avenoli, S., Sessa, F. M., & Steinberg, L. (1999). Family structure, parenting practices, and adolescent adjustment: An ecological examination. In E. M. Hetherington (Ed.), *Coping with divorce, single parenting, and remarriage: A risk and resiliency perspective* (pp. 65–90). Mahwah, NJ: Erlbaum.

Baucom, D., Epstein, N., & LaTaillade, J. L. (2002). Cognitive-behavioral couple therapy, In A. Gurman & N. Jacobson (Eds.), *Clinical handbook of couple therapy* (pp. 26–58). New York: Guilford Press.

Beavers, W. R., & Hampson, R. B. (1990). *Successful families: Assessment and intervention.* New York: Norton.

Berg, I. (1997). *Family-based services: A solution-focused approach.* New York: Norton.

Boscolo, L., Cecchin, G., Hoffman, L., & Penn, P. (1987). *Milan systemic family therapy: Conversations in theory and practice.* New York: Basic Books.

Boss, P. (2001). *Family stress management: A contextual approach.* Thousand Oaks, CA: Sage.

Boszormenyi-Nagy, I. (1987). *Foundations of contextual family therapy.* New York: Brunner/Mazel.

Bowen, M. (1978). *Family therapy in clinical practice.* New York: Jason Aronson.

Bowlby, J. (1988). *A secure base: Parent–child attachment and healthy human development.* New York: Basic Books.

Boyd-Franklin, N. (1989). *Black families in therapy: A multisystems approach.* New York: Guilford Press.

Boyd-Franklin, N., & Bry, B. H. (2000). *Reaching out in family therapy: Home-based, school, and community interventions.* New York: Guilford Press.

Breunlin, D., Schwartz, R., & MacKune-Karrer, B. (1992). *Metaframeworks: Transcending the models of family therapy.* San Francisco: Jossey-Bass.

Byng-Hall, J. (1995). *Rewriting family scripts: Improvisation and systems change.* New York: Guilford Press.

Carter, B., & McGoldrick, M. (1999). *The expanded family life cycle: Individual, family, and social perspectives* (3rd ed.). Needham Heights, MA: Allyn & Bacon.

Carter, B., & McGoldrick, M. (2001). Advances in coaching: Family therapy with one person. *Journal of Marital and Family Therapy, 27,* 281–300.

Cecchin, G. F. (1987). Hypothesizing, circularity, and neutrality revisited: An invitation to curiosity. *Family Process, 26,* 405–414.

Combrinck-Graham, L. (1985). A developmental model for family systems. *Family Process, 24,* 139–150.

deShazer, S. (1988). *Clues: Investigating solutions in brief therapy.* New York: Norton.

Dimidjin, S., Martel, C. R., & Christensen, A. (2002). Integrative behavioral couple therapy. In A. Gurman & N. Jacobson (Eds.), *Clinical handbook of couple therapy* (pp. 251–277). New York: Guilford Press.

Doherty, W. (1995). *Soul searching: Why psychotherapy must promote moral responsibility.* New York: Basic Books.

Doherty, W., Boss, P., LaRossa, R., Schumm, W., & Steinmetz, S. (1993). Family theories and methods: A contextual approach. In P. Boss, W. Doherty, W.

LaRossa, W. Schumm, & S. Steinmetz (Eds.), *Sourcebook of family theories and methods* (pp. 3–30). New York: Plenum Press.

Epstein, N., Bishop, D., & Levin, S. (1978). The McMaster model of family functioning. *Journal of Marriage and Family Counseling. 4,* 19–31.

Epstein, N., & Schlesinger, S. E. (1996). Cognitive-behavioral treatment of family problems. In M. Reineke, F. M. Dattilio, & A. Freeman (Eds.), *Casebook of cognitive-behavioral therapy with children and adolescents.* New York: Guilford Press.

Falicov, C. (1995). Training to think culturally: A multidimensional comparative framework. *Family Process, 34,* 373–388.

Falicov, C. (1998). *Latino families in therapy: A guide to multicultural practice.* New York: Guilford Press.

Fleck, S. (1980). Family functioning and family pathology. *Psychiatric Annals, 10,* 46–57.

Foucault, M. (1980). *Power/knowledge: Selected interviews and other writings.* New York: Pantheon.

Framo, J. (1970). Symptoms from a family transactional viewpoint. In N. Ackerman (Ed.), *Family therapy in transition.* Boston: Little, Brown.

Framo, J. (1992). *Family-of-origin therapy: An intergenerational approach.* New York: Brunner/Mazel.

Freedman, J., & Combs, G. (1996). *Narrative therapy: The social construction of preferred realities.* New York: Norton.

Gilgun, J., Daly, K., & Handel, G. (Eds.). (1993). *Qualitative methods in family research.* Newbury Park, CA: Sage.

Goldner, V. (1985). Feminism and family therapy. *Family Process, 24,* 31–48.

Goldner, V. (1988). Gender and generation: Normative and covert hierarchies. *Family Process, 27,* 17–33.

Gottman, J. (1994). *Why marriages succeed or fail.* New York: Simon & Schuster.

Gralnick, A. (1943). The Carrington family: A psychiatric and social study. *Psychiatric Quarterly, 17,* 294–326.

Green, R.-J., & Werner, P. D. (1996). Intrusiveness and closeness-caregiving: Rethinking the concept of family enmeshment. *Family Process, 33,* 115–136.

Griffith, J., & Griffith, M. (2002). *Encountering the sacred in psychotherapy.* New York: Guilford Press.

Guerney, B. (1991). Marital and family enrichment research: A decade review and look ahead. In A. Booth (Ed.), *Contemporary families.* Minneapolis: National Council on Family Relations.

Haley, J. (1976). *Problem-solving therapy.* San Francisco: Jossey-Bass.

Hardy, K. V., & Laszloffy, T. A. (1995). The cultural genogram: Key to training culturally competent family therapists. *Journal of Marital and Family Therapy, 21,* 227–237.

Hare-Mustin, R. (1986). The problem of gender in family therapy theory. *Family Process, 26,* 15–27.

Henggeler, S. W., Schoenwald, S. K., Borduin, C. M., Rowland, M. D., & Cunningham, P. B. (1998). *Multisystemic treatment of antisocial behavior in children and adolescents.* New York: Guilford Press.

Hoffman, L. (2002). *Family therapy: An intimate journey.* New York: Norton.

Imber-Black, E. (1988). *Families and larger systems.* New York: Guilford Press.

Imber-Black, E., & Roberts, J. (1992). *Rituals for our time.* New York: HarperCollins.

Jackson, D. D. (1977). Family rules: Marital quid pro quo. In P. Watzlawick & J. Weakland (Eds.), *The interactional view*. New York: Norton.

Jacobson, N., & Christensen, A. (1996). *Integrative couple therapy*. New York: Norton.

Johnson, S. (1996). *The practice of emotionally focused couple therapy: Creating connection*. New York: Brunner/Mazel.

Jordan, J., Kaplan, A., Miller, J. B., Stiver, I., & Surrey, J. (1991). *Women's growth in connection: Writings from the Stone Center*. New York: Guilford Press.

Kagan, S., & Weissbourd, B. (1994). *Putting families first*. San Francisco: Jossey-Bass.

Kantor, D., & Lehr, W. (1975). *Inside the family: Toward a theory of family process*. San Francisco: Jossey-Bass.

Karpel, M. (1986). *Family resources: The hidden partner in family therapy*. New York: Guilford Press.

Laird, J. (1998). Family-centered practice in the postmodern era. In C. Franklin & P. Nurius (Eds.), *Constructivism in practice* (pp. 217–233). Milwaukee, WI: Families International, Ltd.

Laird, J., & Green, R.-J. (1996). *Lesbians and gays in families and family therapy*. San Francisco: Jossey-Bass.

Lebow, J. (1997). The integrative revolution in couple and family therapy. *Family Process, 36*(1), 1–17.

Lefley, H. P. (1996). *Family caregiving in mental illness*. Thousand Oaks, CA: Sage.

Lewis, J., Beavers, W. R., Gossett, J., & Phillips, V. (1976). *No single thread: Psychological health in family systems*. New York: Brunner/Mazel.

Luepnitz, D. (2002). *The family interpreted: Feminist theory and clinical practice*. (2nd ed.) New York: Basic Books.

Madanes, C. (1991). Strategic family therapy. In A. Gurman & D. Kniskern (Eds.), *Handbook of family therapy* (Vol. II, New York: Brunner/Mazel.

Markman, H., Renick, M. J., Floyd, F., Stanley, S., &. Clements, M. (1993). Preventing marital distress through communication and conflict management training: A 4- and 5-year follow-up. *Journal of Consulting and Clinical Psychology, 61*, 70–77.

McFarlane, W. (2002). *Multifamily groups in the treatment of severe psychiatric disorders*. New York: Guilford Press.

McGoldrick, M. (Ed.). (1998). *Revisioning family therapy: Race, culture, and gender in clinical practice*. New York: Guilford Press.

McGoldrick, M., Anderson, C., & Walsh, F. (Eds.). (1989). *Women in families: A framework for family therapy*. New York: Norton.

McGoldrick, M., Gerson, R., & Shellenberger, S. (1998). *Genograms: Assessment and intervention* (2nd ed.). New York: Norton.

McGoldrick, M., Giordano, J., & Pearce, J. (Eds.). (1996). *Ethnicity and family therapy* (2nd ed.). New York: Guilford Press.

Minuchin, S. (1974). *Families and family therapy*. Cambridge, MA: Harvard University Press.

Minuchin, P., Colapinto, J., & Minuchin, S. (1998). *Working with families of the poor*. New York: Guilford Press.

Minuchin, S., Montalvo, B., Guerney, B., Rosman, B., & Schumer, F. (1967). *Families of the slums*. New York: Basic Books.

Moos, R., & Moos, B. (1976). A typology of family social environments. *Family Process, 15*, 357–371.

Napier, A., & Whitaker, C. (1978). *The family crucible*. New York: Harper & Row.

Nichols, M., & Schwartz, R. (2001). *Family therapy: Concepts and methods* (5th ed.). Needham Heights, MA: Allyn & Bacon.

O'Hanlon, W., & Weiner-Davis, M. (1989). *In search of solutions: A new direction in psychotherapy*. New York: Norton.

Olson, D. H., Russell, C. S., & Sprenkle, D. H. (1989). *Circumplex model: Systemic assessment and treatment of families*. New York: Haworth.

Patterson, G., Reid, J., Jones, R., & Conger, R. (1975). *A social learning approach to family interaction*. Eugene, OR: Castalia.

Paul, N., & Paul, B. (1975). *A marital puzzle: Transgenerational analysis in marriage*. New York: Norton.

Pinsof, W. (1995). *Integrative problem-centered therapy*. New York: Basic Books.

Rolland, J. (1994). *Families, illness, and disability: An integrative treatment model*. New York: Basic Books.

Satir, V. (1988). *The new peoplemaking*. Palo Alto, CA: Science & Behavior Books.

Scharff, D., & Scharff, J.S. (1987). *Object relations family therapy*. New York: Jason Aronson.

Schumm, W. (1985). Beyond relationship characteristics of strong families: Constructing a model of family strengths. *Family Perspective, 19,* 1–9.

Selvini Palazzoli, M., Boscolo, L., Cecchin, G., & Prata, G. (1980). Hypothesizing, circularity, neutrality: Three guidelines for the conductor of sessions. *Family Process, 19,* 3–12.

Skinner, H., Santa Barbara, J. & Steinhauer, P. (1983). The family assessment measure. *Canadian Journal of Community Mental Health, 2,* 91–105.

Sluzki, C. (1983). Process, structure, and world views in family therapy: Toward and integration of systemic models. *Family Process, 22,* 469–476.

Steinglass, P. (1998). Multiple family discussion groups for patients with chronic medical illness. *Families, Systems, and Health, 16*(1–2), 55–71.

Stierlin, H. (1974). *Separating parents and adolescents*. New York: Aronson.

Stinnett, N., & DeFrain, J. (1985). *Secrets of strong families*. Boston: Little, Brown.

Visher, E., & Visher, J. (1996). *Therapy with stepfamilies*. New York: Brunner/Mazel.

Walsh, F. (1987). The clinical utility of normal family research. *Psychotherapy, 24,* 496–503.

Walsh, F. (1993). Conceptualization of normal family processes. In F. Walsh (Ed.), *Normal family processes* (2nd ed., pp. 3–69). New York: Guilford Press.

Walsh, F. (1996). The concept of family resilience: Crisis and challenge. *Family Process, 35,* 261–281.

Walsh, F. (1998). *Strengthening family resilience*. New York: Guilford Press.

Walsh, F. (1999a). Families in later life: Challenges and opportunities. In B. Carter & M. McGoldrick, (Eds.), *The expanded family life cycle* (3rd ed., pp. 307–326). Needham Heights, MA: Allyn & Bacon.

Walsh, F. (Ed.). (1999b). *Spiritual resources in family therapy*. New York: Guilford Press.

Walsh, F. (2002). A family resilience framework: Innovative practice applications . *Family Relations, 51*(2), 333–355.

Walsh, F., & Anderson, C. (1989). *Chronic disorders and the family*. New York: Haworth.

Walsh, F., & Crosser, C. (Eds.). (2000). Advances in family therapy theory and practice. In P. Allen-Meares & C. Garvin (Eds.), *Handbook of clinical social work* (pp. 301–325). Thousand Oaks, CA: Sage.

Walsh, F., & Scheinkman, M. (1989). (Fe)male: The hidden gender dimension in models of family therapy. In M. McGoldrick, C. Anderson, & F. Walsh (Eds.), *Women in families* (pp. 16–41). New York: Norton.

Weakland, J., Fisch, R., Watzlawick, P., & Bodin, A. (1974). Brief therapy: Focused problem resolution. *Family Process, 13,* 141–168.

Whitaker, C., & Keith, D. (1981). Symbolic–experiential family therapy. In A. Gurman & D. Kniskern (Eds.), *Handbook of family therapy.* New York: Brunner/Mazel.

White, M. (1995). *Re-authoring lives: Interviews and essays.* Australia: Dulwich Centre Publications.

White, M., & Epston, D. (1990). *Narrative means to therapeutic ends.* New York: Norton.

Wood, B. (1985). Proximity and hierarchy: Orthogonal dimensions of family interconnectedness. *Family Process, 24,* 487–507.

Zacks, E., Green, R.-J., & Marrow, J. (1988). Comparing lesbian and heterosexual couples on the Circumplex Model: An initial investigation. *Family Process, 27,* 471–484.

PART II

Varying Family Forms and Challenges

CHAPTER 3

CONTEMPORARY TWO-PARENT FAMILIES
Navigating Work and Family Challenges

Peter Fraenkel

In this chapter I describe the challenges facing contemporary, two-parent families. Framed this way, the task seems enormous: How, in more than cursory fashion, may the multiple sources of stress and opportunity encountered by two-parent families in the 21st century be summarized? Here's a short list:

- Negotiating the transitions incurred by the generic stages of the family life cycle (Chapters 14 and 16) from dating to commitment to marriage; birth of the first child; launching children into school years, adolescence, and independence; retirement and old age; and for many, managing the challenges of divorce and remarriage (see Chapters 4, 5, and 6, this volume), with many possible permutations of this life cycle depending on ethnicity and culture (Chapters 9 and 11), sexual orientation (Chapter 7), religion (Chapter 13), infertility (Diamond, Kezur, Meyers, Scharf, & Weinshel, 1999), and adoption (Chapter 8), among other variables.
- Addressing the common sources of interspousal (Chapter 18), parent–child, and sibling differences, and conflicts that accompany marriage and family life.
- Coping with a whole range of statistically less than normative (for the population as a whole) but nonetheless powerful transitions resulting from onset of acute or chronic illness or disability (Chapter 17); premature death (Rosen, 1998), or the sudden, unexplained disappearance of a spouse or a child (Boss, 2000); and loss or

chronic unavailability of employment (Wilson, 1996), among other circumstances.

- The particular struggles of two-parent families oppressed or marginalized on the basis of race and class (Chapter 10), ethnicity (Chapter 11), immigration status (Chapter 11), sexual orientation (Chapter 7), and advanced age (Mohr, 2000).
- The impact of biologically driven psychological disorders and personality characteristics such as temperament (Chapter 22).
- The impact of the media on self-esteem and body image, especially for children and teens (Gilbert, 1998), contributing to the prevalence of eating disorders (Owen & Laurel-Seller, 2000) and often overriding the influence of parents on how children feel about themselves.
- Rampant advertising and consumerism (Wachtel, 1989), and the ever-growing presence of aggressive and sexual images in the media (Pipher, 1996).
- The effects on families of the ever-diminishing natural resources and wildlife on our planet, and the gradual polluting of what's left (Howard, 1997).
- The multiple challenges faced when both parents work (current chapter; Perry-Jenkins, Repetti, & Crouter, 2000).
- The impact of the phenomenal growth in communication and information technologies (current chapter; Fraenkel, 2001a, 2001b; Imber-Black, 2000).

And the list goes on. Thankfully, the task ahead is bounded by the presence of the other excellent chapters in this book, which focus or at least touch on many of these issues. In this chapter, I focus on one central issue that distinguishes most contemporary two-parent families, namely, the challenges facing families in which both parents work, so-called "dual-earner" families. Since the 1970s, dual-earner families have become the norm (Bond, Galinsky, & Swanberg, 1998), and most two-parent families in the coming decades will continue this pattern.

In discussing dual-earner families, by necessity, I address the multiple challenges of "navigating"[1] (Galinsky, 1999) work and nonwork aspects of life faced by all families, whether two- or one-parent, dual- or single-earner, or headed by heterosexual or same-sex adult partners. I focus on the work–family research conducted with two-parent, heterosexual, married couples, because another chapter of this book focuses on lesbian, gay, and bisexual (LGB) families, and little research has focused on work–family issues in LGB families (Barnett & Hyde, 2001). As much as possible, I note the permutations of work–family patterns and issues that center on differences in race, ethnicity, and social class, although, again, the work–family literature examining these sources of family diversity is still underdeveloped (Barnett & Hyde, 2001).

In addressing work–family issues, it will also be necessary to address the impact on families of technologies that blur the boundary between work and family time (Fraenkel, 2001a, 2001b). Coursing through my discussion of these issues will be a theme increasingly noted in both the professional and popular press: the sense of time pressure and the frantic pace experienced by many contemporary families (Fraenkel, 2001a, 2001b; Fraenkel & Wilson, 2000).

Far from limiting the purview on two-parent families to only one aspect of their lives, a focus on the interface between work and the family nicely refracts a host of central themes: how families organize themselves around the core relational dimensions of gender, power, and connection; how they handle strong emotion; the impact of larger systems and of participation in groups defined by gender, race, ethnicity, and class; and sources of coping and resilience, to name but a few. Over the past decade, an explosion of research on work–family issues has built on the already impressive literature reviewed by Piotrowski and Hughes (1993) in the previous edition of this text. Indeed, that chapter outlined a comprehensive framework for organizing reflection on the relationship between the workplace and families. To honor the authors' contribution and to create a degree of continuity across editions, I loosely adopt their framework, examining the epidemiology of two-parent, dual-earner families, their social–structural, cultural, and developmental contexts, and the nature of their specific challenges. In line with much of the research emerging over the past decade, I add a section on strategies of dual-earner families that view themselves as successful at meeting the many challenges. This chapter draws liberally from several excellent review articles that appeared in the November 2000 issue of the Journal of Marriage and the Family on work and family (Perry-Jenkins et al., 2000), household labor (Coltrane, 2000), economic circumstances (White & Rogers, 2000), poverty (Seccombe, 2000), and family policy (Bogenschneider, 2000).

THE EPIDEMIOLOGY AND STATE OF THE TWO-PARENT, DUAL-EARNER FAMILY

The Two-Parent Family: An Increasingly Rare Family Form

Before launching into the literature on work and the two-parent family, it's worth locating this family composition in terms of its frequency among the increasingly diverse panoply of family forms. The June 2001 report from the United States Bureau of the Census (2001a) indicates that two-parent families, in which a male and a female are married to one another and raise their own children (including shared biological progeny, stepchildren, or adopted children),[2] represent only 23% of all households and less than 50% of family households. Specifically, two-parent married families with children under age 18 constitute 35% of all family households, still slightly higher than the 31% of single-parent households

(U.S. Bureau of the Census, 2001b). If the roughly 1.5 million unmarried, cohabiting couples with children are added to the number of married couples with children, two-parent families with children constitute approximately 37% of all family households. Of the approximately 11% of lesbian or gay cohabiting couples (U.S. Bureau of the Census, 2000b), an unknown percentage are raising children in their household.[3] Finally, the Census does not count as two-parent families those households with children over age 18 living in or out of the home. This may result in a marked underestimation of the viability of the intact two-parent family form.

Thus, although the percentage of married, two-parent families with children is likely larger than some estimates suggest, this family form has certainly declined in numbers over the years, relative to other forms. Although the number of single-mother families increased from 3 million (12%) in 1970 to 10 million (26%) in 2000, and the number of single fathers increased from 393,000 (1%) to 2 million (5%) in the same period, married couples with their own children (again, including step- and adopted children) decreased from 40% to 35% of all families in this period (U.S. Bureau of the Census, 2001a). In addition, the *intact* two-parent family with children (first marriage for both partners, children produced by their sexual union), long lionized in popular culture and viewed as the gold standard of family forms despite the fact that this form never represented a majority of families (Coontz, 2000), is not even a separate category within the U.S. Census or Bureau of Labor Statistics reports, or in major nongovernmental studies such as the National Study of the Changing Workforce (Bond et al., 1998; Galinsky, Bond, & Friedman, 1993).

Increases in the number of single (never-married) parents, and in the rates of long-term unmarried cohabitation, along with the stable and high divorce rate for the last 35 years, in large part accounts for the low frequency of married couples with children. The divorce rate remains close to 50% for first marriages (Goldstein, 1999; Teachman, Tedrow, & Crowder, 2000). Thus, partners who begin as a two-parent, first-marriage family are as likely to remain married as heads are likely to appear more than tails in a coin toss.

For some scholars, clinicians, and social commentators, these statistics suggest a welcome diversification in how families are constructed (Coontz, 2000; Pinsof, 2002; Silverstein & Auerbach, 1999; Stacey, 1996). For others, it virtually signals the social and moral decline of our society (Blankenhorn, 1995; Popenoe, 1996) and/or a major risk for the mental and even physical health of both parents and children (Gottman, 1994; Waite & Gallagher, 2000). Whatever the perspectives on marriage and desires of the partners at the time of divorce, it can be assumed that the current rates of two-parent families represent a markedly different marital outcome than the majority of partners desired when they decided to marry.

A wide range of societal, economic, and relational variables has been proposed as the cause of high divorce rates, including increased lifespan; no-fault divorce laws or at least the changes in social values and decreased stigma of divorce that these laws represent; increased economic empowerment of women and diffusion of contraceptive technology, both giving women more choice; increased levels of poorly managed marital conflict due to economic and work-related stress; reduced access to social support from extended family and community because of increased geographical mobility, and an increased number of adult children of divorce who grew up without models for conflict management and resolution (for reviews, see Greene et al., Chapter 4, this volume; Karney & Bradbury, 1995; Pinsof, 2002; Waite & Gallagher, 2000).

Indeed, there are now many attempts to intervene on some of these variables and thereby increase the number of stable first-time marriages (or at least the odds for those who choose to marry and wish to stay that way). Preventing destructive marital conflict and preserving satisfied marriages has become an ardently pursued goal for some mental health researchers and practitioners (cf. Berger & Hannah, 1999; Markman, Floyd, Stanley, & Storaasli, 1988; Markman, Renick, Floyd, Stanley, & Clements, 1993; Markman, Stanley, & Blumberg, 2001), policy analysts (Ooms, 1998), religious organizations, and even state and federal government. Under George W. Bush's administration, tax laws have been revised to encourage couples to stay married. A number of states have created so-called "covenant marriages" (Bogenschneider, 2000), which make divorce much more difficult to obtain.

Although careful examination of research data suggests that divorce is not in itself inevitably associated with negative effects for adult and child family members (Ahrons, 1995; Guttman, 1993), a growing body of research does identify marital distress, whether or not followed by divorce, as a significant mental and physical health risk factor for adults and children (Fraenkel & Markman, 2002; see Greene et al., Chapter 4, this volume). In addition to the literature on marital processes predictive of distress and divorce, strong arguments and research support the effectiveness of distress prevention programs (Fraenkel & Markman, 2002). However, it is worth noting that although these programs typically work on enhancing partners' coping skills and encouraging examination of their relational beliefs and expectations, they do not focus much on recognizing and intervening in the many challenges two-parent families face at the boundary of the family and the workplace (Bradbury, Fincham, & Beach, 2000; Fraenkel & Markman, 2002).

Prevalence and Economic Status of Dual-Earner Families

Depending on the particular survey, it appears that the rates of two-parent families with two earners has either remained roughly the same over the past decade or increased substantially. The U.S. Bureau of Labor Statistics

(2001) reports that 64.2% of married-couple families with children under 18 are dual earners. The U.S. Bureau of the Census (2001b) reports a slightly higher figure (67%), whereas the most recent National Study of the Changing Workforce (Bond et al., 1998) found that 78% are dual earners, a great increase over the 64% found by an earlier version of this study in 1977.

Given that changes in rates of dual-earner versus single-earner families largely reflect the degree to which women are employed, statistics suggest that women are increasingly well represented in the workforce. Seventy-seven percent of women were employed by 1998 (Perry-Jenkins et al., 2000), and although Latino and Native American mothers were less represented in the workforce than whites, Asian Americans, or African Americans, comparisons with previous decades of women's employment show that the variables of marital status, age, race, and motherhood are having less influence than previously on whether a woman works (Spain & Bianchi, 1996).

However, having a child under the age of 6 in the home continues to affect women's labor participation, and therefore rates of dual earnership. In 2000, the Bureau of Labor Statistics (2001) found that whereas the rates of dual-earner couples rose to 70.3% for families with school-age children only, dual earnership dropped to 56.9% for those with children under age 6. Similar differences (63.9% women working with children under age 6, 78.3% working with children ages 6 to 17) were reported for 1997 by Hayghe (1997). Likewise, although 75% of dual-earner couples both work full-time, when there are children, particularly young children in the home, women are more likely than men to work part-time or to have shorter full-time hours (Bond et al., 1998). Indeed, one of the foremost strategies dual-earner couples use to balance child care needs with employment and career needs is that women temporarily cut back or leave work (Becker & Moen, 1999; Moen & Yu, 2000).

The percentages of dual-earner families are fairly similar across racial/ethnic groups, with slightly lower rates for Latino families. Sixty-four percent of white, 69% of black, 63% of Asian and Pacific Islander, and 51% of Latino families are dual earners (U.S. Bureau of the Census, 2000b). Viewed alone, these statistics suggest greater equality among racial groups in employment rates. Of course, to grasp the relationship between race and families' economic status, it is important also to examine unemployment and income rates. Recent national statistics found black families (all forms, not specifically two-parent) had higher rates of unemployment of at least one member (10.2%) than did Latino families (9%), and both had much higher unemployment rates than did white families (5%) (Bureau of Labor Statistics, 2001). Although unemployment rates for different racial groups may differ for single- versus two-parent families these statistics likely estimate the unequal employment rates for *two-parent* families of different races.

Likewise, average incomes vary dramatically across married-couple families of different races. The mean income in 2000 for white families was $80,767, for black families, $58,143, and for Latino families, $48,367 (U.S. Bureau of the Census, 2001c).

In addition, although employment was up for most groups (White & Rogers, 2000) compared to the prior decade, the much-vaunted economic boom of the late 1990s did not profit all equally. Indeed, the top 20% of earners profited most, especially those in the top 4%, whereas the income of those in the lowest two-fifths of the range actually declined (White & Rogers, 2000). Incomes for adult men without college degrees have declined since the 1960s, whereas income has increased for women irrespective of education (U.S. Bureau of the Census, 1998, as cited in White & Rogers, 2000). However, for white and latino but not black families, men continued to earn more than women (Bond et al., 1998), often for comparable employment. Overall, women's earnings are 73% of men's annual earnings (U.S. Bureau of the Census, 2001d).

Another 1990s phenomenon not specific to two-parent families but certainly affecting them was the dramatic increase in both contingent workers—those without long-term contracts (Rogers, 2000)—and part-time workers (Seccombe, 2000). Temporary agencies employed more persons than any other type of company (Castro, 1993), and the percentage of workers with temporary jobs has doubled over the past decade (Seccombe, 2000). Most often these workers have no or limited benefits through work, resulting in both material and financially determined emotional instability for many families. In the latter part of the decade, a number of emergent publications put a positive spin on this situation, especially for those working in the technology sector, trumpeting the emergence of the "free agent" that worked from home or the road and moved from contract to contract, unfettered by the boring old commitments and daily work rhythms required by traditional company positions (McGovern & Russell, 2001). In addition, many in the technology sector forfeited reasonable salaries for stock options. With the crash of the dot.coms, the free agent rhetoric and the enthusiasm for stock options as a substitute for salary has evaporated, and many dot.com workers are searching for traditional employment or completing education to obtain such jobs (Parnes, 2001).

Thus, although "women, two-earner families, and the college educated benefited the most from the strong economy" in terms of employment (White & Rogers, 2000, p. 1036), taken as a whole, the employment statistics still remind us that white men dominate the workplace, and that the rich still get richer while the poor get poorer. Therefore, in light of recent trends, white, two-parent families, especially well-to-do families, are more likely to do well economically than two-parent families of other racial/ethnic backgrounds.

CHALLENGES AT THE BOUNDARY
OF WORK AND FAMILY

Work Hours and Schedules

It has become almost a truism in the professional and popular literatures that Americans are working longer hours than ever before (Center on Budget and Policy Priorities, 1998; Greenhouse, 1999, 2001), and that this overwork results for many in increased individual and family stress (Schor, 1991). A recent study by the International Labor Organization (2001; Greenhouse, 2001) found that in the 1990s, Americans worked an additional full week per year compared to the 1980s. They worked 3½ weeks more per year than the Japanese, who in earlier decades had been the world's leader in hours worked; and 6½ and 12½ weeks more than British and German workers, respectively. In dual-earner marriages, the average employee reports a work week of 46 hours, with men on average working more hours (50.2) than women (42.4) (Bond et al., 1998). The difference between men's and women's hours is even greater when they are raising children, with men working on average 50.5 hours and women 40.6 hours, and with the largest difference (on average, 11 hours) occurring when children are under 6 years of age (Bond et al., 1998). It is also noteworthy that 13% of salaried employees work an average of 13.2 additional hours at another job, and 83% of these employees do so in addition to a full-time job. Given the previously mentioned finding that in 75% of dual-earner families, both partners work full time, this suggests that partners work a combined average of 91 hours per week. These combined work hours are today substantially higher than 30 years ago: Compared to hours worked in 1970, husbands and wives reported between them an average of 10 hours more work per week (Jacobs & Gerson, 1998).

In addition to regular hours on the job, many employees find the workday expanding around the edges. "Eighteen percent of employees are required to work paid or unpaid overtime hours once a week or more with little or no notice" (Bond et al., 1998, p. 74); 12% of employees spend between one and five nights away from home on business in a 3-month period; and 31% bring work home at least once a week—10% more than took home work in 1977 (Bond et al., 1998).

Although some studies indicate an increase in work hours across class and occupation (Greenhouse, 2001; Schor, 1991), a more fine-grained analysis indicates that work hours varied by class, with stress caused by overwork for some, and by being unable to increase work hours (to make more money) for others (Perry-Jenkins et al., 2000). Increase in work hours appears to be greatest in managerial, professional, and technical occupations (Daly, 2001; Bond et al., 1998). Although most studies have documented increased hours and days of work per year, one study questioning these findings (Robinson & Godbey, 1997) still echoes others that find workers, including those with more job autonomy and control, experiencing work as more hectic and demanding (Bond et al., 1998; Galinsky et al., 1993; Lagerfeld, 1998; Robinson & Godbey, 1997). A recent study by the Families and Work Institute (Galinsky, Kim, & Bond, 2001) found that almost half of employees reported feeling often or very often overworked, overwhelmed by the amount of work they had to do, and/or unable to step back and reflect on their work.

Overall, studies find a strong preference for working fewer hours. In one study, 44% of men and 34% of women reported working more hours than they wished (Clarkberg & Moen, 1999). In another, 63% of employees expressed the desire to work less (Bond et al., 1998), up from 47% in 1992 (Galinsky et al., 1993). Fully 90% of parents were found to prefer a shorter work week (Hewlett & West, 1998). Almost half reported that the main reason they worked more hours than desired was financial need (46%), followed by a sense that they would not be allowed by their companies to reduce their hours (20%), dedication to the company's success (16%), workaholism (5%), and assorted other reasons (13%) (Bond et al., 1998). These numbers suggest that the majority of persons work long hours because they *must,* not by choice—a different conclusion from Hochschild's (1997) finding that parents (especially women) stay longer at work primarily to avoid home life, and different from the popular belief that men's long work hours reflect their sense of entitlement to prioritize their careers over their families (Galinsky, 1999).

More companies now offer flextime, ostensibly allowing more choice in work schedules (Bogenschneider, 2000), and in 1993, the Family and Medical Leave Act (FMLA) was passed, allowing 12 weeks of unpaid leave for childbirth, adoption, or caring for ill family members (Perry-Jenkins et al., 2000). However, these policies often do not translate into real options for workers, for a variety of reasons. For instance, Perry-Jenkins et al. (2000) have pointed out that the FMLA actually is available for only about 50% of workers because it does not apply to small businesses (50 or fewer employees) and is not available for part-time, seasonal, or temp workers, nor for families with same-sex partners. Because it is unpaid leave (unlike the paid leave available in most European countries), it is unfeasible for most lower income workers (Gerstel & McGonagle, 1999).

Likewise, the vast majority of parents support increases in flextime, job sharing, and part-time work with benefits (Hewlett & West, 1998). However, many workers are reluctant to exercise the temporal flexibility provided through these policies because of concerns that they will be regarded by employers and colleagues as not hardworking, increasing their risk of being overlooked for promotions or fired as companies downsize (Fried, 1998; Hochschild, 1997).

Thus, the increase in pressure to work more hours, especially on persons with occupations in which they exercise some control over their time, along with increased provision by companies of opportunities to shape work schedules, psychologically place the "locus of control" (and there-fore, the sense of responsibility) for overwork on the worker rather than on the often subtle or not so subtle messages about expectations and norms within workplace cultures. As a result, many of these workers (and their families) may view their sense of overwork as the result of their own inability to set limits or work efficiently, rather than an understandable at-tempt to survive in an unstable, demanding corporate culture. Locating the problem in the worker rather than the context has also fueled the seemingly insatiable desire for books, software, and systems that promise greater personal efficiency and organization (Covey, Merrill, & Merrill, 1994; Morgenstern, 2000). In a sense, the current tendency to blame work-ers for their out-of-balance work schedules represents for the middle to upper classes a phenomenon parallel to one that has long existed for the underclass when it comes to economic well-being, namely, the myth that failure to move up the economic ladder is due to laziness or lack of talent rather than to a lack of opportunities (Sennett & Cobb, 1972). For many in the middle to upper classes, the sought-after but elusive resource is time, more than money (Bond et al., 1998; Galinsky et al., 1993).

Spending long hours on the job is not the only temporal risk factor in the equation linking work and family stress. Approximately 27% of dual-earner couples have one partner doing shift work (e.g., working other than the usual morning to late afternoon shift). Differences between part-ners in shifts are associated with greater marital distress (Voydanoff, 1988; White & Keith, 1990). Couples in which one partner is a shift worker are between 7 and 11% more at risk for divorce over a 3-year period than cou-ples working the same shift (White & Keith, 1990). Compared to couples working the same shift, couples in which one partner was a shift worker ex-perienced more marital distress, more negative interactions, more dis-agreements, and greater numbers of general sexual and child-related problems (White & Keith, 1990). Importantly, shift work is more likely in families at lower socioeconomic levels (Presser & Cox, 1997; White & Keith, 1990) and for black families over white families, adding yet another stressor to the lives of black families.

Despite documented risks, there may be some benefits to families in-volved in shift work, in that fathers in such families—at least in those fami-lies that cannot or choose not to purchase domestic services—do more child care and housework than fathers in dual-earner families on the same shift (see Coltrane, 2000, for a review). For families that cannot afford good-quality child care, or that strongly value having at least one parent in close contact with the children at all times, shift work allows for two in-comes and "in-family" parenting. On the other hand, one question not an-swered by current research is whether the higher rate of marital distress and divorce in dual-shift couples is partly due to many men's reluctance to do what has traditionally been viewed as "women's work."

Temporal dyssynchronies in parents' work schedules need not be as extreme as shift work in order to create some of the associated challenges (and perhaps, some of the benefits). Differences of as little as 1 or 2 hours in parents' schedules of leaving for and returning from work, when combined with children's wake, bedtime, and school transportation schedules, can result in significantly less or more opportunity to share child care, housework, and family time (see Fraenkel & Wilson, 2000, for a clinical example). The complexity of synchronizing parents' work schedules with one another, and with children's schedules, may be more critical to understanding the experience of time crunch in dual-earner families than long work hours of one or the other parent alone (Jacobs & Gerson, 2001; Presser, 1994).

Technology and the Work–Family Boundary

Whereas some parents struggle with dyssynchronous work shifts, other problems emerge when one or both parents find themselves on one long, endless shift, due to virtually unlimited connectivity to the workplace provided by the explosion of communication and information technologies. Through laptops and other computers, cell phones, pagers, PDAs (personal digital assistants), and wireless Internet access devices, as well as old-fashioned "landline" phones, fax machines, scanners, and home copiers, work can and does occur virtually anywhere, all but erasing the physical boundary between home life and the workplace (Fraenkel, 2001a, 2001b; Fraenkel & Wilson, 2000). Certainly, executives and professionals have long taken work home, at least since the 1950s, when William Hollingsworth Whyte (1957) provided the classic depiction of the American, white-collar employee in *The Organization Man*. However, the availability of multiple means of highly portable electronic linkages to work and the workplace appears to have increased this trend dramatically (Bond et al., 1998) and has to some extent spread it across class and occupations. As a result, an increasing number of couples and families find work invading activities that might otherwise be "work-free zones," such as long-planned romantic dinners, time with kids at the playground, at sporting events and other children's activities, and even vacations. One survey found that 63% of workers had contact with the office during vacation via some form of communication technology (O'Brien, 2000).

As a function of this technology, an increasing number of workers telecommute. By 2000, it was estimated that 21 million people worked at home (Ruhling, 2000), and by 2020, it is estimated that at least 40% of the American workforce will be telecommuters or home office workers. Although advertisements for products related to home offices always depict smiling parents working with relaxed concentration while their kids happily look on (or working on an adjoining desk on their own computer), many parents working at home describe even more intense issues around balancing work and family time than when they worked in out-of-home offices (Belkin, 1999).

This increased connectivity to work can bring benefits as well as problems, depending on how families manage it. On the upside, it can save commuting time. Depending on the demands and structures of the job, telecommuting can allow some people to work part-time and coordinate work flexibly with child and home care (see a case example in Fraenkel, 2001b). When a crisis at work might otherwise have resulted in canceling or delaying a vacation or family event, now a few calls or e-mails initially or periodically allow the work problem to be managed from afar. On the other hand, technology and telecommuting present serious challenges to limiting the encroachment of work on family life (Fraenkel, 2001a, 2001b) and create the conditions for possible temporal exploitation of employees (Friedman, 2001). One study found that 41% of employees frequently use technology for work purposes during nonwork hours and days; 22% reported being required by employers to be accessible through technology; and these employees described themselves as more overworked than employees who rarely or never used technology for work purposes during nonwork hours (Galinsky et al., 2001).

Work Stress and Family Stress: A Complex Relationship

It is clear that Americans work more hours than in recent history, that many feel overworked, and that there is a link between hours on the job and a sense of being overworked (Galinsky et al., 2001). Galinsky and colleagues also found employees' sense of overwork linked to feeling pressured on the job (needing to work fast, hard, and without time to get everything done), to feeling that they often have difficulty focusing on their work, experience many interruptions, have to work on too many tasks at once, and have little control over their work schedules and, consequently, little flexibility with which to meet both work and family responsibilities. Interestingly, all of these contributors to overwork are temporal in nature—variables that I have described as duration, pace, sense of temporal fragmentation, sequence, and daily rhythms (Fraenkel, 1994, 2001b). Compared to persons who do not feel overworked, employees who feel overworked believe they make more mistakes on the job, feel more anger toward employers and more resentment toward colleagues whom they perceive as working less hard, are more likely to look for another job, experience more work–family conflict and less satisfying relationships with family and friends, believe that they do not take good care of themselves, and report more work-related sleep disruption, poorer health, and higher overall levels of stress (Galinsky et al., 2001).

However, the relationship between temporal characteristics of the job and work stress, and between work stress and family difficulties, is not simple or direct. A number of studies suggest that it is the *perception* of overwork, not simply the number of hours per se, and the *experience* of stress, rather than number or intensity of job-related stressors, that determine the degree of linkage between work stress and family distress (see Bogenschneider, 2000; Perry-Jenkins et al., 2000, for reviews). Put differently, work role quality (the degree to which a person experiences fulfillment in work) appears to be more related to overall level of life satisfaction or stress than hours per se (Hyde, Klein, Essex, & Clark, 1995), although at the upper limits, long hours appears to incur anxiety and distress (Bond et al., 1998; Galinsky et al., 2001; Hyde et al., 1995; Voydanoff & Donnelly, 1999). As Galinsky et al. (2001) write, "Every employee reaches a point when increasing work demands simply becomes too much—a point at which personal and family relations, personal health, and the quality of work itself are seriously threatened. Today's 24/7 economy appears to be pushing many employees to and beyond that point" (p. 13).

Research has identified a number of variables that moderate the relationship between work stressors and family life. However, variables traditionally believed to reduce likelihood of job-related stress—for instance, having more control at work—have in other studies been found to predict greater stress. In one study, degree of control over meeting job responsibilities was associated with reduced likelihood of poor health for persons with high self-efficacy, who did not blame themselves for negative work outcomes, but was associated with *increased* likelihood of poor health for those with low self-efficacy and a heightened tendency to blame themselves for negative work outcomes (Schaubroeck, Jones, & Xie, 2001). In addition, some of the same variables that represent end outcomes can also serve as moderators between work variables and other outcomes. For instance, marital quality is both an outcome in itself and a moderator between work stress and other outcomes, such as parent–child conflict. Table 3.1 presents a nonexhaustive list of these moderator variables, along with frequently studied job stressors and family outcomes.

As Perry-Jenkins and colleagues (2000) describe in their review of studies on chronic stress transfer, the link between work stress and a "marital or parent–child relationship outcome was only observed through an individual well-being mediator, such as role strain or emotional distress" (p. 987). They note: "Job stressors have an impact on families when they cause some experience of stress within the individual, such as emotional distress, fatigue, a sense of conflict between work and family roles, or role overload. In the absence of one or more of these intervening links, stress transfer cannot occur" (p. 987).

Another limitation of most existing research noted by Perry-Jenkins et al. (2000) is that it assumes that work-related stress negatively affects individual and family functioning rather than conceptualizing the link between work and family stress as recursive or bidirectional. For instance, a husband's stressful job demands may decrease his availability or emotional

TABLE 3.1. A Model of Variables Influencing Work-Related Family Stress

Work variables	Mediators and moderators	Family impact
Work hours	Perception of work–family	Marital distress
Degree of flexibility	conflict	Conflict with children
of hours	Preference for more or less	and adolescents
Number of roles/	than currently working	Child behavior
responsibilities/	Perceived role overload/	problems
demands	multiple commitments	Spouse's depression/
Interestingness of job	Depression and anxiety in	sense of overload
Too much or too little	stressed or other spouse	
control	Worker emotional distress	
Quality of social climate/	Worker fatigue	
support at work	Commitment to work/career	
Level of occupational	Personality style (Negative	
prestige	affectivity, neuroticism,	
Hour-to-salary ratio	Type A)	
Degree of job security	Coping style	
	Self efficacy and self-esteem	
	Social support	
	Life stage of family/ages of	
	children	
	Child behavior problems	
	Parenting style	
	Number of children	
	Positive or negative marital	
	quality	
	Perceived fairness of	
	housework and child care	
	distribution	
	Gendered beliefs about	
	emotional expression and	
	partner soothing	
	Gender ideology/partners'	
	beliefs about value and	
	acceptability of mother	
	working	
	Race and class	

energy to share responsibilities in family life, leading to the wife's sense of overburden and resentment about carrying his share on top of her own work-related stress and family responsibilities. Both partners may then bring the resulting marital distress back to the workplace, decreasing their focus and effectiveness at work, which in turn contributes to a sense of being overwhelmed with the job's demands. In addition, many studies' findings are confounded because data on individual and family stress and work hours are gathered from the same source, typically, the worker (Perry-Jenkins et al., 2000).

Keeping in mind these important caveats, a number of studies demonstrate relationships between perceived work pressure and increased experience of conflict among multiple family roles and commitments (Crouter, Bumpus, Maguire, & McHale, 1999), as well as emotional distress resulting from conflict between work and family roles (Guelzow, Bird, & Koball, 1991; Paden & Buehler, 1995). Relationships have been found between work stress and likelihood of parent–child conflict and poorer child behavioral and emotional outcomes (Crouter, Bumpus, Head, & McHale, 2001; see Perry-Jenkins et al., 2000, for review); between work stress and decreased parental monitoring and knowledge of children's lives, at least when fathers (but not when mothers) had demanding jobs and there was poor marital quality (Bumpus, Crouter, & McHale, 1999); and between working more hours than desired and a reduced sense of coping ability (Moen & Yu, 2000). Studies of daily stress transfer (Larson & Almeida, 1999; Perry-Jenkins et al., 2000) have found high work stress associated with emotional distress, which is then associated with higher rates of negative marital interactions, increases in physiological arousal, and decreases in mood quality and well-being, and withdrawal from contact with family at the end of the day.

Interestingly, both high and low marital satisfaction may increase the link between workplace stress and family life. Close partners may be more likely to transmit stress to their caregiving partners (Rook, Dooley, & Catalano, 1991), and workers who value their family roles may experience greater conflict between those roles and their work (Wortman, Biernat, & Lang, 1991). Conversely, low marital satisfaction may increase the likelihood that work stress interferes with adequate parenting, possibly by decreasing communication between partners or increasing the total amount of stress to the point that parents withdraw somewhat from their partners as well as their children (Bumpus et al., 1999). In addition, some studies have found a link between marital distress and missed days at work (Forthofer, Markman, Cox, Stanley, & Kessler, 1996).

Studies find important gender differences in the degree to which job stress transfers into negative family processes. Studies of emotion transmission within couples and families generally find that men's emotions affect women's emotions more reliably than the reverse (see Larson & Almeida, 1999, for review). This pattern has been interpreted to reflect and reproduce the typical power difference between men and women, although others argue that it may reflect women's greater responsiveness and their deliberate attempts to elicit their male partners' emotions (Larson & Almeida, 1999). The impact on wives of absorbing negative emotion from the husband's unburdening about work may be exacerbated when husbands fail to show reciprocal interest in their wives' work and other experiences of the day.

Likewise, although, in general, mothers certainly transmit their emotions to their children (Downey, Purdie, & Schaffer-Neitz, 1999), a number of studies indicate that employed fathers transmit more job-related stress to children than do employed mothers (see Larson & Almeida,

1999), although mothers have also been found to withdraw from their preschool children more after stressful workdays (Repetti & Wood, 1997). Thus, although both men and women may experience work stress and transmit it to other family members, men seem particularly likely to do so; women appear to be more skilled at "distress containment" (Downey et al., 1999). Interestingly, more emotional distress is transmitted from the marital to the parent–child subsystem when mothers work full-time than when they work part-time or not at all (Almeida, Wethington, & Chandler, 1999). According to Larson and Almeida (1999), this finding may indicate that a full-time working woman may be less willing to fulfill her husband's explicit or implicit expectation that she will absorb his work-related emotional upset or keep it from reaching the children.

As noted earlier, the relationship between work hours and individual or family stress is complex. Although many experience stress from the increase in work hours and days, many of those at the lower economic rungs of the work ladder—who were more likely to work part-time or 40 hours or less per week—expressed a preference for more work time over family time, especially due to financial pressures (Galinsky et al., 1993; Jacobs & Gerson, 1998; Robinson & Godbey, 1997). In addition, as noted earlier, "underwork" in families can be as stressful and associated with problems as overwork. For instance, families in which fathers worked less than full-time were found to have children with more behavioral difficulties (Parcel & Menaghan, 1994). And the negative effects of poverty on families, and the adults and children in them, are well documented (Seccombe, 2000; Wilson, 1996; White & Rogers, 2000). Even at higher socioeconomic levels, reducing hours of employment can result in challenging trade-offs of career and money for more time with family, and may be more predictive of distress than long hours (Barnett & Gareis, 2000a), suggesting that it is the experienced meaning of reduced work hours rather than hours per se that is most predictive of overall quality of life (Barnett & Gareis, 2000b). Clearly, both ends of the work-hours spectrum can create stress and difficulties for workers and their families.

The Role of Gender in Dual-Earner Lifestyles

Gender plays a role not only in determining income levels, work hours, and the microprocesses of emotion transmission from the workplace into the home but also at every level of the relationship between work and the family (Levner, 2000), as well as in the scientific study of this relationship. A number of authors have argued that both the scientific and popular emphases on the negative effects on families when two parents work represents a barely disguised discomfort with the reality of mothers employed outside the home (Barnett & Rivers, 1998; Holcomb, 1998; Williams, 2000; Galinsky, 1999; Moen & Yu, 2000; Haddock, Zimmerman, Ziemba, & Current, 2001). Barnett and Hyde (2001) persuasively argue that the functionalist, psychodynamic, and sociobiological theories that have informed research in the area of work and family have assumed men's proper place to be at work and women's place to be in the home. The discomfort with women in the workplace persists despite numerous recent findings that reveal the many positive mental and physical health, and relational correlates for both partners when both work (Barnett & Hyde, 2001), and despite the repeated finding that a mother's employment in and of itself does not negatively affect mother–child bonding (Harvey, 1999; National Institute of Child Health and Human Development Early Child Care Research Network, 1997a). In addition, Galinsky's (1999) interviews with children revealed a general sense of enthusiasm for their mothers working, and in her data, "having a working mother [is] *never once predictive* of how children assess their mothers' parenting skills on . . . items that are strongly linked to children's healthy development, school readiness, and school success" (p. xiv, italics in original).

What does matter to children is the degree of stress mothers, *and* fathers, experience about their jobs and working (Galinsky, 1999). Galinsky's data indicate that many children are highly attuned to their parents' degree of work-related stress, and some develop strategies to reduce parents' stress once they are home, or to minimize contact with parents at those times. And how women feel about working depends in part on the degree of support they experience from their spouses about working, including the degree to which this is expressed in sharing of household and child care responsibilities (see my review, below). Thus, fathers/husbands can play an important role in reducing the likelihood of negative spillover from women's employment onto children, just as women have long shielded children from fathers' work-related stress.

In addition to the finding that maternal employment has no significant negative effects on children's development, studies indicate that, overall, nonmaternal child care in the first year of life had no negative effects on children's attachment to their mothers (NICHD Early Child Care Research Network, 1997a). Indeed, for poor children whose families may lack adequate educational resources at home, those who receive high-quality child care demonstrate better academic and social outcomes than those who receive no enriched child care or lower quality care (e.g., see Vandell & Ramanan, 1992; see also the review by Scarr, 1998). High-quality care is defined as a combination of a healthy, safe environment, and age-appropriate educational and social stimulation; warm, responsive interactions between staff and children; age-appropriate staff:child ratios; limited group size; low staff turnover rates; and sufficient staff training in early child education and development (Scarr, 1998).

The findings on impact of quality of child care on children in middle and upper class families are mixed, with some findings of short-term negative effects of lower quality care on cognitive, social, and behavioral outcomes (Scarr, 1998). However, careful analyses suggest that family variables such as the preexisting warmth and sensitivity of the mother toward the child, parenting stress and attitudes, separation anxieties, impact of work stress on family life are much more predictive of child outcomes than quality of nonmaternal care (Scarr, 1998), or at least interact with child care quality to produce negative child outcomes (NICHD Early Child Care Research Network, 1997a). Indeed, family variables confound any findings on impact of child care quality on child outcomes; at least two studies found that family variables such as income, mothers' beliefs about the benefits of maternal employment for children, and mother's personality characteristics correlated with amount and/or quality of child care selected (Bolger & Scarr, 1995; NICHD Early Child Care Research Network, 1997b). However, other researchers caution against either minimizing concern around short-term effects on children of quality of child care or concluding that positive family characteristics will override the impact of lower quality care (Van Horn & Newell, 1999). In general, there is consensus that children who receive good- to high-quality child care do as well or even better than children receiving full-time maternal care, and that there is a need for more good quality, affordable child care (Schulman, 2000).

Barnett and Hyde (2001) garner much evidence for their theory that multiple roles for both partners (parent, partner, and worker) rather than singular roles (typically, men as workers, women as mothers) result in positive health and relational outcomes by buffering the impact of negative events in one or the other role; increasing family income and sharing the responsibility for earning; increasing social support and opportunities in which to experience success, enlarging the number of possible perspectives on one's life, thereby, increasing the complexity of how the self is socially constructed; increasing the number of possible shared experiences for partners to discuss; and challenging partners to confront and disassemble constraining, unidimensional constructions of gender roles. Likewise, the literature reviewed below that documents successful coping strategies of many dual-earner couples represents an important shift that may either herald or reflect a growing adjustment to and enthusiasm for the dual-earner life (Moen & Yu, 2000), and for children, having both parents actively involved in their lives (Galinsky, 1999).

The pattern of larger cultural, social, and economic values, structures, and resources continues to challenge dual-earner couples. Problems (reviewed earlier) include the lack of affordable and reliable child care (Schulman, 2000), limited availability for most employees of the rights guaranteed in the FMLA, limited true support by employers (even when available) for workers utilizing flextime or for translating control over schedules into *reducing*, rather than increasing, hours worked, and a culture that frowns on time off. All these resource deficits and problematic attitudes are derived from the patriarchal breadwinner/homemaker model of family economy that put men in the workforce and women at home (Moen & Yu, 2000). Moen and Yu (2000) refer to this mismatch between the outdated but still dominant work–family model and contemporary employment realities as a "structural lag" that, like other past lags, is in the process of resolution.

Nevertheless, women much more than men end up shouldering the strain of this cultural lag (Hochschild & Machung, 1989; Milkie & Peltola, 1999; Spain & Bianchi, 1996). In addition to needing to reconcile to themselves and justify to others their choice or need to work (Holcomb, 1998), numerous studies have documented that women actually work more hours than men when paid work, housework, and child care are combined (Coltrane, 2000; Galinsky et al., 1993; Hochschild & Machung, 1989; Robinson & Godbey, 1997; Shelton, 1992). And although a number of studies document an increase in men's parenting and recognizing the benefits to themselves, their children, and their marriages (Barnett & Hyde, 2001; Bond et al., 1998), men have been slower to take on a more equal share of housework. Although women's hours of housework have decreased by about one-third from 1965 to 1985, and men's housework hours have doubled (from 2 to 4 hours on average; Robinson & Godbey, 1997), women still do roughly three times more housework than men (Coltrane, 2000). In addition, women are more likely to perform the most time-intensive and routine (daily) household tasks—meal preparation or cooking, housecleaning, shopping for groceries and household goods, washing dishes and cleaning up after meals, and laundry, including washing, ironing, and mending clothes (Blair & Lichter, 1991; Robinson & Godbey, 1997), whereas men gravitate to the less regular and less time-intensive activities of fixing things around the house, yard work, and bills. The time dedicated to routine tasks is approximately 3 hours for every 1 hour of nonroutine tasks (Coltrane, 2000).

Although there are still few studies of racial and ethnic differences in male–female distribution of housework and child care, findings so far show that employed black men do more housework than do employed white men, but employed black women still do at least twice as much housework as their male partners (Coltrane, 2000). Orbuch and Eyster (1997) attribute greater housework sharing between black partners as being due to more egalitarian attitudes and more equal salaries. The findings regarding sharing of housework between Latino partners compared to white partners are mixed (Coltrane, 2000), although Latino partners tend to evaluate distribution of housework less in terms of fairness or unfairness than do white couples.

Interestingly, although men of color may pitch in more with housework than white men, both black and Latino men were less likely than white men to provide care for the children while their wives were working (Brayfield, 1995). Clearly, more research is needed to understand the role of child-rearing ideologies in black and Latino families, and how these beliefs may affect men's involvement in child care.

Overall, the shift in housework distribution between women and men seems attributable to greater percentages of women in the workforce and increasing economic parity; employed women do about one-third less housework than women who are at home full-time (Robinson & Godbey, 1997), and the more equal the earnings between women and men, the more equal the distribution of housework (Coltrane, 2000). A number of studies document the strong relationship between the degree to which women perceive housework as fairly divided with their partner and marital quality, as well as with women's rates of depression (Piña & Bengston, 1994; see review by Coltrane, 2000). In contrast, given the few hours most men devote to housework, it is not surprising that their perceptions of the fairness of housework distribution are unrelated either to their own or their wives' degree of unhappiness or marital distress (Robinson & Spitze, 1992).

Interestingly, women's perceptions of unfairness about housework distribution persist even in studies that find total hours of work (paid and unpaid at home) for men and women roughly equal when men's generally longer job hours are factored in (Coltrane, 2000). This highlights the difference between these two forms of work: Paid work is typically linked to one's education and career interests, is a major source of self-esteem and self-definition, and is often carried out in contexts in which it accrues social as well as financial rewards, whereas housework is unrelated to education or career, accrues little appreciation, and is often viewed as something that must be done, and not as a valued aspect of self (Hochschild, 1997). Couple therapists are often faced with men who argue that, because of their long work hours, they should not be expected to do more of the routine housework. Therapists may find it useful to point out the distinction between the experienced value and rewards of paid work versus housework and child care, as a prelude to suggesting that in the interest of fairness to their female partners (and improving wives' marital satisfaction), men may need to do more around the house. If more persuasion is needed, the therapist might quote Scott Coltrane, a (male) expert on the role of housework in marital relationships, who writes, "The single most important predictor of a wife's fairness evaluation is what portion of the housework her husband contributes," and that "marital satisfaction increases in relation to the amount of routine housework that is shared by spouses" (Coltrane, 2000, p. 1225). Likewise, in rigorous prospective studies, Gottman (1994) has found men's doing of housework significantly related to future marital satisfaction and lower likelihood of divorce.

In addition to doing more housework, women carry more of the load of the connections between the family and extended family, and between the family and the various services needed to sustain the family's well-being. Women are significantly more likely than men to attend to the needs of the older generation (Henderson & Allen, 1991; Neal, Chapman, Ingersoll-Dayton, & Emlen, 1993), potentially fueling women's sense of resentment and resulting in conflict between partners (Scharlach, 1994).

Women, more than men, include within their commute to and from work complex sequences of children's appointments and chores, a phenomenon known as "trip chaining" (Rosenbloom, 1998). And even when families are able to afford domestic and child care assistants, it is women more than men who supervise their work (Coltrane, 2000).

Although the temporal conditions created by two working parents might be expected to have led to a widespread shift in the younger, post-feminist generation from the traditional male–female divisions regarding responsibility for the home and care of children and elders, this does not yet seem generally to be the case (Galinsky et al., 1993). And although many younger couples may ascribe to and practice a peer marriage (Schwartz, 1994) prior to having a child, the vast majority settle into a neo-traditional arrangement after the birth of the first child, with men typically working longer hours and women taking or shifting to employment that allows them to fulfill home and child-rearing responsibilities. Those who refuse to travel, relocate, or work overtime, typically sacrifice long-term career advancement—the so-called "mommy track" (Moen & Yu, 2000). Designating attempts to "balance" work and family life as women's issues tends to reinforce traditional biases, when children and families would benefit from more balanced time and commitment from both parents.

Walsh (1989) suggests that a combination of biological and socialization factors result in mothers rather than fathers cutting back. Biologically influenced aspects of attachment[4] and the wish to breast-feed, along with still-powerful cultural scripts noted earlier about parenting and about men's and women's proper roles regarding employment versus family, may lead a woman to prefer staying home at least part-time with the infant. The decision is often cinched by the man's higher earning potential and then encouraged, because men typically earn even more when their wives stay at home than when they work (Chun & Lee, 1999; Friedman & Greenhaus, 2000). With the woman home more, it typically falls on her to do more housework as well as the arranging of preschools, after-school educational activities, and play dates, even though the many examples of full-time working mothers (both married and single) who handle these chores and arrangements along with a job indicate that men could take on some or all of these responsibilities. Gradually the couple slides into at least an approximation of the traditional male breadwinner–female homemaker roles (Walsh, 1989), even when the partners initially ascribed to a more equitable sharing of household and child care responsibilities.

However, a number of studies suggest that dual-earner families do best when adult partners hold flexible gender role assumptions (Barnett & Hyde, 2001). For instance, marital quality is negatively affected by wives earning more than their husbands only when husbands attach great self-definitional and emotional value to their earning power, as many men still do (Brennan, Barnett, & Gareis, 2001). Earnings and job status were found to be less influential on marital quality than beliefs about gender roles (Vannoy & Philliber, 1992). Interestingly, mothers' sex role attitudes about women may be as important if not more so than men's attitudes about women in enhancing their ability to navigate the multiple demands of work and family life. One study found that a mother's but not a father's sex role attitudes about women's roles predicted the degree to which the mother's work was viewed by women as providing an overall gain for family life (Marshall & Barnett, 1993). Another found that when women believe they must be home full-time with children, they benefit less psychologically from their work lives (Hoffman, 1989). Of course, from a feminist perspective, women's beliefs about their proper roles derive from the larger set of patriarchal cultural values and mores, especially when reinforced by spouses, extended families, and the media.

By choosing one frequently adopted strategy of avoiding work–family conflicts—delaying pregnancy until well into one's 30s or even 40s (Moen & Yu, 2000)—women potentially incur health problems, and couples commonly experience emotional distress if they encounter fertility difficulties (Diamond et al., 1999). Given the higher rates of multiple births linked to fertility-enhancing medical procedures, couples that delay having a child may end up with a larger child care load all at once.

In summary, at many levels, the lives of male and female dual-earner partners differ, and both partners' beliefs about gender are deeply embedded in how they approach and feel about navigating the challenges of blending work and family life.

SUCCESSFUL COPING IN DUAL-EARNER FAMILIES

Although much work remains to identify the pathways that lead from work stress to individual and family distress (and vice versa), it is equally important to examine these pathways from a positive-coping, family resilience (Walsh, 1998) perspective. Without contributing to the described tendency of our culture to place responsibility for how well families cope solely on the degree of resourcefulness of working parents and their families, research must identify the variables associated with navigating work and family life in a manner that contributes to the well being of all family members. Indeed, although some studies suggest that few couples believe they manage all their work and family roles well (Hochschild, 1997), several other studies indicate that a large number of dual-earner families cope fairly successfully and even thrive (Barnett & Hyde, 2001; Barnett & Rivers, 1998; Galinsky, 1999; Haddock et al., 2001; Marshall & Barnett, 1993; Moen & Yu, 2000). Importantly, this conclusion emerges not only from research with adult family members but also from research with children (Galinsky, 1999). Indeed, as noted earlier, Barnett and Hyde (2001) have proposed an "expansionist" theory of work and the family that better captures much of the emerging data showing the physical and mental health, and relational benefits that accrue when men and women inhabit multiple roles (parent, spouse, worker) and the negative outcomes associated with the absence of, or time constraints on, particular roles (especially the absence of parenting for men, working for women).

One limitation to note from the outset is that, like many of the studies referenced earlier, studies on successful coping with dual earnership have almost entirely sampled white families in the middle class or above. Despite this limitation, interesting findings have emerged on successful coping. The Haddock et al. (2001) study interviewed 47 mostly white, well-educated, middle-class couples that viewed themselves as benefiting more than not from a dual-earner lifestyle, and as having developed means of achieving a successful blend between work and family life. Philosophies and practices reported by these couples included prioritizing family time and well-being (e.g., in making decisions about work hours and career advancement, setting boundaries on work time); emphasizing equality and partnership in the marital relationship (through joint responsibility for household tasks and child rearing, joint decision making, mutual appreciation and support); maximizing play and fun at home; concentrating on work while at the workplace; taking pride in their family and in how they are balancing multiple roles and responsibilities, and believing the family benefits from both parents working (rather than absorbing the dominant cultural narrative that it harms the children); living simply—including limiting activities that impede active family engagement, such as watching television and unnecessary expenditures; adopting high but realistic expectations about household management; employing planning strategies that save time; being proactive in decision making; and remaining conscious of time as a valuable resource.

Drawing on her 1998 phone survey and questionnaire study of parents and children, Galinsky (1999) outlined a number of approaches to navigating the "transition from home to work and from work to home" (p. 299). Her suggestions to parents include getting organized the night before; setting wake-up times that decrease rush; creating rituals for saying good-bye to children and for reengaging with them after work; expecting the reconnection phase to include children expressing in words or behavior their problems from the day; finding trustworthy child care and educators; creating standing backup child care plans; creating transitional rituals to switch into and out of work, maintaining both focused, uninterrupted time with kids and time just to "hang out," and after particularly stressful work days, explicitly letting children know that they need some brief time alone. She also emphasizes the need for parents to talk "intentionally," not apologetically, about their work, giving them a sense of their enjoyment and excitement about it, as well as the challenges.

Other studies (Becker & Moen, 1999) have found that dual-earner couples cope by "scaling back" commitment to paid work, with mothers doing most of the scaling back. As shown by the previously cited data on

differences in men's and women's work hours, scaling-back strategies interact with the family's life cycle: A common pattern was that women curtail work for the period of infancy and early childhood, returning to more
full-time work once the child enters school. Although some couples trade
off between partners the balance of family versus paid work over the life
cycle (Becker & Moen, 1999), the majority that scale back take on a more
traditional gender arrangement.

Over the past decade of working clinically with dual-earner families
and conducting psychoeducational distress-prevention workshops for
nondistressed couples (Fraenkel, Markman, & Stanley, 1997), I have developed a number of attitude shifts and practices that decrease stress and
maintain positive connection between couple partners, which then benefit
their interactions with children (Fraenkel, 1994, 1996, 1998a, 1998b,
2001a, 2001b; Fraenkel & Wilson, 2000). In terms of attitudes, I have previously identified three myths (and here add one more) that interfere with
realistic coping with time constraints: the myth of spontaneity, of the need
to completely separate housework from family fun, of infinite perfectibility, and of total control. The myth of spontaneity holds that no matter how
fast-paced, demanding, and mismatched family members' individual
schedules, time for fun and connection should not be scheduled, but
rather should occur spontaneously. This myth essentially precludes time
for connection. Rather, families must dedicate and preserve a place in
their schedules for time together, which may take the form of rituals that
imbue the activities with particular meaning (Imber-Black & Roberts,
1998), or simply rhythms and routines that accrue greater emotional and
relational significance over time and repetition (Fraenkel, 1994). Within
the time set aside for connection, couples and families can invite a great
deal of spontaneity and serendipity.

The second myth holds that fun and pleasurable family activities must
not involve work. One danger of emphasizing the intrusion of work time
on family and couple time, and of casting homemaking activities as work,
is that a wide range of otherwise boring tasks are overlooked as opportunities for pleasurable family connection. This work/family pleasure distinction puts more pressure on the limited time left when work in and out of
the home is done. Many chores associated with upkeep of the home can
be more enjoyably completed as family activities—the fairly routinized,
"mindless" tasks of washing dishes, cooking meals, folding laundry, and
running errands can all become opportunities for talking, affection, and
playfulness. Men, who may avoid taking on more of the housework in
favor of spending nonwork time with the children, can learn to combine
the two, taking more of the burden of both off women.

The third myth, that of "infinite perfectibility," views the family time
crunch as wholly resolvable through better time management and holds
that no compromises need be made in the number of activities families
take on. The belief that "you can have it all"—two-careers on full tilt and

lots of family quality time, and that children must be provided as wide a variety of enriching classes and other extracurricular activities as possible, coupled with well-marketed time management books and tools—leads many families to experience a frantic imperative to fit it all in. The harried pace that results diminishes pleasure in all activities and results in families experiencing even the time they have as inadequate (Daly, 2001). To act against this myth, families need to make choices that reflect their priorities and values, and to view their lives as having different periods stretching into the future, during which they can plan to achieve certain goals and engage in certain activities rather than trying to do everything at once. For instance, rather than fretting about never getting out of the house on Saturday nights as they used to, because of difficulties finding a babysitter, couples with very young children can view this period of their lives as more "centripetal" (Combrinck-Graham, 1985) and home-focused, and see it as an opportunity to discover and nurture togetherness activities that can be done at home.

The fourth myth, which builds on the third, holds that families' time and quality of life is totally under their control. Thus, if one partner is feeling pressured to work long hours despite a desire to cut back, the other partner blames her or him (or the worker blames him- or herself). This myth represents the flip side of the broader American myth, mentioned earlier, in which a family's economic well-being is viewed simply as a function of the workers' hard work, dedication, and ability to take advantage of society's limitless opportunities (Sennett & Cobb, 1972), and ignores the powerful impact of realistic workplace and economic pressures to spend more hours on the job lest the employee be fired or not promoted. Operating outside the influence of this myth requires that partners appraise the real power of social and economic contexts to shape their lives, and set realistic goals for the present and future to balance work and family time.

To decrease the transmission of negative affect from work into the home and family interactions, I recommend a practice called the Decompression Chamber (Fraenkel, 1998a). Larson and Almeida's (1999) research-based recommendation that families pay particular attention to managing the negative spillover from work to home that occurs for many between 5 and 7 P.M. supports the usefulness of this particular practice. Each partner makes a list of the kinds of after-work activities (both solo or conjoint) he or she finds best help him or her to relax and to make the transition into the rest of the evening. Common activities include: taking a shower, reading the paper, watching a bit of television, exercise, yoga and meditation, playing with the children, and talking about the events of the day with one's partner. The partners then compare their lists and develop a "decompressing sequence" that accommodates one another's needs as much as possible and also recognizes the need to accomplish various child care and home care tasks. The couple is then encouraged to test the sequence out and refine it as necessary. The exercise is helpful in normalizing, as stressful, this transition between the workday and after-workday, and in resolving frequently unspoken struggles between partners about getting their individual needs met. It also often provides an opening for partners to talk about their longings for more soothing and care from one another—an aspect of interaction found highly predictive of relationship satisfaction and stability (Gottman, Coan, Carrere, & Swanson, 1998)—as well as to reveal their needs for "alone time." In many cases, I've found it also a useful entree into conversations about each partner's beliefs and expectations, borne from both past experience and family and culture of origin, about how to handle difficult emotions emerging from work.

To increase the sense of connection between partners across busy days and hours of being apart, I recommend a practice called the "sixty-second pleasure point" (Fraenkel, 1998b). Partners first make a list of all the fun, pleasurable, and even sensual activities they can do with one another that each last 60 seconds or less. Partners are encouraged to consider activities that can be done when physically together as well as apart (using a variety of technological means of communication). Frequently mentioned activities include short massages, a hug or kiss, talking about something funny or interesting, leaving little notes in each other's wallets, sharing a snack, sending an erotic e-mail, and planning what to do when they have more time. Couples are then encouraged to enact two such 60-second pleasure points in the morning before they leave for work, two more when they are both at work, and two more when they reunite in the evening, with partners sharing responsibility for initiating the pleasure points. Couples that utilize this technique typically report an enhanced sense of connection across the day, which in turn decreases their anxiety about reconnecting at day's end, taking pressure off this transition. Although I have not conducted research on this technique, it is supported by the Gottman et al. (1998) findings about the positive, long-term effects on marital satisfaction and stability of partners' initiating and responding to each other's bids for often-short periods of attention.

More important than any specific technique or practice, I have found it critical that for families to thrive in a dual-earner lifestyle, members, especially adult partners, need to maintain an open and ongoing dialogue about the challenges they face. This includes a recognition of the powerful influences on their experience of personal financial conditions and global economics, the impact of the cultures of the adult partners' respective workplaces and of the broader set of cultural beliefs about work, gender roles, and the good life, some of which they may inherit from their families of origin, and some of which they encounter simply as members of society. Recognizing the real power of these conditions, contexts, and belief systems to shape individual and family experience can allow family members to sustain a nonblaming attitude that engenders mutual support and allows them to direct energies toward active coping and maximal enjoyment of the dual-earner life. Finally, recognizing that they are not alone in the struggle to balance work and home may lead to new dialogues and action within workplaces, communities, and political arenas that promote more widespread, family-friendly policies regarding maternity–paternity leave, flextime, longer vacations, and other measures that decrease the stress of needing to choose between more time at work and more time with family. For healthy family functioning and the satisfaction of all members, changes in the mores of the work and broader culture are essential in order for employees to avail themselves of these policies. Ultimately, the domains of work and family life should not be set in competition with one another, but rather should blend together and contribute to each other's well being.

ACKNOWLEDGMENTS

Preparation of this chapter was supported in part by grants from the Ruth Perl Kahn Research Fund and the Louis and Anne Abrons Foundation to the Ackerman Institute/City College of New York Center for Time, Work, and the Family. I wish to thank Skye Wilson and Jody Brandt for their assistance in assembling the literature and demographic data, and Terry Bond of the Families and Work Institute for conducting some additional analyses of the data from the National Study of the Changing Workforce to answer questions pertinent to this chapter.

NOTES

1. Ellen Galinsky, a pioneer in this area of research, argues that the term "balancing" work and family creates an either–or frame in which an increase in time and energy devoted to one domain is viewed as automatically depleting the other domain. She suggests the notion of "navigating work and family life" (Galinsky, 1999, p. xvi) to capture better the need for flexibility in moving between these domains, and to emphasize the goal of maximizing positive mutual influence ("positive spillover") and minimizing negative mutual influence ("negative spillover"). I suggest and use in this chapter an additional, complementary term, "successful blending," to capture and positively connote the inevitable interrelatedness of the two domains.
2. Reports from the U.S. Census and U.S. Bureau of Labor Statistics both define families with "own children" as including biological, step-, and adopted children. Data on the nature of the relationship of children to the householder are available, but do not report the children's relationship to the spouse. Likewise, in reporting on married couples, these reports do not distinguish between first-marriage and remarriage families.
3. The U.S. Census does collect some data on unmarried, same-sex partners in its long form, but in accordance with the 1996 Federal Defense of Marriage Act, it does not consider same-sex couples identifying themselves as married to constitute married family households. There are several unreliable estimates of the number of lesbian and gay parents and their number of children in the litera-

ture. In data cited by Stacey and Biblarz (2001), there are between 800,000 to 7 million lesbian or gay parents between ages 18 and 59. They estimate that between 1 and 12% of children (between 1 and 9 million children) have a lesbian or gay parent, but these authors state that the majority of these children came from heterosexual marriages in which one parent later identified her- or himself as lesbian or gay. (As a result of increased acceptance of homosexuality, and lesbian and gay parenting, these authors suggest that in the future, there will be fewer children born to lesbian or gay parents who are initially in heterosexual marriages, and more born in LGB families.) Thus, it may be assumed that some percentage of the 3.7% of households that describe themselves to be cohabiting are gay or lesbian, and that some percentage of the 40.9% of cohabiting couples with children are gay or lesbian.

4. Of course, men also experience attachment to their infants that is in part biologically based. However, they are socialized to disregard these feelings and express their nurturance by getting back to work and making more money.

REFERENCES

Ahrons, C. (1995). *The good divorce: Keeping your family together when your marriage comes apart.* New York: HarperCollins.

Almeida, D. M., Wethington, E., & Chandler, A. L. (1999). Daily transmission of tensions between marital dyads and parent–child dyads. *Journal of Marriage and the Family, 61,* 49–61.

Barnett, R. C., & Gareis, K. C. (2000a). Reduced-hours employment: The relationship between difficulty of trade-offs and quality of life. *Work and Occupations, 27,* 168–187.

Barnett, R. C., & Gareis, K. C. (2000b). Reduced-hours, job-role quality and life satisfaction among married women physicians with children. *Psychology of Women Quarterly, 24,* 358–364.

Barnett, R. C., & Hyde, J. S. (2001). Women, men, work, and family. *American Psychologist, 56,* 781–796.

Barnett, R. C., & Rivers, C. (1998). *She works/he works: How two-income families are happy, healthy, and thriving.* New York: HarperCollins.

Becker, P. E., & Moen, P. (1999). Scaling back: Dual-earner couples' work–family strategies. *Journal of Marriage and the Family, 61,* 995–1007.

Belkin, L. (September 29, 1999). A wild ride on the swivel chair. *The New York Times,* p. G1.

Berger, R., & Hannah, M. T. (Eds.). (1999). *Preventive approaches in couples therapy.* Philadelphia, PA: Brunner/Mazel.

Blair, S. L., & Lichter, D. T. (1991). Measuring the division of household labor: Gender segregation of housework among American couples. *Journal of Family Issues, 12,* 91–113.

Blankenhorn, D. (1995). *Fatherless America: Confronting our most urgent social problem.* New York: Basic Books.

Bogenschneider, K. (2000). Has family policy come of age? A decade review of the state of U.S. family policy in the 1990s. *Journal of Marriage and the Family, 62,* 1136–1159.

Bolger, K. E., & Scarr, S. (1995). Not so far from home: How family characteristics predict child care quality. *Early Development and Parenting, 4,* 103–112.

Bond, J. T., Galinsky, E., & Swanberg, J. E. (1998). *The 1997 national study of the changing workforce.* New York: Families and Work Institute.

Boss, P. (2000). *Ambiguous loss: Learning to live with unresolved grief.* Cambridge, MA: Harvard University Press.

Bradbury, T. N., Fincham, F. D., & Beach, S. R. H. (2000). Research on the nature and determinants of marital satisfaction: A decade in review. *Journal of Marriage and the Family, 62,* 964–980.

Brayfield, A. (1995). Juggling jobs and kids: The impact of employment schedules on fathers' caring for children. *Journal of Marriage and the Family, 57,* 321–332.

Brennan, R. T., Barnett, R. C., & Gareis, K. C. (2001). When she earns more than he does: A longitudinal study of dual-earner couples. *Journal of Marriage and Family, 63,* 168–182.

Bumpus, M. F., Crouter, A. C., & McHale, S. M. (1999). Work demands of dual-earner couples: Implications for parents' knowledge about children's daily lives in middle childhood. *Journal of Marriage and the Family, 61,* 465–475.

Castro, J. (March 29, 1993). Disposable workers. *Time,* pp. 43–47.

Center on Budget and Policy Priorities. (1998). *Poverty rates fall, but remain high for a period with such low unemployment.* Washington, DC: Center on Budget and Policy Priorities. [Available online: www. cbpp. org/9–24–98pov. htm]

Chun, H., & Lee, I. (2001). Why do married men earn more: Productivity or marriage selection. *Economic Inquiry, 39,* 307–319.

Clarkberg, M., & Moen, P. (1999, January). *The time-squeeze: The mismatch between work-hours patterns and preferences* (BLCC Working Paper No. 99-04). Ithaca, NY: Cornell University, Bronfenbrenner Life Course Center.

Coltrane, S. (2000). Research on household labor: Modeling and measuring the social embeddedness of routine family work. *Journal of Marriage and the Family, 62,* 1208–1233.

Combrinck-Graham, L. (1985). A developmental model for family systems. *Family Process, 24,* 139–150.

Coontz, S. (2000). *The way we never were: American families and the nostalgia trap.* New York. Basic Books.

Covey, S. R., Merrill, A. R., & Merrill, R. R. (1994). *First things first: To live, to love, to learn, to leave a legacy.* New York: Fireside.

Crouter, A. C., Bumpus, M. F., Head, M. R., & McHale, S. M. (2001). Implications of overwork and overload for the quality of men's family relationships. *Journal of Marriage and Family, 63,* 404–416.

Crouter, A. C., Bumpus, M. F., Maguire, M. C., & McHale, S. M. (1999). Linking parents' work pressure and adolescents' well-being: Insights into dynamics in dual-earner families. *Developmental Psychology, 35,* 1453–1461.

Daly, K. J. (2001). Deconstructing family time: From ideology to lived experience. *Journal of Marriage and Family, 63,* 283–294.

Diamond, R., Kezur, D., Meyers, M., Scharf, C. N., & Weinshel, M. (1999). *Couple therapy for infertility.* New York: Guilford Press.

Downey, G., Purdie, V., & Schaffer-Neitz, R. (1999). Anger transmission from mother to child: A comparison of mothers in chronic pain and well mothers. *Journal of Marriage and the Family, 61,* 62–73.

Forthofer, M. S., Markman, H. J., Cox, M., Stanley, S., & Kessler, R. C. (1996). Associations between marital distress and work loss in a national sample. *Journal of Marriage and the Family, 58,* 597–605.

Fraenkel, P. (1994). Time and rhythm in couples. *Family Process, 33,* 37–51.

Fraenkel, P. (1998a). Time and couples: Part I. The decompression chamber. In T. Nelson & T. Trepper (Eds.), *101 interventions in family therapy* (Vol. II, pp. 140–144). West Hazleton, PA: Haworth Press.

Fraenkel, P. (1998b). Time and couples: Part II. The sixty second pleasure point. In T. Nelson & T. Trepper (Eds.), *101 interventions in family therapy* (Vol. II, pp. 145–149). West Hazleton, PA: Haworth Press.

Fraenkel, P. (2001a). The beeper in the bedroom: Technology has become a therapeutic issue. *Psychotherapy Networker, 25,* 22–65.

Fraenkel, P. (2001b). The place of time in couple and family therapy. In K. Daly (Ed.), *Minding the time in family experience: Emerging perspectives and issues* (pp. 283–310). London: JAI.

Fraenkel, P., & Markman, H. J. (2002). Prevention of marital disorders. In D. Glenwick & L. Jason (Eds.), *Innovative strategies for promoting health and mental health across the lifespan* (pp. 245–271). New York: Springer.

Fraenkel, P., Markman, H., & Stanley, S. (1997). The prevention approach to relationship problems. *Sexual and Marital Therapy, 12,* 249–258.

Fraenkel, P., & Wilson, S. (2000). Clocks, calendars, and couples: Time and the rhythms of relationships. In P. Papp (Ed.), *Couples on the fault line: New directions for therapists* (pp. 63–103). New York: Guilford Press.

Fried, M. (1998). *Taking time: Parental leave policy and corporate culture.* Philadelphia: Temple University Press.

Friedman, S. D., & Greehaus, J. H. (2000). *Work and family—Allies or enemies?* New York: Oxford University Press.

Friedman, T. L. (January 30, 2001). Cyber-serfdom. *The New York Times,* p. A23.

Galinsky, E. (1999). *Ask the children: What America's children really think about working parents.* New York: Morrow.

Galinsky, E., Bond, J. T., & Friedman, D. E. (1993). *The changing workforce: Highlights of the national study.* New York: Families and Work Institute.

Galinsky, E., Kim, S. S., & Bond, J. T. (2001). *Feeling overworked: When work becomes too much.* New York: Families and Work Institute.

Gerstel, N., & McGonagle, K. (1999). Job leaves and the limits of the Family and Medical Leave Act: The effects of gender, race, and family. *Work and Occupations, 26,* 1208–1233.

Gilbert, K. (1998). The body, young children, and popular culture. In N. Yelland (Ed.), *Gender in early childhood* (pp. 55–71). Florence, KY: Taylor & Francis/Routledge.

Goldstein, J. R. (1999). The leveling of divorce in the United States. *Demography, 36,* 409–414.

Gottman, J. M. (1994). *What predicts divorce: The relationship between marital processes and marital outcomes.* Hillsdale, NJ: Erlbaum.

Gottman, J. M., Coan, J., Carrere, S., & Swanson, C. (1998). Predicting marital happiness and stability from newlywed interactions. *Journal of Marriage and the Family, 60,* 5–22.

Greenhouse, S. (September 5, 1999). So much work, so little time. *The New York Times,* Sect. 4 (Week In Review), p. 1.

Greenhouse, S. (September 1, 2001). Americans' international lead in hours worked grew in 90s, report shows. *The New York Times*, p. A8.

Guelzow, M. G., Bird, G. W., & Koball, E. H. (1991). An exploratory path analysis of the stress process for dual-career men and women. *Journal of Marriage and the Family, 53*, 141–164.

Guttman, J. (1993). *Divorce in psychosocial perspective: Theory and research*. Hillsdale, NJ: Erlbaum.

Haddock, S. A., Zimmerman, T. S., Ziemba, S. J., & Current, L. R. (2001). Ten adaptive strategies for family and work balance: Advice from successful families. *Journal of Marital and Family Therapy, 27*, 445–458.

Harvey, E. (1999). Short-term and long-term effects of parental employment on children of the National Longitudinal Survey of Youth. *Developmental Psychology, 35*, 445–459.

Hayghe, H. V. (1997, September). Developments in women's labor force participation. *Monthly Labor Force Review*, pp. 41–46.

Henderson, K. A., & Allen, K. R. (1991). The ethic of care: Leisure possibilities and constraints for women. *Society and Leisure, 14*, 97–113.

Hewlett, S. A., & West, C. (1998). *The war against parents: What we can do for America's beleaguered moms and dads*. New York: Houghton Mifflin.

Hochschild, A. R. (1997). *The time bind: When work becomes home and home becomes work*. New York: Holt.

Hochschild, A. R., & Machung, A. (1989). *The second shift*. New York: Avon.

Hoffman, L. W. (1989). Effects of maternal employment in the two-parent family. *American Psychologist, 44*, 283–292.

Holcomb, L. W. (1998). *Not guilty: The good news about working mothers*. New York: Scribner.

Howard, G. S. (1997). *Ecological psychology: Creating a more earth-friendly human nature*. Notre Dame, IN: University of Notre-Dame Press.

Hyde, J. S., Klein, M. H., Essex, M. J., & Clark, R. (1995). Maternity leave and women's mental health. *Psychology of Women Quarterly, 19*, 257–285.

Imber-Black, E. (2000). The new triangle: Couples and technology. In P. Papp (Ed.), *Couples on the fault line: New directions for therapists* (pp. 48–62). New York: Guilford Press.

Imber-Black, E., & Roberts, J. (1998). *Rituals for our times: Celebrating, healing, and changing our lives and our relationships*. New York: Jason Aronson.

International Labor Organization press release. (August 31, 2001). New ILO study shows U.S. workers put in longest hours. Key Indicators of the Labor Market 2001–2002 due to be released November 2001. [Available online: us. ilo. org/news/prsrls/20010831_kilm. html]

Jacobs, J. A., & Gerson, K. (1998). Who are the overworked Americans? *Review of Social Economy, 4*, 442–459.

Jacobs, J. A., & Gerson, K. (2001). Overworked individuals or overworked families?: Explaining trends in work, leisure, and family time. *Work and Occupations, 28*, 40–63.

Karney, B. R., & Bradbury, T. N. (1995). The longitudinal course of marital quality and stability: A review of theory, method, and research. *Psychological Bulletin, 118*, 3–34.

Lagerfeld, S. (1998). Who knows where the time goes? *Wilson Quarterly, 22*, 58–70.

Larson, R. W., & Almeida, D. M. (1999). Emotional transmission in the daily lives of families: A new paradigm for studying family process. *Journal of Marriage and the Family, 61,* 5–20.

Levner, L. (2000). The three-career family. In P. Papp (Ed.), *Couples on the fault line: New directions for therapists* (pp. 29–47). New York: Guilford.

Markman, H. J., Floyd, F. J., Stanley, S. M., & Storaasli, R. D. (1988). Prevention of marital distress: A longitudinal investigation. *Journal of Consulting and Clinical Psychology, 56,* 210–217.

Markman, H. J., Renick, M. J., Floyd, F. J., Stanley, S. M., & Clements, M. (1993). Preventing marital distress through communication and conflict management training: A 4- and 5-year follow-up. *Journal of Consulting and Clinical Psychology, 61,* 70–77.

Markman, H. J., Stanley, S. M., & Blumberg, S. L. (2001). *Fighting for your marriage: Positive steps for preventing divorce and preserving a lasting love.* San Francisco: Jossey-Bass.

Marshall, N. L., & Barnett, R. C. (1993). Work-family strains and gains among two-earner couples. *Journal of Community Psychology, 21,* 64–77.

McGovern, M., & Russell, D. (2001). *A new brand of expertise: How independent consultants, free agents, and interim managers are transforming the world of work.* New York: Butterworth-Heineman.

Milkie, M. A., & Peltola, P. (1999). Playing all the roles: Gender and the work–family balancing act. *Journal of Marriage and the Family, 61,* 476–490.

Moen, P., & Yu, Y. (2000). Effective work/life strategies: Working couples, work conditions, gender, and life quality. *Social Problems, 47,* 291–326.

Mohr, R. (2000). Reflections on golden pond. In P. Papp (Ed.), *Couples on the fault line: New directions for therapists* (pp. 312–334). New York: Guilford Press.

Morgenstern, J. (2000). *Time management from the inside out: The foolproof system for taking control of your schedule—and your life.* New York: Holt.

Neal, M. B., Chapman, N. J., Ingersoll-Dayton, B., & Emlen, A. C. (1993). *Balancing work and caregiving for children, adults, and elders.* Newbury Park, CA: Sage.

National Institute of Child Health and Human Development [NICHD] Early Child Care Research Network. (1997a). The effects of infant child care on infant–mother attachment security: Results of the NICHD Study of Early Child Care. *Child Development, 68,* 860–879.

National Institute of Child Health and Human Development [NICHD] Early Child Care Research Network. (1997b). Familial factors associated with the characteristics of nonmaternal care for infants. *Journal of Marriage and the Family, 59,* 389–408.

O'Brien, K. (September 20, 2000). On the next vacation, don't forget the laptop. *The New York Times,* p. G1.

Ooms, T. (1998). *Toward more perfect unions: Putting marriage on the public agenda.* Washington, DC: Family Impact Seminar.

Orbuch, T. L., & Eyster, S. L. (1997). Division of household labor among black couples and white couples. *Social Forces, 76,* 301–332.

Owen, P. R., & Laurel-Seller, E. (2000). Weight and shape ideals: Thin is dangerously in. *Journal of Applied Social Psychology, 30,* 979–990.

Paden, S. L., & Buehler, C. (1995). Coping with the dual-income lifestyle. *Journal of Marriage and the Family, 57,* 101–110.

Parcel, T. L., & Menaghan, E. G. (1994). *Parents' jobs and children's lives.* New York: Aldine de Gruyter.

Parnes, A. (September 5, 2001). Dot-commers trade options for books. *The New York Times,* (Workplace Section), p. G1.

Perry-Jenkins, M., Repetti, R. L., & Crouter, A. C. (2000). Work and family in the 1990s. *Journal of Marriage and the Family, 62,* 981–998.

Piña, D. L., & Bengston, V. L. (1993). The division of household labor and wive's happiness—Ideology, employment, and perceptions of support. *Journal of Marriage and the Family, 55,* 901–912.

Pinsof, W. M. (2002). The death of "till death do us part": The transformation of pair-bonding in the 20th century. *Family Process, 41,* 135–157.

Piotrkowski, C. S., & Hughes, D. (1993). Dual-earner families in context: Managing family and work systems. In F. Walsh, (Ed.), *Normal family processes: Emerging family forms and challenges* (pp. 185–207). New York: Guilford Press.

Pipher, M. (1996). *The shelter of each other: Rebuilding our families.* New York: Ballantine.

Popenoe, D. (1996). *Life without father: Compelling new evidence that fatherhood and marriage are indispensable for the good of children and society.* Cambridge, MA: Harvard University Press.

Presser, H. B. (1994). Employment schedules among dual-earner spouses and the division of household labor by gender. *American Sociological Review, 59,* 348–364.

Presser, H. B., & Cox, A. G. (1997, April). The work schedules of low-educated American women and welfare reform. *Monthly Labor Review,* pp. 25–33.

Repetti, R. L., & Wood, J. (1997). Effects of daily stress at work on mothers' interactions with preschoolers. *Journal of Family Psychology, 11,* 90–108.

Robinson, J., & Godbey, G. (1997). *Time for life: The surprising ways Americans use their time.* University Park: Pennsylvania State University Press.

Robinson, J., & Spitze, G. (1992). Whistle while you work?: The effect of household task performance on women's and men's well-being. *Social Science Quarterly, 73,* 844–861.

Rogers, J. (2000). *Temps.* Ithaca, NY: Cornell University Press.

Rook, K., Dooley, D., & Catalano, R. (1991). Stress transmission: The effects of husbands' job stressors on the emotional health of their wives. *Journal of Marriage and the Family, 53,* 165–177.

Rosen, E. (1998). *Families facing death* (2nd ed.). San Francisco: Jossey-Bass.

Rosenbloom, S. (1998). *Transit markets of the future: The challenge of change. Report 28.* Washington, DC: National Academy Press.

Ruhling, N. A. (2000, June). Home is where the office is. *American Demographics,* pp. 54–60.

Scarr, S. (1998). American child care today. *American Psychologist, 53,* 95–108.

Scharlach, A. E. (1994). Caregiving and employment: Competing or complementary roles? *Gerontologist, 34,* 378–385.

Schaubroeck, J., Jones, J. R., & Xie, J. L. (2001). Individual differences in utilizing control to cope with job demands: Effects on susceptibility to infectious disease. *Journal of Applied Psychology, 86,* 265–278.

Schor, J. B. (1991). *The overworked American.* New York: Basic Books.

Schulman, K. (2000). *The high cost of child care puts quality care out of reach for many families.* Washington, DC: Children's Defense Fund.

Schwartz, P. (1994). *Peer marriage: How love between equals really works.* New York: Free Press.

Scott, J. (August 31, 2001). In 90s economy, middle class stayed put, analysis suggests. *The New York Times*, pp. A1, B7.

Seccombe, K. (2000). Families in poverty in the 1990s: Trends, causes, consequences, and lessons learned. *Journal of Marriage and the Family, 62*, 1094–1113.

Sennett, R., & Cobb, J. (1972). *The hidden injuries of class*. New York: Norton.

Shelton, B. A. (1992). *Women, men and time: Gender differences in paid work, housework, and leisure* (Contributions in Women's Studies 127). New York: Greenwood Press.

Silverstein, L. B., & Auerbach, C. F. (1999). Deconstructing the essential father. *American Psychologist, 54*, 397–407.

Spain, D., & Bianchi, S. M. (1996). *Balancing act: Motherhood, marriage, and employment among American women*. New York: Russell Sage Foundation.

Stacey, J. (1996). *In the name of the family: Rethinking family values in the post-modern age*. Boston: Beacon.

Stacey, J., & Biblarz, T. J. (2001). (How) does the sexual orientation of parents matter? *American Sociological Review, 66*, 159–183.

Teachman, J. D., Tedrow, L. M., & Crowder, K. D. (2000). The changing demography of America's families. *Journal of Marriage and the Family, 62*, 1234–1246.

U.S. Bureau of the Census. (1998). *Current population reports, P60-203, measuring 50 years of economic change using the March Current Population Survey*. Washington, DC: U.S. Government Printing Office.

U.S. Bureau of the Census. (2000a). *Table FG1: Married couple family groups, by labor force status of both spouses, and race and Hispanic origin/1 of the reference person: March 2000*. [Available online: www.census.gov/population/socdemo/hh-fam/p20-537/2000/tab/fg1. pdf]

U.S. Bureau of the Census. (2000b). *Note on same-sex unmarried partner data from the 1990 and 2000 censuses*. [Available online: www.census.gov/population/www/cen2000/samesex. html]

U.S. Bureau of the Census. (June 2001a). Fields, J., & Casper, L. M. America's families and living arrangements: March 2000. *Current Population Reports*, Series P20-537. [Available online: www.census.gov/prod/2001pubs/p20-537.pdf]

U.S. Bureau of the Census. (July, 2001b). *Table MC1: Married couples by labor force status of spouses: 1986 to present*. [Available online: www.census.gov/population/socdemo/hh-fam/tabMC-1. txt]

U.S. Bureau of the Census. (September, 2001c). *Table FINC-03: Presence of related children under 18 years old—all families by total money income in 2000, type of family, work experience in 2000, race and Hispanic origin of reference person*. [Available online: http://ferret.bls.census.gov/macro/032001/faminc/new03_031.htm]

U.S. Bureau of the Census. (2001d). *Little progress on closing wage gap in 2000* (Current Population Survey). Washington, DC: Government Printing Office.

U.S. Bureau of Labor Statistics. (1998). *Labor force statistics from the Current Population Survey (Table A-2): Employment status of the civilian population by race, sex, age, and Hispanic origin*. [Available online: www.bls.gov/webapps/legacy/cpsatab2.htm]

U.S. Bureau of Labor Statistics. (2001). *Employment characteristics of families in 2000*. [Available online: http://stats.bls.gov/newsrels.htm]

Van Horn, M. L., & Newell, W. (1999). Costs and benefits of quality child care. *American Psychologist, 54*, 142–143.

Vandell, D. L., & Ramanan, J. (1992). Effects of early and recent maternal employment on children from low-income families. *Child Development, 63,* 938–949.

Vannoy, D., & Philliber, W. W. (1992). Wife's employment and quality of marriage. *Journal of Marriage and the Family, 54,* 387–398.

Voydanoff, P. (1988). Work role characteristics, family structure demands, and work–family conflict. *Journal of Marriage and the Family, 50,* 749–761.

Voydanoff, P., & Donnelly, B. W. (1999). Multiple roles and psychological distress: The intersection of the paid worker, spouse, and parent roles with the role of the adult child. *Journal of Marriage and the Family, 61,* 725–738.

Wachtel, P. L. (1989). *The poverty of affluence: A psychological portrait of the American way of life.* Philadelphia: New Society.

Waite, L. J., & Gallagher, M. (2000). *The case for marriage: Why married people are happier, healthier, and better off financially.* New York: Doubleday.

Walsh, F. (1998). *Strengthening family resilience.* New York: Guilford Press.

Walsh, F. (1989). Reconsidering gender in the "marital quid pro quo." In M. McGoldrick, C. Anderson, & F. Walsh (Eds.), *Women in families: A framework for family therapy* (267–285). New York: Norton.

White, L., & Keith, B. (1990). The effect of shift work on the quality and stability of marital relations. *Journal of Marriage and the Family, 52,* 453–462.

White, L., & Rogers, S. J. (2000). Economic circumstances and family outcomes: A review of the 1990s. *Journal of Marriage and the Family, 62,* 1035–1051.

Whyte, W. H. (1957). *The organization man.* New York: Doubleday Anchor.

Williams, J. (2000). *Unbending gender: Why family and work conflict and what to do about it.* New York: Oxford University Press.

Wilson, W. J. (1996). *When work disappears: The world of the new urban poor.* New York: Knopf.

Wortman, C., Biernat, M., & Lang, E. (1991). Coping with role overload. In M. Frankenhaeuser, U. Lundberg, & M. Chesney (Eds.), *Women, work, and health: Stress and opportunities* (pp. 85–110). New York: Plenum.

CHAPTER 4

RISK AND RESILIENCE AFTER DIVORCE

Shannon M. Greene
Edward R. Anderson
E. Mavis Hetherington
Marion S. Forgatch
David S. DeGarmo

Divorce and life in a single-parent household have become common experiences for growing numbers of parents and children in contemporary American society. The purpose of this chapter is to provide an overview of the kinds of stresses and adaptive challenges that adults and children face when confronting transitions that surround divorce. We start by placing the topic in a broader perspective by examining the prevalence of divorce and its related transitions, along with factors that increase the risk of marital instability. Then we explore concomitant changes in family processes, relationships, and life experiences, including a consideration of the ways in which parents and children cope with their newly evolving family situations. We conclude with a brief focus on postdivorce parental repartnering, in other words, how courtship and nonmarital cohabitation affect family processes and the well-being of individual family members. The final section is brief, not because of a lack of importance, but due to a current gap in the literature. Indeed, research that addresses the formation and quality of newly emerging intimate relationships is a critical part of better understanding the aftermath and impact of divorce, as well as the success of any eventual remarriages. Visher et al., Chapter 6, this volume, examine the related topic of remarriage in detail.

PREVALENCE OF DIVORCE AND
RELATED TRANSITIONS

Divorce is a common transition for families in the United States, with over 1 million decrees granted each year (U.S. Bureau of the Census, 1998). Rates of divorce have more than tripled in the past 50 years, and although there has been a modest decline in recent decades, the lifetime probability of a first marriage ending in divorce still approaches 50% (Goldstein, 1999; Teachman, Tedrow, & Crowder, 2000). In fact, 43% of first marriages end within the first 15 years of the relationship (Bramlett & Mosher, 2001). The overall increase in rates of divorce reflects a combination of factors. Recent gains in economic self-sufficiency for women and erosion of earnings for men without college degrees may leave wives less dependent on the marriage for purely financial reasons (Cherlin, 1998). Although the vast majority of adults still view marriage as desirable, growing numbers question whether it is essential for happiness (Seltzer, 2000). These changing views are reflected in a narrowing gap over the past three decades for reports of happiness and well-being that historically have favored married over single individuals (Hetherington & Kelly, 2002; Waite & Gallagher, 2000). It also has been proposed that contemporary couples may enter marriage with less commitment to building a mutually satisfying, enduring relationship, instead emphasizing personal gratification, while placing unrealistic demands for emotional fulfillment on their spouse (Waite & Gallagher, 2000). Divorce itself is viewed increasingly as an acceptable solution to an unsatisfying marriage (Cherlin, 1998), as evidenced by the introduction of no-fault divorce and the easing of related laws. Finally, as more individuals achieve greater longevity (and thus spend a proportionally smaller part of their overall lifespan dedicated to the task of raising children), changing circumstances and personal values may strain existing relationships and increase risk for dissolution. In support, while risk for divorce remains highest in the first decade of marriage, greater numbers of middle-aged and elderly couples are now breaking up (U.S. Bureau of the Census, 1998).

About half of all dissolving marital unions consist of families with children (U.S. Bureau of the Census, 1998). In the United States, 40% of all children experience a parental divorce, with nearly 90% placed primarily in the physical custody of their biological mother. These single-parent arrangements are often short-lived given that half of all divorced individuals remarry within 4 years. Respective remarriage rates vary by gender: 65% for women and 75% for men. Thus, one-third of American children eventually will become members of a stepfamily. A focus on only formal changes in union formation such as divorce and remarriage is likely to underestimate substantially the number of transitions and reorganizations that children and parents experience as part of postdivorce family life. Informal arrangements in the form of nonmarital cohabitation have become an increasingly common antecedent or even an alternative to remarriage. In fact, about one-fourth of all stepfamilies consist of these nonmarital cohabiting unions (Bumpass, Raley, & Sweet, 1995). Proportionally greater numbers of postdivorce couples choose to cohabitate, with about three-fourths of adults cohabitating before a second marriage, in contrast to one-third before a first marriage. Cohabitation effectively cuts in half the time a child will spend in a truly single-parent postdivorce household, dropping the median duration from 7 to 3.7 years before the family is joined by a live-in partner (Bumpass & Raley, 1995). Half of these cohabiting unions are short-lived, ending within a year either through separation or remarriage, although rates of marriage following cohabitation are decreasing (Seltzer, 2000). Thus, whereas about 20% of children experience the dissolution of their parents' second marriage, many more will encounter multiple family transitions relating to changes in nonmarital cohabitating arrangements. Collectively, these events have important potential implications for adjustment, because multiple transitions increase the adaptive challenges that confront parents and children (Capaldi & Patterson, 1991).

RISK FACTORS THAT CONTRIBUTE TO MARITAL INSTABILITY

Relative risk for experiencing divorce depends on a variety of factors. With respect to ethnicity, the general historical trend of rising divorce rates, along with increases in cohabitation and decreases in rates of remarriage, are found for non-Hispanic whites, African Americans, and Hispanic whites. These groups differ, however, by absolute level, with African Americans remaining single longer and less likely to marry. African Americans also are more likely to separate, to divorce, to remain separated without seeking a divorce, but less likely to remarry (Teachman et al., 2000). Socioeconomic factors and related stressors likely play a part in explaining these ethnic differences in divorce given that African Americans on average are less educated, poorer, and more often unemployed than whites.

Risk for divorce in a first marriage doubles for couples living together prior to marriage and is 25% higher for those whose own parents divorced (Sweet & Bumpass, 1992). Risk also reflects age at marriage, such that 59% of women who marry as minors will divorce before reaching their 20th anniversary (Bramlett & Mosher, 2001). Relative risk drops by 30% for those who marry in their early 20s, and an additional 10% for those who marry at ages 25 and above, although the steepest drop in risk is realized when comparing those who marry during what is essentially still childhood— under age 18—versus early adulthood. Education is related inversely to risk for divorce, in part because educated individuals are more likely to come from nondivorced family backgrounds and to marry at later ages (Sweet & Bumpass, 1992).

The likelihood of divorce also is associated with patterns of interaction and personal characteristics of married adults. Couples are at higher risk for divorce if their interaction involves escalation or reciprocation of negative affect, disengagement, stonewalling, contempt, denial, and blaming (Gottman & Notarius, 2001; Hetherington, 1999b; Hetherington & Kelly, 2002). Relatedly, risk increases if couples differ on their views of family life, and if they share few interests or friends (Hetherington, 1999b; Notarius & Vanzetti, 1983). Sexual dissatisfaction contributes more to risk of instability for men than for women (Hetherington & Kelly, 2002; also see Walsh, Chapter 2, this volume), although the finding is stronger for white than for African American men (Orbuch, Veroff, & Hunter, 1999). Additionally, risk is associated with preexisting levels of personal adjustment, such as antisocial behavior, depression, alcohol/substance abuse, and impulsivity. Individuals with a history of these kinds of problems are more likely to encounter stressful life events, to experience relationship distress that ends in divorce, and to be deficient in parenting skills (Capaldi & Patterson, 1991; Hetherington, 1999b; Kitson, 1992; Kurdek, 1990). Antisocial individuals also are more likely to select an antisocial partner (Amato, 2000; Hetherington & Kelly, 2002), thereby compounding any relationship problems.

Finally, some researchers have proposed a potential genetic component to risk for divorce that underlies links between adult adjustment problems, inadequate parenting practices, and child behavior problems. In support, rates of concordance for divorce and similarity on adult adjustment problems that erode both marital and parent–child relationships (e.g., antisocial or impulsive behavior) are greater for identical than for fraternal twins (Jocklin, McGue, & Lykken, 1996; McGue & Lykken, 1992). Although genetics may contribute to risk, longitudinal studies show that the experience of an unhappy marriage and eventual divorce exerts adverse effects, at least temporarily, on the mental and physical health of adults and children; this experience also leads to emergence of problems in parenting (Amato, 2000; Hetherington, 1993; McLanahan, 1999). We turn next to a theoretical consideration of adjustment to divorce.

A PROCESS MODEL OF DIVORCE

The most commonly accepted theoretical model of divorce involves a process perspective that addresses stress, risk, and resilience. In this model, divorce is viewed as a cascade of potentially stressful changes and disruptions in the social and physical environments of adults and children, rather than as reactions to a single negative event (e.g., Amato, 2000; Hetherington, 1993; Hetherington, Bridges, & Insabella, 1998; Simons & Associates, 1996). Thus, marital instability and divorce introduce a complex chain of marital transitions and family reorganizations that alter roles and relationships, and affect individual adjustment. Each transition presents new adaptive challenges, and the response to these challenges is influenced by previous family functioning and experiences. The roles and relationships developed in the first marriage will shape the response to divorce and life in a single-parent family, and previous family experiences will affect the adaptation of family members to postdivorce changes such as cohabitation or remarriage (Amato, 2000; Hetherington, 1993, 1999a, 1999b; Hetherington & Kelly, 2002).

The success with which individuals cope with these stressors depends on the activation of protective factors (i.e., those that buffer the person or promote resilience in coping with the challenges of divorce) and vulnerability factors (i.e., those that increase the likelihood of adverse consequences). Protective and vulnerability factors include personal characteristics of the individual, family processes and relationships, and ecological systems external to the family, such as friends, extended family, school, the workplace, and the larger neighborhood. Developmental factors also play a central role in the adjustment of children and adults to marital transitions. Individuals may be more sensitive to stresses and opportunities presented by marital transitions at specific developmental periods; some challenges may trigger delayed adjustment effects to divorce (i.e., so-called "sleeper" effects). In addition to the normative challenges associated with changes in age, family members must confront non-normative challenges associated with the event of divorce (e.g., adjusting to life in a single-parent household, parental dating, remarriage). Thus, this model underscores the importance of studying the postdivorce adjustment of parents and children over time as marital transitions and family reorganizations unfold. Moreover, although risks associated with divorce have been emphasized most often in the literature, divorce may offer parents and children potential benefits: an escape from an unhappy, conflictual family situation; the opportunity to build more fulfilling relationships; and the potential for personal development. In other words, what is perhaps most striking about this model is not the inevitability but the *diversity* of responses for parents and children who face the challenges of divorce. We turn next to a consideration of empirical research on divorce adjustment for parents and children.

EFFECTS OF DIVORCE ON ADJUSTMENT

Adult Adjustment

Divorce is one of the most stressful events that an individual may experience. Some stress is inevitable given resulting transformations in marriage and family relationships, and shifts in daily routines, roles, activities, and social relationships. There may be challenges to the way that people view themselves, with some reporting a sense of being off-balance or adrift, no longer certain of who they are or what they want (Hetherington & Kelly, 2002). Even those who are relieved to be free of an unhappy marriage may be apprehensive about the future and the many stressors they are encountering.

A primary source of stress concerns inadequate levels of income. Divorce typically leads to a dramatic reduction in the custodial parent's household income, especially that of custodial mothers (Gongla & Thomson, 1987), with per capita declines averaging 13–35% in national populations (Cherlin, 1998; Peterson, 1996). Reduced income contributes to other potentially stressful circumstances, such as changes in employment, education, and residence (DeGarmo & Forgatch, 1999; Forgatch, Patterson, & Ray, 1996; Lorenz et al., 1997; McLanahan, 1999; Patterson & Forgatch, 1990). Stress usually dissipates with time (DeGarmo & Forgatch, 1997; Forgatch et al., 1996; Hetherington, 1993; Lorenz et al., 1997), although those with lower incomes generally experience greater numbers of disruptive events. If income remains low, stress often persists. Correlations between income and happiness/life satisfaction are generally small, however, with social relationships and emotional support largely moderating adverse effects of economic distress on family relations and adjustment following divorce (Hetherington & Kelly, 2002; Simons & Associates, 1996).

Given the challenges surrounding marital dissolution, it is not surprising that individuals report a host of related adjustment problems. As compared to the nondivorced, individuals who separate or divorce have higher incidence of motor vehicle accidents, increased risk of psychopathology, and elevated drinking and drug use, alcoholism, suicide, and even death (see reviews by Amato, 2000; Burman & Margolin, 1992; Hetherington et al., 1998). Those with a shorter separation time and greater emotional attachment to the former spouse have significantly poorer immune functioning and higher levels of health problems and depression (Hetherington & Kelly, 2002; Kiecolt-Glaser et al., 1988). Separated and divorced populations are overrepresented in both inpatient and outpatient psychiatric populations, with admission rates approximately six times higher than for married individuals. Prospective studies show that at least some adjustment problems, such as decrements in psychological well-being and increased alcohol and substance use and depression, result from the experience of divorce itself rather than from preexisting conditions (e.g., Aseltine & Kessler, 1993; Doherty & Needle, 1991; Hope, Rodgers, & Power, 1999; Marks & Lambert, 1998). There may also be a lingering sense of anger toward the ex-spouse and problems with loneliness. Collectively, these kinds of problems may explain why many individuals report difficulties in performing even routine tasks associated with their jobs after a divorce (Hetherington & Kelly, 2002).

Not all postdivorce changes are negative. A few studies that have explored potentially positive effects found that after a divorce, some individuals report improvements in autonomy, overall happiness, social involvement, and career development (Acock & Demo, 1994; Hetherington, 1993; Hetherington & Kelly, 2002; Kitson, 1992). Relative gain or loss in functioning appears to be rooted in the prior history of the marital relationship. Those who were previously unhappy in their marriage are more likely to report gains in psychological functioning after the divorce, as opposed to those who previously viewed their marriage as happy (Hetherington & Kelly, 2002; Wheaton, 1990). There are scattered findings of improved adjustment in men following divorce (Riessmann, 1990), although improved adjustment generally may favor women over men, given that women are more adversely affected by the presence of a distressed marriage, whereas men are more adversely affected by being unmarried (Hetherington & Kelly, 2002). Married men, for example, typically report better health, wealth, happiness, and social integration than those who remain single (Nock, 1998). Alternately, women at 2 years postdivorce are less depressed, and more healthy and competent at parenting than those who remain in unhappy, conflictual marriages (Hetherington, 1993; Hetherington & Kelly, 2002). Women also often remark on fulfillment, independence, confidence, and new competencies that they've developed in the 2 years since divorcing (Acock & Demo, 1994; Hetherington, 1993; Hetherington & Kelly, 2002; Kitson, 1992; Riessmann, 1990). Yet the experiences of divorced women are extremely diverse; some report unhappiness and social isolation, whereas others are overrepresented in a group of exceptional achievers—those with high self-esteem who excel in work, social relations, and parenting (Hetherington, 1993; Hetherington & Kelly, 2002). Coping strategies also have implications for adjustment. Resilience appears to be enhanced when individuals use active planning and effective problem solving, and seek social support rather than distraction and avoidance (Hetherington & Kelly, 2002; Sandler, Tein, & West, 1994).

With respect to custodial parents, those who have difficulties in adapting to stressful changes also show evidence of problematic relationships with their children; those problematic relationships, in turn, interfere with adjustment in children (Bank, Forgatch, Patterson, & Fetrow, 1993; Forgatch & DeGarmo, 1997b; Simons & Johnson, 1996; Wolchik et al., 2000). Thus, within the context of the divorced family, parental adjustment assumes a critical role given that child adjustment typically follows from how well adults in the household manage any stress (Hetherington et al., 1992; Patterson & Bank, 1989; Simons & Associates, 1996). Of course, children's own adjustment difficulties contribute to the custodial parent's level of stress and quality of parenting (Forgatch et al., 1996). Thus, processes operating between the custodial parent and child contribute to the long-term adjustment of both family members (Forgatch et al., 1996; Greene & Anderson, 1999; Hetherington et al., 1998; Patterson & Bank, 1989).

Child Adjustment

The relation between divorce and child adjustment is well established, although controversy arises over how best to integrate the findings. Readers may encounter, for example, the following seemingly incongruent statements:

1. Children of divorce are at serious risk for maladaptation.
2. Most children display no serious difficulties after their parent's divorce.
3. Substantial numbers of children of divorce are better adjusted than those from nondivorced households.
4. Some children's lives are enhanced by their parent's divorce.
5. Negative effects of divorce on children generally resolve soon afterward.
6. Children may be adversely affected even into adulthood by parental divorce.
7. Many of the negative effects associated with divorce exist well before the marriage ends.

Interestingly, each statement correctly summarizes a part of the literature relating to children of divorce. These statements further comprise two broad domains: (1) descriptions of the overall risk associated with divorce (statements 1–4); and (2) changes in adjustment over time (statements 5–7).

Overall Risk

Studies of divorce generally find that approximately 20–25% of children in divorced families experience high levels of problem behaviors versus 10% of children from nondivorced households (e.g., Forgatch et al., 1996; Hetherington et al., 1992; McLanahan & Sandefur, 1994; Simons & Associates, 1996; Zill, Morrison, & Coiro, 1993). Select studies produce larger differences between children from divorced and nondivorced households (e.g., 48% vs. 15%; Stolberg & Mahler, 1994), although meta-analyses come closer to the first set of figures (17% vs. 10%; Amato & Keith, 1991b; Amato, 2000). Using the 20% versus 10% figures for ease of calculation, we could correctly conclude that the experience of parental divorce essentially doubles the risk of serious problems for children (support for statement 1). We could also correctly conclude that the overwhelming majority of children (i.e., the 80% without behavioral problems) show no serious difficulties in relation to their parent's divorce (support for statement 2). Both conclusions are supported by the data, although the former emphasizes risk, whereas the latter emphasizes resilience. Furthermore, with substantial overlap in the distribution of adjustment between the children from divorced versus nondivorced families, we also could correctly conclude that a substantial number of children of divorce (i.e., about 40%), are better adjusted than their nondivorced counterparts (support for statement 3).

Some researchers have argued that the divorce itself is but a marker for other factors that create problematic adjustment in children. One potential factor involves parental conflict, such that children appear to be better off in cases in which the divorce substantially reduces levels of parental conflict (support for statement 4) (Amato, Loomis, & Booth, 1995; Booth & Amato, 2001; Jekielek, 1998). Children from the most conflicted homes also are more likely to report feeling relieved that their parents divorced, although those from less conflicted homes are more likely to report distress after their parents' divorce (Amato & Booth, 1997). Many children, in fact, initially respond to divorce with confusion, anxiety, and anger, but over time are able to adjust, with the support and involvement of a caring, competent adult. In summary, we can find empirical support for the four statements of overall risk presented earlier; each provides a different emphasis of the same body of literature—just as any "sound bite" comprises a condensed but often only partial version of the facts.

Adjustment over Time

Evidence suggests that for children of divorce, some adjustment problems may be transitory, others may persist, and still others may be present long before the actual dissolution occurs. Longitudinal studies (e.g., Guidubaldi, Perry, & Nastasi, 1987; Hetherington, Cox, & Cox, 1982) find, for example, that many problems dissipate within the 1–2 years following a divorce, as families adjust to their new life situation (support for statement 5). In other cases, effects of divorce persist over time. Hetherington (1993) found that boys who experience parental divorce while in preschool continue to show significant elevations in externalizing behavior than their nondivorced counterparts, with differences maintained into adolescence. In fact, elevations in externalizing were reported consistently across source (boys, mothers, teachers, peers, and trained observers). With respect to early adolescence, Hetherington et al. (1992) reported that, regardless of gender, children demonstrated difficulties in school and home settings even 4–6 years after the divorce. In a meta-analysis of 37 studies linking parental divorce in childhood with eventual adjustment in adulthood, Amato and Keith (1991a) found moderately sized negative effects for depression, diminished life satisfaction, and lower marital quality, educational attainment, income, occupational prestige, and physical health (support for statement 6). As married adults, children of divorce also are more likely than those from nondivorced backgrounds to display reciprocally negative and escalating exchanges with their spouses and to demonstrate less effective problem solving (Hetherington, 1999b). Divorce rates are higher as well, at 70% for the first 5 years of marriage for those from divorced family backgrounds (Bumpass, Martin, & Sweet, 1991). Selection of a stable, supportive spouse from a nondivorced family, however, can essentially eliminate the risk of marital instability associated with having divorced parents (Hetherington, 1999b; Hetherington & Kelly, 2002).

In part, long-term effects may persist because of disruptions in normal developmental trajectories during the period of adolescence. Chase-Lansdale, Cherlin, and Keirnan (1995) found, for example, that effects in adulthood were mediated by problems arising in adolescence. The kinds of problems that children of divorce encounter as adolescents also are potentially more disruptive to their lives, such as school dropout, early parenthood, and elevated drug use (Furstenberg & Teitler, 1994; Needle, Su, & Doherty, 1990; Newcomer & Udry, 1987; Zill et al., 1993). In addition, a confluence of risk factors may occur in adolescent girls from divorced families. Girls from divorced and remarried families achieve physical signs of puberty earlier, which, when combined with association with older male peers, poor parental monitoring and control, and an overtly sexually active divorced mother, leads to early initiation of sexual activities, more sexual partners, and higher rates of sexually transmitted diseases and pregnancy (Hetherington, 1993; Hetherington & Kelly, 2002).

Despite evidence for long-term difficulties, some problems stem not from the divorce itself but from earlier deteriorating conditions in the family (support for statement 7). Block, Block, and Gjerde (1986) found that behavioral problems, particularly in boys, existed up to 11 years before the divorce. Chase-Lansdale and colleagues (1995) showed that by controlling for predivorce functioning at age 7, effects of divorce at age 11 were substantially reduced, particularly for boys. Other prospective studies, however, find that effects of divorce remain significant even after controlling for predivorce functioning (e.g., Furstenberg & Teitler, 1994; Hetherington, 1999a; Needle et al., 1990; Zill et al., 1993). Chase-Lansdale et al. (1995) reported, for example, that after controlling for problems at age 7, children of divorce still demonstrate a 39% increase in clinical levels of psychological problems in young adulthood.

In an effort to synthesize the literature on divorce, researchers increasingly are adopting a perspective that emphasizes diversity in children's responses (Amato, 2000; Hetherington et al., 1998; Hetherington & Kelly, 2002). Relatedly, there is growing interest in identifying the conditions that influence risk versus resilience, such as the child's own temperament (e.g., Hetherington, 1991), although resilience does not mean that children are invulnerable to effects of divorce (Emery, 1999). Although divorce generally exerts only a moderately negative—and in many cases temporary—effect on children, the differences are far from trivial for the families involved. Most families avoid the more calamitous outcomes, such as school dropout and unwed pregnancy. But avoiding calamity is not the equivalent of having achieved success. Emery (1999) describes the concerns of many parents who worry that their children, while not necessarily demonstrating clinically significant levels of problems, still show some level of behavioral problems or emotional distress from having experienced the divorce. Many families seek help in addressing these concerns, with children of divorce being twice as likely as those from nondivorced homes to receive psychological treatment (Zill et al., 1993). Some of what they seek to repair or bolster in treatment may be key family relationships. Thus, the diversity of postdivorce outcomes for children reflects various unique qualities of the family, to be discussed in the following section.

EFFECTS OF DIVORCE ON FAMILY RELATIONSHIPS

Although custodial-father families are among the fastest growing arrangements in the United States (U.S. Bureau of the Census, 1998), research on postdivorce relationships between parents and children typically concerns the more prevalent family arrangement of custodial mothers and noncustodial fathers. Such arrangements were once called "father-absent" families, terminology that is becoming increasingly outdated as many fathers assume a larger role in their children's lives after a divorce.

Relationships between Divorced Spouses

After a divorce, overall levels of physical contact, conflict, and emotional attachment between spouses typically diminish rapidly. Men are more likely, however, to have lingering emotional attachment to the ex-spouse and to entertain thoughts of reconciliation, although, ironically, men also are quicker to remarry. In cases where their ex-spouse remarries, women commonly report sustained anger, resentment, and competitiveness toward the new wife (Hetherington & Kelly, 2002). If violence arises, it is most likely to occur in the time during the decision to divorce and immediately after the separation, with highest risk for couples in which wives have initiated the divorce. By 6 years postdivorce, most adults have moved on to build reasonably satisfying lives, and intense emotions associated with the breakup have faded. About 25% of divorced parents exhibit sustained or even increased conflict that usually concerns finances and relations with the children (Buchanan, Maccoby, & Dornbusch, 1996; Maccoby & Mnookin, 1992; Tschann, Johnson, Kline, & Wallerstein, 1990). Some children may feel "caught" between parental loyalties or think that they are to blame for these arguments; in such situations, boys are more likely to engage in noncompliant, angry, acting-out behaviors, whereas girls are more likely to respond with guilt and anxiety (Hetherington, 1999a).

Ideal postdivorce family life would seemingly involve minimal conflict between parents who are able to engage in a cooperative, supportive role with regard to each other's involvement with the child. Such a situation characterizes only about one-fourth of divorced households. Instead, most ex-spouses develop a pattern of disengaged or parallel parenting, characterized by little collaboration or communication but, fortunately, with few instances of active undermining of the other parent (Ahrons, 1999; Buchanan et al., 1996; Hetherington, 1999a; Hetherington & Kelly, 2002).

Relationships between Custodial Parents and Children

In the early years after divorce, custodial mothers and fathers often struggle with task overload and question their adequacy as parents; they also experience health problems associated with a lowered immune system and report psychological distress such as anxiety, depression, and loneliness (Hetherington, 1993; Hetherington & Kelly, 2002; Kiecolt-Glaser et al., 1988; Simons & Associates, 1996). Custodial parents often are preoccupied with their own adjustment problems, and demonstrate irritability and a lack of emotional support toward the children. Discipline may be erratic and punitive, while monitoring of children's whereabouts and behaviors typically diminishes (Forgatch et al., 1996; Hetherington, 1993). As a consequence, children generally display increased noncompliance, anger, and dependence during this time. Relationships involving custodial mothers and their sons may be especially disturbed, as demonstrated by the presence of escalating, mutually coercive interactions (DeGarmo & Forgatch, 1999; Hetherington, 1993; Hetherington et al., 1992). By 2 years postdivorce, many of these problems have diminished, although the custodial mother–son relationship continues to be more distressed than those in nondivorced families. In contrast, after an initial period of perturbation, relationships involving custodial mothers and their daughters often are characterized as warm, close, and companionate.

Additional problems may surface during adolescence. As daughters reach puberty, their relationships with mothers may become strained, particularly in cases where early-maturing daughters demonstrate precocious sexual or acting-out behaviors. Maternal attempts to correct for these problems by increasing parental monitoring and control of the adolescent daughter generally are unsuccessful (Hetherington, 1993; Hetherington et al., 1992). About one-third of children of divorce also disengage from their families earlier than counterparts in nondivorced families. If familial influence is replaced with involvement in an antisocial peer group, risk for delinquent behavior may increase; alternatively, development of a supportive relationship with a competent adult (e.g., a grandparent, teacher, or neighbor) may buffer negative effects of this early familial disengagement (Hetherington, 1993).

Although custodial mothers and fathers demonstrate similarities in the pattern of deterioration and recovery of competent parenting, some differences remain. Custodial mothers communicate and self-disclose more openly with their children and are more active in monitoring children's activities and knowing their friends. Custodial fathers report less child-rearing stress than do mothers and tend to have fewer problems with discipline or control. Additionally, divorce appears to undermine opposite-gender relationships more than same-gender relationships, such that mothers and daughters are considerably more affectionate and close than daughters and fathers, or mothers and sons. Sons in divorced families have less contact with fathers and feel less affectionate toward them than sons in nondivorced families, although the differences are relatively small (Amato & Booth, 1997).

Consistent with findings for nondivorced households, the parenting style that works well in divorced households is authoritative, characterized by warmth, support, responsiveness, and consistent control and monitoring. In contrast to disengaged, authoritarian, or permissive parenting styles, children raised with an authoritative parenting style have higher levels of social and academic competence, and lower levels of psychopathology (Anderson, Lindner, & Bennion, 1992; Avenoli, Sessa, & Steinberg, 1999; Hetherington, 1993; Hetherington & Kelly, 2002). Divorced parents are less likely than those in nondivorced households to use an authoritative parenting style, however (Hetherington, 1993; Hetherington & Kelly, 2002; Simons & Associates, 1996; Thomson, McLanahan, & Curtin, 1992), and mean levels of problem behaviors are still higher in divorced versus nondivorced families, even when authoritative parenting is used (Anderson et al., 1992). It is important also to note that much of the research on divorced families is based on white, middle-class samples, with little known about whether variations in process or outcome differ by ethnic group or setting.

Relationships between Noncustodial Parents and Children

Following divorce, noncustodial parents experience grief and anger over being less involved in their children's lives; their contact with children also diminishes rapidly (Arditti, 1992; Arendell, 1986, 1995; Furstenberg & Nord, 1987; Hetherington, 1993; Lindner-Gunnoe, 1993). Not surprisingly, the child's relationship with the custodial parent often is closer than that with the noncustodial parent (Amato, 2000; Hetherington & Stanley Hagan, 2002). Although rates of contact between noncustodial fathers and their children are increasing (Amato & Gilbreth, 1999), about 20% of children have no contact or contact limited to only a few times a year (Hetherington et al., 1998); only one-fourth to one-third have weekly visits (Hetherington et al., 1998; Maccoby & Mnookin, 1992). Decreased noncustodial involvement is related to low socioeconomic status, residential distance, and remarriage. Contact is more likely to be maintained in situations in which mediation is used, when there is low parental conflict, when the noncustodial parent believes he or she has some control in decisions affecting the child, and when the child is a boy (Amato, 2000; Amato & Gilbreth, 1999; Braver et al., 1993; Maccoby & Mnookin, 1992).

Many noncustodial fathers use their visitation primarily for recreation with their children (Amato & Gilbreth, 1999; Furstenberg & Nord, 1987) and tend to be relatively permissive (Hetherington & Jodl, 1994). Fathers may be reluctant to use their visits to set firm rules, to monitor or discipline their children's behavior, or to help with homework (Amato & Gilbreth, 1999; Furstenberg & Nord, 1987; Hetherington & Stanley Hagan, 2002). Instead, noncustodial father–child relationships often are friendly and egalitarian in nature (Arendell, 1986; Furstenberg & Nord, 1987; Hetherington & Stanley Hagan, 2002).

In contrast to noncustodial fathers, noncustodial mothers are more likely to sustain and facilitate contact with their children, and are less likely to diminish contact when either parent remarries. Although they are less authoritative than custodial mothers or mothers in nondivorced families, noncustodial mothers are more likely to make efforts at monitoring and controlling their children's behavior, and to be more supportive and sensitive to their children's needs. Children report feeling closer to noncustodial mothers than to noncustodial fathers, and noncustodial mothers are more influential in the adjustment of their children, particularly in relation to their daughters (Furstenberg & Nord, 1987; Hetherington, 1993; Hetherington & Kelly, 2002; Lindner-Gunnoe, 1993). The greater involvement and closeness of noncustodial mothers may interfere with the formation of close bonds with a stepmother (Hetherington & Kelly, 2002).

A central goal of legal policies such as joint custody and mediation, as well as therapeutic interventions designed to target postdivorce parenting, has been to help families maintain the child's contact with both parents following divorce (Emery, Kitzmann, & Waldron, 1999). It has been puzzling, therefore, that frequency of contact with the noncustodial parent only rarely demonstrates positive child effects (Amato, 2000; Amato & Gilbreth, 1999). Rather, the conditions of visitation and the quality of parent–child relations are important predictors for child adjustment. Under conditions of low interparental conflict, visits from an authoritative, stable, noncustodial parent benefit children and adolescents (Amato & Gilbreth, 1999; Hetherington, 1993; McLanahan & Sandefur, 1994; Simons & Associates, 1996). Under conditions of high conflict, or with an inept, abusive, or severely maladjusted or alcoholic parent, visits may be harmful (Johnston, Kline, & Tschann, 1989). This may explain why although joint custody and mediation increase child support and contact with noncustodial parents, they seldom show advantages in the adjustment of children (Emery et al., 1999; Maccoby & Mnookin, 1992). Such situations may be encouraging even highly contentious parents to remain involved (Johnston et al., 1989).

Relationships between Siblings

In contrast to the postdivorce research on parent–child relationships, studies of siblings are rare. The few studies in this area show that sibling relationships following parental divorce are generally distressed, marked by patterns of conflict and negativity, as well as disengagement and avoidance (Conger & Conger, 1996; Hetherington, 1993; Hetherington & Kelly, 2002; MacKinnon, 1989). Within 4–6 years after divorce, many of these differences have abated, although, consistent with the research on parent–child relationships, sibling relationships in divorced families continue to be more negative compared to those in nondivorced families (Anderson & Rice, 1992). Patterns of disengagement and avoidance may explain why child adjustment is less strongly related to sibling relationship quality in divorced versus nondivorced families (Anderson et al., 1992).

Research in this area also provides evidence for a spillover effect with other family relationships. More negative sibling relationships are related to higher levels of conflict occurring between divorced spouses, and between parents and children (Conger & Conger, 1996; Hetherington, 1993; Hetherington & Kelly, 2002; MacKinnon, 1989). Over time, the presence of a sibling may introduce the potential for differential treatment by parents, and differential involvement in parental disputes (Greene & Anderson, 1999). When sibling relationships are positive, they may buffer the effects of a conflictual relationship with a parent (Hetherington, 1993), although boys appear to receive less sibling support than do girls (Anderson & Rice, 1992; Conger & Conger, 1996; Hetherington, 1993). Even in adulthood, it is mothers and female siblings who promote more family cohesion through phone calls, organizing joint activities or celebrations, and coming together at vacations (Hetherington, 1999a).

Relationships with Grandparents

Following divorce, a strengthening of ties with blood relatives often occurs (Gongla & Thomson, 1987). Many divorced mothers turn to their own parents for economic assistance; about one-fourth of divorced women live with their parents at some point after the divorce (Hetherington & Kelly, 2002). Many custodial mothers and fathers also rely on their family of origin for child care and emotional support. In African American families, help is more likely to take the form of providing services, in contrast to the economic support provided in white families (Cherlin & Furstenberg, 1994).

Related research findings on the role of grandparents in protecting children from the adverse effects of parental divorce have been mixed. Some have found that children, especially African Americans in mother-headed homes, may benefit from the presence of a grandmother in the home (Kellam, Adams, Brown, & Ensminger, 1982); however, family stress may increase in situations where residential grandmothers and divorced mothers conflict on views of control and discipline of children, the divorced mother's social life, and level of independence (Hetherington, 1989). Moreover, when support from grandparents comes with unwanted advice, costs, and restrictions, it is unhelpful to parents or children (Amato, 2000; Cherlin & Furstenberg, 1994; Hetherington, 1989; Kitson, 1992; Miller, Smerglia, Gaudet, & Kitson, 1998). When the presence of a grandparent has advantageous effects on children, it is because the grandmother's support leads to improved maternal parenting (Hetherington, 1989). Although there is little research on the impact of grandfathers on children's adjustment, some evidence indicates that an involved, competent, residential grandfather in a divorced family can decrease antisocial behavior and increase achievement in grandsons (Hetherington, 1989).

EXTRAFAMILIAL RELATIONSHIPS AND DIVORCE

In addition to family ties, relationships external to the family have the potential to exert influence on adjustment after divorce. In fact, this influence may occur even before the actual breakup: About 75% of those who initiate a divorce report that either an adult confidant (e.g., a friend, or family member) or new romantic partner played a major role in their decision to leave the marriage (Hetherington & Kelly, 2002). In the aftermath of divorce, parents seem likely to continue seeking contact from these adults for support and assistance.

Relationships with Adult Confidants

The presence of a caring adult or confidant may help promote healthy adult postdivorce adjustment, thereby benefiting parenting during the postdivorce period. Unfortunately, marital breakups may undermine adult relationships and thus diminish available social support (Rands, 1988). Reduced access to supportive social relationships may be an important determinant of the emotional distress and disrupted parenting that typically manifests in divorced persons (Gongla & Thomson, 1987). These disruptions and the concomitant loss of support may be greatest for those who are most distressed and depressed, and whose problem-solving skills have deteriorated severely (DeGarmo & Forgatch, 1997; Gongla & Thomson, 1987; Patterson & Forgatch, 1990). In fact, stress and negative affect have been shown to interfere with the quality of relational support and problem solving demonstrated between custodial parents and adults from their social network (DeGarmo & Forgatch, 1997, 1999; Forgatch & DeGarmo, 1997a; Patterson & Forgatch, 1990).

Relationships with Romantic Partners

Along with the divorce comes the legally and socially sanctioned potential to form new romantic attachments with other adults. In fact, the strongest contributor to a divorced adult's well-being and happiness is the eventual formation of a supportive, mutually caring, intimate relationship (Hetherington, 1993; Hetherington & Kelly, 2002). About one-third of parents already have such a relationship in place at the point of filing for divorce, and most will begin to date in the first year following the filing (Anderson et al., 2001). Moreover, situations in which the romantic partner is residential may provide more immediate support than nonresidential partners, or nonresidential friends and relatives (DeGarmo & Forgatch, 1997; Simons & Johnson, 1996). Unlike a live-in partner, who is available to offer encouragement, advice, and actual help with child rearing, nonresidential partners, friends, and relatives, even if supportive, may not be present to assist with everyday duties, and thus exert little influence on the quality of parenting.

Ironically, the potential for a new partner to offer emotional and social support to the family is not always reflected in improved child outcomes. The adjustment of children in cohabiting families may be worse than that in divorced, single-parent households (Buchanan et al., 1996; Cherlin & Furstenberg, 1994; Seltzer, 2000). It may be that the stresses and challenges in forming successful cohabiting relationships (e.g., ambiguity of the new partner's parental role, uncertainty of a long-term commitment) at times outweigh the benefits of possible support, or that the adverse effects of divorce are pervasive and long-lasting (Anderson, Greene, Hetherington, & Clingempeel, 1999; Buchanan et al., 1996; Cherlin & Furstenberg, 1994). Yet many postdivorce families are able over time to establish gratifying relationships and a salutary environment in which competent children can develop (Hetherington et al., 1998; Seltzer, 2000; Thomson et al., 1992). Given that cohabitation is such a common experience for postdivorce families, we turn next to a consideration of the available literature.

REPARTNERING AND NONMARITAL COHABITATING RELATIONSHIPS

Nonmarital cohabitation appears to be a difficult transition for many families. Buchanan et al. (1996) have found, for example, that boys in cohabitating postdivorce households scored higher on almost every problem measured, including substance use, school deviance, antisocial behavior, poor grades, and problem peer relations compared to remarried families. Girls in cohabitating families were more likely than those whose parents were remarried or romantically noninvolved to have strained relations with the custodial parent. Additionally, parenting was problematic in dating and cohabitating families as opposed to remarried families. Nonmarital cohabitation has adverse potential effects for adult adjustment as well; the risk of physical abuse to adults in cohabitating relationships is three times greater than that for married couples, 15% versus 5% (Waite, 2000). Perhaps because of uncertainty in the cohabitating state, couples are less likely to pool income, although income sharing increases when a child is born into the union.

Compared to stepfathers or nondivorced fathers with biological children, the cohabiting romantic partner is likely to be less financially and emotionally invested in any residential children. The cohabiting romantic partner's relationships and parenting style with residential children are more problematic, with the partner typically devoting less time to youth-oriented activities at school or in community or religious organizations (Thomson et al., 1992). When cohabitating families experience strain between the romantic partner and child, it can spill over into distressed relations between the custodial parent and child, particularly daughters (Buchanan et al., 1996).

Given the challenges inherent in adjusting to divorce, along with the likelihood that many of these families eventually will remarry, which factors contribute to successful repartnering? Although literature on the topic of postdivorce repartnering at present is limited, it seems likely that the period prior to actual legal remarriage comprises a time of potentially dramatic levels of change, as the custodial parent, the new romantic partner, and any residential children meet one another and begin to form the basis for new relationships and efforts toward forging a new family system. Specifically, repartnering success may be dependent on how well custodial parents handle three central challenges in the repartnering process: (1) developing effective decision-making strategies for dating others, (2) serving as gatekeepers or regulators of information to children concerning their own repartnering and their ex-spouse's repartnering; and (3) acting as managers of emerging relationships in repartnered families.

As part of the first challenge, developing decision-making strategies in dating, custodial parents must evaluate their personal readiness to begin the dating process; some already have begun the process of repartnering even as the marriage dissolved, whereas others may not be ready for months or even years after the divorce. Parents also must decide on their selection criteria for the new romantic partner, including the strategies used to meet others, such as the dating arena or specific setting that they select as a way to access a potential source of eligible partners (e.g., work, bars and clubs, religious organizations, personal ads, the Internet, contact with friends or relatives). Finally, parents must determine the extent to which considerations about the child affect the process of dating, including the child's own level of readiness and individual adjustment. The little available research suggests that positive child adjustment, in fact, may accelerate the repartnering process (Forgatch et al., 1996; Montgomery, Anderson, Hetherington, & Clingempeel, 1992).

With respect to the second challenge, custodial parents must serve in the role as gatekeeper, by orchestrating whether, when, and how to disclose information relating to the romantic relationship itself (e.g., the extent of this disclosure, its timing and level of developmental appropriateness). For example, they must decide how to handle the child's exposure to any implied sexual involvement between the parent and partner, such as the frequency and timing of sleepovers. The success with which the custodial parent is able to manage such situations has important potential implications for children given that inappropriate levels of exposure may lead to precocious sexual knowledge (Hetherington, Cox, & Cox, 1978; Wallerstein & Kelly, 1980).

With the third challenge, managing emerging relationships, custodial parents must incorporate the new romantic partner into the existing system with the child, such as deciding on the level of the partner's involvement in disciplining the residential children. There also must be opportunities for joint activities shared between children and the new romantic partner. Shared activities may influence how well families adapt over the long term to the new romantic partner (Montgomery et al., 1992). Relatedly, the adjustment of families to postdivorce events such as parental repartnering takes place against a backdrop of mutual and recursive influence among family members. The ways in which the custodial parent responds to the interaction between the new romantic partner and the child provides, for example, a signal to the child as to how to interpret and further react to the partner's behavior. The child's response to overtures made by the new romantic partner may provide the custodial parent with a means to gauge the successful integration of the partner into the family and, thus, an indirect assessment of the long-term prospects for the repartnered relationship. Moreover, whereas much of this discussion on postdivorce parental repartnering has concerned the custodial parent, the little available research demonstrates that even changes in the *non*custodial parent's romantic life exert effects on child development (Anderson et al., 1999). In summary, the negotiation of family transitions around postdivorce repartnering has important implications for adult and child adjustment and parental functioning. Further research is needed to identify the putative mechanisms involved in successful repartnering and to inform theory, as well as interventions, with divorced populations.

SUMMARY

The breakdown of a marriage initiates a series of notable changes in the lives of parents and children. As emerging challenges are met, new relationships formed, and family roles and processes altered, most adults and children experience considerable stress. Whereas about one-fourth experience lasting problems in adjustment, it should be underscored that most are resilient, able to move on and lead satisfying new lives. Postdivorce resilience largely depends on the ability of parents and children to build close, constructive, mutually supportive relationships that play a profound role in buffering families from effects of related adversity.

REFERENCES

Acock, A. C., & Demo, D. H. (1994). *Family diversity and well-being.* Thousand Oaks, CA: Sage.

Ahrons, C. R. (1999). Divorce: An unscheduled family transition. In B. Carter & M. McGoldrick (Eds.), *The expanded family life cycle: Individual, family, and social perspectives* (pp. 381–397). Boston: Allyn & Bacon.

Amato, P. R. (2000). The consequences of divorce for adults and children. *Journal of Marriage and the Family, 62,* 1269–1287.

Amato, P. R., & Booth, A. (1997). *A generation at risk: Growing up in an era of family upheaval.* Cambridge, MA: Harvard University Press.

Amato, P. R., & Gilbreth, J. G. (1999). Nonresident fathers and children's well-being: A meta-analysis. *Journal of Marriage and the Family, 61,* 557–575.

Amato, P. R., & Keith, B. (1991a). Parental divorce and adult well-being: A meta-analysis. *Journal of Marriage and the Family, 53,* 43–58.

Amato, P. R., & Keith, B. (1991b). Parental divorce and the well-being of children: A meta-analysis. *Psychological Bulletin, 110,* 26–46.

Amato, P. R., Loomis, L. S., & Booth, A. (1995). Parental divorce, marital conflict, and offspring well-being in early adulthood. *Social Forces, 73,* 895–916.

Anderson, E. R., Greene, S. M., Forgatch, M. S., DeGarmo, D. S., Walker, L., & Malerba, C. (2001). *Patterns of repartnering after divorce.* Unpublished manuscript, University of Texas at Austin.

Anderson, E. R., Greene, S. M., Hetherington, E. M., & Clingempeel, W. G. (1999). The dynamics of parental remarriage: Adolescent, parent, and sibling influences. In E. M. Hetherington (Ed.), *Coping with divorce, single parenting, and remarriage: A risk and resiliency perspective* (pp. 295–319). Mahwah, NJ: Erlbaum

Anderson, E. R., Lindner, M. S., & Bennion, L. D. (1992). The effect of family relationships on adolescent development during family reorganization. *Monographs of the Society for Research in Child Development, 57*(2–3, Serial No. 227), 178–200.

Anderson, E. R., & Rice, A. M. (1992). Sibling relationships during remarriage. *Monographs of the Society for Research in Child Development, 57*(2–3, Serial No. 227), 149–177.

Arditti, J. A. (1992). Differences between fathers with joint custody and noncustodial fathers. *American Journal of Orthopsychiatry, 62*(2), 186–195.

Arendell, T. (1986). *Mothers and divorce: Legal, economic and social dilemmas.* Berkeley: University of California Press.

Arendell, T. (1995). *Fathers and divorce.* Thousand Oaks, CA: Sage.

Aseltine, R. H., & Kessler, R. C. (1993). Marital disruption and depression in a community sample. *Journal of Health and Social Behavior, 34,* 237–251.

Avenoli, S., Sessa, F. M., & Steinberg, L. (1999). Family structure, parenting practices, and adolescent adjustment: An ecological examination. In E. M. Hetherington (Ed.), *Coping with divorce, single parenting and remarriage: A risk and resiliency perspective* (pp. 65–90). Mahwah, NJ: Erlbaum.

Bank, L., Forgatch, M. S., Patterson, G. R., & Fetrow, R. A. (1993). Parenting practices of single mothers: Mediators of negative contextual factors. *Journal of Marriage and the Family, 55,* 371–384.

Block, J. H., Block, J., & Gjerde, P. F. (1986). The personality of children prior to divorce: A prospective study. *Child Development, 57,* 827–840.

Booth, A., & Amato, P. R. (2001). Parental divorce relations and offspring postdivorce well-being. *Journal of Marriage and the Family, 63,* 197–212.

Bramlett, M. D., & Mosher, W. D. (2001). *First marriage dissolution, divorce, and remarriage in the United States: Advance data from vital and health statistics.* Hyattsville, MD: National Center for Health Statistics.

Braver, S. L., Wolchick, S. A., Sandler, I. N., Sheets, V. L., Fogas, B., & Bay, R. C. (1993). A longitudinal study of nonresidential parents: Parents without children. *Journal of Family Psychology, 7*(1), 9–23.

Buchanan, C. M., Maccoby, E. E., & Dornbusch, S. M. (1996). *Adolescents after divorce.* Cambridge, MA: Harvard University Press.

Bumpass, L. L., Martin, T. C., & Sweet, J. A. (1991). The impact of family background and early marital factors on marital disruption. *Journal of Family Issues, 12,* 22–42.

Bumpass, L. L., & Raley, R. K. (1995). Redefining single-parent families: Cohabitation and changing family reality. *Demography, 32,* 97–109.

Bumpass, L. L., Raley, R. K., & Sweet, J. A. (1995). The changing character of stepfamilies: Implications of cohabitation and nonmarital childbearing. *Demography, 32,* 425–436.

Burman, B., & Margolin, G. (1992). Analysis of the association between marital relationships and health problems: An interactional perspective. *Psychological Bulletin, 112*(1), 39–63.

Capaldi, D. M., & Patterson, G. R. (1991). Relation of parental transitions to boys' adjustment problems: I. A linear hypothesis. II. Mothers at risk for transitions and unskilled parenting. *Developmental Psychology, 27,* 489–504.

Chase-Lansdale, P. L., Cherlin, A. J., & Keirnan, K. E. (1995). The long-term effects of parental divorce on the mental health of young adults: A developmental perspective. *Child Development, 66,* 1614–1634.

Cherlin, A. J. (1998). Marriage and marital dissolution among black Americans. *Journal of Comparative Family Studies, 29,* 147–158.

Cherlin, A. J., & Furstenberg, F. F. (1994). Stepfamilies in the United States. *Review of Sociology, 20,* 359–381.

Conger, R. D., & Conger, K. J. (1996). Sibling relationships. In R. L. Simons & Associates (Eds.), *Understanding differences between divorced and intact families* (pp. 104–121). Thousand Oaks, CA: Sage.

DeGarmo, D. S., & Forgatch, M. S. (1997). Determinants of observed confidant support. *Journal of Personality and Social Psychology, 72,* 336–345.

DeGarmo, D. S., & Forgatch, M. S. (1999). Contexts as predictors of changing maternal parenting practices in diverse family structures: A social interactional perspective of risk and resilience. In E. M. Hetherington (Ed.), *Coping with divorce, single parenting and remarriage: A risk and resiliency perspective* (pp. 227–252). Mahwah, NJ: Erlbaum.

Doherty, W. J., & Needle, R. H. (1991). Psychological adjustment and substance use among adolescents before and after a parental divorce. *Child Development, 62,* 328–337.

Emery, R. E. (1999). Postdivorce family life for children: An overview of research and some implications for policy. In R. A. Thompson & P. R. Amato (Eds.), *The postdivorce family: Children, parenting, and society* (pp. 3–27). Thousand Oaks, CA: Sage.

Emery, R. E., Kitzmann, K. M., & Waldron, M. (1999). Psychological interventions for separated and divorced families. In E. M. Hetherington (Ed.), *Coping with divorce, single parenting and remarriage: A risk and resiliency perspective* (pp. 332–344). Mahwah, NJ: Erlbaum.

Forgatch, M. S., & DeGarmo, D. S. (1997a). Adult problem solving: Contributor to parenting and child outcomes in divorced families. *Social Development, 6*(2), 238–254.

Forgatch, M. S., & DeGarmo, D. S. (1997b). Confidant contributions to parenting and child outcomes. *Social Development, 6,* 237–253.

Forgatch, M. S., Patterson, G. R., & Ray, J. A. (1996). Divorce and boys' adjustment problems: Two paths with a single model. In E. M. Hetherington & E. A. Blechman (Eds.), *Stress, coping, and resiliency in children and the family* (pp. 67–105). Mahwah, NJ: Erlbaum.

Furstenberg, F. F., & Nord, C. W. (1987). Parenting apart: Patterns of childrearing after marital disruption. *Journal of Marriage and the Family, 47,* 893–904.

Furstenberg, F. F., Jr., & Teitler, J. O. (1994). Reconsidering the effects of marital disruption: What happens to children of divorce in early adulthood? *Journal of Family Issues, 15*(2), 173–190.

Goldstein, J. R. (1999). The leveling of divorce in the United States. *Demography, 36*(6), 409–414.

Gongla, P. A., & Thomson, E. H. (1987). Single-parent families. In M. B. Sussman & S. K. Steinmetz (Eds.), *Handbook of marriage and the family* (pp. 297–418). New York: Plenum Press.

Gottman, J. M., & Notarius, C. T. (2001). Decade review: Observing marital interaction. *Journal of Marriage and the Family, 62,* 146–166.

Greene, S. M., & Anderson, E. R. (1999). Observed negativity in large family systems: Incidents and reactions. *Journal of Family Psychology, 13,* 372–392.

Guidubaldi, J., Perry, J. D., & Nastasi, B. K. (1987). Assessment and intervention for children of divorce: Implications of the NASP-KSU nationwide survey. In J. Vincent (Ed.), *Advances in family intervention, assessment, and theory* (Vol. 4, pp. 109–151). New York: Plenum Press.

Hetherington, E. M. (1989). Coping with family transitions: Winners, losers, and survivors. *Child Development, 60,* 1–14.

Hetherington, E. M. (1991). The role of individual differences and family relationships in children coping with divorce and remarriage. In P. Cowan & E. M. Hetherington (Eds.), *Family transitions* (pp. 165–174). Hillsdale, NJ: Erlbaum.

Hetherington, E. M. (1993). An overview of the Virginia longitudinal study of divorce and remarriage with a focus on early adolescence. *Journal of Family Psychology, 7*(1), 39–56.

Hetherington, E. M. (1999a). Should we stay together for the sake of our children? In E. M. Hetherington (Ed.), *Coping with divorce, single parenting and remarriage: A risk and resiliency perspective* (pp. 93–116). Mahwah, NJ: Erlbaum.

Hetherington, E. M., (1999b). Social capital and the development of youth from nondivorced, divorced, and remarried families. In A. Collins (Ed.), *Relationships as developmental contexts: The 29th Minnesota Symposium on Child Psychology.* Hillsdale, NJ: Erlbaum.

Hetherington, E. M., Bridges, M., & Insabella, B. M. (1998). What matters? What does not?: Five perspectives on the association between marital transitions and children's adjustment. *American Psychologist, 53,* 167–184.

Hetherington, E. M., & Clingempeel, W. G., in collaboration with Anderson, E. R.,

Deal, J. E., Stanley Hagan, M., Hollier, E. A., & Lindner, M. S. (1992). Coping with marital transitions: A family systems perspective. *Monographs of the Society for Research in Child Development, 57*(2–3, Serial No. 227).

Hetherington, E. M., Cox, M., & Cox, R. (1978). The aftermath of divorce. In J. H. Stevens, Jr., & M. Mathews (Eds.), *Mother–child, father–child relations* (pp. 148–176). Washington, DC: National Association for the Education of Young Children.

Hetherington, E. M., Cox, M., & Cox, R. (1982). Effects of divorce on parents and children. In M. Lamb (Ed.), *Nontraditional families* (pp. 233–288). Hillsdale, NJ: Erlbaum.

Hetherington, E. M., & Jodl, K. (1994). Stepfamilies as settings for development. In A. Booth & J. Dunn (Eds.), *Stepfamilies* (pp. 55–80). Cambridge, MA: Harvard University Press.

Hetherington, E. M., & Kelly, J. (2002). *For better or for worse: Divorce reconsidered.* New York: Norton.

Hetherington, E. M., & Stanley Hagan, M. (2002). Parenting in divorced and remarried families. In M. Bornstein (Ed.), *Handbook of parenting* (2nd ed., pp. 287–315). Mahwah, NJ: Erlbaum.

Hope, S., Rodgers, B., & Power, C. (1999). Marital status transitions and psychological distress: Longitudinal evidence from a national population sample. *Psychological Medicine, 29,* 381–389.

Jekielek, S. (1998). Parental conflict, marital disruption and children's emotional well-being. *Social Forces, 76,* 905–936.

Jocklin, V., McGue, M., & Lykken, D. T. (1996). Personality and divorce: A genetic analysis. *Journal of Personality and Social Psychology, 71,* 288–299.

Johnston, J. R., Kline, M., & Tschann, J. (1989). Ongoing post-divorce conflict in families contesting custody: Effects on children of joint custody and frequent access. *American Journal of Orthopsychiatry, 59,* 576–592.

Kellam, S. G., Adams, R. G., Brown, C. H., & Ensminger, M. A. (1982). The long-term evolution of the family structure of teenage and older mothers. *Journal of Marriage and the Family, 4,* 539–554.

Kiecolt-Glaser, J. K., Kennedy, S., Malkoff, S., Fisher, L. D., Speicher, C. E., & Glaser, R. (1988). Marital discord and immunity in males. *Psychosomatic Medicine, 50,* 213–229.

Kitson, G. C. (1992). *Portrait of divorce: Adjustment to marital breakdown.* New York: Guilford Press.

Kurdek, L. A. (1990). Divorce history and self-reported psychological distress in husbands and wives. *Journal of Marriage and the Family, 52,* 701–708.

Lindner-Gunnoe, M. (1993). *Noncustodial mothers' and fathers' contributions to the adjustment of adolescent stepchildren.* Unpublished doctoral dissertation, University of Virginia, Charlottesville.

Lorenz, F. O., Simons, R. L., Conger, R. D., Elder, G. H. J., Johnson, C., & Chao, W. (1997). Married and recently divorced mothers' stressful events and distress: Tracing change across time. *Journal of Marriage and the Family, 59,* 219–232.

Maccoby, E. E., & Mnookin, R. H. (1992). *Dividing the child: Social and legal dilemmas of custody.* Cambridge, MA: Harvard University Press.

MacKinnon, C. E. (1989). An observational investigation of sibling interactions in married and divorced families. *Developmental Psychology, 25,* 36–44.

Marks, N. F., & Lambert, J. D. (1998). Marital status, continuity, and change among young and midlife adults. *Journal of Marriage and the Family, 53,* 103–110.

McGue, M., & Lykken, D. T. (1992). Genetic influence on risk of divorce. *Psychological Science, 6,* 368–373.

McLanahan, S. (1999). Father absence and the welfare of children. In E. M. Hetherington (Ed.), *Coping with divorce, single parenting and remarriage: A risk and resiliency perspective* (pp. 117–146). Mahwah, NJ: Erlbaum.

McLanahan, S., & Sandefur, G. (1994). *Growing up with a single parent: What hurts, what helps?* Cambridge, MA: Harvard University Press.

Miller, N. B., Smerglia, V. L., Gaudet, D. S., & Kitson, G. C. (1998). Stressful life events, social support, and the distress of widowed and divorced women. *Journal of Family Issues, 19,* 181–203.

Montgomery, M. J., Anderson, E. R., Hetherington, E. M., & Clingempeel, W. G. (1992). Patterns of courtship for remarriage: Implications for child adjustment and parent–child relationships. *Journal of Marriage and the Family, 54,* 686–698.

Needle, R. H., Su, S. S., & Doherty, W. J. (1990). Divorce, remarriage, and adolescent substance use: A prospective longitudinal study. *Journal of Marriage and the Family, 52,* 157–196.

Newcomer, S., & Udry, J. R. (1987). Parental marital status effects on adolescent sexual behavior. *Journal of Marriage and the Family, 49,* 235–240.

Nock, S. L. (1998). *Marriage in men's lives.* New York: Oxford University Press.

Notarius, C. I., & Vanzetti, N. A. (1983). The marital agenda as protocol. In E. E. Filsinger (Ed.), *Marriage and family assessment* (pp. 209–227). Beverly Hills, CA: Sage.

Orbuch, T. L., Veroff, J., & Hunter, A. G. (1999). Black couples, white couples: The early years of marriage. In E. M. Hetherington (Ed.), *Coping with divorce, single parenting and remarriage: A risk and resiliency perspective* (pp. 23–46). Mahwah, NJ: Erlbaum.

Patterson, G. R., & Bank, L. (1989). Some amplifying mechanisms for pathologic processes in families. In M. R. Gunnar & E. Thelen (Eds.), *Systems and development: The Minnesota Symposia on Child Psychology* (Vol. 22; pp. 167–209). Hillsdale, NJ: Erlbaum.

Patterson, G. R., & Forgatch, M. S. (1990). Initiation and maintenance of process disrupting single-mother families. In G. R. Patterson (Ed.), *Depression and aggression in family interaction* (pp. 209–245). Hillsdale, NJ: Erlbaum.

Peterson, R. R. (1996). A re-evaluation of the economic consequences of divorce. *American Sociological Review, 61,* 528–536.

Rands, M. (1988). Changes in social networks following marital separation and divorce. In R. M. Milardo (Ed.), *Families and social networks* (pp. 127–146). Newbury Park, CA: Sage.

Riessmann, C. K. (1990). *Divorce talk: Women and men make sense of personal relationships.* New Brunswick, NJ: Rutgers University Press.

Sandler, I. N., Tein, J. Y., & West, S. G. (1994). Coping, stress, and the psychological symptoms of children of divorce: A cross-sectional and longitudinal study. *Child Development, 65,* 1744–1763.

Seltzer, J. A. (2000). Families formed outside of marriage. *Journal of Marriage and the Family, 62,* 1247–1268.

Simons, R. L., & Associates. (1996). *Understanding differences between divorced and intact families: Stress, interaction, and child outcome.* Thousand Oaks, CA: Sage.

Simons, R. L., & Johnson, C. (1996). The impact of marital and social network support on quality of parenting. In G. R. Pierce, B. R. Sarason, & J. G. Sarason (Eds.), *Handbook of social support and the family* (pp. 269–287). New York: Plenum Press.

Stolberg, A. L., & Mahler, J. (1994). Enhancing treatment gains in a school-based intervention for children of divorce through skill training, parental involvement and transfer procedures. *Journal of Consulting and Clinical Psychology, 62,* 147–156.

Sweet, J. A., & Bumpass, L. L. (1992). Disruptions of marital and cohabitation relationships: A social demographic perspective. In T. L. Orbuch (Ed.), *Close relationship loss: Theoretical approaches* (pp. 67–89). New York: Springer-Verlag.

Thomson, E., McLanahan, S. S., & Curtin, R. B. (1992). Family structure, gender, and parental socialization. *Journal of Marriage and the Family, 54,* 368–378.

Thornton, A. (1977). Children and marital stability. *Journal of Marriage and the Family, 39,* 531–540.

Teachman, J. D., Tedrow, L. M., & Crowder, K. D. (2000). The changing demography of America's families. *Journal of Marriage and the Family, 62,* 1234–1246.

Tschann, J. M., Johnston, J. R., Kline, M., & Wallerstein, J. (1990). Conflict, loss, change, and parent–child relationships: Predicting children's adjustment during divorce. *Journal of Divorce and Remarriage, 13,* 1–22.

U.S. Bureau of the Census. (1998). Marital status and living arrangements: March 1996. *Current Population Reports,* Series P20-496. Washington, DC: U.S. Government Printing Office.

Waite, L. J. (2000). Trends in men's and women's well-being in marriage. In L. J. Waite (Ed.), *The ties that bind: Perspectives on marriage and cohabitation* (pp. 268–392). New York: Aldine de Gruyter.

Waite, L. J., & Gallagher, M. (2000). *The case for marriage: Why married people are happier, healthier, and better off financially.* New York: Doubleday.

Wallerstein, J. S., & Kelly, J. B. (1980). *Surviving the breakup: How children and parents cope with divorce.* New York: Basic Books.

Wheaton, B. (1990). Life transitions, role histories, and mental health. *American Sociological Review, 55,* 209–223.

Wolchik, S. A., West, S. G., Sandler, I. N., Tein, J. Y., Coatsworth, D., Lengua, L., Weiss, L., Anderson, E. R., Greene, S. M., & Griffin, W. (2000). An experimental evaluation of theory-based mother and mother–child programs for children of divorce. *Journal of Consulting and Clinical Psychology, 68,* 843–856.

Zill, N., Morrison, D. R., & Coiro, M. J. (1993). Long-term effects of parental divorce on parent–child relationships, adjustment, and achievement in young adulthood. *Journal of Family Psychology, 7,* 91–103.

CHAPTER 5

THE DIVERSITY, STRENGTHS, AND CHALLENGES OF SINGLE-PARENT HOUSEHOLDS

Carol Anderson

Single-parent households make up 26% of all American families with children under the age of 18, a dramatic 58% increase since 1970. There are now over 12 million single-parent households, approximately 10 million of which are maintained by mothers (U.S. Census Bureau, 2001). Even though many divorced single parents are likely to remarry, over half of the children born in the 1990s will spend some or all of their childhood in a single-parent household (Furstenberg & Cherlin, 1991; Lamb, Sternberg, & Thompson, 1997).

Given the prevalence of the single-parent family form, gaining an understanding of the needs, strengths, and challenges of single parents and their children is crucial. It is, however, a more complex task, because the category "one-parent household" is an increasingly heterogeneous one (Garfinkel & McLanahan, 1986). Some single parents are well off, others are poor. Some have the financial support and involvement of the other parent; others do not. Some have always been single; others are divorced or widowed. Some have an extensive network of supportive family and friends; others are relatively isolated. Some work; some do not. Some choose to be single parents and may have additional challenges associated with adoption; others are single parents as the result of a lost relationship or at least the lost dream of a relationship. Some live alone with their children; others live with parents, and still others have another adult in the home. Certainly, the category includes an increasing number of never-married poor and minority women struggling to raise two or three children as they are pressured to move from welfare to work, but single parenthood is also growing across all socioeconomic groups, with the greatest increase among the affluent and well educated. Today, there are never-married celebrities; career women with high incomes, who can afford private schools and full-time child care; gay and lesbian parents with biological or adopted children; and a small but increasing number of fathers with primary responsibility for their children.

These groups have some issues in common, but many more issues that are especially characteristic of their particular form of single-parent family. For instance, African American single parents are more likely to be impoverished, with the attendant risks for negative outcomes, but they also often have a more supportive kinship system than is commonly found in other nuclear family structures (Murry, Bynum, Brody, Willert, & Stephens, 2001; McAdoo, 1997; Chatters, Taylor, & Jayakody, 1994). How well single-parent families function is not only the result of the family structure or composition, but also a range of complex, interacting individual, familial, and community factors of risk and resilience (Hetheringon, Bridges, & Insabella, 1998; Hetherington & Stanley Hagan, 2000).

PATHWAYS TO SINGLE PARENTHOOD

An increasing number of women and men choose to become single parents through adoption, an uncommitted relationship, or artificial insemination by a friendly or anonymous donor. These particular increases in the prevalence and variety of single parents generate cries of alarm from some who fear that marriage is in danger of going out of style. This is highly unlikely. Even though single parents can and do create satisfying lives on their own, most would prefer to be parents in the context of a marriage or a long-term, loving relationship. Thus, the pathway that brings individuals to single parenthood often evolves by default (i.e., they had no such intimate relationship, or it was terminated through separation, divorce, or death of a partner). In other words, many single-parent families are built on a foundation of loss, whether the loss of a partner or the loss of a dream. A relationship has not worked or a marriage has ended, often for very good, and painful, reasons. Whether the terminated relationships involved abuse, betrayal, or unresolved conflict, single parents and their children almost certainly have had to mourn a loss or deal with the fallout of anger and disappointment.

Single-parent mothers often have the additional burden of feeling that they have failed at what is seen as any woman's prime mission, that of holding on to her partner and maintaining a nuclear family unit—an assumption often reinforced by negative feedback from family and friends. The impact of this personal and social baggage is a backdrop for both never-married and divorced parents as they enter single parenthood, taking on constant, primary responsibility. All of these factors (i.e., parental social or psychological characteristics, the reasons and pathways to single parenthood), contribute to the level of life satisfaction of single parents and their ability to parent. They also influence the psychological health and development of their children.

THE SPECIAL CHALLENGES OF SINGLE-PARENT FAMILIES

In contrast to the stereotyped view of single-parent households as inherently deficient, most single parents provide the structure, values, and nurturance that their children need, despite the challenges and criticisms they encounter (Hawkins & Eggebeen, 1991). Their homes are not "broken," their lives are not miserable, and their children may have problems, but most eventually thrive.

Financial hardship, however, is frequently noted to be the most significant challenge. Many low-income single parents live competently on the edge of crisis, keeping the balls in the air, but acutely aware that some emergency need for increased funds, some break in the routine, can push a carefully organized but marginal system over the edge into chaos. Certainly, the basic tasks of everyday survival are likely to take a greater proportion of the single parents' waking energies than those of parents in two parent families. Many single parents complain that they rarely have periods of respite, and that there is no time in the day, week, or year that they are not performing chores or responsibilities, or worrying about them. They must manage their children, a household, a job, and at least a marginal social life without going under, and without the assistance of a partner to help with minor and major emergencies.

Going it alone, coping with the loss of a relationship, and enduring financial hardship are common tasks that leave single parents and their children more psychologically vulnerable (Acock & Demo, 1994; Arendell, 1986; Belle, 1990; Hall, Gurley, Sachs, & Kryscio, 1991; Hetherington, Cox, & Cox, 1978; Furstenberg & Cherlin, 1991; Kalter, 1990; Simons & Johnson, 1996; Shaw & Emery, 1987; Wallerstein & Blakeslee, 1989). Compared to their married counterparts, they work longer hours, face more stressful life changes, are more frequently depressed, and have more economic problems and less emotional support in performing their parental role (Burden, 1986; Compas & Williams, 1990; Gringlas & Weinraub, 1995; McLanahan & Sanderfur, 1994; McLoyd 1993; 1998; McLoyd & Wilson, 1991; Stack, 1989; Travato & Lauris, 1989; Tschann, Johnston, & Wallerstein, 1989). Single parents are also more physically vulnerable. A very large Scandinavian study of mostly urban single mothers demonstrated a 70% higher risk of premature death, a vulnerability that remained at a 24% higher rate even when the findings were adjusted for seocioeconomic status, number of children, previous severe medical and psychiatric history, and housing (Weitoft, Haglund, & Rosen, 2000). These at-risk families that live on a financial and social edge are seen most frequently by therapists, particularly in mental health centers of inner cities.

What is known about the well-being of children raised in single-parent families is complex, with considerable disagreement as to what impact there is and whether it is lasting (Allison & Furstenberg, 1989; Demo & Acock, 1988; Holloway & Machida, 1992; Hetherington 1999a, 1999b). Certainly, as a group, the children of single parents have more than their fair share of behavioral or emotional problems. They have lower academic performance, lower self-esteem, more acting out, and/or more difficulties with peers (Amato & Keith, 1991; Conger et al., 1992; Fursternberg, Brooks-Gunn, & Morgan, 1987; Gringlas & Weinraub, 1995; Hetherington, 1999b; McLanahan & Sandefur, 1994; Zill, 1990; Samuelsson, 1994; Simons, Lorenz, Conger, & Wu, 1992; Wallerstein, 1987). The conclusion often is that children who grow up in a household with only one biological parent are worse off, on average, than children who grow up in a household with two parents, regardless of the parents' race or educational background (McLanahan & Sandefur, 1994). Unfortunately, research documenting the specific tribulations of single parents and their children is flawed. Many studies are based on a cultural deficit model that fails to address individual differences among single parents, some of whom are successfully raising children. A sole focus on deficits gives a skewed view of single-parent families and does not help us to understand and/or maximize their resilience and strengths, or increase our understanding of the factors that make it possible for some parents to respond well to the unique problems and tasks of single parenthood (Brodsky, 1999; McLoyd, 1990; Spencer, 1990).

In addition, although considerable data show that single parents in comparison to their married counterparts are more likely to be depressed and to have children who are more likely to have social and emotional problems, many of these studies do not address the relative impact of poverty (Edin & Lein, 1997), whether there is a history of living in a dysfunctional or abusive nuclear family (Cherlin, Chase-Lansdale, & McRae, 1998; Demo & Acock, 1988; Hetherington & Stanley Hagan, 1995), the stage of adjustment to divorce (Ahrons & Miller, 1993; Hetherington, 1989), or the relative impact of having become a single-parent household by choice, divorce, or unwed and/or teen parenthood. Although divorce and living in a single-parent household can have a long-term impact that carries into adulthood (Chase-Lansdale, Cherlin, & Kiernan, 1995; Cherlin et al., 1998; Hetherington, 1999a, 1999b), there is also evidence that much of the negative impact of divorce on children does not necessarily hold in the long term, especially if children continue to be cared for by a supportive adult (Amato, 1993; Blechman, 1982; Elder, Conger, Foster, &

Ardelt, 1992; Friedman & Andrews, 1990; McLanahan & Booth, 1989). It is also difficult to draw conclusions about the well-being of all single-parent families without considering that many households are single in name only. A parent may be officially alone but actually reside with extended family, friends, or a long-term, intimate partner who is in some way involved in helping with household tasks or child rearing. In addition, many noncustodial parents are actively involved with their child and may provide the primary parent with financial and emotional support. These relationships, often invisible to researchers and clinicians, confound any conclusions about the impact of single parenting, father absence, mother aloneness (Kellam, Ensiminger, & Turner, 1977), or other vital aspects of family functioning and processes (Billingsley & Morrison-Rodriguez, 1998).

THE CIRCULAR INFLUENCE OF POVERTY, STRESSFUL LIFE EVENTS, AND PARENTAL FUNCTIONING: POVERTY IS BAD FOR PARENTAL AND CHILD MENTAL HEALTH

Although numerous studies show an association between financial strain, maternal psychological problems, child development, and family functioning (Belle, 1990; Conger et al., 1992; Downey & Coyne, 1990; Kessler & Neighbors, 1986; McLoyd, 1990), it is difficult to disentangle the relative stress of poverty, class, racial discrimination, parenting behavior, and child outcome. Poverty is perhaps the most overwhelming influence on single parents and their children and is crucial in interpreting studies of the needs and problems of single-parent households. In fact, studies suggest that it accounts for more of the variance in both child outcomes and parental functioning than single parenthood per se (Brooks-Gunn & Duncan, 1997; Chase-Lansdale & Brooks-Gunn, 1995; Duncan & Brooks-Gunn, 1997). Poverty is correlated with lower school achievement and a higher incidence of behavior problems, even when factors such as mother's age at the child's birth, family structure, and community disadvantage are taken into account. About 25% of children under age 6 live in poverty (Brooks-Gunn & Duncan, 1997; Hernandez, 1997), and many poor families have been dependent solely on rapidly evaporating welfare for support (Blank, 1997). It is often asserted that young, single African American mothers are less functional, but they are also disproportionately poor (Duncan, 1991; Wilson, 1987; 1996). They are also more likely to have become parents as teenagers and to be exposed to stressful life events that put them at increased risk for psychological distress (Belle, 1990; Kessler & Neighbors, 1986; McLoyd, 1990; McLanahan, 1983). Some have found that financial strain is associated with higher levels of depressive symptoms in parents, which directly and negatively influence the quality of their child rearing

(Eamon & Zuehl, 2001; Jackson, Brooks-Gunn, Huang, & Glassman, 2000). Others have found that depression is associated with diminished nurturance of children (Crinc & Greenberg, 1987; Downey & Coyne, 1990; McLoyd & Wilson, 1991). Thus, poor, single, frequently depressed mothers often must deal with higher rates of child problems while coping with the impact of poverty itself, a known influence on parental psychological functioning, child functioning, and family relationships (Duncan & Brooks-Gunn, 1997; Hope, Power, & Rodgers, 1999; Jackson et al., 2000).

Yet poverty is associated with many factors beyond single parenthood. Poor parents are more likely to have less education, fewer resources, less helpful support networks, and to live in more troubled communities (Hall et al., 1991; Simons, 1996), all factors that influence parental stress, disempowerment, satisfaction, and the development of children. Living in troubled communities, moreover, frequently requires that single parents be more vigilant about rules and supervision to ensure the safety of their children (Elder et al., 1992; Furstenberg, 1993; Garbarino & Kostelny, 1993). Poverty is destructive not only because of the lack of resources to meet basic needs, but also because parents have to tolerate external authorities and agencies intruding into their lives and judging their decisions; it means experiencing a lack of respect from schools, landlords, and community contacts, and having so few resources that parents accept poor treatment in relationships that they otherwise would reject.

One of the more malignant aspects of poverty may be its contribution to a mother's depression, self-esteem, independence, and the decisions she makes about staying or leaving abusive or neglectful relationships. Without the assurance that she can survive financially on her own, a woman is more likely gradually to lose her sense of self, to learn to tolerate abuse or neglect, and to become increasingly psychologically vulnerable. In turn, these maternal stresses can have an impact on family functioning, child-rearing practices, and children's development.

In summary, poverty is such a strong determinant of well-being that it accounts for about half of the disadvantage in children's lower achievement, and when its influence is factored out, the differences between the adjustment of children in one- and two-parent families all but disappear (Blechman, 1982; Duncan & Brooks-Gunn, 1997).

SPECIAL ISSUES IN LOW-INCOME
AND MINORITY SINGLE PARENTHOOD

Close to 75% of all single-parent families are minorities. Over 71% of all African American families are maintained by single parents, 65% of whom have never married (U.S. Bureau of the Census, 2001). In fact, African Americans have higher rates of teen parenthood and are less likely to marry, more likely to separate, and less likely to remarry (Cherlin, 1998a).

Poor women of any race who become single mothers as teenagers have a special set of problems and tasks. A teenager who has a child so that someone will love her is often shocked by the unrelenting and constricting aspects of child rearing. Because many of the children of teen parents are the product of relatively transient relationships, fathers are less likely to marry or to take responsibility for the child (Wilson, 1987).

Although low-income single-parents are likely to have more stress and a fragmented or chaotic household, even these parents and children can learn how to get their needs met within their networks. With support from extended family, both maternal well-being and parenting behaviors can be facilitated, providing more time and available energy to monitor children, more effective limit setting and nurturance, and more useful connections with community members and teachers on the behalf of children. The tradition of grandparents and other family members being willing to step in to help is a serious benefit that may provide the support and child care that allows these mothers to finish high school, work, and have a social life. Fortunately, consistent with "the tradition that has no name" (the acceptance of responsibility by the wider network maintained in African American communities), households frequently contain many other relatives, and beyond the household, active family networks provide frequent contact, social support, and mutual aid (Hatchett, Cochran, & Jackson, 1991). These provisions are often key to single-parent survival (Hatchett & Jackson, 1993; Jayakody & Chatters, 1997; Malson, 1986; McAdoo, 1980; Taylor, Jackson, & Quick, 1982; Thompson & Peebles-Wilkens, 1992). However, even with this tradition of rich connectedness, mothers who need the most support (those with the least income and education, and the most psychological difficulties) tend to have smaller networks and to receive less help from them (Caldwell, 1996; Hatchett & Jackson, 1993).

In addition, living in a household with three generations often provides the support teen mothers and children need, even though such households have their own set of strains, difficulties, and complicated relationship and generational boundary issues. The addition of a new generation to an existing family household requires fundamental changes in the way the whole family is structured and the way roles are defined, with an ongoing need to sort out child care tasks and adult responsibilities. The time when a teen naturally seeks more independence becomes a time when she needs increased support from her family to help with her child (Stolba & Amato, 1993); in some areas, she must defer authority, usually to her own mother (while taking charge of her child and maintaining her own credibility as the child's parent). At the same time, her parents must continue the life-cycle task of launching and letting go, which is more difficult if they must also provide continued financial and emotional support to a daughter they do not see as responsible (Hines et al., 1999).

Many families of teenage girls find it particularly difficult to support the ongoing involvement of the baby's father with their daughter, her baby, and their family life (Johnson, 2001). Some resent him and consider his participation to be either irrelevant or troublesome. Still, if they can support his involvement, they can help to create the important bond between father and child, and contribute to the psychological well-being of the adolescent mother (Thompson & Peebles-Wilkens, 1992) and the maintenance of family ties. Whether fathers remain involved with the child depends to a great extent on their own experience of being fathered, whether they have an ongoing relationship with the child's mother, and whether they have a history of drug use or other antisocial behavior (Florsheim, Moore, Zollinger, MacDonald, & Sumida, 1999; Furstenberg & Weiss, 2000). Research indicates that a main predictor for teen fatherhood involvement is employability (Wilson, 1987). Those young men who lacked education and job prospects due to racial discrimination and disadvantaged inner-city neighborhoods were less likely to take and sustain responsibility for the children they fathered, whereas those who had better job prospects and were able to support a family were more likely to do so (Wilson, 1987).

Facilitating the continued involvement of teen fathers deserves special attention, because it is so important and so difficult (Lehr & MacMillan, 2001). Since it is relatively easy for them to be ignored and to abandon contact with their child, it is important to reach out to them, to establish rapport and assist them in the process of becoming or continuing to be responsible parents (Kiselica, Stroud, & Rotzien, 1999; Lane & Clay, 2000). Some young fathers have reported that barriers to their ongoing involvement with their child include their relationship with the mother, her extended family, and the activities of agencies (Allen & Doherty, 1998).

Therapists can facilitate their ongoing contact with the child by helping both the mother and her family to see that it is in the best interests of the child. Whether or not the father continues to be involved, it is important to strengthen the child's network by minimizing the loss of extended family members and family friends, and increasing the involvement of community supports. Teachers, soccer coaches, Big Brothers, and activity group leaders can be considered possible network resources for children. Males in this wider network of adults can be recruited to provide contacts and activities to minimize the impact of the loss of those fathers who do not remain involved. Even if no single individuals are able to make a major or permanent commitment to the child, each can offer a portion of what is needed.

POSTDIVORCE SINGLE PARENTHOOD

The transition to single parenthood postdivorce is a particularly difficult time that requires single parents to address issues of loss, decreased financial viability, and changed relationships with friends and family, while also finding reasonable ways to support or at least tolerate the ongoing involvement of their child's noncustodial parent. Postdivorce, mothers in particular confront a serious decrease in income and suffer the strains of managing on limited funds. Whether or not a father assumes ongoing parental responsibility depends on such factors as age, education, employment, and financial status (Johnson, 2001). Although they know it is important, most divorced mothers report that the process of negotiating a workable relationship with an ex-spouse for the sake of their child is a considerable strain.

An adult single parent who returns to live with her family of origin after a divorce may be able to receive child care and financial help, but often at the cost of her independence. These once-autonomous mothers commonly find it frustrating when they become caught in conflicts with their own parents over how to manage their children, and they struggle to maintain a sense of themselves as competent adults in the face of increased parental involvement and control (Isaacs & Lean, 1987; Chase-Lansdale, Brooks-Gunn, & Zamsky, 1994). When intergenerational conflicts are minimized, these arrangements can provide enriching opportunities for all family members: Grandparents can have stronger connections with their grandchildren, single parents can have times of genuine respite, knowing that the children are being cared for by family members who love them, and children can have a variety of adult caretakers and sibling-like relationships with cousins. In fact, such expanded families can provide a sense of belonging that transcends what is provided by many intact, but more isolated, nuclear families.

Following divorce, children need supportive adults who function well enough to provide fairly consistent nurturance, values, and limits. These children are less likely to experience their families as either predictable or normal, but they can and do adjust to their circumstances. They are more likely to have irregular contact with their noncustodial parent and his or her network, to have parents who cannot agree on visitation arrangements, and to be at greater risk for mental health problems as adults (Cherlin et al., 1998). Therapists must assess the potential impact of these multiple factors on a given family and help family members to use their strengths and their network of family and friends to manage these problems. One of the major challenges facing single parents is the need to be two parents in one. Following a divorce, this entails reorganizing the family system, so that children can take on greater age-appropriate responsibilities while the custodial parent combines nurturing and disciplinary roles, and provides both financial and socioemotional support.

Clinicians often do not consider, however, that many noncustodial fathers are actively involved with their children or would prefer to be (Danzinger & Radin, 1990), which makes the term "single-parent family" (rather than single-parent household) a misnomer. When the noncustodial divorced parent, usually the father, has not remarried, and especially if there is shared custody, there may actually be two single-parent households to consider. This fact is often neglected in our focus on the family unit living together. Even in never-married families, there is evidence that fathers who are romantically involved with a child's mother, especially if the two are cohabiting, are involved with their child(ren), at least initially (Johnson, 2001). Unfortunately, father involvement decreases if this romantic relationship terminates (Arendell, 1996; Perkins & Davis, 1996), perhaps in part, because fathers appear to need the mothers of their children as mediators of their relationships with their children (Cherlin, 1998b), or because they have difficulty tolerating the mother's new romantic relationship(s).

For many postdivorce families, a single-parent household is a temporary state: Eventually a remarriage or a live-in partner enters the picture. This may or may not contribute to less stress for the single parent. It may mean more conflict over child-rearing practices, competition for parental time and energy. For mothers with the extra problem of an unrelated male adult in the home, who may be less tolerant of normal child behaviors or more seductive with daughters, the risk of child abuse might be an added source of concern. However, it also may provide intimacy and emotional support, help with both parental and household tasks, extra income to mitigate financial strain, and possible connections to an additional network.

SINGLE-PARENT FATHERS

Single-parent father households are a small but growing subgroup of one-parent families. Single-father families now make up 5% of all single-parent families, up from 1% in 1970 (U.S. Bureau of the Census, 2000). Fathers who have sole custody of their children have different ways of coping and are seen differently by their communities than single-parent mothers. These fathers are more likely to be employed and reasonably financially secure (Barber & Eccles, 1992). Compared to single mothers who are heads of households, they are less likely to be criticized, but are rather seen as noble. On the other hand, single mothers are also more likely to have an available network to provide psychological support; single fathers are more emotionally isolated. Fortunately, custodial fathers more readily draw on extended family members or girlfriends to provide practical support and child care, and noncustodial mothers are more likely to stay involved and carry parenting responsibilities. Still, single fathers have their own problems. Some complain of not having role models to normalize their experiences, of having to deal with traditional male socialization, which complicates nurturing and balancing work, family, and socializing (Greif, 1995a, 1995b, 1996). Others report not feeling welcome in some child care groups or school activities, or even report being regarded with suspicion as potential sexual predators by other parents, who resist allowing their children to play or have slumber parties in male-headed homes.

More frequently, therapists encounter single-parent fathers who have dual or partial custody as a result of a parental divorce. It is important to recognize that many of these men are caring fathers who would like to be seriously involved in the lives of their children, not necessarily the stereotyped "deadbeat dads," who don't want contact with their children (Johnson, 2001). Their financial support and physical contact with their children may have diminished over the process of a bitter divorce, which may in turn cause mothers to withhold child contact or influence children to reject their fathers out of loyalty to their mothers. This, of course, can become a vicious cycle of each parent withholding what the other needs. Furthermore, ambivalence about contact with children often contributes to a lack of follow-through with promised plans and visits, stirring children's feelings of abandonment and anger at their noncustodial parent's lack of reliability. This anger is often taken out on custodial mothers, who may act from a desire to protect their child from repeated disappointments.

Invisible or unavailable fathers may well desire more contact and be willing to take on more responsibility for the sake of their children, but often fathers who could be helped to become more involved are ignored by therapists, and overstressed and ambivalent mothers may find it impossible to address the task of increasing father involvement. Noncustodial fathers should be contacted to assess their current and potential contributions to their children's emotional and financial support (Amato & Gilbreth, 1999). By recognizing that parents, as well as children, may be caught in a vicious cycle reinforcing the cutoff, therapists can avoid placing blame and can work to help each individual move toward creating a better relationship. Custodial mothers can be helped to appreciate that an involved father is a benefit to the whole family, and likely includes financial support for the children.

Still, father involvement in the child's network is important enough to invest time and energy to find ways not only to maintain it but also to ensure its substance. If the father has not remarried, he too is a single parent, perhaps with less daily responsibility, but with significant single-parenting tasks of his own. If he has remarried, he may need help in balancing the needs of his children and his new family. The most common problems are losing contact, or maintaining contacts that are not just brief, unnatural play dates. Single-parent fathers may need help in behaving as a parent not a friend (Arendell, 1986; Furstenberg & Nord, 1985; Simons & Beaman, 1996; Whitbeck, Simons, & Kao, 1994). It is clear that children tend to do better if their father continues to actually participate as a father (Simons, Whitbeck, Beaman, & Conger, 1994), but little evidence shows that father visitation per se has any impact at all (Amato, 1993; Emery, 1988; Furstenberg & Cherlin, 1991; Simons & Beaman,

1996). The bottom line is that children do better when both parents are active participants in their lives. Therefore, both parents should be helped to cooperate with regard to the best interests of their child (Ahrons, 1994; Lamb et al., 1997). Divorced single parents who can each maintain an active parenting role, without becoming overly combative with each other, provide children with the possibility of two loving homes and themselves with welcome periods of respite.

INFLUENCES CONTRIBUTING TO SUCCESS
IN SINGLE-PARENT HOUSEHOLDS

The single most important factor contributing to successful single-parent households is adequate income to meet the needs of parent, child, and household. Beyond this basic and overriding issue, several factors amenable to therapeutic intervention also contribute to the success of single-parent households, especially adequate attention to parental social and psychological needs, maternal employment, a strong and predictable family structure, strong networks, and the positive involvement of the noncustodial parent with the child. Maternal well-being increases the ability to raise children successfully in single-parent households. Mothers who are stressed, depressed, and overwhelmed are less able to provide the nurturance and structure children need, so attention to the needs of single parents is crucial. Good self-esteem contributes to good parenting; it is a serious problem that many women and men become single parents without much self-confidence or self-esteem. Some got involved with their partners because they had little esteem; others lost their sense of self in a neglectful or abusive relationship, and still others have never lived long enough on their own to develop an independent sense of self-worth. Although employment and social or family obligation can take away time that mothers might otherwise have spent with their children, recent studies find that the resultant increase in self-esteem and decrease in depressive symptomatology contribute to improved parenting (Jackson & Huang, 2000).

Employment contributes significantly not only to available household resources but also to maternal self-esteem, a key factor in the ability of single parents to accomplish the tasks that face them (Holloway & Machida, 1992). There is evidence that it improves to the well-being of both single mothers and their children (Jackson & Huang, 2000; Jackson, Gyamfi, Brooks-Gunn, & Blake, 1998), perhaps in part because it contributes to the maintenance of family structure and offers mothers some respite from constant child care. Employed mothers who are able to obtain more resources for their families and have more satisfying networks are less punitive with their children (McLoyd, 1990). Also, children of employed mothers have better developmental outcomes than low-income, unemployed mothers (Desai, Chase-Lansdale, & Michael, 1989; Vandell & Ramanan, 1992).

A strong family organization with clear generational boundaries creates a more predictable environment. Also, at least for sons (who appear more vulnerable to the impact of marital dissolution), the maintenance of family routines appears buffer stress and contribute to a sense of control and security in the family (Jackson, 1998; Jackson & Huang, 2000; Morrison & Cherlin, 1995). The predictability provided by routines and limits appears to contribute to better family functioning, more optimal child outcomes, and better functioning during a crisis. Because there is a natural tendency for depressed or overwhelmed parents to neglect routine household maintenance, single parents may need support to keep alive family rituals, such as holidays and birthday celebrations. Daily routines, such as dinner together or age-appropriate bedtimes for children, are especially important to sustain. Often, an exhausted parent has difficulty getting children to bed; in turn, children become overtired and are likely to become emotionally overloaded, increasing the likelihood of concentration difficulties in school. Family therapists, rather than overburdening a mother, can draw on older children to assist more with daily chores and bedtime routines. Also, these routine activities, such as bedtimes, can become an opportunity for close, quiet time together. Such small structural family therapy interventions can bring a measure of order and relief to a disorganized family system.

Support networks are also crucial for the maintenance of successful single-parent households. Single-parent families are profoundly influenced by the social context in which they spend their lives, whether this is a supportive network of biological and legal family members, chosen family and friends, or an isolated existence in a judgmental community. Single-parent families embedded in a fabric of social and instrumental support are less vulnerable than those without such support (Belsky, 1984; Edin & Lein, 1997; Gladov & Ray, 1986; Koeske & Koeske, 1990; Malson, 1986; McLoyd, Jayarantne, Ceballo, & Borquez, 1994; Taylor, Chatters, & Jackson, 1997). Many single-parent families are well connected outside the home, have support from a nonresident parent (Amato & Gilbreth, 1999), contain other adult family members within the household, or have a live-in significant partner (Simons, 1996). Supportive live-in relatives or partners are important, because single-parent mothers who live independently often suffer greater financial and child care strains, and sometimes greater social isolation. Also, psychoeducational and support groups help single parents find emotional and social resources away from or in the absence of family networks.

CLINICAL IMPLICATIONS/INTERVENTIONS

In working with single-parent families, it is important to maintain a respectful stance, and a strengths- and resilience-based approach, while remaining alert to the common challenges family members face and the symptoms of distress they are likely to exhibit. Therapists should keep in mind the following themes: that single parent families are a diverse group; that they are likely coping with experiences of loss and overwhelmed with practical management tasks that leave them running on empty; that they are likely to have diminished income or financial hardship and to be struggling with issues of self-esteem; that they have problems in maintaining consistency and authority without support; and that they may be at risk of neglecting their own needs. It is crucial to understand the challenges and problems they face, without wavering from a recognition and appreciation of their strengths. Suggestions for practical management strategies are helpful, but more importantly, the needs of single parents must be appreciated while they are being encouraged to find their own solutions. If parents' needs are not met, they are more likely to become both overwhelmed and depressed, and less patient and more punitive in parenting (McLoyd, 1990; McLoyd et al., 1994). These parents need support in limit setting, child management, and attending to their own needs; assistance in negotiating workable and cooperative relationships with the children's father and members of the extended family; and help with time management.

Because parents often put their own needs last, the most difficult therapeutic task of all is to help parents recognize the need for self-nurturance, in order to be able to cope over the long haul. When single parents maintain that the needs of their children come first, they sometimes need to hear that what their children need most is a parent who is not overstressed. Therapists also are urged to take a longitudinal perspective that emphasizes the capabilities of parents and children for resilience and adaptation. Using this perspective, therapists can help single parents to decrease risks and overcome the immediate challenges they face, by affirming their ability to parent their children, and by helping them to mobilize supportive aspects of their community.

The most crucial mistake therapists of any theoretical model can make is implicitly to blame single parents for their children's problems. These "therapeutic" behaviors are all the more problematic given that single-parent families are most likely to come for help at three very sensitive points in time: immediately after a divorce, when the family is working to manage reactions to loss and to create a new structure (Kissman & Allen, 1993); when parent coping has been compromised by depression or overwork (Betchen, 1992); and, most frequently, when children encounter academic and behavioral difficulties (Westcot & Dries, 1990). To engage single parents at these times, the therapist should pay special attention to their experiences on the journey to single-parent status and acknowledge their current efforts to succeed at raising children without the sanction of a marriage or in the face of a marriage, that was not viable. This acknowledgment and recognition lays the groundwork for an approach to working with single-parent families that emphasizes their social context, structure, and longitudinal development.

Engaging Single-Parent Families

It is crucial to spend time connecting with the single parent. Not surprisingly, there is evidence that attention to parental needs, even when the presenting complaint is focused entirely on the child, improves engagement and outcome (Prinz & Miller, 1994). Given what we know about single parents' history and current reality, it would seem obvious and inevitable that therapists address parents' well-being as a major target of assessment and intervention. This is the case. In part, this may be the result of society's view of a normal family as a two-parent unit, and its stigmatization of single-parent households as "broken" and "fatherless." Additionally, the field of mental health tends to blame mothers and to focus on their deficiencies when their children have difficulties, believing that mothers should meet needs, not have them. It may also be, however, that parents frequently do not seek or accept help for themselves (Dover, Leahy, & Foreman, 1994). It is important to emphasize that the significance of maternal well-being is not raised here to again blame mothers, but to emphasize the importance of addressing their needs. In the context of busy schedules and task overload, these mothers may view therapy as just one more time consuming burden (Kazdin, 2000). They may believe that they would not be so stressed if only their children were better behaved, and fear that they will lose their children if they acknowledge problems. However, like a perverse game of dominos, a mother's coping influences her child's adjustment, and if a mother's needs are not addressed, there is a negative impact on her child's mental health and response to therapy (Brent et al., 1997; Dover et al., 1994; Hall et al., 1991; Holloway & Machida, 1992; Shear, Anderson, & Greeno, 1997). Although there are no data on this issue for single fathers, it seems logical that the pattern would be the same.

Effective management of immediate challenges will helps to increase the self-esteem of parents and children, so that they gain the skills and courage to reach out to extended family and friends, and build bridges of competence to the future. It is a challenge for many therapists to work positively and effectively with single-parent families, because societal views are reinforced by the pervasive focus on pathology in clinical training. The presence of problems in single-parent families is not necessarily evidence of individual inadequacies, moral weaknesses, or intrapsychic turmoil. There are very real individual problems within many of these families, and our caseloads contain a disproportionate number of single parents requesting help. But these parents and children also have strengths and resilience, both of which must be appreciated and acknowledged before we can see their lives in perspective and help them address the challenges they face, whatever the causes.

Recognizing and Mobilizing Strengths

A primary focus on the strengths and potential of single parents that make survival and adjustment possible supports them in their efforts to be responsible and loving with their children (Walsh, 1998). All single-parent families have strengths that can be mobilized to solve the problems of family members. If conducted in the context of recognizing single-parent strengths and resources, therapy can help to increase parental confidence and empower parents, normalizing the struggles of single parenthood as predictable stresses rather than personal failures. An emphasis on parental competence, along with problems that the parent can control and change, is a good place to start. Helping single parents to see their experience through a cultural and developmental lens lays the groundwork for helping them cope more effectively (Holloway & Machida, 1992). From the perspective of an increased awareness that all single parents have similar challenges, that all suffer from a deficit of societal support, and that there are even benefits to single parenthood, these parents are likely to feel less alone (Arditti & Madden-Derlich, 1995). Such information can be woven into discussions with single parents about their history and current circumstances, thereby helping them to become anthropologists of their own system (Black, 1996; 2000), and providing the distance from daily struggles that can help generate specific strategies to combat parental or child vulnerabilities.

Although a consistent effort should be made to help single parents recognize their competencies, it is important to acknowledge the burdens they carry. Sometimes, out of eagerness to be supportive to parents and to avoid pathologizing them, well-intentioned friends and professionals imply that there is nothing the parents can't handle. Unfortunately, this message can close down topics about which the mother wants to talk, areas about which she does not feel good, competent, or wise. For instance, one mother described not wanting to see a therapist because she felt the pressure to be "constantly wonderful." Thus, in attempting to affirm a single parent's strengths, it is important to include some discussion of her problems, so that she does not feel dismissed or patronized. Only after listening to a parent's story should the therapist make an effort to affirm the resilience and courage he or she generates on a daily basis in the face of those challenges (Walsh, 1998).

Too frequently, women internalize the societal message that satisfaction and fulfillment require a marital partner. At the same time, living with and raising children alone can be lonely and overwhelming. Only after parents really believe that the therapist understands the difficulties of "going it alone" should they be reminded that they can be happy and fulfilled, even without a spouse, and feel proud of their accomplishments in raising their children. Discussion of the risks, and especially the benefits, of single parenthood can help parents to see that many of the things they are being forced to learn will in time become valued strengths. Benefits include the increased closeness that occurs between single parents and their children; the accelerated growth and development of children who function in helping roles; the early acquisition of independence and a wide range of survival skills, including the ability to cope with loss and adapt to change; and the increased appreciation of the need for connections with people, resulting in links to a rich, diverse, and flexible network of friends, neighbors, extended family, and religious groups. The effective coping of children also should be affirmed, because many of them come to grips with issues that would challenge many adults, and they make important contributions to the family's well-being.

Mobilizing strengths often requires that therapists address the issue of the single parent's sense of self-worth. For very young single mothers, increasing self-esteem may require practical help in discovering who they are, in caring for their child, in managing their ambivalence about the loss of their teenage freedoms, without neglecting their responsibilities, becoming resentful, or feeling bad about themselves. For newly divorced single mothers, increasing self-esteem sometimes involves helping them to feel less responsible for the failure of their marriage, helping them to see they can survive outside the bounds of the social and financial structure provided by a marriage, and cultivating in them a view of themselves as capable of "flying solo" or reconnecting, if they so desire (Anderson & Stewart, 1994). Therapists can help to increase the self-esteem of those women who tend to be self-sacrificing by helping them to avoid neglecting their own needs. They must be encouraged to focus a little of their energies on nurturing themselves, even when their initiative is low, if not for their own good, then for the good of their children. For example, it is important to validate the need to set reasonable boundaries on child care demands. Appropriate bedtimes for children, delegation of child care responsibilities to older children for short periods of time, or alternation of child care responsibilities with a sibling or friend benefits mothers by giving them quiet time for themselves. Structuring weekly time alone and setting up clear boundaries provide respite and decrease the all-or-none dilemma of escape fantasies.

If parents suffer from depression, low self-esteem, or simply task overload, it certainly isn't their fault, and the demoralizing impact of these forces must be countered to enable single parents to provide for the needs of their children. Therapists can facilitate this process by working with the parent to create webs of support, affirming strengths and reinforcing the parent's role as family executive. Particular care must be taken by therapists to avoid exacerbating any parental sense of deficiency by falling into the trap of trying to ingratiate themselves with children at parental expense, getting caught in a triangle between the parent and child, or even between the parent and the family of origin. In addition, whereas improving family structure and generational boundaries can be helpful, care must be taken to avoid setting up charts and token economies that require an unrealistic amount of monitoring that overtaxes already overburdened parental resources.

Reinforcing Structure, Routines, and Parental Authority

Forming a new family, or reorganizing from a two-parent family, requires that the single parent gain credibility and assume power as the primary executor of the family system. This task may be particularly difficult for parents who have never lived independently, who have tended to rely on their spouses to provide discipline or nurturance, and/or who are temporarily immobilized by depression or loss. Because this new family structure must be created at a time of high stress, when the new single parent may feel least prepared, a significant amount of support may be necessary.

The central challenges for teen mothers are learning to take responsibility consistently and enforce rules that protect their children in disadvantaged communities. This is complicated by the unpredictable stresses in their own lives. When it isn't clear who is in charge in multigenerational homes (e.g., the teen or her parents), children can become confused or learn to play one adult against another to get what they want. A common problem for many divorced parents is too great a tolerance for a child's negative behaviors and a tendency to become overly permissive in attempts to make up for the losses and damage they think their children have suffered because of the divorce or lack of father involvment. Because some data suggest that low income and fewer resources are associated with an increase in maternal violence (Margolin, 1992), it is also crucial to draw the line carefully between the need for firm limits and overly punitive parental reaction.

All children, especially distressed children who have experienced traumatic life transitions, need the security of structure, predictability, and stability. Clear boundaries and limits, key elements in maintaining family structure, are also important for maintaining parental sanity. At the most basic level, it is important to define who is in and who is out of the family, who comes to sessions, and who has the right to make household rules. For single mothers living in the homes of their own parents, or for women who have men living with them for relatively short periods of time, these roles and boundaries shift and are often unclear. Helping the single parent to negotiate issues of power, rules, and responsibilities with her parents, lover, and children is sometimes the most important task of therapy, because it lays the groundwork to help everyone live together.

When overwhelmed, single parents sometimes lose the ability to set effective limits, unless a crisis is in progress. They frequently find themselves exhausted by unproductive standoffs with their children (Hetherington & Clingempeel, 1992; Herz, 1988; Morawetz & Walker, 1984) that leave them angry, discouraged, and exhausted. One way to avoid negative family interaction is to help parents work out a more equitable division of labor that provides them with help and respite. Therapists can help by sorting out tasks that a parent can reasonably delegate to children, depending on their age and family circumstances. The mother's ability to be in charge of her family can be complicated by her need for older children to take some responsibility for younger siblings and household chores. These chores should be clearly delegated, not abdicated, by a parent clearly in charge of the household. Also, it is important that therapists help families to avoid labeling children with titles such as "man of the house," which implies that a son has taken his father's place.

In some families, mothers allow children to have so much authority that their own is compromised. Therapists can help mothers to retain their status as the ultimate authority and keep a direct line to each child even as they delegate more than the usual number of responsibilities to their older children. Mothers who worry that increased responsibility may do damage to their older children can be reassured that this will not be the case, unless the child is totally deprived of a childhood. When a mother has problems establishing herself as the family executive, therapists can repeatedly reinforce her authority in front of her children and serve as a model by limiting children effectively in the sessions. The therapist can also help a parent to involve extended family members and the other adults in her life to support her efforts.

Establishing predictability in family life is not just a matter of creating rules and setting limits. Family stability and parental authority also can be reinforced by maintaining family routines and rituals that contribute to the comfort of predictability. Some single parents become so overwhelmed with day-to-day survival issues that they neglect the need for routines and rituals, forgetting the comfort and sense of continuity they provide. In fact, after a death, or a divorce, some families avoid even the most basic rituals, such as regular family dinners, not to mention Sunday outings, birthday parties, or other holiday celebrations. Some parents admit to feeling that rituals are not relevant, because there is no longer a "real" family. It is essential that therapists explore and challenge views that single-parent families are abnormal or deficient based on societal norms that reify the intact family. Reestablishing rituals and routines can reassure children by reinforcing the feeling that theirs is a normal family.

Dealing with Live-In Partners

One common "solution" mothers choose for these problems, in part out of fear of being alone, is to bring a romantic partner into their household, even when they are less than certain he is an appropriate choice. In effect, they "barter" with him to provide for some of their financial, sexual, or psychological needs in a quid pro quo arrangement, with or without real companionship or commitment. Researchers have noted that the support of a confidant, usually a boyfriend, protects adult women from depression in the face of stressful life events (Brown & Moran, 1997). Under the best of circumstances, these limited relationships can meet some important needs and even develop into supportive and lasting ties.

The contributions of some live-in partners are not always positive. Many compete with the children for the single parent's time and attention, undermine maternal authority and rule setting, or get intensely involved with both parent and child, only to leave precipitously. Additionally, men who do not have a biological/genetic bond to a child are more likely to be physically and sexually abusive (Margolin, 1992). Single mothers who are psychologically or financially insecure often find themselves struggling with conflicting loyalties to their children and to their partner. They also find it difficult to establish the boundaries necessary to protect their children from these partners for fear of being left without the support they desperately need. These women many be in the greatest need of help to expand their adult support network.

Complicated negotiations may be needed when live-in boyfriends who espouse traditional gender norms expect to establish family rules when they have neither the mandate nor the credibility to make them, and when they contribute little practical or financial help. Their attempts to wield authority are frequently rebuffed, especially by adolescents. Negotiating stylistic differences in authority between mothers and boyfriends creates tensions of its own. Because some single mothers have trouble standing up for their rights, or even knowing that it is appropriate to do so, therapists can help by making it clear to male partners that their role is not that of parent, but that of a support and backup for the mother in her efforts to care for and discipline her children.

Building on Natural Connections

Because the context of single-parent households is so vital, assessment of the number and quality of supports available to single parents forms one of the cornerstones of treatment. An assessment of existing and potential kin and social networks lays the groundwork for beginning to broaden parents' sense of connectedness. It is essential to determine the quality of these contacts, because stress-laden social networks can be associated with increased conflict, maternal depression, and parenting problems (Olson, Kieschnick, Banyard, & Ceballo, 1994; Richardson, Barbour, & Bubenzer, 1991). Single mothers who do have intense and frequent contact with their family, for instance, report mixed blessings. Extended family members may be the source of increased stress through their disapproval of maternal behavior, alignments with children, split loyalties after divorce, need for elder care, or requests for help for a variety of other family troubles (Dakof & Taylor, 1990). Family therapy may be helpful in reconciling conflictual or estranged relationships and interrupting destructive triangles. In families with serious dysfunction or abuse, therapy may be more helpful in building extrafamilial resources.

For instance, one young mother who worked hard to support her 9-month-old daughter in a community day care preferred to turn to her "family" of friends rather than her crack-addicted sister and alcoholic mother, who both asked for money and criticized her for neglecting her child by taking a job instead of seeking public assistance. In such extreme cases, friendship networks are lifelines to be cultivated.

Therapist can help to alleviate problems in single-parent households by facilitating a web of support beyond the household. This includes encouraging a range of positive connections for both the parent and child, including an interrelated archipelago of individuals and groups that provide a context of reciprocal support and mutual responsibility. Network interventions should be planned with a wide-angle lens, addressing the needs of each family member for both a sense of belonging and concrete assistance. Therapists can help single parents begin to mobilize their networks by first attending to others living in the home. Next, they should attend to close family and friends outside the home who are actively involved in important aspects of family life, and those network members who might be available, if asked. Finally, therapists should help single parents to build new connections for companionship, as well as support. Once it is determined which friends and members of the extended family might be available, moves can be made to facilitate connections, and, if necessary, plan interventions to decrease tensions in stressful relationships.

In postdivorce single parent families, predivorce networks sometimes assume that the single parent would be uncomfortable in gatherings of couples or intact families, while others may be uneasy about seeming to choose one partner's side over the other in the divorce. Recently divorced single mothers may also be seen as a threat to intact marriages. Thus, friends they had when they were married may no longer be available, unless they work to keep these contacts. It is possible, with effort, to sort out, maintain, and strengthen most of these ties, but single mothers may need to be strongly encouraged to tolerate the risk of rejection or the discomfort of going alone to social gatherings. Helping single parents to redefine relationships with their families of origin may be especially important for those who have difficulty accepting or understanding a divorce or a choice to become a single parent. For some, it is important to explore religious or cultural taboos against divorce or single parenthood.

However, there are times when a single parent's network cannot provide the right kind of help or support: Ties may have been weakened or disrupted by divorce or relocation; existing network members may be insensitive to the problems of single parents and their children; those single parents who need them most may not have the skills to develop and maintain helpful relationships; and many single parents find it exceedingly difficult to ask available extended family or friends to pitch in with practical, financial, or emotional support. Their pride, fear of becoming a burden, fear of rejection, or even fear of loss of custody, make it hard to ask for help. Developing new strands of support can also seem like just one more chore to an overextended, overstressed single parent. Many single parents would rather collapse on the couch after a trying day than take the initiative to connect, especially with people they don't know well. Therapists need to be empathetic with the challenges, without sinking in the parent's sense of hopelessness and helplessness. It takes encouragement and coaching to get network development off the ground.

In addition, other sources of social support in the community can be tapped: established community groups, religious congregations, and workplace contacts. For a single parent, connections with groups such as "Mother's Day Out," craft classes, church groups, and so on, can help her to develop new relationships and meet some of her needs for activities and respite. If single parents can join the workplace, they not only increase their support network, they also become self-sufficient, develop improved self-esteem, and experience positive fallout in their children's behavior (Hofferth, Smith, McLoyd, & Finkelstein, 2000). To address the particular need for relationships with people in similar circumstances, parents can be encourages to join or form groups for single parents. Such groups are inherently supportive, providing mothers with the opportunity for activities and discussions that can make them feel less isolated and stigmatized. In addition, they can provide opportunities for maternal respite through trade-off of child care responsibilities, transportation to children's activities, or information about community resources.

Children's networks also require attention. Only children may need a variety of connections to balance the intensity of the single-parent–child relationship, and siblings competing for limited parental resources may need other adults to fill the gaps in what any one parent, however competent, cannot provide. Even though we now know that divorce also has positive effects (Arditti & Madden-Derlich, 1995; Barber & Eccles, 1992; Waite & Berryman, 1986), the loss of contact with a father and his network causes pain and has serious network ramifications (Amato & Keith, 1991; Furstenberg et al., 1987; Gringlas & Weinraub, 1995; Hetherington et al., 1978; Zill, 1990). It has been suggested that as much as 70% of the social network may be disrupted in a divorce, so, for children, the loss experienced extends beyond the lost parent (Hetherington et al., 1978). If possible, therapists should work to involve the father as an ongoing part of the child's network. If the relationship with an ex-spouse is conflictual or the risk of abuse precludes contact with the children, continued involvement with the child's grandparents, aunts, uncles, and cousins may still be possible.

DISCUSSION AND CONCLUSIONS

Given that parenting is one of the most difficult life tasks even with two parents working together, it's easy to understand the difficulties of single parents attempting to maintain healthy families, raise their children, and have a satisfying adult life for themselves in the context of unsupportive communities. Four guidelines can help to keep the work with single-parent families on the right track.

1. Remember that the family unit is not only those who live in a household but can also include a noncustodial parent and extended family members. Expand your view of family resources beyond a myopic view of the system, even if that view is currently accepted by the parent.

2. For some, becoming a single parent is traumatic; for others, it is a blessing. It is important to listen to the perceptions of the single parent in order to intervene effectively and help with the tasks or problems of greatest concern.

3. Ongoing relationships with a noncustodial parent can be stressful to the custodial parent. With some work, however, they can also be managed and of help to the child and, ultimately, useful in providing more financial support and respite for the primary parent.

4. Single parents have an overload of child care and household chores, limited time and energy for their own interests, and, frequently, insufficient money to cover their own basic needs and those of their children. Single mothers in particular tend to neglect their own needs, even when this is called to their attention. Some feel that the only legitimate reason to take care of themselves is that it is important for their child(ren). This is often an effective way to present the issue to mothers who defer to the needs of everyone else at their own expense.

5. Finally, symptoms in single-parent families may be less the result of personal inadequacy than of social stigma and the inadequacy of the service systems that should be supporting them. Society's failure to provide single-parent families with a financial, social, or psychological safety net not only contributes to their distress but also requires that each individually address and conquer problems that could be better addressed collectively. What they need from society and from therapists is understanding, support, and help in mobilizing their strengths and networks to create and

manage a workable life in the face of multiple competing and complex challenges.

REFERENCES

Acock, A. C., & Demo, D. H. (1994). *Family diversity and well-being.* Thousand Oaks, CA: Sage.

Ahrons, C. (1994). *The good divorce: Keeping your family together when your marriage comes apart.* New York: HarperCollins.

Ahrons, C. R., & Miller, R. B. (1993). The effect of the post divorce relationship on paternal involvement: A longitudinal analysis. *American Journal of Orthopsychiatry, 63*(3), 441–450.

Allen, W. D., & Doherty, W. J. (1998) "Being there": The perception of fatherhood among a group of African American adolescent fathers. In H. I. McCubbin, E. A. Thompson, A. I. Thompson, & J. E. Fromer (Eds.), *Resiliency in African American families* (Vol. 3, pp. 207–244). Thousand Oaks, CA: Sage.

Allison, P. D., & Furstenberg, F. F. (1989). How marital dissolution affects children: Variations by age and sex. *Developmental Psychology, 25,* 540–549.

Amato, P. R. (1993). Children's adjustment to divorce: Theories, hypotheses, and empirical support. *Journal of Marriage and the Family, 55,* 23–38.

Amato, P. R., & Gilbreth, J. G. (1999). Nonresident fathers and children's well-being: A meta-analysis. *Journal of Marriage and the Family, 61,* 557–573

Amato, P. R., & Keith, B. (1991). Parental divorce and the well-being of children: A meta-analysis. *Psychological Bulletin, 110,* 26–46.

Anderson, C. M., Stewart, S., & Dimidjian, S. (1994). *Flying Solo: Single Women in Midlife.* New York: Norton.

Arditti, J. A., & Madden-Derdich, D. (1995). No regrets: Custodial mothers' accounts of the difficulties and benefits of divorce. *Contemporary Family Therapy, 17*(2), 229–248.

Arendell, T. (1986). *Mothers and divorce: Legal, economic, and social dilemmas.* Berkeley: University of California Press.

Arendell, T. (1996). *Co-parenting: A review of the literature.* Commissioned paper for the National Center on Fathers and Families. Philadelphia: University of Pennsylvania Press.

Barber, B. L., & Eccles, J. S. (1992). Long-term influence of divorce and single parenting on adolescent family- and work-related values, behaviors, and aspirations. *Psychological Bulletin, 111*(1), 108–126.

Belle, D. (1990). Poverty and women's mental health. *American Psychologist, 45,* 385–387.

Belsky, J. (1984). The determinants of parenting: A process model. *Child Development, 55,* 83–96.

Betchen, S. J. (1992). Short-term psychodynamic therapy with a divorced single mother. *Family in Society, 73*(2), 116–121.

Billingsley, A., & Morrison-Rodriguez, B. (1999). The black family in the 21st century and the church as an action system: A macro perspective. In L. A. See (Ed.), *Human behavior in the social environment from an African American perspective* (pp. 31–47). Binghamton, NY: Haworth Press.

Black, L. (1996). Families of African origin: An overview. In M. McGoldrick, J. Giordano, et al. (Eds.), *Ethnicity and family therapy* (2nd ed., pp. 57–65). New York: Guilford Press.

Black, L. (2000). Therapy with African American couples. In P. Papp (Ed.), *Couples on the fault line: New directions for therapists* (pp. 205–221). New York: Guilford Press.

Blank, R. M. (1997). *It takes a nation: A new agenda for fighting poverty.* Princeton, NJ: Princeton University Press.

Blechman, E. (1982). Are children with one parent at psychological risk?: A methodological review. *Journal of Marriage and the Family, 44,* 179–198.

Brent, D. A., Holder, D., Kolko, D., Birmaher, B., Baugher, M., Roth, C., Iyengas, S., & Johnson, B. A. (1997). A clinical trial for adolescent depression comparing cognitive, family and supportive psychotherapy. *Archives of General Psychiatry, 54*(9), 877–855.

Brodsky, A. E. (1999). Making it: The components and process of resistance among urban African American single mothers. *American Journal of Orthopsychiatry, 69*(2), 148–160.

Brooks-Gunn, J. (1990). Identifying the vulnerable young child. In D. E. Rogers & E. Ginzberg (Eds.), *Improving the life chances of children at risk* (pp. 15–35). Boulder, CO: Westview Press.

Brooks-Gunn, J., & Duncan, G. (1997). The effects of poverty on children and youth. *The Future of Children, 7,* 55–71.

Brown, G. W., & Moran, P. M. (1997). Single mothers, poverty, and psychiatric status. *Psychological Medicine, 27,* 21–33.

Burden, D. S. (1986). Single parents and the work setting: The impact of multiple job and homelife responsibilities [Special issue]. *Family Relations, 35,* 37–43.

Caldwell, C. H. (1996). Predisposing, enabling and need factors related to patterns of help-seeking among African American women. In H. W. Neighbors & J. S. Jackson (Eds.), *Mental health in Black America* (pp. 146–160). Thousand Oaks, CA: Sage.

Chase-Lansdale, P. L., & Brooks-Gunn, J. (1995). *Escape from poverty: What makes a difference?* New York: Cambridge University Press.

Chase-Lansdale, P. L., Brooks-Gunn, J., & Zamsky, E. S. (1994). Young African-American multigenerational families in poverty: The quality of mothering and grandmothering. *Child Development, 65,* 373–393.

Chase-Lansdale, P. L., Cherlin, A. J., & Kiernan, K. K. (1995). The long term effects of parental divorce on the mental health of young adults: A developmental perspective. *Child Development, 66*(6), 1614–1634.

Chatters, L. M., Taylor, R. J., & Jayakody, R. (1994). Fictive kinship relations in black extended families. *Journal of Comparative Family Studies, 25*(3), 297–312.

Cherlin, A. J. (1998a). Marriage and marital dissolution among black Americans, *Journal of Comparative Family Studies, 29*(1), 147–158.

Cherlin, A. J. (1998b). On the flexibility of fatherhood. In A. Booth & A. C. Crouter (Eds.), *Men in families: When do they get involved? What difference does it make?* (pp. 41–46). Mahwah NJ: Erlbaum.

Cherlin, A. J., Chase-Lansdale, L. P., & McRae, C. (1998). Effects of parental divorce on mental health throughout the life cycle. *American Sociological Review, 63*(2), 239–249.

Compas, B. E., & Williams, R. A. (1990). Stress, coping, and adjustment in mothers and young adolescents in single and two-parent families. *American Journal of Community Psychology, 18,* 525–545.

Conger, R. D., Conger, K. J., Elder, G. H., Jr., Lorenz, F. O., Simons, R. L., & Whitbeck, L. B. (1992). A family process model of economic hardship and adjustment of early adolescent boys. *Child Development, 63,* 526–541.

Crinc, K., & Greenberg, M. (1987). Maternal stress, social support, and coping: Influences on early mother–child relationship. In C. Boukydis (Ed.), *Research on support for parents and infants in the postnatal period* (pp. 25–40). Norwood, NJ: Ablex.

Dakof, G. A., & Taylor, S. E. (1990). Victim's perceptions of social support: What is helpful from whom. *Journal of Personality and Social Psychology, 58,* 80–89.

Danzinger, S., & Radin, N. (1990). Absent does not equal uninvolved: Predictors of fathering in teen mother families. *Journal of Marriage and the Family, 52,* 636–642.

Demo, D. H., & Acock, A. C. (1988). The impact of divorce on children. *Journal of Marriage and the Family, 50,* 619–648.

Desai, S., Chase-Lansdale, P. L., & Michael, R. T. (1989). Mother or market?: Effects of maternal employment on the intellectual ability of four-year-old children. *Demography, 26,* 545–561.

Dover, S. J., Leahy, A., & Foreman, D. (1994). Parental psychiatric disorder: Clinical prevalence and effects on default from treatment. *Child Care, Health and Development, 20*(3), 137–143.

Downey, G., & Coyne, J. (1990). Children of depressed parents: An integrative review. *Psychological Bulletin, 108,* 50–76.

Duncan, G. J. (1991). The economic environment of children. In A. Huston (Ed.), *Children in poverty: Child development and public policy* (pp. 23–50). New York: Cambridge University Press.

Duncan, G. J., & Brooks-Gunn, J. (1997). *Consequences of growing up poor.* New York: Russell Sage Foundation.

Eamon, M. K., & Zuehl, R. M. (2001). Maternal depression and physical punishment as mediators of the effect of poverty on socioemotional problems of children in single-mother families. *American Journal of Orthopsychiatry, 71*(2), 218–226.

Edin, K., & Lein, L. (1997). *Making ends meet: How single mothers survive welfare and low-wage work.* New York: Russell Sage Foundation.

Elder, G. H., Jr., Conger, R. D., Foster, E. M., & Ardelt, M. (1992). Families under economic pressure. *Journal of Family Issues, 13,* 5–37.

Emery, R. E. (1988). *Marriage, divorce, and children's adjustment.* Beverly Hills, CA: Sage.

Florsheim, P., Moore, D., Zollinger, L., MacDonald, J., & Sumida, E. (1999). The transition to parenthood among adolescent fathers and their partners: Does antisocial behavior predict problems in parenting? *Applied Developmental Science, 3*(3), 178–191.

Friedeman, M. L., & Andrews, M. (1990). Family support and child adjustment in single-parent families. *Issues in Comprehensive Pediatric Nursing, 13,* 289–301.

Furstenberg, F. F. (1993) How families manage risk and opportunity in dangerous neighborhoods. In W. J. Wilson (Ed.), *Sociology and the public agenda* (pp. 231–258). Newbury Park, CA: Sage.

Furstenberg, F. F., Brooks-Gunn, J., & Morgan, S. P. (1987). *Adolescent mothers in later life.* Cambridge, UK: Cambridge University Press.

Furstenberg, F. F., & Cherlin, A. J. (1991). *Divided families: What happens to children when parents part.* Cambridge, MA: Harvard University Press.

Furstenberg, F. F., & Nord, C. W. (1985). Parenting apart: Patterns of child-rearing after marital disruption. *Journal of Marriage and the Family, 47,* 893–904.

Furstenberg, F. F., & Weiss, C. C. (2000). Intergenerational transmission of fathering roles in at risk families. *Marriage and Family Review, 29*(2–3), 181–201.

Garbarino, J., & Kostelny, K. (1993). Neighborhood and community influences on parenting. In T. Luster & L. Okagaki (Eds.), *Parenting: An ecological perspective* (pp. 203–226). Hillsdale, NJ: Erlbaum.

Garfinkel, I., & McLanahan, S. S. (1986). *Single mothers and their children: New American dilemma.* Washington, DC: Urban Institute Press.

Gladov, N. W., & Ray, M. P. (1986). The impact of informal support systems on the well-being of low income single parents. *Family Relations, 35,* 113–123.

Greif, G. L. (1995a). On becoming a single father with custody. In J. E. Shapiro, M. J. Diamond, M. Greenberg (Eds.), *Becoming a father: Contemporary, social, developmental, and clinical perspectives.* New York: Springer.

Greif, G. L. (1995b). Single fathers with custody following separation and divorce. *Marriage and Family Review, 20,* 1–2, 213–231.

Greif, G. L. (1996). Working with families headed by single fathers. *The Hatherleigh Guide to Marriage and Family Therapy* [The Hatherleigh Guide Series, 6]. New York: Hatherleigh Press.

Gringlas, M., & Weinraub, M. (1995). The more things change . . .: Single parenting revisited. *Journal of Family Issues, 16*(1), 29–52.

Hall, L. A., Gurley, D. N., Sachs, B., & Kryscio, R. J. (1991). Psychosocial predictors of maternal depressive symptoms, parenting attitudes, and child behavior in single-parent families. *Nursing Research, 40*(4), 214–220.

Hatchett, S. J., Cochran, D. L., & Jackson, J. S. (1991). Family life. In J. S. Jackson (Ed.), *Life in Black America* (pp. 46–83). Newbury Park, CA: Sage Publications.

Hatchett, S., & Jackson, J. S. (1993). African American extended kin systems: An assessment. In HP McAdoo (Ed.), *Family ethnicity: Strength in diversity* (pp. 90–108). Thousand Oaks, CA: Sage.

Hawkins, A. J., Eggebeen, D. J. (1991). Are fathers fungible? Patterns of coresident adult men in maritally disrupted families and young children's well-being. *Journal of Marriage and the Family, 53*(4), 958–972.

Hernandez, D. J. (1997). Poverty trends. In G. J. Duncan & J. Brooks-Gunn (Eds.), *Consequences of growing up poor* (pp. 18–34). New York: Russell Sage Foundation.

Hetherington, E. M. (1989). Coping with family transitions: Winners, losers, and survivors. *Child Development, 60,* 1–14.

Hetherington, E. M. (1999a). Should we stay together for the sake of the children? In M. E. Hetherington (Ed.), *Coping with divorce, single parenting, and remarriage: A risk and resiliency perspective* (pp. 93–116). Mahwah, NJ: Erlbaum.

Hetherington, E. M. (1999b). Social capital and the development of youth from nondivorced, divorced and remarried families. In A. W. Collins & B. Laursen (Eds.), *Relationships as developmental contexts: The Minnesota Symposium on Child Psychology.* Mahwah, NJ: Erlbaum.

Hetherington, E. M., Bridges, M., & Insabella, G. M. (1998). What matters? What does not?: Five perspectives on the association between marital transitions and children's adjustment. *American Psychologist, 53*(2), 167–184.

Hetherington, E. M., & Clingempeel, W. G. (1992). Coping with marital transitions. *Monographs of the Society for Research in Child Development, 57* (2–3, Serial No. 227).

Hetherington, E. M., Cox, M., & Cox, R. (1978). The aftermath of divorce. In J. Stevens & M. Mathews (Eds.), *Mother/child father/child relationships* (pp. 149–176). Washington, DC: National Association for the Education of Young Children.

Hetherington, M. E., & Stanley Hagan, M. (1995). Parenting in divorced and remarried families. In M. H. Bornstein (Ed.), *Handbook of parenting: Vol 3. Status and social conditions of parenting* (pp. 233–254). Hillsdale, NJ: Erlbaum.

Hetherington, M. E., & Stanley Hagan, M. (2000). Diversity among stepfamilies In D. H. Demo, K. R. Allen, & M. A. Fine (Eds.), *Handbook of family diversity.* New York: Oxford University Press.

Herz, F. B. (1988). The post divorce family. In B. Carter & M. McGoldrick (Eds.), *The changing family life cycle* New York: Gardner Press. 372–398.

Hines, P. M., Garcia-Preto, N., McGoldrick, M., Almeida, R., Weltman, S. (1999). Culture and the Family Life Cycle. In B. Carter & M. McGoldrick (Eds.), *The expanded life cycle: Individual, family and social perspectives* (3rd ed., pp. 69–87). Boston: Allyn & Bacon.

Hofferth, S. L., Smith, J., McLoyd, V. C., Finkelstein, J. (2000). Achievement and behavior among children of welfare recipients, welfare leavers, and low-income single mothers. *Journal of Social Issues, 56*(4), 747–774.

Holloway, S. D., & Machida, S. (1992). Maternal child-rearing beliefs and coping strategies: Consequences for divorced mothers and their children. In I. E. Sigel, A. V. McGillicuddy-DeLisi, & J. J. Goodnow (Eds.), *Parental belief systems: The psychological consequences for children* (2nd ed., pp. 249–265). Hillsdale, NJ: Erlbaum.

Holloway, S. D., & Machida, S. (1991). Child-rearing effectiveness of divorced mothers: Relationship to coping strategies and social support. *Journal of Divorce and Remarriage, 14*(3–4), 179–201.

Hope, S., Power, C., & Rodgers, B. (1999). Does financial hardship account for elevated psychological distress in lone mothers? *Social Science and Medicine, 49,* 1637–1649.

Isaacs, M. B., & Lean, G. H. (1987). Social networks divorce, and adjustment: A tale of three generations. *Journal of Divorce, 9,* 1–16.

Jackson, A. P. (1998). The role of social support in parenting for low-income, single, black mothers. *Social Service Review, 72,* 365–378.

Jackson, A. P., Brooks-Gunn, J., Huang, C., & Glassman, M. (2000). Single mothers in low-wage jobs: Financial strain, parenting, and preschoolers' outcomes. *Child Development, 71,* 1409–1423.

Jackson, A. P., Gyamfi, P., Brooks-Gunn, J., & Blake, M. (1998). Employment status, psychological well-being, social support, and physical discipline practices of single black mothers. *Journal of Marriage and the Family, 60,* 894–902.

Jackson, A. P., & Huang, C. C. (2000). Parenting stress and behavior among single mothers of preschoolers: The mediating role of self-efficacy. *Journal of Social Service Research, 26,* 29–42.

Jayakody, R., & Chatters, L. M. (1997). Differences among African American single mothers: Marital status, living arrangements, and family support. In R. J. Taylor, J. S. Jackson, & L. M. Chatters (Eds.), *Family life in black America* (pp. 167–184). Thousand Oaks, CA: Sage.

Johnson, W. E. (2001). Paternal involvement among unwed fathers. *Children and Youth Services Review, 23*(6–7), 513–536.

Kalter, N. (1990). *Growing up with divorce: Helping your child avoid immediate and later emotional problems*. New York: Free Press.

Kazdin, A. E. (2000). Perceived barriers to treatment participation and treatment acceptability among antisocial children and their families. *Journal of Child and Family Studies, 9*(2), 157–174.

Kellam, S. G., Ensiminger, M. E., Turner, R. J. (1977). Family structure and the mental health of children concurrent and longitudinal community wide studies. *Archives of General Psychiatry, 34*(9), 1012–1022.

Kessler, R., & Neighbors, H. (1986). A new perspective on the relationships among race, social class, and psychological distress. *Journal of Health and Social Behavior, 27*, 107–115.

Kiselica, M. S., Stroud, J., & Rotzien, A. (1999). Counseling the forgotten client: The teen father. *Journal of Mental Health Counseling, 14*(3), 338–350.

Kissman, K., & Allen, J. A. (1993). *Single parent families*. Newbury Park, CA: Sage.

Koeske, G. F., & Koeske, R. D. (1990). The buffering effect of social support on parental stress. *American Journal of Orthopsychiatry, 60*(3), 440–451.

Lamb, M., Sternberg, K., & Thompson, R. (1997). The effects of divorce and custody arrangements on children's behavior, development, and adjustment. *Family and Conciliation Courts Review, 35*, 393–404.

Lane, T. S., & Clay, C. (2000). Meeting the service needs of young fathers. *Child and Adolescent Social Work Journal, 17*(1), 35–54.

Lehr, R. & MacMillan, P. (2001). The psychological and emotional impact of divorce: The noncustodial fathers' perspective. *Families in Society, 82*(4), 373–382.

Malson, M. R. (1986). The black working mother as role model. *Radcliffe Quarterly, 72*, 24–25.

Margolin, L. (1992). Child abuse by mothers' boyfriends: Why the overrepresentation? *Child Abuse and Neglect, 16*(4), 541–551.

McAdoo, H. P. (1980). Black mothers and the extended family support network. In L. F. Rodgers-Rose (Ed.), *The black woman* (pp. 125–144). Newbury Park, CA: Sage.

McAdoo, H. P. (1997). *Black Families* (3rd Ed.). Thousand Oaks, CA: Sage.

McLanahan, S. (1983). Family structure and stress: A longitudinal comparison of two-parent and female-headed families. *Journal of Marriage and the Family, 45*, 347–357.

McLanahan, S., & Booth, K. (1989). Mother-only families: Problems, prospects, and policies. *Journal of Marriage and the Family, 51*, 557–580.

McLanahan, S., & Sanderfur, M. J. (1994). *Growing up with a single parent: What hurts and what helps*. Cambridge, MA: Harvard University Press.

McLoyd, V. C. (1990). The impact of economic hardship on black families and children: Psychological distress, parenting, and socioemotional development. *Child Development, 61*, 311–346.

McLoyd, V. C. (1993). Employment among African-American mothers in dual-earner families: Antecedents and consequences for family life and child development. In J. Frankel (Ed.), *The employed mother and the family context* (pp. 180–226). New York: Springer.

McLoyd, V. C. (1998). Socioeconomic disadvantage and child development. *American Psychologist, 53*, 185–204.

McLoyd, V. C., Jayarantne, T. E., Ceballo, R., & Borquez, J. (1994). Unemployment and work interruption among African-American single mothers: Effects on parenting and adolescent socio-emotional functioning. *Child Development, 65,* 562–589.

McLoyd, V. C., & Wilson, L. (1991). The strain of living poor: Parenting, social support, and child mental health. In A. C. Huston (Ed.), *Children in poverty: Child development and public policy* (pp. 105–135). New York: Cambridge University Press.

Morawetz, A., & Walker, G. (1984). *Brief therapy with single-parent families.* New York: Brunner/Mazel.

Morrison, D. R., & Cherlin, A. J. (1995). The divorce process and young children's well-being: A prospective analysis. *Journal of Marriage and the Family, 57*(3), 800–812.

Murry, V. M., Bynum, M. S., Brody, G. H., Willert, A., & Stephens, D. (2001). African American single mothers and children in context: A review of studies on risk and resilience. *Clinical Child and Family Psychology Review, 4,* 133–155.

Olson, S. L., Kieschnick, E., Banyard, V., & Ceballo, R. (1994). Socioenvironmental and individual correlates of psychological adjustment in low-income single mothers. *American Journal of Orthopsychiatry, 64*(2), 317–330.

Perkins, W., & Davis, J. (1996). *Fathers care: A review of the literature.* Commissioned paper for the National Center on Fathers and Families. Philadelphia: University of Pennsylvania Press.

Prinz, J., & Miller, G. E. (1994). Family-based treatment for childhood antisocial behavior: Experimental influences on dropout and engagement. *Journal of Consulting and Clinical Psychology, 62*(3), 645–650.

Richardson, R., Barbour, N. B., & Bubenzer, D. L. (1991). Bittersweet connections: Informal networks as sources of support and interference for adolescent mothers. *Family Relations, 40,* 430–434.

Samuelsson, M. A. K. (1994). Associations between the mental health and social networks of children and parents in single-parent families: A comparison between a clinical group and a control group. *Acta Psychiatrica Scandinavica, 90,* 438–445.

Shaw, D. S., & Emery. R. E. (1987). Parental conflict and other correlates of the adjustment of school-age children whose parents have separated. *Journal of Abnormal Child Psychology, 15,* 269–281.

Shear, M. K., Anderson, C. M., & Greeno, K. (1997, July). *Psychiatric illness in mothers who bring children for mental health care.* Paper presented at the NIMH meeting, Improving the Condition of People with Mental Illness: The Role of Services Research, Washington, DC.

Simons, R. L. (1996). *Understanding differences between divorced and intact families: Stress, interaction, and child outcome.* Thousand Oaks, CA: Sage.

Simons, R. L., & Beaman, J. (1996). Father's parenting. In R. L. Simons (Ed.), *Understanding differences between divorced and intact families: Stress, interaction, and child outcome* (pp. 94–103). Thousand Oaks, CA: Sage.

Simons, R. L., & Johnson, C. (1996). Mother's parenting. In R. L. Simons (Ed.), *Understanding differences between divorced and intact families: Stress, interaction, and child outcome* (pp. 81–93). Thousand Oaks, CA: Sage.

Simons, R. L., Lorenz, F. O., Conger, R. D., & Wu, C. (1992). Support from spouse as mediator and moderator of the disruptive influence of economic strain on parenting. *Developmental Psychology, 29,* 368–381.

Simons, R. L., Whitbeck, L. B., Beaman, J., & Conger, R. D. (1994). The impact of mothers' parenting, involvement by nonresidential fathers, and parental conflict on adjustment of adolescent children. *Journal of Marriage and the Family, 56,* 356–374.

Spencer, B. (1990). Development of minority children: An introduction. *Child Development, 61,* 267–268.

Stack, S. (1989). The impact of divorce on suicide in Norway, 1951–1980. *Journal of Marriage and the Family, 51,* 229–238.

Stolba, A., & Amato, P. R. (1993). Extended single-parent households and children's behavior. *Sociological Quarterly, 34*(3), 543–549.

Taylor, R. J., Chatters, L. M., Jackson, J. S. (1997). Changes over time in support network involvement among Black Americans. In R. J. Taylor, J. S. Jackson, & L. M. Chatters (Eds.), *Family life in black America* (pp. 293–316). Thousand Oaks, CA: Sage.

Taylor, R. J., Jackson, J. S., & Quick, A. D. (1982). The frequency of social support among black Americans: Preliminary findings from the National Survey of Black Americans. *Urban Research Review, 8*(2), 1–4.

Thompson, M. S., & Peebles-Wilkens, W. (1992). The impact of formal, informal, and societal support networks on the psychological well-being of black adolescent mothers. *Social Work, 37*(4), 322–328.

Thornberry, T. P., Smith, C. A., & Howard, G. J. (1997). Risk factors for teenage fatherhood. *Journal of Marriage and the Family, 59*(3), 505–522.

Travato, F., & Lauris, G. (1989). Marital status and mortality in Canada: 1951–81. *Journal of Marriage and the Family, 51,* 907–922.

Tschann, J. M., Johnston, J. R., & Wallerstein, J. S. (1989). Resources, stresses and attachment as predictors of adult adjustment to divorce: A longitudinal study. *Journal of Marriage and the Family, 51,* 1033–1046.

U.S. Bureau of the Census. (2001). America's families and living arrangements: Population characteristics. Washington, DC: U.S. Department of Commerce.

U.S. Census Bureau. (2001). America's Families and Living Arrangements: Population Characteristics. Washington DC: US Department of Commerce.

Vandell, D. L., & Ramanan, J. (1992). Effects of early and recent maternal employment on children from low-income families. *Child Development, 63,* 938–949.

Waite, L. J., & Berryman, S. F. (1986). Job stability among young women: A comparison of traditional and nontraditional occupations. *American Journal of Sociology, 92*(3), 568–595.

Wallerstein, J. S. (1987). Children of divorce: A ten-year study. In E. M. Hetherington & J. D. Arasteh (Eds.), *The impact of divorce, single parenting and stepparenting on children* (pp. 197–214). Hillsdale, NJ: Erlbaum.

Wallerstein, J. S., & Blakeslee, S. (1989). *Second chances, men, women, and children a decade after divorce.* New York: Ticknor & Fields.

Walsh, F. (1996). The concept of family resilience: Crisis and challenge. *Family Process, 35*(3), 261–281.

Weitoft, R. G., Haglund, B., & Rosen, M. (2000). Mortality among lone mothers in Sweden: A population study. *Lancet, 355,* 1215–1219.

Westcot, M., & Dries, R. (1990). Has family therapy adapted to the single-parent family? *American Journal of Family Therapy, 18*(4), 353–372.

Whitbeck, L., Simons, R., & Kao, M. (1994). The effects of divorced single mothers' dating and sexual attitudes on the sexual attitudes and behaviors of their adolescent children. *Journal of Marriage and the Family, 56,* 615–621.

Wilson, W. J. (1987). *The truly disadvantaged: The inner city, the underclass, and public policy.* Chicago: University of Chicago Press.

Wilson, W. J. (1996). *When work disappears: The world of the new urban poor.* New York: Knopf.

Zill, N. (1990). *U.S. children and their families: Current conditions and recent trends.* Report of the Select Committee on Children, Youth and Families, U.S. House of Representatives, Washington, DC.

CHAPTER 6

REMARRIAGE FAMILIES AND STEPPARENTING

Emily B. Visher
John S. Visher
Kay Pasley

Stepfamilies are now a part of everyday family life in America. Since 1970, the number of households that include stepparents and stepchildren has increased dramatically. In fact, using a broad definition of a stepfamily (a household containing a child who is biologically related to only one of the adults), our best estimates suggest that at least one-third of all children under 18 who reside with two adults in the United States were in step situations (Bumpass, Raley, & Sweet, 1995; Fields, 2001; Seltzer, 1994). However, these estimates fail to take into account two other groups of children: (1) those who live with a single parent and have contact with the nonresident parent who is remarried or partnered, and (2) those who are older than 18, with remarried or partnered parents. Thus, our best estimates simply underestimate the step population (Pasley, 2001). Although remarriage rates have dropped somewhat, cohabitation rates have increased especially among divorced persons, and cohabitation is a viable alternative to remarriage except for those in the oldest generation (Bumpass et al., 1996; Teachman, Tedrow, & Crowder, 2000, U.S. Census Bureau, 1995; Chevan, 1996). Because many individuals have lived at one or more times in stepfamily situations that ended, and others will experience stepfamily life in their futures, most scholars agree with demographer Paul Glick (1991), who said, "In this perspective, it would not be unreasonable to expect that more than half of all Americans alive today have been, are now, or will eventually be in one or more step situations before they die."

American institutions, such as the law (e.g., Fine & Fine, 1992; Mahoney, 2000; Mason & Mauldon, 1997, Ramsey, 1995), the schools (e.g., Crosbie-Burnett, 1995), and the church (e.g., Young, 2001), as well as society in general, have not kept pace with the reality of these important family changes. As such, the general perception of "family" continues to be a mom, a dad, two children, and a dog. Any family form that deviates from this perception is devalued.

Although certainly there is more recognition today of stepfamilies, they continue to exist under a cloud of negative stereotyping (Ganong & Coleman, 1997), and the term "stepchild" is still used to connote less than adequate attention. This uncomfortable status no doubt contributes to the search for bland and neutral synonyms such as "reconstituted," "blended," or "remarriage" family in place of the more descriptive term: stepfamily. Our impression is that it will take many more years for society to overcome the influence of the old fairy tales and the bias in favor of the first-marriage family, before divorce, remarriage and the idealization of marriages other than first marriages will be assumed to be positive, albeit challenging, life-cycle stages.

It is in this current problematic milieu that stepfamilies are created and attempt to move toward successful integration. Although estimates vary, most scholars agree that between 40 and 52% of all first marriage end in divorce (Bramlett & Mosher, 2001; National Center for Health Statistics [NCHS], 2001; Norton & Miller, 1993), and about half of all marriages are a remarriage for at least one of the adults (Norton & Miller, 1993; NCHS, 2001). Unfortunately, about 60% of remarriages end in divorce (Bramlett & Mosher, 2001; Norton & Miller, 1993), especially when remarried couples have stepchildren (Booth & Edwards, 1992). In addition, about 20% of American children will experience more than one parental divorce before they become adults (Booth & Edwards, 1992; Coleman, Ganong, & Fine, 2000). In addition to divorce, widowhood is another avenue through which parents become single and may eventually remarry.

Research is helpful in suggesting that it is not the structure per se of remarried families that is responsible for these divorces; as with other types of families, family processes and the quality of the relationships between the individuals in the family determine success (Demo & Cox, 2000; Lansford, Cebello, Abbey, & Stewart, 2001). However, within the more complex stepfamily structure, developing effective interaction skills and forming satisfactory relationships often are difficult, and the uneasy interface between stepfamilies and the culture does not help with this process. A stepmother's words may mirror those of other stepparents when she says, "I feel as though everyone I know is looking over my shoulder waiting for me to screw up."

Unfortunately family pathologizing remains prevalent in American society. A recent cartoon shows a large auditorium with a banner overhead that identifies the gathering as the "Annual Convention of Adult Children of Normal Parents." Only two seats are occupied; the rest of the auditorium is empty. For stepfamilies, as for other families, societal validation and support are important ingredients for the maximization of individual and family potential. If this affirmation does develop, it could lead stepfamilies to value their type of family more fully and view themselves as making a positive contribution to the diversity of family life in America.

STEPFAMILY RESEARCH

Over the past 20 years, empirical research concerned with stepfamily life has flourished in both quantity and quality (see the decade reviews by Coleman & Ganong, 1990; Coleman et al., 2000). To date, most normative stepfamily research concerns three types of remarriage families: (1) families in which the wife has children in the household; (2) those in which the husband has children in the household; and (3) families in which both adults have children in the household. Stepfamilies with a mutual child also have received some, albeit limited, attention. We discuss findings that have been corroborated by several studies, including citations as examples rather than attempting to be exhaustive.

Stepfather Families

Stepfather families are one of the most common stepfamily structures, with about 15% of all children under age 18 residing with their mother and her spouse or partner (U.S. Census Bureau, 1995). Studies indicate that this type of stepfamily tends to experience less stress than other stepfamilies, especially when the stepchildren are younger (Hetherington, 1993; MacDonald & DeMaris, 1996). Boys respond more favorably than girls to having a stepfather in the household (Bray & Kelly, 1998; Hetherington, 1993; Hetherington & Clingempeel, 1992), and many children develop satisfying relationships with their stepfathers over time (Ganong & Coleman, 1994). Acceptance by stepchildren is fostered when stepfathers engage in less discipline and control behaviors (Bray & Kelly, 1998; Ganong, Coleman, Fine, & Martin, 1999) and are more supportive (Bray & Kelly, 1998; Hetherington & Clingempeel, 1992). In fact, there is some evidence that stepfathers who engage in and maintain affinity-seeking behaviors develop warmer and closer relationships with their stepchildren than do those whose affinity-seeking behaviors diminish over time (Ganong et al., 1999). When stepchildren ignore the overtures of stepfathers early, stepfathers are more likely to withdraw from such interaction (Hetherington & Clingempeel, 1992). Thus, the reciprocal nature of interaction between stepfathers and stepchildren affects the quality of the relationship that is developed and maintained over time (Hetherington, 1993; O'Connor, Hetherington, & Clingempeel, 1997).

Stepmother Families

Stepmother families, in which the woman is the stepparent, tend to report more stress than do stepfather families (Nielson, 1999). Children, particularly girls, also experience higher stress when living with their father and stepmother than with their mother and stepfather. These consistent, important findings indicate situational dynamics at work that create special relationship problems for stepmother families. Because stepmother families are usually defined as stepfamilies in which the father has physical custody of at least one of his children, it may be that disturbances in mother–child bonding patterns, particularly mother–daughter bonding, are more upsetting to children than disturbances in the father–child relationship during and after divorce. Difficulty between the children's mother and stepmother also has been mentioned as a possible contribution to the greater stress in stepmother families (Ahrons, 1994; Bray & Depner, 1993; Nielson, 1999; Norwood & Wingender, 1999), although little empirical research explores the relationship between same-sex nonresident parent and resident stepparent.

The fact that women are still expected to set the emotional tone for the family probably contributes strongly to the differences in functioning between stepfather and stepmother families (Nielson, 1999). In addition, research shows that fathers abdicate child-rearing responsibilities to their new wives, and many stepmothers assume such responsibilities because of their perceptions of the stepchildren's best interests (Norwood & Wingender, 1999).

It is not uncommon for resident stepmothers to not be mothers themselves (Nielson, 1999); as such, they may have limited parenting experience and more unrealistic expectations for the stepparent role. Evidence suggests that stepparents (both stepfathers and stepmothers) who lack prior parenting experience have more difficulty adjust to living with stepchildren (Ihinger-Tallman & Pasley, 1997). However, because societal expectations are that women should assume more child care and child-rearing responsibilities, such expectations can become internalized by stepmothers. When they find themselves ineffective with their stepchildren, especially when the children are older, stepmothers' sense of competence and value is diminished (Nielson, 1999; Quick, McKenry, & Newman, 1995).

Another factor that may contribute to these differences is that in the United States, fathers, as a rule, move out after a divorce, and boys lose the person with whom they can most readily share interest and identify. Because 85% of the time children live with their mother after a remarriage (U.S. Census Bureau, 1995), boys have gained an important male figure, whereas girls have retained their relationship with their mother and now need to share her with a new partner. Girls also may become competitive with their mothers for the attention of their stepfather (Hetherington, 1993). In families where divorced parents share custody, and these are growing in number, many children live at least part of the time in both stepfather and stepmother family households, if both parents remarry.

Complex Stepfamilies

Complex stepfamilies, in which both adults have children from a previous marriage living in the household, account for approximately 7% of stepfamilies (White & Booth, 1985). Evidence shows that the greatest likelihood of redivorce is in complex stepfamilies (Coleman et al., 2000; Ihinger-Tallman & Pasley, 1997). Indeed, the greater the number of children, the more likely the couple will divorce (Hetherington, 1993). The challenges of working out these complex households are further complicated by dynamics in the relationships among stepsiblings and new rivalries with shifts in their positions from oldest to youngest, or to only girl or boy.

Stepfamilies with a Mutual Child

About half of all remarriages have an "ours" child typically within the first 2 years (Wineberg, 1992). Although not all people who remarry bring a child from the prior marriage into the new household (Pasley & Ihinger-Tallman, 1997), estimates suggest that about 5% of all remarried households do include three sets of children—his, hers, and "ours" (Coleman et al., 2000).

Clearly, the addition of a mutual child can complicate the integration of stepfamily members, although little empirical evidence is available on these families. A notable exception is the study by Bernstein (1989), who interviewed 150 people from 55 stepfamilies with a mutual child born during the remarriage. In general, if the child was born prior to successful stepfamily integration, there was likely to be increased stress and difficulty. For example, following the birth of a mutual child, a stepmother who had no prior children of her own tended to devote more loving attention to her new biological child than to her stepchildren. The husband, the parent of all the children, felt upset about these differences in overt expression of feelings and emotional attachments. This created severe tension between the couple.

A child conceived early in the stepfamily integration process in an attempt to make a failing relationship work, in fact, may have an opposite effect, as is true for first-marriage families. However, in most instances, if the child was born after the couple formed a solid relationship, the parents believed that the birth of the child contributed positively to the integration of the family (Bernstein, 1989).

Other research (Wineberg, 1992) shows the buffering effect of a mutual child on the likelihood of divorce. Specifically, we know that over half of all remarriages end in divorce, and 50% of these occur in the first 5 years. However, partners who have a mutual child are less likely to divorce in the first 10 years than those without a child born to the remarriage (this also includes remarriages without any children present). After 10 years, the rate of divorce is similar for remarriages with and without a mutual child.

Knowing what is common in different types of stepfamilies can provide involved individuals with some understanding of the typical sources of stress in their particular stepfamily. This knowledge can enable them to deal more effectively with situations that arise and also enhance their self-esteem and coping skills by giving them a helpful perspective of common behaviors and situations. They can then experience the difficulties as normative challenges rather than as signals that the family is not successful.

THE INTEGRATION PROCESS

Remarriage means families are in transition from life in the former households to an integrated stepfamily household, a process that takes time (Papernow, 1993)—and may be likened to the acculturation process of immigrating families as they move to a new country (See Falicov, Chapter 11, this volume). In fact, the early work of Landau-Stanton (1985) with such families identified important similarities: There are many necessary adjustments to be made, and individuals and subgroups in the extended family often move toward acculturation at differing rates. This discrepancy of movement can lead to stressful interpersonal relations. Scholars agree that many of these symptoms are related to transitional difficulties rather than being manifestations of serious intrapsychic problems (Bray & Kelly, 1998; O'Connor, Hetherington, & Reiss, 1998; Visher & Visher, 1988).

Although everyone in stepfamilies must make many adjustments to new situations, children frequently have additional complexities because they retain "dual citizenship" (M. Weston, personal communication, September 20, 1985) in two households and cultures, with different languages, different foods, and many different customs and ways of doing things. Not surprisingly, there is often tension as they pack to leave, unpack when they arrive, or overstep the unwritten proprieties of a particular family culture. There is richness in the diversity, too, but it takes acceptance, tolerance, understanding, and familiarity for children to experience the special rewards of each family. Parents and stepparents who allow their children to enjoy these varied experiences reduce the children's loyalty conflicts and contribute much toward creating their own successful families (McGoldrick & Carter, 1999). Slowly, former alliances and ways of doing things become transformed as stepfamily members move from having little or no emotional connections between them to the establishment of bonds that give them a greater sense of acceptance and belonging together as a family unit developing a sense of "we-ness."

Papernow (1993) described seven emotional and developmental stages in the integration process. In the beginning stages of Fantasy, followed by Immersion, then Awareness, the household tends to split apart along biological lines when tensions appear. Only gradually do the adults become aware that relationship changes need to occur. In the middle stages, Mobilization and Action, the tensions become acute, and it is at this point that many stepfamily couples divorce, because the two adults are unable to resolve their many differences and work together as a team. For many families, it may take 5–6 years before the adults form a solid couple bond and work as a team to meet the challenges of stepfamily life. The final stages, Contact and Resolution, mark a time of deepening stepparent–stepchild relationships and a growing recognition that the stepfamily has achieved stability as a unit. Even the frequent household changes resulting from the dual citizenship of the children, who spend time in both households, can feel more natural and normal. Ultimately, remarriage families achieve satisfactory bonding between the couple and steprelatives, so that family members feel connected and find satisfaction in their relationships. Although discussed in different terms, more recent evidence (Bray & Kelly, 1998) supports Papernow's idea that the Fantasy stage is an overriding starting point for many stepfamilies. Thus, the task of many remarried families is to confront their unrealistic expectations to develop a lifestyle that fits for them.

Relatedly, research shows that the development of a mutually satisfying relationship between the stepparent and the stepchildren is the strongest predictor of family integration, harmony, and stability (Bray & Kelly, 1998). We are not alone in believing that the quality of the stepparent–stepchild relationship serves as the barometer of the quality and stability of the marriage and family. Papernow (1993) also found that satisfactory steprelationships follow the establishment of a good couple relationship. Thus, satisfactory family integration requires the development of good step relationships, as well as the creation of a solid couple bond. Taken together, these studies suggest that, unlike many first-marriage families, couples in stepfamilies may form good couple bonds, but good stepparent–stepchild relationships do not necessarily follow. Indeed, couples often may divorce even when the two adults are happy together, because they have not been able to form satisfactory stepparent–stepchild relationships. Research suggests that these new relationships are relatively independent of one another and need to be developed separately. The usual pattern is for the couple first to learn to work together, which then provides a foundation with enough stability for the development of satisfactory relationships between stepparent and stepchildren (Papernow, 1993).

DYNAMIC ISSUES IN STEPFAMILY SYSTEMS

As family systems, stepfamilies are more complex in their structure, with a greater number of built-in subsystems and more ambiguity than is found in first-marriage families (see Pasley & Ihinger-Tallman, 1997). Boundaries are less clear and homeostatic stability is lacking because of potentially constant fluctuations within the membership of the household. "We have an accordion family," said one parent/stepparent, "One day there are the two of us; the next, there are nine." There are continual transitions that can result in greater stress and less cohesiveness. We believe that these households must deal with the following major dynamic issues:

1. Outsiders versus insiders
2. Boundary disputes
3. Power issues
4. Conflicting loyalties
5. Rigid, unproductive triangles
6. Unity versus fragmentation of the new couple relationship

Outsiders versus Insiders

Although individuals in first-marriage families may experience being "left out," in stepfamilies with the many types of "mergers" taking place, there is a constant problem of helping outsiders to become insiders, if there is to be household unity. Often the outsider is a stepfather joining an ongoing group, a mother and her children; or it may be a woman marrying a man who has custody of his children; or children coming to stay in the household on weekends or for the summer; or an adolescent changing residence from the mother and stepfather's household to the father and stepmother's household. Being a newcomer in any type of group can cause confusion that results in discomfort, both for the person or persons trying to be "one of the gang" and for the original group, who may feel intruded on and protective of the status quo. In the newness of these relationships and the less "neutral" emotional climate of the stepfamily group, the feelings of exclusion, intrusion, rejection, and resultant anger and depression can become amplified. Working out ways of dealing with the shifts and transitions takes time and understanding, patience, and tolerance for ambiguity (Pasley & Dollahite, 1995).

Boundary Disputes

Because children are often members of two separate households, the stepfamily boundaries can get blurred, as the adults in the two households discuss and negotiate the arrangements involving the children. However, it is necessary in most instances, for each household to recognize the boundaries to that particular unit. The adults in each household do have control over how they decide to deal with the individuals and events that take place within that sphere. In fact, if there is not some separation between the two households, there is little chance for a stepfamily to develop any sense of cohesiveness and unity.

Within the household, there also can be many "turf" problems that must be worked out: who sleeps where; what personal privacy is possible; what space can be reserved for whom. For example, consider the stepfamily in which the husband's three children rejoined the household every 3–4 days for a few days at a time. The house was small, and the mother's three children who lived there had to shift where they slept, where they put their clothes, and where they could go to relax or to be alone—all necessary changes to make space to accommodate the "extra" family members. Bedrooms became dormitories, and the continual chaos created tension and instability for everyone. This family needed to work out ways in which to ameliorate the impact of such major changes, so "property rights" became clear and consistent, and there was a stable place for each person.

Unfortunately, little empirical evidence supports the clinical evidence noted here. Research does show that stepmother families experience the greatest boundary ambiguity, but that such ambiguity is not associated with marital adjustment (Pasley, 1987; Pasley & Ihinger-Tallman, 1989). It may well be that ambiguity plays out less in the marital relationship than in other key step relationships, such as that of the stepparent and stepchild.

Power Issues

Power issues in stepfamilies can be exaggerated for many reasons. Women, who have been on their own for some time because of a divorce or the death of a husband, and who take pride in having "proved" their capabilities, frequently have no desire to return to a relationship that is not egalitarian and may seek out relationships where they have more power (Burgoyne & Morrison, 1997; Pyke & Coltrane, 1996). They have discovered that they can take care of themselves and their children. Many are wary of sharing this newfound control or power with another adult for fear of falling back into previously dissatisfying patterns.

Often money is equated with power, and divorced and remarried men can often feel that they have been robbed of their power and control and have become "walking wallets" to their former family (Arendell, 1995). The outlay of resources to a prior family means there is less for the remarried family. Also, both partners may be secretive about financial matters (Engel, 1999), which often exacerbates power issues that affect many relationship areas.

In stepfamilies, children can gain power in the age-old game of "divide and conquer"—a game also played in first-marriage families. However, because their biological parents now live in separate households and typically do not interact on a daily basis, there is greater opportunity to be successful at this game. If, in addition, the parents maintain only minimal and hostile contact with each other, there exists a built-in system that makes it extremely easy for children to gain tremendous power. "If you don't treat me right, I'll go live with my Dad." "You are really mean! My mother lets me watch TV until midnight." Although children want and need to feel a sense of mastery and power, they also need and want to know that there are stronger adults on whom they can depend.

Conflicting Loyalties

Loyalty conflicts can hardly be avoided. In a biological family, children may feel more comfortable with one parent than with the other, but they are not placed in the position of choosing whom to ask to a special event or to spend the weekend. They are part of each parent and feel torn apart when their parents are no longer together, with divided loyalties that perhaps increase when another adult enters the picture through parental remarriage. The more amicable the relationships between all the parental figures, the fewer the children's loyalty conflicts. Adolescents in stepfamilies report that loyalty conflicts are particularly stressful (Kennedy, 1985; Lutz, 1983).

When one parent has died and the surviving parent remarries, the remarriage can be seen by the children as a betrayal of the former spouse (McGoldrick & Carter, 1999). It may appear to the children that the new couple relationship negates the former relationship. Therefore, the stepparent stirs many strong emotions, particularly in older children who have lived with their other biological parent longer, and it can be difficult for the children to accept their new stepparent.

As for remarried parents, because the parent–child relationships have preceded the new couple relationship, adults often feel caught between their children and their new partners (Clingempeel, Coyler, & Hetherington, 1995). It may, indeed, seem to remarried parents that the new primary adult relationship is a betrayal of the older parent–child bonds. However, a satisfactory couple bond is usually necessary for a remarriage to succeed. Therefore, if a new primary couple bond is not established, it is likely that the children in the stepfamily will experience still more loss and disruption in their lives as their second family breaks apart.

Rigid and Unproductive Triangles

Triangles exist in all families. However, the subgroupings present in stepfamilies can produce particularly rigid, unproductive triangles. Unproductive triangles involve three individuals in a struggle in which clear, dyadic relationships are not possible. Important triangles in stepfamilies include the following:

1. Remarried parent in the middle, not allowing a direct relationship between a stepparent and a stepchild.
2. Remarried parent and stepparent standing united against a former spouse.
3. Child caught in the middle between hostile former spouses.
4. Child caught in the middle between mother and stepmother or father and stepfather.

Because of the complexity of the subgroups in a stepfamily and the heightened emotions involved and the long duration of some of the relationships, it can be difficult to break down these groupings so simple and more direct dyadic relationships are possible.

Unity versus Fragmentation of the New Couple Relationship

Many of the internal and external pulls on the new couple relationship have already been mentioned, such as the feelings of betrayal at the formation of a primary couple relationship, and the pull of grandparents who have difficulty adjusting to the new branches grafted onto their family tree (Pasley & Ihinger-Tallman, 1997). Still others may include the divisiveness of children who still hope disruption will lead to their biological parents' reunion; the insecurity of being a "second" spouse and perhaps not being seen by others as the "real" mate; and, initially, the absence of a shared family history or way of doing things (McGoldrick & Carter, 1999).

The interface between the stepfamily and the community can also produce tensions that strain the couple. Schools, churches, legal and health care systems, and social institutions of all types continue to consider the biological parents as the legitimate voice for children and points of contact. As such, stepparents are left out, even though they have been primary parental figures in children's lives for many years. Human flexibility exceeds that of institutions, and the broader social system is slow to respond to the need for many changes in these areas.

CHARACTERISTICS OF SUCCESSFUL
REMARRIED FAMILIES

Only recently has research begun to move away from a "deficit model" of stepfamilies (Coleman & Ganong, 1990) to look at what makes a remarriage family successful. Although this work remains in its infancy, important characteristics of successful stepfamilies are emerging. This knowledge provides supportive goals that give the adults a direction in which to move the family. As with any type of family, there is a range within which family members find satisfaction and a sense of well-being; it is not as though the family must achieve the "ideal" to be successful. As Kelly

(1995) stated, "The concept of healthy or good family functioning is a relative concept. . . . Families act in more or less functional ways at different times under different circumstances." The following characteristics are observed and reported by remarriage families in which children and adults experience warm interpersonal relationships and satisfaction with their lives.

Expectations Are Realistic

With few exceptions, individuals in successful stepfamilies are realistic about what they can expect for their families (Bray & Kelly, 1998), and they do not accept the common misconceptions about stepfamily life—the expectation of instant love and adjustment, or that stepfamilies should be the same as first-marriage families. They are aware that love and caring take time to achieve and that there are differences between remarriage families and first-marriage families. They do not attempt to force their family into a first-marriage family mold.

They recognize that instant love or adjustment is an unrealistic expectation because relationships take time to grow and cannot be forced (Pasley, Rhoden, Visher, & Visher, 1996; Visher, Visher, & Pasley, 1997). In all families, parent–child relationships run from hot to cold, and to expect reciprocal caring from individuals who suddenly find themselves living together after remarriage can lead to feelings of disappointment, insecurity, and anger (Bray & Kelly, 1998).

Successful stepfamilies realize that satisfactory ways of doing things can be worked out much faster than can emotional bonding between people; they relax and let the children set the pace for the new relationships (Papernow, 1993; Bray & Kelly, 1998). They accept the fact that younger children can more easily develop relationships with stepparents than adolescents can, who are struggling with their own sense of identity and already growing away emotionally from their family or families (Pasley, Dollahite, & Ihinger-Tallman, 1993). As one adolescent in a stepfamily put it, "Two parents are more than enough. I don't need another telling me what to do."

Often, because of their strong desire to erase past hurts for themselves and their children, remarried parents and stepparents cling to the expectation for "instant love." They frequently feel guilty about their children's reactions to the divorce or death of a parent (Arendell, 1995; Bray & Kelly, 1998), and they wish to make up for the children's pain. However, the pressure to feel a certain way, and then be unable to do so, can create feelings of confusion, anger, and guilt for stepparents and stepchildren. Attempts to force friendship and caring cause pressure that usually leads to just the opposite. If everyone tries too hard or "pussyfoots" around issues and finds it impossible to relax, then anger rather than positive regard results. In successful remarriage families, this expectation of instant love is understood and rejected; the stepfamily members relax their expectations about their feelings, and often relationships slowly blossom into caring bonds that last (Bray & Kelly, 1998; Papernow, 1993).

A closely related expectation is that stepfamilies will operate the same as first-marriage families. Children in remarriage families usually are acutely aware of differences, and almost universally, the adults in well-functioning stepfamilies at some psychological level recognize and accept that many stepfamily characteristics are not shared by those in first-marriage families. First identified by Visher and Visher in 1979, many of the following characteristics hold true today:

1. Stepfamilies are formed following many losses and changes. Parent–child relationships have been altered, with marriage dreams shattered, and many changes have occurred in living arrangements.
2. The members of a stepfamily come together at different phases in their individual, marital, and family life cycles. As a result, they often experience competing developmental needs. For example, the marital priorities of woman who has not been previously married may compete with the needs to care for her husband's three children, or the needs of an adolescent for growing independence and time with peers may compete with the new remarriage family's need for cohesion.
3. Both children and adults have experienced differing traditions and ways of doing things in previous families in which they have lived. As a result, they may have many different values and convictions about how families "should" operate.
4. Parent–child relationships precede rather than follow the relationship between the couple. Therefore, numerous alliances are already in existence when the stepfamily is formed.
5. The children have a parent elsewhere, in reality or in memory (if their parent has died or disappeared). As such, there is an important person to the children in another household.
6. Although estimates vary, we know that after divorce, many children have some contact with their nonresident parent (Braver & O'-Connell, 1998; Seltzer, 1994), which means that there are shifts in household membership when children move between parental households.
7. Stepparents have few legal rights (Mahoney, 2000; Ramsey, 1995). This can lead to uncomfortable situations in which stepparents cannot sign consent forms for their stepchildren, include them in insurance policies, or have rights for visitation after a divorce or death of their spouse. Such exclusion can pose problems in stepfamilies of long duration where the stepparent and stepchild have developed a strong bond.

With the acknowledgment of these complexities and mastery of the challenges, stepfamilies can find the special rewards available in this more complex remarriage family structure. For example, more parenting adults can share child-rearing responsibilities, and couples can have time to themselves when the children are in their other household.

Losses Can Be Mourned

We often say that stepfamilies are families "born of loss," because they are formed following a death or a divorce. Even adults who wanted to divorce have lost a relationship that they had expected to continue. For the partner who has not been married before, losses come from a discrepancy between fantasies of what their marriage would be like and the realities of stepfamily life, with a former spouse and stepchildren immediately part of their lives (Bray & Kelly, 1998; Papernow, 1993). When these and other losses are acknowledged and grieved, unrecognized sadness does not prevent and block embracing the process of moving toward satisfying step relationships.

In well-functioning remarriage families, the adults are sensitive to the sadness when children are upset and depressed (Pasley & Ihinger-Tallman, 1997), partly because they have not had control over these major changes in their lives. The adults support the children in the verbal expression of their feelings—their fears, their anticipations, and their anger—and allow the children time to adjust to the many changes. Maintaining extended family bonds, especially with grandparents, aunts and uncles, and cousins, provides a network of continuity for children in the face of loss and change.

There Is a Strong Couple Relationship

The presence of a strong couple, with partners working together as a team, is an important characteristic of successful stepfamilies, just as it is in first-marriage families. Scholars agree that successful stepfamilies are less cohesive than are first-marriage families (Coleman et al., 2000), and successful stepfamilies retain stronger parent–child alliances than exist in successful first-marriage families (Anderson & White, 1986; Brown, Green, & Druckman, 1990). Such findings are not surprising when we considers the structural characteristics of this type of family. It is important to note that although these differences are statistically significant they are so small as to have little practical meaning (Coleman et al., 2000). According to Bray (1999) these difference may simply reflect developmental variations in families. Less cohesion and stronger alliances does not mean dysfunction.

The adults in well-functioning stepfamilies understand the importance of providing an atmosphere of stability. Although they continue to pay attention to the needs of their children, they do not consider it a betrayal of their earlier relationship with them to form a primary relationship with their new partner. Not only does their new couple relationship bring happiness to the adults, but it can also reduce the children's anxiety about another parental breakup, create an atmosphere in which maintaining parent–child relationship can be respected by the stepparent, and encourage supportive and warm steprelationships. It also can provides the children with a model of partners who are happy together and work as a team to meet family challenges; this is an important model for children as they grow to adulthood and form their own couple relationships.

Satisfactory Step Relationships Have Formed

Relationships within most first-marriage families tend to be satisfying if the couple relationship is good. Because this does not necessarily follow in remarriage families, particular attention in needed for the development of interpersonal relationships between stepparent and stepchildren and between/among stepsiblings. For the stepfamily to be successful as a family, steprelationships are of great importance, and, as a rule, well-functioning stepfamilies illustrate the validity of guidelines for successful integration (Bray & Kelly, 1998).

The stepparent enters into a parenting role slowly and gradually (Bray, Berger, & Boethel, 1995; Bray & Kelly, 1998; Pasley & Ihinger-Tallman, 1997). This is important because a new stepparent has little or no authority so far as the children are concerned, unless they are young. For a stepparent, status with the children in a stepfamily is "earned," not "acquired," as is the status of the biological parent.

Successful stepparents do not "come in like the cheerleader of the Western World," as one initially unsuccessful stepmother said. Instead, they gradually build relationships with their stepchildren and slowly take on disciplinary functions (Bray & Kelly, 1998). If the stepchildren are adolescents when the integration process begins, they may be on their own before the stepparent has taken on a parent-like role. The successful partners will work together as a team, with the parent initially taking the active parent role with his or her children, and the stepparent supporting this behavior through monitoring stepchildren's behavior on behalf of the parent. Roles are not based on society's stereotypes of the traditional nurturing mother and financially responsible, disciplinary father. The relationship is basically egalitarian, and role function is determined by parenthood rather than by gender. As the stepparent is able to form a satisfactory relationship with the children, a parenting role may become appropriate.

Some remarried parents are able to form good couple relationships, but they find it difficult to encourage and support stepparent–stepchild bonding, which usually requires a shift in the parent–child relationship to occur. Initially, as the couple becomes solidified, the parent is actively supportive of the stepparent's relationship with stepchildren. Next, caring and respectful relationships are developed between the stepparent and stepchildren. Then, as connections solidify between adults and children, the household can function satisfactorily.

In well-functioning remarriage families, the relationship between a stepparent and a stepchild can be quite diverse and need not become a parental role (Bray & Kelly, 1998; Erera-Weatherly, 1996). Having the freedom to form varied types of interpersonal relationships is satisfying both to the adult and to each child. One young person was thankful for her stepfather, saying, "I really love my stepfather, and I appreciate the fact that he is a good companion to me, a confidante and friend to my brother, and a parent to my little sister" (Visher & Visher, 1990, p. 10).

At times, step relationships between stepsiblings may not be particularly warm (Hetherington & Clingempeel, 1992). It takes effort from each person to develop a bond, and children sometimes are reluctant to make this type of commitment. Even when the adults are fair to all the children, adequately meet their individual needs, and avert jealousies, stepsiblings may differ greatly in their styles and values, and never form close relationships. Similarly, stepparents and stepchildren, for a variety of reasons, may not develop warm interpersonal ties. In these families, tolerance and respect for differences enable such individuals to live together until the children mature and live on their own (Pasley et al., 1993). Well-functioning remarriage families often remain open to the possibility of building positive relationships in later years, when the stresses of earlier relationships shift to warmth and caring.

Satisfying Routines and Rituals Are Established

Stepfamily members come together from different family backgrounds. Indeed, if both adults have been married once previously, their marriage represents a seventh household forged from the six previous family systems experienced by the two adults:

Wife	*Husband*
Family of origin	Family of origin
First-marriage family	First-marriage family
Single-parent household	Single-parent household
Present stepfamily household	

This household also represents the third family unit experienced by each child. A fourth unit is experienced if the other parent remarries.

The difficult challenge in all these family experiences is the need to recognize that there is more than one way to do the laundry, cook a turkey, or celebrate a holiday. It is not a matter of one right or wrong way.

The positive side of past family experiences is the opportunity for members to share and decide from diverse and varied backgrounds what ways of doing things and rituals the new unit would like to adopt (Whiteside, 1988; Pasley et al., 1993). It may mean devising a way to celebrate Thanksgiving that combines (1) previous ways of sharing household tasks, (2) an entirely new method of doing things together, or (3) innovative ways to combine valued elements of former methods.

The flexibility and creativity that flow from the necessity of actually working out such arrangements can bring rewards to all involved. A stepfather put it this way: "I used to be a pretty rigid guy, but I've had to be more flexible, and this has helped me at work as well as at home." Successful stepfamilies have worked out positive rituals and appreciate the creativity and cooperation that accompanies these decisions.

The Separate Households Cooperate

Well-functioning stepfamilies also develops satisfactory arrangements between the children's multiple households. This is important, because when the two households cooperate rather than compete in raising the children, the young people experience less intense loyalty conflicts, and they and the adults are more able to relax and enjoy family life. Formation of a "parenting coalition" (Visher & Visher, 1989) can occur when all the adults directly involved with the children acknowledge and appreciate the special attributes and skills that each has to offer the children. Sharing parental responsibility allows the adults to have more time for themselves than is possible when children are in the household on a full-time basis, and it gives the children an opportunity for more diverse interpersonal experiences.

As a rule, it takes time to work out this type of cooperation (Ahrons, 1994). The couple relationship needs to have developed, so that both partners feel secure in their relationship, and parents and stepparents need the security that comes from recognizing how important they are to their children and stepchildren. Then, it becomes possible to view the other household in neutral terms rather than as a threat of more loss of the children. Some remarriage families become friendly with each other and come together frequently (Bray & Kelly, 1998). However, this is not the usual situation, and it certainly is not a necessary foundation for cooperating. Whatever the amount of contact, successful stepfamilies feel independent of the other household and, at the same time, feel connected through the children. For many, it is a "business relationship" that allows the households to cooperate in matters dealing with the children. This is invaluable when family events take place—holidays, graduations, weddings. These important times can then be pleasant and fulfilling times for all.

THERAPEUTIC IMPLICATIONS

Many stepfamily members need education and support to assist them in their journey together. Educational and mutual self-help groups around the country answer this need. In addition, organizations have been formed to provide ongoing education and/or support networks for stepfamilies.

A growing number of individuals in stepfamilies also seek professional help. Some research in which members of stepfamilies were asked about their experiences in therapy (Pasley et al., 1996; Visher et al., 1997) has demonstrated that not all therapeutic strategies are perceived as helpful. Although the basic therapeutic skills are used with stepfamilies and other families, a few specific guidelines make a great deal of difference when working with stepfamily members, either individually, in different subgroup combinations, or as a family unit (Visher & Visher, 1988, Pasley et al., 1993; Browning, 1995; Papernow, 1993; Pasley & Dollahite, 1995):

1. It is difficult but extremely important to overcome the emotional concept of the "ideal" American family, so that there is no futile attempt to fit a stepfamily into a first-marriage family mold.

2. It is helpful to assess stepfamilies differently than first-marriage families. Because of cultural and structural characteristics that produce added external stress, individuals in stepfamilies may seem to be more emotionally upset. Seeing the entire family together initially may increase emotional tension (Browning, 1995) and discourage them immediately. Starting with the couple relationship can be effective, strengthening the newest and most fragile subsystem.

3. Unlike similar behavioral characteristics of individuals in first-marriage families, these increased emotional tension and behaviors in stepfamily members may simply indicate their need for support and validation of their experience. They need help to increase self-esteem, confidence, and the ability to make productive choices. As they begin to experience a sense of mastery, the chaos tends to be controlled. Deeper couple or individual issues may emerge that are in need of attention. In most cases, child behavior problems improve dramatically as remarried family tasks are accomplished.

4. In a study of successful stepfamily therapy, Pasley et al. (1996) and Visher et al. (1997) reported that the most helpful therapeutic interventions are validation of feelings and clarifications that lead to greater understanding of other members' perceptions, especially regarding stepchildren. Both strategies require knowledge of normative stepfamily development.

5. Together with the new couple, it may be important at times to include the other parent, grandparents, or other significant adults in the therapeutic process. The focus of the meeting needs to be clearly stated

ahead of time: It should be limited to issues involving the children and not serve as an attempt to resolve former spousal relationships. Such meetings occur most frequently in regard to custody and visitation questions. Meetings need to include stepparents to validate their position and to solidify the remarriage family unit.

6. Countertransference, both positive and negative, can be particularly difficult to deal with the complex dynamics of stepfamily situations in which the therapist's feelings may be strong. For this reason, consultation or the use of cotherapists can be extremely valuable.

SUMMARY

As society changes, new patterns are evolving. However, at the present time, we have discussed characteristics of stepfamilies that have been validated by clinical observation and empirical research. Stepfamilies are families emerging out of hope. Remarried parents or stepparents are different than parents in a first-marriage family, and growing up in a stepfamily can be more complicated than growing up in a biological family. Successful stepfamilies accept and understand these differences and allow themselves the necessary time to accomplish the tasks that lead to successful integration. They understand that their transitional difficulties are predictable and not due to personal inadequacies, and that actions they take can lead to happiness and satisfaction for all members of the family unit. They also understand that the task they have set for themselves is challenging but not impossible, and that "second chances" may ultimately work for everyone.

REFERENCES

Ahrons, C. R. (1994). *The good divorce.* New York: HarperCollins.

Anderson, J. Z., & White, G. D. (1986). An empirical investigation of interaction and relationship patterns in functional and dysfunctional nuclear families and stepfamilies. *Family Process, 25,* 407–422.

Arendell, T. (1995). *Fathers and divorce.* Thousand Oaks, CA: Sage.

Bernstein, A. C. (1989). *Yours, mine and ours: How families change when remarried parents have a child together.* New York: Scribners.

Booth, A., & Edwards, J. N. (1992). Starting over: Why remarriages are more stable. *Journal of Family Issues, 13,* 179–194.

Bramlett, M. D., & Mosher, W. D. (2001). *First marriage dissolution, divorce, and remarriage: United States: Advance data from vital and health statistics, No. 323.* Hyattsville, MD: National Center for Health Statistics.

Braver, S., & O'Connell, D. (1998). *Divorced dads: Shattering the myths.* New York: Putnam.

Bray, J. H. (1999). Stepfamilies: The intersection of culture, context, and biology

[Commentary]. *Monographs for the Society of Research on Child Development (Series 259), 64*(4), 210–218.

Bray, J. H., Berger, S. H., & Boethel, C. L. (1995). Role integration and marital adjustment in stepfather families. In K. Pasley & M. Ihinger-Tallman (Eds.), *Stepparenting: Issues in theory, research, and practice* (pp. 253–279). Westport, CT: Praeger.

Bray, J. H., & Depner, S. (Eds.). (1993). *Nonresidential parenting: New vistas in family living.* Newbury Park, CA: Sage.

Bray, J. H., & Kelly, J. (1998). *Stepfamilies: Love, marriage, and parenting in the first decade.* New York: Broadway Books.

Brown, A. C., Green, R. J., & Druckman, J. (1990). A comparison of stepfamilies with and without child-focused problems. *American Journal of Orthopsychiatry, 60*, 556–566.

Browning, S. (1995). Treating stepfamilies: Alternatives to traditional family therapy. In K. Pasley & M. Ihinger-Tallman (Eds.), *Stepparenting: Issues in theory, research, and practice* (pp. 175–198). Westport, CT: Praeger.

Bumpass, L. L., Raley, R. K., & Sweet, J. A. (1996). The changing character of stepfamilies: Implications of cohabitation and nonmarital childbearing. *Demography, 32*, 425–436.

Burgoyne, C. B., & Morrison, V. (1997). Money and remarriage: Keeping things simple and separate. *Sociological Review, 45*, 363–394.

Chevan, A. (1996). As cheaply as one: Cohabitation in the older population. *Journal of Marriage and the Family, 58*, 656–667.

Clingempeel, W. G., Coyler, J. J., & Hetherington, E. M. (1995). Toward a dissonance conceptualization of stepchildren and biological children loyalty conflicts: A construct validity study. In K. Pasley & M. Ihinger-Tallman (Eds.), *Stepparenting: Issues in theory, research, and practice* (pp. 151–174). Westport, CT: Praeger.

Coleman, M., & Ganong, L. H. (1990). Remarriage and stepfamily research in the 1980s: Increased interest in an old family form. *Journal of Marriage and the Family, 52*, 925–940.

Coleman, M., Ganong, L., & Fine, M. A. (2000). Reinvestigating remarriage: Another decade of progress. *Journal of Marriage and the Family, 62*, 1288–1307.

Crosbie-Burnett, M. (1995). The interface between stepparent families and schools: Research, theory, policy and practice. In K. Pasley & M. Ihinger-Tallman (Eds.), *Stepparenting: Issues in theory, research, and practice* (pp. 199–216). Westport, CT: Praeger.

Demo, D. H., & Cox, M. J. (2000). Families with young children: A review of research in the 1990s. *Journal of Marriage and the Family, 62*, 867–895.

Engel, M. (1999). Pockets of poverty: The second wives club—examining the financial [in]security of women in remarriage. *William and Mary Journal of Women and the Law, 5*(2), 309–381.

Erera-Weatherly, P. (1996). On becoming a stepparent: Factors associated with the adoption of alternative stepparenting styles. *Journal of Divorce and Remarriage, 25*(3/4), 155–174.

Field, J. (2001). Living arrangements of children: Fall 1996. *Current Population Reports, P70–74.* Washington, DC: U.S. Census Bureau.

Fine, M. A., & Fine, D. R. (1992). Recent changes in the laws affecting stepfamilies: Suggestions for legal reform. *Family Relations, 41*, 334–340.

Ganong, L., & Coleman, M. (1994). *Remarried family relationships.* Newbury Park, CA: Sage.

Ganong, L., & Coleman, M. (1997). How society views stepfamilies. *Marriage and Family Review, 26*(1/2), 85–106.

Ganong, L., Coleman, M., Fine, M. A., & Martin, C. (1999). Stepparents affinity-seeking and affinity-maintaining strategies with stepchildren. *Journal of Family Issues, 20,* 299–327.

Glick, P. C. (1991, October). *A demographic perspective of stepfamilies.* Address to the annual conference of the Stepfamily Association of America, Lincoln, NE.

Hetherington, E. M. (1993). An overview of the Virginia longitudinal study of divorce and remarriage with a focus on early adolescence. *Journal of Family Psychology, 7,* 39–56.

Hetherington, E. M., & Clingempeel, W. G. (1992). Coping with marital transitions: A family systems perspective. *Monographs of the Society for Research on Child Development, 57* (2/3, Serial No. 227), 1–242.

Ihinger-Tallman, M., & Pasley, K. (1997). Stepfamilies in 1984 and today—a scholarly perspective. *Marriage and Family Review, 26*(1/2), 19–40.

Kelly, P. (1995). *Developing healthy step families: Twenty families tell their stories.* Binghamton, NY: Haworth Press.

Kennedy, G. E. (1985). Family relations as perceived by college students from single-parent, blended, and intact families. *Family Perspective, 19,* 117–129.

Landau-Stanton, J. K. (1985). Adolescents, families and cultural transitions: A treatment model. In M. P. Mirkin & S. Koman (Eds.), *Handbook of adolescent and family therapy* (pp. 363–381). New York: Gardner Press.

Lansford, J. E., Ceballo, R., Abbey, A., & Stewart, A. (2001). Does family structure matter: A comparison of adoptive, two-parent biological, single-mother, step-father, and stepmother households. *Journal of Marriage and Family, 63,* 840–851.

Lutz, E. P. (1983). The stepfamily: An adolescent perspective. *Family Relations, 32,* 261–280.

MacDonald, W. L., & DeMaris, A. (1996). Parenting stepchildren and biological children: The effects of stepparent's gender and new biological children. *Journal of Family Issues, 17,* 5–25.

Mahoney, M. M. (2000). The rights and duties of stepparents at the time of divorce. *American Journal of Family Law, 14,* 252–256.

Mason, M. A., & Mauldon, J. (1997). The new stepfamily requires new public policy. *Journal of Social Issues, 52*(3), 11–27.

McGoldrick, M., & Carter, B. (1999). Remarried families. In B. Carter & M. McGoldrick (Eds.), *The expanded family life cycle* (3rd ed., pp. 417–435). Boston: Allyn & Bacon.

Nielson, L. (1999). Stepmothers: Why so much stress? *Journal of Divorce and Remarriage, 30*(1/2), 115–148.

Norwood, P. K., & Wingender, T. (1999). *The enlightened stepmother: Revolutionizing the role.* New York: Avon.

Norton, A. J., & Miller, L. F. (1993). Marriage, divorce and remarriage in the 1990's. *Current Population Reports, P 23-180.* Washington, DC: U.S. Census Bureau.

O'Connor, T. G., Hetherington, E. M., & Clingempeel, W. G. (1997). Systems and bidirectional influences in families. *Journal of Social and Personal Relationships, 14,* 491–504.

O'Connor, T. G., Hetherington, E. M., & Reiss, D. (1998). Family systems and adolescent development: Shared and nonshared risk and protective factors in nondivorced and remarried families. *Development and Psychopathology, 10,* 353–375.

Papernow, P. (1993). *Becoming a stepfamily: Patterns of development in remarried families.* New York: Gardner.

Pasley, K. (1987). Family boundary ambiguity: Perceptions of adult remarried family members. In K. Pasley & M. Ihinger-Tallman (Eds.), *Remarriage and stepparenting: Current research and theory* (pp. 206–224). New York: Guilford Press.

Pasley, K. (2001, February). *Changing face of American stepfamilies.* Invited address to the First National Conference on Stepfamilies, New Orleans, LA.

Pasley, K., & Dollahite, D. (1995). The nine Rs of stepparenting adolescents: Research-based recommendations for clinicians. In D. K. Huntley (Ed.), *Understanding stepfamilies: Implications for assessment and treatment* (pp. 87–100). Alexandria, VA: American Counseling Association.

Pasley, K., Dollahite, D., & Ihinger-Tallman, M. (1993). Bridging the gap: Clinical applications of research findings on the spouse and stepparent roles in remarriage. *Family Relations, 42,* 315–322.

Pasley, K., & Ihinger-Tallman, M. (1989). Boundary ambiguity in remarriage: Does ambiguity differentiate degrees of marital adjustment and integration. *Family Relations, 38,* 46–52.

Pasley, K., & Ihinger-Tallman, M. (1997). Stepfamilies: Continuing challenges for the schools. In T. W. Fairchild (Ed.), *Crisis intervention for school-based helpers* (2nd ed., pp. 60–100). New York: Schribner & Sons.

Pasley, K., Rhoden, J. L.,Visher, E. B., & Visher, J. S. (1996). Successful stepfamily therapy: Clients' perspectives. *Journal of Marriage and Family Therapy, 22,* 319–333.

Pyke, K., & Coltrane, S. (1996). Entitlement, obligation and gratitude in family work. *Journal of Family Issues, 17,* 60–82.

Quick, D. S., McKenry, P. C., & Newman, B. (1995). Stepmothers and their adolescent children: Adjustment to new family roles. In K. Pasley & M. Ihinger-Tallman (Eds.), *Stepparenting: Issues in theory, research, and practice* (pp. 105–126). Westport, CT: Praeger.

Ramsey, S. H. (1995). Stepparents and the law: A nebulous status and need for reform. In K. Pasley & M. Ihinger-Tallman (Eds.), *Stepparenting: Issues in theory, research, and practice* (pp. 217–238). Westport, CT: Praeger.

Seltzer, J. A. (1994). Intergenerational ties in adulthood and childhood experiences. In A. Booth & J. Dunn (Eds.), *Stepfamilies: Who benefits? Who does not?* (pp. 153–163). Hillsdale, NJ: Erlbaum.

Teachman, J., Tedrow, L. C., & Crowder, K. D. (2000). The changing demography of America's families. *Journal of Marriage and the Family, 62,* 1234–1246.

U.S. Bureau of the Census. (1995). *Statistical abstract of the United States: 1995* (115th ed.). Washington, DC: U.S. Government Printing Office.

Visher, E. B., & Visher, J. S. (1979). *Stepfamilies: A guide to working with stepparents and stepchildren.* New York: Brunner/Mazel.

Visher, E. B., & Visher, J. S. (1988). *Old families, new ties: Therapeutic strategies with stepfamilies.* New York: Brunner/Mazel.

Visher, E. B., & Visher, J. S. (1989). Parenting coalitions after remarriage: Dynamics and therapeutic guidelines. *Family Relations, 38,* 65–70.

Visher, E. B., & Visher, J. S. (1990). Dynamics of successful stepfamilies. *Journal of Divorce and Remarriage, 14*(1), 3–12.

Visher, E. B., Visher, J. S., & Pasley, K. (1997). Stepfamily therapy from the client's perspective. *Marriage and Family Review, 26*(1/2), 191–213.

White, L. K., & Booth, A. (1985). The quality and stability of remarriage: The role of stepchildren. *American Sociological Review, 50,* 689–698.

Whiteside, M. G. (1988). Creation of family identity through ritual performance in early remarriage. In E. Imber-Black, J. Roberts, & R. A. Whiting (Eds.), *Rituals in families and family therapy* (pp. 276–304). New York: Norton.

Wineberg, H. (1992). Childbearing and dissolution of the second marriage. *Journal of Marriage and the Family, 54,* 879–887. Lesbian and Gay Families.

Young, J. B. (2001). Remarried Catholics: Searching for church belonging. In K. Scott & M. Warren (Eds.), *Perspectives on marriage: A reader* (2nd ed., pp. 387–393). New York: Oxford University Press.

CHAPTER 7

LESBIAN AND GAY FAMILIES

Joan Laird

T here have been remarkable changes in the sociopolitical context surrounding lesbian and gay families[1] over the past decade. In many ways, those changes seem to be positive and progressive for the gay and lesbian population—families, couples, and individuals. The sea changes in gay visibility in popular culture—film, television, theater, and the written media—signal a profound shift in public discourse. Gay and lesbian characters, references, and jokes abound in television dramas and comedies. Several have featured gay "marriages" or commitment ceremonies. A few gay actors have come out, and major, presumably heterosexual, stars have risked playing gay or lesbian roles. A small but growing number of public figures in politics, the arts, and other fields began to publicly come out and, in the Clinton administration, a number of openly gay persons were appointed to public office.

However, many scholars and commentators are skeptical about the political and social meanings of this increased visibility for both the heterosexual and gay populations, and note the contradictions and paradoxes facing what seems to be "acceptance." Walters (2001) argued, in her comprehensive documentation of the increasing and unprecedented visibility of lesbians and gays in the 1990s, that this is a historic moment in American society, but one that is rife with paradox. Lesbians and gays are simultaneously depicted as chic and pioneering, and as a major sign of social deterioration and the source of the destruction of the family as we know it.

Society's ambivalence is reflected, for instance, in "don't ask; don't tell," a compromise policy that allows only closeted gays to serve in the military. In a most ironic turn of events, after the September 11, 2001, terror-ist attacks, the U.S. government decided that openly gay persons can serve in the military during the national crisis, yet left unclear whether they would then be discharged after the conflicts cease. At the same time that a growing number of lesbians and gay men enjoy both expanded antidis-crimination and fair employment laws, and domestic partner benefits, vio-lence against gay men and lesbians has escalated. In spite of growing safe school initiatives, many young people continue to face the ravages of het-erosexism and homophobia in their family and peer contexts. Openly gay males cannot serve in leadership positions in the Boy Scouts. In some states, gay men and lesbians are still losing custody of their birth children and are prevented from adopting or foster parenting. Partners of gay and lesbian birth or adoptive parents are still unable in most parts of the coun-try to adopt children they may have cared for and supported since infancy, and may have to forfeit all rights if the couple separates or the biological parent dies, or becomes incapacitated. Massachusetts still has an anti-sodomy law on the books. In general, it remains the case that lesbians and gay men possess limited civil and legal rights, and face opportunity barri-ers, accusations of immorality, nonwelcoming and unsafe environments, and, at times, violent attacks against persons and property. In a less tangi-ble sense, they swim in a sea of heterosexist language and practice, always marked by "difference" in many life settings, and always marginal and mar-ginalized.

Goffman (1963) defined "normality" as the absence of stigma. From this viewpoint, because gay men and lesbians constitute one of the most, if not *the* most, stigmatized groups in this society, we cannot consider such individuals "normal," whether or not they live in formations that resemble or may be defined as American families. On the other hand, these families seem to carry out successfully what have traditionally been conceptualized as family functions in this society. In my view, "normality" is a sociocultural and political construction, its definitions shaped and represented by vari-ous coalitions of definers who have greater influence over public discourse in this area. Thus, "normality" should not be seen as a characteristic of person or family but rather as compliance with accepted, socially con-structed norms or sets of rules for living.

In both the social science and family therapy fields, the notions of "gay" or "lesbian," and that of "family," have, at least until very recently, been mutually exclusive concepts. This failure to allow into public con-sciousness a definition of family that might refer to same-sex couples living alone or with children, or to solo lesbian or gay parents has accounted in part for the striking lack of attention to these families in family research, in the clinical literature in general, and in the family therapy field in par-ticular. Allen and Demo (1995) and Clark and Serovich (1997), in their reviews of the marriage and family literature, found that gay, lesbian, and bisexual issues are generally ignored.

DEFINING THE SAME-SEX FAMILY

Up to this point, the gay or lesbian family has not been defined, a task central to any discussion of family, yet one as amorphous and complex as determining the meaning of "heterosexual" or "homosexual." Definitions of family are political and ideological, created and re-created in social discourse and shaped in social relations of power. Particular definitions gradually assume the strength of conventionality. In the United States, common definitions of family have been built on symbols of law and nature, legal marriage, and blood relatedness. However, in recent decades, some theorists have argued for broader definitions of family that encompass ideas of "household," a notion incorporated in Mary Richmond's (1930) idea that a family consisted of "all who share a common table." Such broader, less restrictive, definitions imply that what constitutes a family is a movable feast on the one hand, shaped by codifications in law or religion, and on the other by groups of individuals who share particular kinds of commitments and roles.

Definitions of gay and lesbian families defy cultural assumptions about the meaning of "family," cross over family definitions organized by blood and legality and, in blood terms, make for a genealogical nightmare. They are families formed from lovers, friends, biological and adopted children, blood relatives, stepchildren, and even ex-lovers, families that do not necessarily share a common household. In fact, in some lesbian communities, the boundaries between family, kinship, and community become quite diffuse. Although it has been said, "You can't pick your relatives," in fact, that is exactly what gay families, in devising a new system of kinship, do. They "choose" their families, retaining the familiar symbol of blood, and combining it with symbols of love and choice. It is important to recognize, as Weston (1991) points out, that there is no uniform or normative definition for the "gay family" any more than there is for the "American family." Furthermore, there is no normative structure for the gay or lesbian family. These families, like all families, come in many sizes and shapes. Some consist of couples without children and others of groups of adults, some of whom may be partnered. Families with children may be headed by a single parent, a same-sex couple, or a multiple-parent extended family arrangement. Some lesbian families incorporate biological or, for want of a better word, "fictive" fathers. They are rich and poor, black and white; Jewish, Christian, and Muslim, Italian and Armenian. Except for the fact that one or more members are lesbian or gay, these families cross cut the same social categories as other families. In fact, there is no clear demarcation between heterosexual and gay families, because heterosexual families usually have one or more gay members and, similarly, gay or lesbian families usually have one or more heterosexual members.

Family therapists, in their research, theoretical, and practice writing, have generally unquestioningly incorporated prevailing cultural conceptions of family grounded in metaphors of blood and law. To unpack the first of these notions, that of blood, in this society and in Western culture, we have largely assumed that biological relatedness is at the heart of family formation. This idea, a definitional process and not a "reality," makes procreation the heart of family life. Conceptions of the family life course, for example, have typically been child-centered, beginning with legal marriage and following the course of children's growth and separation through various stages. The prevailing biological metaphor leads to the notion that any family not blood-related is "fictive," a substitute, family-like alternative to the "real" family—a father-headed, mother-supported, nuclear family with children. Weston (1991) suggests that all kinship is in some sense fictional—"that is, meaningfully constituted rather than 'out there' in a positivist sense" (p. 105). Genes and blood, then, are merely symbols "implicated in one culturally specific way of demarcating and calculating relationships" (p. 105).

The notion of biological family in the family field has been strengthened by structural and functional notions about how families should be organized, what their central roles and tasks are, and how they should be carried out. These templates are organized by age and sex. Central to structural conceptions of family are normative notions concerning hierarchy, internal and external boundaries, and degrees of separateness and connectedness. Both the feminist and postmodern critiques in family therapy have stimulated a reexamination of our assumptions about family structure and process, bringing history, the cultural context, and the politics of gender and heterosexual relationships into the theoretical and definitional arena.[2]

The current phenomenon of same-sex couples choosing and forming families, pioneering and innovating family forms in which legal marriage and heterosexual partnering and, in many cases, procreation, are not the organizing metaphors, like feminism, offers a rich resource for reexamining and perhaps reshaping family therapy assumptions about family and kinship. These families are generating new ideas not only about the formation and structure of families but also about how couples and families may operate as they pioneer new ways to conceptualize and practice parenting, couple relationships, and role and task divisions. With their relatively fluid boundaries and varied memberships, their patterns of nonhierarchical decision making, their innovative divisions of labor, and the relative weight given to friendship as well as blood relatedness, such families offer further challenge to dominant notions of family structure and function, and present an opportunity for mental health professionals to assess the limitations in current definitions of family and kinship.

Clearly, the long-standing silence about family diversity is being disturbed these days. In addition to an increasing focus on divorced, remarried, single-parent, multigenerational, cohabiting heterosexual, and other "nontraditional" family forms, more and more research and other scholarly work is becoming available on lesbian- or gay-headed families and their children. Most of this work, whether carried out by heterosexual, lesbian, gay, or bisexual researchers, is highly affirming of the relative success of gay family arrangements.

Research on gay and lesbian couples and families can teach us important things about all families—about couple satisfaction, egalitarianism, gender and sexuality relationships, creative parenting, children raised in nontraditional homes, adaptation to tensions in this society, and especially about strength and resilience (Anderson & Sussex, 1999). It is interesting that in spite of the still pervasive and profound stigmatization of gay life, lesbian and gay men are building stable and satisfying couple relationships and forming families that seem to be doing at least as well as other kinds of families in carrying out their sociologically defined family roles and tasks. In fact, some researchers are predicting that this will be the decade of the gay family. However, the fact that these families are still so marginalized makes it more difficult to study and describe them in the same manner as other nontraditional or alternative families. The bulk of lesbian and gay couple and family research focuses on couple relationships and satisfaction, lesbian mothers, and the well-being of children of (primarily) lesbian and gay parents. Most of these studies are quantitative in nature, and frequently use personality or self-assessment measures, exploring one or more characteristics of the couples or individuals of interest, and/or comparing lesbian and gay families or family members to heterosexual populations. The samples are usually small, and it has been extremely difficult to recruit cross-cultural or representative samples. Other sources, such as clinical case reports (e.g., Bepko & Johnson, 2000; Crawford, 1987, 1988; Goodrich, Rampage, Ellman, & Halstead, 1988; Krestan, 1988; Krestan & Bepko, 1980; Laird, 1988, 1989, 1993a, 1999; Roth, 1989; Roth & Murphy, 1986), journalistic accounts (Benkov, 1994; Miller, 1989), oral histories and indigenous accounts (Hall Carpenter Ardhives, 1989a, 1989b), culture and kinship studies (Herdt, 1992a; Weston, 1991), and qualitative studies take us inside the everyday lives of gay and lesbian families, giving us brief glimpses. A few ethnographic studies of gay and lesbian family life have appeared in recent years, providing a fuller sense of the complexity and richness of everyday life in these couples and families (e.g., Carrington, 1999; Lewin, 1993; Weston, 1996). Tasker and Golombok (1997), in the only longitudinal study to date, followed 25 individuals born in heterosexual unions to mothers who later entered lesbian relationships, from childhood to adulthood, comparing them with children raised in heterosexual-headed families.

While the rhetoric rages, on the one hand, the same-sex marriage movement gathers supporters and legal cases challenging traditional family forms, and norms proliferate; on the other hand, family values adherents step up their efforts to promote the "normal" family and to punish the aberrant family. In the midst of this cultural war, ordinary people continue to find unique and diverse ways of constructing families that they believe meet their needs and enhance their opportunities for personal fulfillment and for coping with the challenges of the complex and puzzling world of the 21st century. People are writing their own family narratives in spite of widespread pressure to return to the idealized and nostalgic "way we never were" (Coontz, 1992, Stacey, 1996). These narratives feed the flames of the debate over who has the right to define "family" and "normal family" in this society. It is the lesbian or gay family that finds itself at the very center of this national debate that, for a variety of reasons, heated up in the 1990s. In a sense, it is the lesbian (and thus fatherless) family that serves as the central scapegoat in guarding against family "breakup" and promoting the return of women to the home.

THE CURRENT SOCIAL POLICY CONTEXT

Local, state, and national governments, through social and family policies, determine the rights, rules, and benefits for families, thus sanctioning certain kinds of families and ignoring or actively discriminating against others (see Hartman, Chapter 23, this volume). For instance, President Bush's campaign to tie welfare benefits to legal heterosexual marriage is a powerful example of how the federal government can influence family formation, rewarding certain families at the expense of others. Similarly, states, communities, institutions, courts, corporations, and other structures can provide or withhold benefits and privileges such as employment, health insurance, or inheritance rights, in the process encouraging some family forms and discouraging others.

At the same time that the family values movement seems to gain more influence with recent changes in political power at the national level, lesbians and gay men are stepping up their battle for various kinds of civil rights and domestic benefits. The most dramatic and divisive initiative of the last decade has been the same-sex marriage movement, which has sparked a passionate public debate. The now famous Hawaii case, in which two couples sought but ultimately failed to win the right to marry, has nevertheless encouraged many other lesbians and gay men to seek to have their relationships legally and/or religiously sanctioned (Sullivan, 1997). Although lesbians and gays may have registered partnerships and child custody rights in some European nations and, in the Netherlands the right to legally marry, the closest we have come to similar rights in the United States is the controversial and still contested "civil union" legislation enacted in Vermont. When it looked for a period of time that the Hawaiian case for marriage rights might succeed, a powerful backlash developed. Some states enacted legislation banning the recognition of same-sex marriage, and in 1996, Congress quickly adopted, and President Clinton signed, the Defense of Marriage Act, which would allow Congress to override state marriage laws. Some consider this yet uncontested act unconstitutional. But the same-sex marriage cause has also served as a stimulus and justification for antigay stances taken by the family values, marriage, and fatherhood movements, efforts supported most vocally by not only the religious right and other ultraconservative groups but also by many centrists (Stacey, 1996). For example, no major candidate for President or Vice-President in the 2000 national election publicly supported same-sex marriage rights, a stance most consider political suicide. Marriage, it was proclaimed, should be reserved for the union between a man and a woman. This fiery and continuing national debate has nothing to do with the success, mental or social health, or social responsibility of lesbian or gay couples and their children. It has everything to do with cultural struggles over the meaning of "family," and protecting and preserving heterosexual marriage and the power of heterosexual fatherhood.

Another lively policy issue at the beginning of the new millenium is gay adoption, most recently endorsed by the prestigious American Academy of Pediatrics (Tanner, 2002). At present, approximately half the states allow gay adoption, whereas a few expressly forbid it.

IS THE LESBIAN OR GAY FAMILY A "THREAT"?

Before the late 1970s, most gay and lesbian families with children were headed by men and women whose children had been born or adopted in a heterosexual marriage or coupling. Then, lesbians began to *choose* to give birth to and adopt children outside the context of legal marriage. Gradually, news of a "lesbian baby boom" has trickled into the media, as increasing numbers of lesbians, with or without partners, have chosen to have children (Patterson, 1992). This phenomenon poses a major contradiction to the widely accepted notion that every child needs a father and undoubtedly has helped to fuel the "fatherhood" and family values movements. Some gay men are serving as custodial parents for their children, a few have been able to adopt, and a smaller number have successfully engaged surrogate mothers to bear their children.

Actually, in terms of sheer numbers, how much of a "threat" is the lesbian and gay family? Scholars for years have been making widely variant estimates on the numbers of lesbians, gay men, and children of gay or lesbian parents. Estimates range from 1 to 5 million lesbian mothers and 1 to 3 million gay fathers, and various researchers have posited anywhere from 6 to 14 million children of lesbian or gay parents (cf. Patterson, 1996). But these numbers are highly speculative, because the gay population has been virtually unidentified and uncounted in the U.S. census. The 1996 Federal Defense of Marriage Act (H.R. 3396) instructs all federal agencies to recognize only opposite-sex marriages for the purposes of enacting any agency programs, including the national census. Thus, those responses that indicate same-sex spouse were invalidated in the 1990 and 2000 censuses. However, in the 2000 census, these responses were reallocated to the "unmarried partner" category. In conjunction with an additional question regarding the sex of the unmarried partner, it begins to be possible to estimate roughly the number of gay households. There is no way of knowing just how accurate these figures are, but for the first time, gay and lesbian couples are being counted in some fashion. Whatever the numbers, it is clear that gay and lesbian expressions of family and kinship are having profound effects on the larger society's construction of these categories (Weston, 1991).

LESBIAN AND GAY FAMILIES IN SPACE AND TIME

The next sections are organized using a time–space diagram (see Figure 7.1) that also served as the organizing conception for an earlier work (Hartman & Laird, 1983). First, I comment on the larger social and cultural contexts in which gays and lesbians have been and are defined by others and by themselves.

Second, gay and lesbian families, like all families, are viewed intergenerationally. Each family member is influenced by and must come to terms with the specific history and culture of his or her own family of origin in its

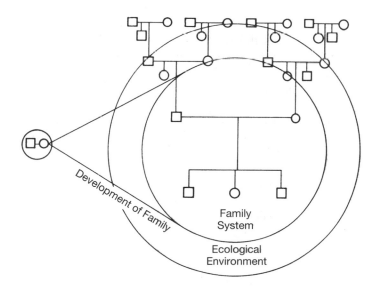

FIGURE 7.1. The family in space and time. From Hartman and Laird (1983, p. 113). Copyright 1983 by The Free Press, a Division of Macmillan, Inc. Reprinted by permission.

sociocultural context. Each new family must determine how it will fit on the extended family tree and how it will negotiate family-of-origin issues. This can be particularly difficult, complex, and painful when neither legal nor biological relationships, prevailing determinants of family relatedness, constitute necessary norms for gay or lesbian coupling or parenthood.

Third, in family therapy, life-cycle "stage" theories have been central (e.g., Carter & McGoldrick, 1999). These metaphors have dominated study of individual gay and lesbian identity and development as well, especially around the phenomenon of "coming out." Some attention has more recently turned to the life cycle of the gay couple and of the lesbian family. Is the life-cycle model useful, and what are its limitations for describing the life course of gay and lesbian families?

Then, moving inside the lesbian and gay family, some of the dimensions and metaphors that have been of interest to family theorists are considered. What can we say at present about family structure and process, and about how these families are doing? How relevant are concepts such as boundary, enmeshment, fusion, and cohesion? What can these families teach us about heterosexual families, about gender identity and relationships? About courage under fire and resilience? Do such families have special strengths? Do they have unique kinds of problems? The chapter concludes with a brief commentary on what I see as current practice and research priorities.

SOCIOCULTURAL CONTEXT

In the previous edition of this volume, I discussed whether homosexuality should be viewed as an essential or constructed identity (Laird, 1993a). Whether or not that controversial debate will ever be resolved, it is clear that whatever biological predispositions for homosexuality may eventually be found, biology is always shaped and experienced in social context. From a narrative/constructionist point of view, once persons at any age find themselves attracted sexually to members of the same sex or engage in sexual relations, they begin to seek understanding and to give meaning to these experiences. Some would argue that experiences or events have no meanings until they are named or given language. Once the label "gay" or "lesbian" or "homosexual" is attached to such experiences, individuals may recast their pasts, restorying their self-narratives to make sense of current feelings, thoughts, and behaviors. Thus, the typical adolescent "crush" of a young girl for her female teacher may become reconstructed in young adulthood as "an early lesbian attraction." Whether or not we believe that homosexuality is an "essential" part of being, or a personal narrative that can only be understood in historical and sociocultural context, many of those who identify themselves as lesbian or gay see homosexuality as a core, fundamental, or essential part of their being, of "who they really are." For many, it does not seem a matter of choice or political belief, but rather a matter of "accepting" and coming to terms with the inevitable, of developing strategies for survival.

However, it is clear that gays and lesbians are as diverse in their individual adaptations and cultural performances as heterosexuals. What virtually every researcher sympathetic to and affirming of gay and lesbian identity and behavior seems to agree upon is the importance of addressing the influences of societal homophobia and heterosexism in terms of their impact on individual psychological and familial functioning. Although certain patterns of cultural or subcultural expression may be observed and certain patterns of stress and adaptation traced, not only do individuals and families experience and cope with societal homophobia differently, but there is also increasing evidence that time and space are crucial variables in the making of the American gay or lesbian. In other words, in contrast to the focus on identity and coming out, Herdt (1992b) believes that the more important and neglected questions are (1) What does a gay man [or lesbian] come out *to?* and (2) What does a gay man [or lesbian] come out *to be?*

In his view, being gay signifies identity and role, familiar notions, but more than that, a "distinctive system of rules, norms, attitudes . . . and beliefs from which the culture of gay men is made, a culture that sustains the social relations of same-sex desire" (p. 5). Gay, in his view, can no longer be seen as merely a sexual matter, or a lifestyle, or an enclave.

The Gay Liberation Movement and the gradual rise of cultural symbols and institutions (music and music festivals, bookstores, local and national newspapers and periodicals, films, plays, community and social groups, centers for gay adolescents, social networks, the Gay Pride Day March, and so on) signal the rise of not only a sense of *communitas*, or of *Gemeinschaft*, but also of a larger national culture, or *Gesellschaft*. Interestingly, AIDS has had an important role in welding together gay men and lesbians into a common cause, part of the crystallization of "a new moral order of gay prosocial attitudes and political activism across the country" (Herdt, 1992b, p. 11). These and other changes are making possible a meaningful and rich cultural life to come out to, a life course for the lesbian and the gay man, and presumably for the lesbian and the gay family as well, that will be quite different from the possibilities just a generation ago (Faderman, 1991).

Furthermore, gay and lesbian couples and families may have very different experiences depending on factors such as the culture and availability of gay and lesbian communities, their ethnic and family-of-origin ties and loyalties, and their social class positions. Some lesbian and gay couples and families live in (and, contrary to conventional wisdom, are quite contented and well functioning) cultural milieus that are almost entirely heterosexual and afford little access to the symbols and organizations of gay community. The latter may be for some an assimilationist choice. At the other extreme, some lesbian and gay families may choose to locate in areas with very strong lesbian or gay communities, adopting a more separatist strategy and socializing almost exclusively with other gays and lesbians. Krieger (1982) argued that, at times, lesbian (and presumably gay male) communities can threaten as well as affirm individual identity. Like all communities, groups, and families, they can provide a haven from a hostile or nonaccepting outside world, or they can constrain individuality in their zeal for political unity.

Gay families vary tremendously in how they live and story their lives. For example, Lynch (1992), in his study of "nonghetto" gays, found that suburban homosexuals were more circumspect, more fearful of exposure, anticipated more intolerance and discrimination, and had fewer homosexual relations, less homosexual sex, less social involvement with homosexuals, and more social involvements with heterosexuals than their urban counterparts. Although the same-sex behaviors of black men and women have rarely been studied (the overwhelming profile of the subject in most research has been the young, white, well-educated, middle-class male), there seems to be widespread agreement that there are even stronger anti-homosexual attitudes in groups oppressed on the basis of color (Greene & Boyd-Franklin, 1996, Liu & Chan, 1996; Morales, 1996). Peterson (1992) finds no distinct gay culture in the black community and suggests that many black men experience racism and prejudice not only from the larger society but also in the white gay community. Oppressed ethnic minorities confront troubling conflict between their ethnic loyalties and their sexual orientations; to endorse gay identity may mean to betray ethnic and family loyalties.

One other issue should be addressed here. It is common to argue that gay and lesbian individuals and families have no role models, no guidelines or social prescriptions for how to live their lives. It seems to me that two assumptions are implicit in this stance. The first is that gays and lesbians somehow cast off or eschew American culture or are *different* cultural beings from heterosexuals. In my view, to take this stance is to make what Hare-Mustin (1987) terms the "alpha error," that is, in this case, to exaggerate the differences between gay persons and their heterosexual counterparts. Most gay men and lesbians are raised in families headed by opposite-sex parents, where they are taught to be males and females, and to embrace American cultural values, as well as the norms and beliefs in their particular families, religions, and ethnic groups—what might be called "family culture." Their families of origin and the families they form must deal with all the same issues as any family, as is powerfully documented in the Blumstein and Schwartz (1983) study of American couples.

Although gay culture is frequently contrasted to American "heterosexual" culture, to adopt gay symbols, to join gay organizations, to identify to self and others as gay is not to abandon American culture. Heterosexuals do not "own" American culture, and gay families, like other families, crosscut all social classes, ethnic and religious groups, and political affiliations, mixing gay symbols with many of the same symbols and ritual aspects important to most American families. Lesbian and gay couples may reject some of the more traditional notions of gender roles learned in their families of origin, as do many heterosexual couples, but they carry on other family traditions, relational patterns, parenting models, and values about morality or politics or career choices. Like many heterosexual American couples these days, gay and lesbian families are searching for new ways to make families work, to share home and career responsibilities, and are questioning traditional ways of handling money, sex, and power. If lesbian couples are in the midst of a "baby boom" and are organizing their families around child rearing, many heterosexual couples today are choosing *not* to marry or have children. In other words, "choice" rather than "tradition" has become the clarion call for both straights and gays; heterosexual couples, too, perhaps as a response to geographic dispersal, have formed extended families and social support networks based on friendship and common interests. Lukes and Land (1990) suggest that the concept of "biculturality" (or multiculturality) offers a more useful construction in thinking about gay and lesbian culture than "difference."

Furthermore, gay and lesbian communities are just as diverse as other kinds of communities; it is crucial not to assume from experience with one community that we understand gay or lesbian "culture" or "norms" for all such communities, or that all gays or lesbians in a particular community are similarly encultured to what seem to be local gay or lesbian cultural norms. Differences are mediated by class, gender, ethnicity, historical experience, and other sociocultural variables. As clinicians, it is essential to understand overarching cultural themes for gays and lesbians, the particular community context in which our clients live, as well as their relationships with that community. Gay culture, like all culture, is emergent, improvised, performed, and always changing (Laird, 1998).

Many students of gay and lesbian life have argued that the lack of accessible gay and lesbian models casts gay individuals and families adrift, without any stars or charts to follow. Many lesbians and gays, however, are actively involved in their communities and move easily back and forth between their gay networks and extended kinship groups, and the larger community. In one sense, gay and lesbian families may be freer to choose from the best of both the straight and gay worlds, innovating in those areas where neither community practices nor family traditions meet their visions. The Gay and Lesbian Movement, like the Black Pride Movement, at times has had an investment in highlighting and maintaining "difference," and has gone through several different phases in defining "political correctness." In the early days of the modern Women's Movement, radical lesbian feminists tended to see forming families with children and even coupling as imitations of oppressive, patriarchal, heterosexual marriage. Lesbian single mothers or couples with children often found themselves unwelcome in certain gay communities. Whatever the political pulls and community pressures, it is likely that for many gay and lesbian people, gay culture is only one of many resources, albeit an important one, for anchoring one's identity and for seeking cultural guidance.

THE FAMILY OVER TIME

How then, if many of these families are not bound by legal marriage or organized by biological procreation and parenting, are we to understand them in intergenerational terms? What is the meaning of "family of origin," and how important are blood relationships? For some time, biological metaphors dominated family therapy theory, particularly in Bowen's (1978) central concepts of "differentiation" and "fusion," and his "family of origin" theory, where blood/origin relationships imply great power throughout life. Individual and family problems are attributed to lack of sufficient differentiation, and therapy focuses on becoming "unstuck," or at least less stuck, in the undifferentiated family ego mass. There is little room in the original theory for considering more fluid notions of family organized by choice and constructed in various ways, for such families question the primacy of the biological metaphor.

A second assumption implicit in family theory has to do not only with the power but also the importance of the blood family. It is assumed that people *need* their families of origin. Loyalty and cohesiveness are fostered through this discourse; blood families are seen as crucial to survival for the child and retain their emotional power over the adult. As an individual, it is believed one must come to terms with the family of origin, if only to rid oneself of troubling emotional baggage, and the couple must renegotiate relationships and boundaries with both families of origin (Bowen, 1978; Carter & McGoldrick, 1999; Hartman & Laird, 1983). Many gays and lesbians living with partners for many years are still defined as single by their families, their families of choice unrecognized in a homophobic silence that serves to obliterate the competition for the loyalty of a son or daughter.

"Coming out" to self and others has been seen as essential to the development of a coherent sense of self, of self-esteem, and of healthy homosexuality, so "coming out" to family has also been seen as essential to the gay family. Certainly, much of the clinical and indigenous literature on relationships between gays and lesbians and their families of origin is replete with stories of harsh and rejecting responses of parents to their children's gay sexual orientation and choice of relationships (Saghir & Robins, 1973; Chafetz, Sampson, Beck, & West, 1974; Savin-Williams, 1996). Some gay persons have been "disowned," whereas others have had to make serious personal compromises and relational sacrifices in order to maintain their contact with parents, siblings, and other family-of-origin members. Even with increased visibility and acceptance, it is still the case that many choose to keep their sexual identities secret from the family of origin, whereas others make tacit agreements not to talk about it and to keep that part of their lives entirely separate. This conspiracy of denial, many believe, may preserve family harmony and maintain connection, but it can dilute intimacy and undermine authenticity in family relationships. In some cases, it may allow the family of origin to tyrannize its adult offspring emotionally and may exact heavy costs to the psychological well-being and personal integrity of the gay child or adult.

It is not clear, however, that we "need" our families of origin to function well, or that emotional cutoffs from families doom us to loneliness and isolation, haunted by invisible loyalties and stuck in the undifferentiated family ego mass. Recent researchers have begun to challenge some of these assumptions. For example, Green, Bettinger, and Zacks (1996), in a 2-year longitudinal study of 48 lesbian couples, found that whether or not partners were out to family-of-origin members was unrelated to couple satisfaction at the beginning or end of the period under study. Nor did satisfaction vary between couples who stayed together and those who separated. Savin-Williams (2001) found that whereas 10 to 15% of parents reject their child, 70 to 75% show varying degrees of acceptance, and the rest become fully accepting. Green and Mitchell (2002) are critical of the prevalent notion in family theory that it is necessarily healthy for lesbian and gay clients to come out to their families of origin. As they argue, there can be many constructive reasons for maintaining secrecy, which may have to do with sociocultural issues of ethnic identity and community, physical safety, economic survival, or significant differences in fundamental values. Secrecy and silence are not always negative or destructive phenomena, but may be indicative of personal strength or part of a strategy for being true to one's own life narrative. Ponse (1978), for example, argues for the importance of secrecy to the very existence and cohesiveness of many lesbian communities, whereas Laird (1993b, 1998) maintains that secrecy for lesbians can serve the important purposes of fostering a common language and traditions, and a sense of "we-ness" or specialness. Secrecy, used by resistance movements everywhere, is often needed to help combat oppression.

Although the family of origin is an important part of the context surrounding gays and lesbians and is also important in understanding individual, couple, and family dynamics, it should be pointed out that we know very little about the ways that gay and lesbian offspring who do defy their families' proscriptions and do incur rejection forge their lives apart from their families. Can the friendship networks and innovative kinship systems many gays and lesbians build offer a context for not only familiness but also continued personal growth? Kurdek (1988), based on his study of the perceived social supports of gay and lesbian couples, concludes that partners and friends, not family-of-origin members, are the primary providers of support for most gays and lesbians, a conclusion supported by Levy's (1989) research. Kurdek and Schmitt (1987) also found that the frequency of support from family members was not related to the psychological adjustment of the gay or lesbian. In the Savin-Williams (1989) study of 317 gay and lesbian youths, a lesbian was more comfortable with her sexual orientation if her parents accepted her homosexuality, but these variables did not predict her level of self-esteem. Among gay males, parental acceptance predicted the gay youth's comfort with his sexual orientation only if the parents were perceived as important components of his self-worth. Family rifts and emotional cutoffs occur for many reasons. As Friedman (1988) points out, the family's rejection of a child's choice of partner or spouse for reasons of religion or ethnicity can camouflage efforts to keep a son or daughter closely bound. Homosexuality also offers a convenient excuse for demanding such loyalty.

My own ethnographic interviews with a nonclinical sample of 19 lesbians of widely varying ages, as well as many years of clinical and personal experience, suggest that lesbians develop any number of creative strategies for dealing with homophobic and rejecting families, without necessarily sacrificing their own integrity. Some lesbians very consciously choose to allow a certain level of family denial; they accept it and dislike it but do not let it or family emotional distance dominate their lives. There is reason to believe that for many, the process of constructing a lesbian identity and facing the adversities of family outrage and community homophobia can be enriching and strengthening. Perhaps to take the path less traveled can widen one's intellectual and emotional horizons, as those who study resilience have learned. None of the women I interviewed was completely cut off from family of origin, and some enjoyed close and accepting relationships. Nevertheless, several wished their families were more accepting and even overtly proud of their lesbian choices. But these women, without exception, have constructed narratives to explain their relationships and uses of language with their blood families that are not self-shaming or self-blaming. They believe they have made good choices and regret that their families cannot be more joyful about their lives (Laird, 1996).

Several students of gay and lesbian families have noted that families mourn multiple losses when their children declare a gay orientation (e.g., Sanders, 1993), including mourning the loss of some of the dreams and expectations they may have had for their children and themselves, based on the assumed heterosexuality of their children, such as a long-held wish for a son- or daughter-in-law, or grandchildren. Their stories about their gay children must be stringently edited in a homophobic world, and they must make difficult decisions about how to explain that man standing next to their son in the family photo album. Ordinary kinship language will not suffice. Many gays and lesbians who have children from former heterosexual partnerships, or lesbians who choose to have biological children with a known or unknown donor, or to adopt, have found that the lure of the grandchildren often helps to soften family homophobia, linking family of blood and family of choice (Lewin, 1993). In some cases, the nonbiological grandparents maintain close relationships with the grandchildren even after a lesbian couple has separated.

Families of origin also live in a sociocultural context that is heterosexist and homophobic. Most loving parents want to accept their gay children, but many face their own confusion and homophobia, and may feel responsible, blaming themselves for their child's sexual identity. Some may even feel contaminated by the offspring's homosexuality. Most families of origin do not have the same kind of "alternative" cultures or extended support networks that their gay or lesbian offspring can turn to in times of stress; they often have no one with whom they can share their confusion and hurt. Indeed, many face church condemnation, and some may be actively shunned by others, a particularly painful experience for parents of HIV-infected gay men, who may be ostracized from the very communities whose support they desperately need.

Two of the many ways families socialize their young are through family story and ritual. Imber-Black (1989), Laird (1988), Roth (1989), and Slater and Mencher (1991) have pointed out that many of our most important cultural rituals and celebrations are not easily available to gays and lesbians, and, frequently, the creative rituals they devise are not enacted in conjunction with families of origin or in contexts of societal recognition and support. Furthermore, women's stories and the narrative genres available to women in general and lesbians in particular are constrained in patriarchal societies and in the patriarchal family (Laird, 1989). Lesbians and gay men may feel extremely invisible and isolated at heterosexual rituals such as weddings or anniversary parties, but at the same time, gay cultural experiences are typically not shared or celebrated in or with families of origin. Thus, it seems important to ask what place gays and lesbians, and *their* new couple and family experiences occupy in the ongoing ritual life, folklore, and mythology of the extended family. Do their cultural experiences become part of the larger biological family folklore? Or does the gay–lesbian branch break off the family tree? Increasingly, lesbian and gay couples are having public commitment ceremonies and other kinds of family-only and more public ritual celebrations that include family-of-origin members, as well as creating new rituals characterized as gay or lesbian, whereas some families are becoming more sensitive to and changing the heterosexist languages and practices in many rituals. Lesbian and gay rituals usually draw upon, incorporate, and revise symbols and practices from larger cultural traditions, religious or spiritual beliefs, and so on, as well as include new elements that reforge their ritual lives in ways that are gay affirming and even transformative.

THE FAMILY LIFE CYCLE

Stage and life cycle theories, central in individual developmental theory and in family therapy (e.g., Carter & McGoldrick, 1999), have also been central in gay and lesbian studies. The "coming out" process (the evolution of an individual's gay identity), the stages of couple development, the stages that families learning they have a gay child go through and, most recently, the lesbian family life cycle have all been scrutinized using a "stage" conception.

DeVine (1984) posited a five-stage developmental model to explain the systemic changes families undergo as they try to cope with their children's homosexual preferences. He argues that the family experiences a crisis that destabilizes its equilibrium. In the first three stages, which he labels subliminal awareness, impact, and adjustment, the family attempts to maintain some level of homeostasis. In the last two stages, the family moves toward resolution and integration, meaning that it changes its structure to accommodate the life-cycle movements of the focal member. Outcomes depend on, he believes, the degree of family cohesion, the nature of its regulative structure, and particular family themes. Herdt and Koff (2000) have written a useful guide for families on the road they travel when a child is gay.

Slater and Mencher (1991) applied family life-cycle notions to what they term the "lesbian family life cycle." Pointing out that Carter and McGoldrick's original conception of the family life cycle is child-centered and occurs in a context of social validation and support, they argue that the lesbian life cycle is typically and traditionally not child-centered and not affirmed in the larger society. Although they believe that lesbian family life experience may parallel heterosexual experiences in some ways, they see the lesbian family as largely bereft of useful role models. This, then, is a situation that can at times lead to greater flexibility, liberating the couple from more rigid constraints on role performance, but one that may introduce more uncertainty and complexity into role negotiation.

Just as gay and lesbian family life-cycle models are making their way into the family therapy literature, stage models in general, and gay and lesbian life cycle models in particular, are coming under increasing criticism. Sophie (1985/1986), for example, examined six theories of lesbian identity development through repeated interviews with 14 women undergoing change with respect to their sexual orientation. She found some support for a general stage theory but also marked discrepancies, concluding that the process of lesbian identity development is highly sensitive to the social/historical context.

Historian Lillian Faderman (1984/1985) argued that Minton and McDonald's (1983/1984) three-stage model of progression toward homosexual identity did not generally fit lesbian experience. She believes that the process for women who came out through the radical feminist movement occurred in reverse order; coming out is highly influenced by historical circumstance. Many women came to view heterosexuality as detrimental to their freedom, often assuming a lesbian identity before they had had a lesbian sexual experience. In their discussion of the "coming out" of gay and lesbian youth today, Boxer and Cohler (1989) questioned the validity of developmental research in general. Most such research relies on respondents' recollections of their childhood and adolescence, leading to a "developmental psychology of the remembered past" (p. 316). Much of the research, they argue, fails to account for the discontinuities and changes that characterize the lives of many gay and lesbian adults, and the changing social contexts that "dramatically affect the lives of persons within a specific generation or age-linked cohort" (p. 319). Boxer and Cohler believe that the issues of vulnerability and resistance, that is, the capacity of gay and lesbian youth to remain resilient when confronted by adverse circumstances, are crucial to understanding the life course. Predictive approaches must

> be complemented by a narrative or interpretive approach that is concerned with the manner in which persons experience and interpret or "make sense" of these life changes. Little is known of the manner in which persons create a narrative that renders adversity coherent in terms of experienced life history, or the manner in which presently constructed meanings of life changes may be altered in order to maintain a sense of personal integration. . . . For some persons, the experience of adverse life events may be used as an explanation for the failure to realize personal goals. For others, this misfortune becomes the impetus for increased effort in order to attain these goals. (pp. 319–320)

Longitudinal studies show that lives are not as predictable over time as often assumed. Age, without cultural and historical knowledge, is an "empty" variable in the study of lives.

Modernist views of "coming out" contain the essentialist notion that there is a closeted, "real" homosexual self that the individual must come to recognize and accept. Interestingly, the bisexual is often defined as someone who has not accepted his or her real, homosexual self, even though his or her heterosexual experiences may be emotionally and sexually satisfying and may predominate. Several decades of literature on "coming out" in marriage encouraged the view that heterosexually married people who have same-sex sexual or emotional relationships need to work toward embracing their "true" homosexual selves. Modernist views of self and sexuality, however, ignore the fact that many people change their sexual orientations and sexual habits over time, and many are equally comfortable, in differing ways, in emotional and sexual relationships with same- or opposite-sex partners (Kitzinger & Wilkinson, 1997; Tiefer, 1995). In postmodern thought, the "self" is seen as socially constructed, an ongoing and changing narrative (Gergen, 1991); thus, the main issues for heterosexually partnered couples in which one may have same-sex attractions may have far more to do with their views of relationship and partnership, of monogamy and nonmonogamy, and their meanings of commitment rather than a revelation of a new core sexual self.

Families hand down much more than particular family structures or heterosexist role divisions. Has the heritage of the traditional heterosexual couple been lost when a child chooses a gay or lesbian family, any more than when a heterosexual adult child chooses to remain single or becomes divorced or adopts children? Or when their heterosexual children experiment with new and more flexible balances of home and work lives? Must we either be identical to our parents or repudiate all of their teachings? It is far more likely that gays and lesbians, like everyone else, emerge from their families, taking with them some blend of the life patterns and values with which they have grown up. A gay man may not choose to form his most intimate relationship with someone just like Mom but, on the other hand, he may choose someone sensitive, flexible, resilient, and assertive like his mother, and socially conscious and risk-taking like his father. And, if he has children, he may consider these important qualities to hand down the generations.

Although stage models can contribute to our knowledge of gay and lesbian family culture, it is important to point out that there are enormous differences in the social, historical, and community contexts in which gays have formed and are forming families, that gays come out at widely varying ages over the life span, and that there are also wide variations in family pattern, form, and membership. It is challenging even to map who is inside and who is outside in some gay and lesbian families, for example. More useful will be a search for the unique narratives such families construct to give meaning to their lives, longitudinal studies that capture changes over time as the social context changes, descriptions of the varied and complex ways they go about family life, and especially the strategies they develop to cope with homophobia and heterosexism. It is important to *begin* with the gay and lesbian experience in all of its many variations.

INSIDE THE FAMILY

Lesbian and Gay Couples

Lesbian and gay couples and families are in most respects like all families. They must negotiate their relationships with the larger community and their families of origin, forging social networks and establishing boundaries between themselves and the outside world, as well as negotiating relationships and roles, developing problem-solving strategies, mediating conflicts, and marking boundaries inside the family. They must decide who will do what, when, where, and how, in order to meet the particular needs of the family as a whole and of individual family members, whose interests at times may conflict or compete. Like all families, they face possibilities for conflict over divisions of labor; the use of money, space, and time; their sexual and intimate relationships; and issues of closeness and distance, dominance and subordination, child-rearing ideologies, and so on.

However, these families differ from others in at least two important ways. First, they are usually headed by solo parents who identify as lesbian or gay, or are headed by same-sex couples. Some contain multiple parenting figures; and some may include close friends who are not sexually involved with each other, grandparents, and biological or nonbiological children. Same-sex couples with children from former marriages resemble stepfamilies and encounter many of the same special issues, whereas gay and lesbian families headed by single parents face the same shortage of resources as most single-parent families do. Second, these families function in a world that may not recognize or accept their family commitment and definition, and must manage a "spoiled identity" (Goffman, 1963).

A number of researchers have compared same-sex couples to heterosexual and/or cohabiting couples along a number of relationship dimensions. Such research, presumably, can shed light not only on what same-sex "marriage" relationships are like but, as Blumstein and Schwartz (1983), Carrington (1999), Green, Bettinger, and Zacks (1996), Kurdek and Schmitt (1987), and others have pointed out, can also highlight the effects of gender on relationship quality. The most comprehensive research project on American couples was carried out by Philip Blumstein and Pepper Schwartz (1983) two decades ago. They studied heterosexual married, heterosexual cohabiting, gay male, and lesbian couples along the dimensions of money, sex, and power. Using both quantitative and qualitative data (over 12,000 returned questionnaires, as well as intensive interviews with 300 couples), they investigated the relational complexities in these marital and nonmarital family forms. They found many similarities across family forms. What *American Couples* achieves is a close and comprehensive look at how gender and sexual orientation affect the ways couples choose to live their lives, the kinds of rewards they encounter, the problems they confront, and the problem-solving strategies they adopt. Blumstein and Schwartz conclude, as we might suspect, that there are many coupling issues in which gender "sameness" can be valuable and other areas in which it can generate problems. Similarly, the issue of gender "differentness" can enrich a couple's life or tear it asunder. For example, Gottman and Levenson (1999) find that same-sex couples handle conflicts better than similar heterosexual couples, whereas Zacks, Green, and Marrow (1988) find that lesbian couples have significantly higher levels of cohesion and adaptability than heterosexual couples. Because heterosexual marriage is considered the norm, it offers social rules, rituals, standards, and practices, as well as social sanctions for continuance. These aspects help to "keep people together and help to make an orderly exit if the relationship ends" (Blumstein & Schwartz, 1983, p. 318). Lesbian and gay cultures contain no such clear prescriptions, except perhaps a common emphasis on egalitarianism. Green and Mitchell (2002) apply Boss's (1999) concepts of "boundary ambiguity" and "ambiguous loss" to the kinds of challenges of ambiguity that lesbian and gay individuals and couples face. For instance, they lack timetables, clear rules, or public or even private ritual marking for transitions to committing or dissolving a relationship. It is amazing, then, that lesbian and gay couple relationships are as stable as they are.

Many issues of interest concerning lesbian and gay families might be discussed here. I briefly address three issues that are prominent in mythology, clinical reporting, and research: fusion in lesbian couples, monogamy or sexual promiscuity in gay male households, and role division, or what Carrington (1999) calls "the myth of egalitarianism."

Fusion in Lesbian Couples

For a long time, scholars and clinicians seemed to agree that "fusion," defined by Burch (1982, 1986) as a state of psychic unity in which ego boundaries are crossed and two individuals experience a sense of oneness, and by Karpel (1976) as undifferentiation within the relational context, was the predominant relational quality in lesbian relationships. Merger or fusion is seen as an important part of sexual and emotional intimacy, but it has also been marked as the primary cause of tension and conflict. Writers differ, however, on what they see as the root causes of fusion. Krestan and Bepko (1980), in their pioneering paper, hypothesized that because the larger society both stigmatizes the relationship and fails to respect couple boundaries, lesbian couples "tend to rigidify those boundaries further and to turn in on themselves, adopting what has been described as a 'two against a threatening world' posture" (p. 278). They also introduce the notion that because women have been socialized to deny self, neither partner in a lesbian couple "has had much practice at self-definition and autonomy in a relational context" (p. 284). Fusion, in turn, is blamed for diminishing sexual interest, many other relationship difficulties, and the major cause of relationship termination.

Several scholars have argued that the norms for relationship and sexuality are primarily male-dominated; thus, the emotional intensity of female–female relationships can be misunderstood or interpreted pathologically, when in fact it may be normative for female couples. Goodrich et al. (1988) pointed out that the concept of fusion is highly gendered, arguing that lesbian couples intend a different relational vision, one based not on power politics, but on intimacy, mutuality, interdependence, and equality. Mencher (1990) takes the argument a step further, grounding the notion of fusion in contemporary self-in-relation theories of women's development and relational capacities, and casting a more positive, strengths-oriented light on the meaning of fusion in lesbian relationships. The very qualities that are pathologized, such as intense intimacy, are often seen by lesbians themselves as relational advantages, creating a greater sense of safety and trust, and thus greater self-actualization and risk taking. To the best of my knowledge, there is no definitive research on fusion levels in lesbian couples, and no clear notion of what levels of fusion or differentiation may be normative for couples in general or lesbian couples in particular.

Monogamy

If the specter of fusion and myths about women's sexuality haunt the thinking on lesbian relationships, the gay couple is tainted by social images that portray gay males as promiscuous, flamboyant, and bar hopping; couplehood itself is an anomaly. Several researchers have attempted to move beyond the stereotypes, examining more closely what the relationships and sexual behaviors of gay male couples are like. For example, McWhirter and Mattison (1984), who studied 156 couples from the San Diego area, concluded that "openness" in terms of extracouple relationships seemed to enhance couple longevity, because all of the couples together longer than 5 years had open relationships. Harry (1984), studying a large sample of gay men (774) in Chicago, found similar patterns, whereas Bell and Weinberg (1978), who compared closed and open couples from San Francisco, found that open couples attributed more importance to the partner, were more liberal politically, and had higher rates of self-acceptance. Peplau and Cochrane (1981) found no differences between open and closed couples together 3 years or longer in terms of intimacy, satisfaction, security, or commitment, and Kurdek and Schmitt (1985), who compared gay men in monogamous and nonmonogamous relationships, found more longevity in open relationships but no differences in psychological adjustment.

Ideas such as promiscuity or monogamy are concepts that are highly value laden. What is important is what these concepts mean to the couples themselves. For some couples, an extracouple sexual encounter or affair may feel like the ultimate betrayal; for others, it may be interpreted as an experience that has little to do with and does not contaminate the couple relationship. Blumstein and Schwartz (1983) concluded that women, whether in heterosexual marriage, cohabiting, or same-sex couples, have fewer outside partners than men. Thirty-three percent of the heterosexual men and 82% of the gay males in their sample had been nonmonogamous since the beginning of the relationship compared to 26% of cohabiting women, 21% of married women, and 28% of lesbians. Although lesbians had been slightly less monogamous than female cohabitors or marrieds, they had had fewer outside partners than any of the other groups, their affairs often a one-time event or single affair. Gay men, Blumstein and

Schwartz report, do commonly have sex with strangers. What they call the "trick mentality" has been a social institution within the gay male world for a long time. Tricking allows men to have sex without emotional involvement—one reason, in their opinion, that gay male couples can tolerate very high rates of nonmonogamy without serious threat to the relationship. Outside sex is not related to gay men's overall happiness or commitment to the relationship. However, Green and Mitchell (2002) point out that a large number of gay men do have monogamous relationships and view extrarelational sex as betrayal. They cite a recent study (Campbell, 2000) in which 70% of gay male partners reported being in a monogamous relationship. There is some evidence that AIDS has fostered a move toward more monogamy and longevity in gay relationships. Forstein (1986) and Herdt (1992b) are among those who have pointed out that AIDS has shaped a trend toward more sexual exclusivity and more stability in gay male couple relationships.

Two prominent changes have occurred in lesbian political and cultural norms over the last two decades. Many lesbians, distancing from earlier antifamily feminism, have increasingly chosen to birth or adopt children either as single women or in the context of lesbian couplehood. Other (particularly younger) lesbians have revitalized the antimonogamy stance, arguing against monogamy as the emblem of patriarchy, and are endorsing concurrent relationships with multiple partners of the same or opposite sex.

Egalitarianism

It has been commonly assumed that the outstanding feature of lesbian and gay relationships is egalitarianism, that is, a relatively equal division of labor inside and outside of the home. Blumstein and Schwartz (1983) concluded that lesbians "[were in] the vanguard in changing women's roles in the 1980s" (p. 329). Like most women, they value companionship and they want their relationships at the center of their lives. They do not wish either to dominate or to be dependent or subordinate; they want their partners to share both domestic life and work, and to succeed in the outside world of work. Carrington (1999) offers a different view: that egalitarianism in lesbian and gay families is to some extent a myth, and that couples develop narratives that camouflage the actual inequalities and differences to conform to larger social notions of femininity and masculinity. Who does what in lesbian and gay families, he finds, varies significantly by class, gender, race, geographic location, and other variables.

CHILDREN OF LESBIAN AND GAY PARENTS[3]

The last two decades have also brought a substantial number of studies devoted to the psychological growth and social adjustment of children of gay parents. Patterson (1996), in a comprehensive review of this research, suggests that this trend has been motivated by several factors, including (1) the need on the part of gays and lesbians considering parenthood to understand the issues and challenges they may face, (2) the concerns of social scientists with how such families and their children cope with oppression, (3) the impact of this nontraditional family form on psychosocial development, and (4) the provision of more accurate information to a legal system that has been uneven at best and discriminatory at worst in determining the fates of lesbian and gay parents and their children.

Estimates of how many children live with lesbian or gay parents fluctuate widely, from 6 to 14 million. In a recent statement supporting second-parent adoption in lesbian and gay families, the American Academy of Pediatrics (Tanner, 2002) reported that as many as 9 million children in the United States have at least one gay parent. There is some reason to believe that, with greater visibility, changes in the politics of family in the lesbian and gay community, the current "lesbian baby boom" (Patterson, 1991), and advances in reproductive technology, these figures will continue to increase. Yet, as Stacey and Biblarz (2001) point out, with more people coming out at earlier ages, it is also possible that fewer lesbian and gay persons will be pressured into marriage, a trend that could reduce the actual numbers of children of gay and lesbian parents. Formerly married gay or lesbian parents may have full custody, shared custody, or visitation rights, or may, in fact, have been denied any access, solely on the basis of sexual orientation. The gay parent may be single or in a couple relationship in which one or both partners have brought children from their heterosexual alliances into the newly formed family. Today, many more lesbians and lesbian couples are intentionally choosing to have biological children through known or unknown donor insemination, and in some instances, both partners may choose to bear children (Morningstar, 1999). Some gay men serve as sperm donors, sometimes sharing parenting with the mother, although a few have used a surrogate mother.

Adoption of children by gay and lesbian persons has been a highly controversial social and legal issue. One state (Florida) bans gay and lesbian adoption altogether, and two states ban such couples from adopting. About half of the states have allowed second-parent adoption in cases in which one partner is the legal parent. In many instances, one partner has adopted or become a foster parent by not disclosing sexual orientation; in other situations, child and family workers, desperate to find good homes, look the other way (Ricketts & Achtenberg, 1989). Although these are pragmatic strategies, such practices do little to help dispel the various social myths concerning parenting by gays. Furthermore, the coparent not only has no legal rights in relation to the child but also is essentially invisible. Other couples avoid adoption establishment channels in the United States, seeking children from other countries, where infants are available and not too many questions are asked.

One theme that dominates the literature is that children of these relationships are raised in a world in which they will likely face social discrimination and perhaps even ridicule and isolation. Crawford (1987) is among those who have called attention to the problem of language, to the fact that there are no socially approved terms that define the couple relationship or name the role of the coparent. Not only do children not have an accepted or comfortable language to describe their families but also because of external threats from ex-husbands, ex-wives, grandparents, and others, they are sometimes enjoined from talking about their families at all. Adolescents, often insecure about their own only partially resolved sexual identities, are particularly vulnerable to peer pressure and harassment in social climates in which "faggot" is the ultimate putdown for the male, and "dyke" for the female. Children may be embarrassed to bring friends to their homes or to have to explain that other woman who comes to Parent's Night at school or visits them in the hospital. And school or other important community figures in the lives of children may project their own homophobic fears onto children of gay families, offering them little support or understanding. Others may not only insist on silence and invisibility but may also may allow and even subtly encourage violence. The news is not entirely negative, however. Some schools, from preschool and upward, teach their classes that children come from many kinds of families, and that all are to be valued. Some school systems have allowed and even encouraged gay and lesbian student alliances or support groups, include gay and lesbian educational topics, and may sponsor antiharassment programs.

Interestingly, in spite of widespread agreement about the special difficulties children in gay families face, to date, a convergence of studies over three decades suggests that the mental and social health, the peer and other social relationships of children of lesbian and gay parents, do not differ significantly from those of children in heterosexual families (Allen & Burrell, 1996; Bigner, 1996; Bozett, 1987; Flaks, Ficher, Masterpasqua, & Joseph, 1995; Patterson, 1992, 1996; Stacey & Biblarz, 2001). Topics of interest to researchers include gender identity, sex-role behavior, sexual orientation, various personality dimensions, behavioral and emotional health, self-concept, moral judgment, and intelligence of children of gay and lesbian parents. There is even some evidence to suggest that lesbian mothers are more concerned than single heterosexual mothers that their children have opportunities for male role models and good relationships with adult men, including divorced fathers (Kirkpatrick, Smith, & Roy, 1981; Golombok, Spencer, & Rutter, 1983).

Others, such as Wardle (1997), have faulted the research and argued that homosexuality is detrimental to children, a stance that has already had influence in legal decision making. A primary concern in a heterosexist, homophobic society is that children of gay and lesbian parents will themselves become gay or lesbian. Another is that daughters will be more masculine and sons more feminine than children from "normal" families. Stacey and Biblarz (2001), in response to Wardle, review the research to date and present their own critique. What they uncover is a "politics" of research that they feel does not truly advance social science or make the best use of the research opportunities the study of lesbian and gay families might provide. First, numerous flaws in this body of research should not be overlooked. Virtually all studies of gay and lesbian families have concluded that the adult sexual orientations of children of gay or lesbian parents do not differ from those whose parents are heterosexual. This seems to make sense, because it is equally clear that most homosexual adults were themselves reared in heterosexual families. Neither do children of lesbian mothers differ in terms of gender-role identity. Patterson (1992) states that "although studies have assessed over 300 offspring of gay or lesbian parents in 12 different samples, no evidence has been found for significant disturbances of any kind in the development of sexual identity among these individuals" (pp. 25–26). In her view, prevailing fears that children of gay and lesbian parents will have sexual identity problems are groundless. She concludes:

> The picture of lesbian mothers' children which emerges from results of existing research is thus one of general engagement in social life with peers, with fathers, and with mothers' adult friends—both male and female, both heterosexual and homosexual. Insofar as one can tell from the existing research literature, then, fears about children of lesbians and gay men being sexually abused by adults, ostracized by peers, or isolated in single-sex homosexual communities are unfounded. (p. 34)

Stacey and Biblarz (2001), however, believe that parental gender and sexual orientation do account for some differences between children of heterosexual and lesbian and gay families. They predict that "children who derive their principal source of love, discipline, protection, responsibility, and identification from women . . . should develop less stereotypical symbolic, emotional, practical, and behavioral gender repertoires" (p. 177). Furthermore, other factors, such as the fact that lesbians and gays who become parents are likely to be older, urban, educated, and self-aware, and tend to live in diverse, relatively tolerant communities, tend to bias the social science research in favor of positive effects on their children. Gay and lesbian parents are apt to be more conscious and affirming of issues of child sexual development. Because such children grow up in contexts of marginality and tolerance for difference, Stacey and Biblarz predict, counter to the conclusions of most scholars, that we would expect these children to be more open to sexual experimentation with both sexes and to a homosexual identity. In fact, they argue, although the research to date does show only a very slight increase in the percentages of children who may become gay or lesbian, there is evidence to suggest that more children experiment with their sexuality.

Stacey and Biblarz (2001) urge that, as social scientists, we not capitulate to heterosexist ideology. They state, "the case for granting equal rights to non-heterosexual parents should not require finding their children identical to those reared by heterosexuals" (p. 178). Whereas they disagree with those who take a "no differences" stance, they "unequivocally endorse their conclusion that social science research provides no grounds for taking sexual orientation into account in the political distribution of family rights and responsibilities. . . . Paradoxically, if the sexual orientation of parents were to come to matter less for political rights, it could matter more for social theory" (p. 179). Sexual differences are not deficits.

A number of important questions remain unanswered. For instance, although much is made of fusion in lesbian relationships, might there not be beneficial effects for children raised in families that are not structured along patriarchal lines, with no rigid, sex-linked role divisions that circumscribe the potentials for male or female children, a family in which both parents may have been socialized to be nurturing and emotionally expressive? Interestingly, if lesbian couples do indeed experience more intense intimacy and togetherness, perhaps the emotional needs of the couple are more likely to be met in the relationship rather than through the children. Do children of lesbian parents do better with lovingness, connectedness, and intimacy but perhaps worse with anger, competition, and conflict than children from heterosexual families? What are the gender development issues for children when both parents have been socialized to be men?

Family systems concepts are as useful or as limited and problematic in studying lesbian and gay families as in studying any families. They are concepts that grow out of particular cultural constructions and may or may not be particularly relevant to any one family's own narratives, to its understanding of its own experiences, or to its kinship patterns. We need always to be sensitive to the cultural, sexist, heterosexist, and other biases in the templates we use, and with whatever families we are studying. In terms of gay and lesbian life, we are a long way from understanding whether there is something we can call gay culture and what it looks like, and what "normative patterns" for gay and lesbian family and kinship may be. In this postmodern era, perhaps concepts that lead us to search for the essential parts of kinship and culture, and make assumptions about normality are not the most useful tools we might employ for family research.

CONCLUSION

Gay and lesbian families are extremely diverse, both like and different from other families. Earlier scholars searched for "cause" and thus for "cure," whereas, since the late 1960s, the effort has been primarily one of demonstrating that gays, lesbians, their children, and their families are not only as "normal" and "healthy" as everyone else but also very much like other families. Problems are almost always attributed to the noxious heterosexist and homophobic environment.

Researchers, depending on their personal politics, have often assumed an attacking or defensive bias that has not served the best or most creative aims of social science research. Some researchers identified with the family values movement and/or the religious right have portrayed homosexual coupling and parenthood as dangerous to society, children, and the future of the family. Other scholars have noted the pioneering efforts these families have made in building nurturing and satisfying couple relationships, and in fashioning family contexts that facilitate the health, well-being, and gender flexibility of their children. However, only a few researchers have commented on or attempted to explain the success of these families and their amazing levels of resilience, in spite of the fact they often must confront individuals, institutions, and governmental systems that neither respect them nor are willing to grant them ordinary civil rights. The current body of feminist theory and research, and the growing body of interesting and rich work on African American culture offer meaningful contrasts to the predominant deficit perspective in gay and lesbian studies. It takes time, as scholars from other oppressed groups have learned, to move from a reactive to a more proactive stance. "Pride," of course, brings its own set of complexities. It also can mean exaggerating difference and uniqueness, political separatism, and the heightening of "essentialist" notions, another force keeping gay and lesbian studies out of the postmodern era.

Part of the reason we do not know as much as we might has to do with the fact, in my view, that as students and as researchers we have started from the standpoint of majority culture and have attempted to measure deviation/difference, which fails to get us "inside" the lives and meanings of those we study. We have too often started with templates of structure, process, and developmental stage, as well as sexist and heterosexist definitions of family and of kinship, using them to map the data. Experience that does not fit these maps is not included, and we have rarely listened to the unfettered voices of those we study.

The research challenge is made more difficult by the secrecy and invisibility that continues to characterize many aspects of gay and lesbian life. It has been next to impossible to obtain random or representative samples. Another problem, as in much of social science, and particularly in psychological research, is that the great majority of work has centered on white, middle-class, well-educated, often male populations, usually from large urban areas, where there are known gay communities and thus a pool of informants. We know very little about lesbians and gays of color, and how they fare in their ethnic communities and in the white gay or lesbian worlds; about lesbians and gays who are less well educated or financially secure; and about those who live in largely heterosexual suburbia or in small towns and rural areas.

Our field continues to need detailed, holistic accounts of the daily lives of gay and lesbian families, studies that might reveal the complexity, the richness, and the diversity of their experiences. Much of what looks like gay "culture" to students of gay and lesbian life has more to do with societal homophobia or with the conscious and adaptive mockery of conservative cultural prescriptions around sexual behavior and object choice by lesbians and gays themselves. Studies need to be done in many different contexts that include lesbians and gays in all of their own diversities (e.g., Weston, 1991, 1996). We need studies that privilege their narratives, their meanings and beliefs; studies that bracket prior theories rather than produce what we expect to see.

Family and kinship, as we have become aware, are much more complex cultural categories than early leaders in the family therapy movement or in the family social sciences might have envisioned. What is more, the meanings of family and of kinship keep shifting and are reconstructed in social discourse to meet the needs of a changing world. Lesbian and gay families are taking an active and creative role in that reconstruction.

NOTES

1. In this chapter I use the term "gay family" and "lesbian family" to refer to same-sex couples and to families with children headed by a gay or lesbian couple, or gay or lesbian solo parent. In am indebted to Robert-Jay Green for pointing out that some of the families I refer to are composed of both gay and/or lesbian and heterosexual members and, strictly speaking, deserve some new terminology such as "mixed gay/straight" or "dual orientation" families.
2. See, for example, Goldner (1985, 1988); Goodrich, Rampage, Ellman, and Halstead (1988); Hare-Mustin (1978, 1987); Lerner (1988); Luepnitz (1988); McGoldrick, Anderson, and Walsh (1989); and Walters, Carter, Papp, and Silverstein (1988).
3. One topic, which deserves a paper of its own, is not covered here, namely the special issues concerning concerning gay and lesbian children and youth of heterosexual or gay/lesbian parents. Savin-Williams (1989, 1996, 2001) is an excellent resource.

REFERENCES

Allen, K. R., & Demo, D. H. (1995). The families of lesbian and gay men: A new frontier in family research. *Journal of Marriage and the Family, 57*, 1–17.

Allen, M., & Burrell, N. (1996). Comparing the impact of homosexual and heterosexual parents on children: Meta-analysis of existing research. *Journal of Homosexuality, 32*, 19–35.

Anderson, S., & Sussex, B. (1999). Resilience in lesbians: An exploratory study. In J. Laird (Ed.), *Lesbians and lesbian families: Reflections on theory and practice* (pp. 305–329). New York: Columbia University Press.

Bell, A. P., & Weinberg, M. S. (1978). *Homosexualities: A study of diversity among men and women.* New York: Simon & Schuster.

Benkov, L. (1997). *Reinventing the family: The emerging story of lesbian and gay parents.* New York: Crown.

Bepko, C., & Johnson, T. (2000). Gay and lesbian couples in therapy: perspectives for the contemporary family therapist. *Journal of Marital and Family Therapy, 26,* 409–419.

Bigner, J. (1996). Working with gay fathers: Developmental, postdivorce parenting, and therapeutic issues. In J. Laird & R.-J. Green (Eds.), *Lesbians and gays in couples and families: A handbook for therapists.* San Francisco: Jossey-Bass.

Blumstein, P., & Schwartz, P. (1983). *American couples: Money, work, sex.* New York: Morrow.

Boss, P. (1999). *Ambiguous loss: Learning to live with unresolved grief.* Cambridge, MA: Harvard University Press.

Bowen, M. (1978). *Family therapy in clinical practice.* New York: Jason Aronson.

Boxer, A. M., & Cohler, B. J. (1989). The life course of gay and lesbian youth: An immodest proposal for the study of lives. *Journal of Homosexuality, 17*(3/4), 355.

Bozett, F. W. (1987). Children of gay fathers. In F. W. Bozett (Ed.), *Gay and lesbian parents* (pp. 39–57). New York: Praeger.

Burch, B. (1982). Psychological merger in lesbian couples: A joint ego psychological and systems approach. *Family Therapy, 9*(3), 201–277.

Burch, B. (1986). Psychotherapy and the dynamics of merger in lesbian couples. In T. S. Stein & C. J. Cohen (Eds.), *Contemporary perspectives on psychotherapy with lesbians and gay men* (pp. 57–71). New York: Plenum Press.

Campbell, K. M. (2000). *Relationship characteristics, social support, masculine ideologies and psychological functioning of gay men in couples.* Unpublished doctoral dissertation, California School of Professional Psychology, Alameda, CA.

Carrington, C. (1999). *No place like home: Relationships and family life among lesbians and gay men.* Chicago: University of Chicago Press.

Carter, B., & McGoldrick, M. (1999). *The expanded family life cycle.* Boston: Allyn & Bacon.

Chafetz, J. S., Sampson, P., Beck, P., & West, J. (1974). A study of homosexual women. *Social Work, 19,* 714–723.

Clark, W. M., & Serovich, J. M. (1997). Twenty years and still in the dark?: Content analysis of articles pertaining to gay, lesbian, and bisexual issues in marriage and family therapy journals. *Journal of Marital and Family Therapy, 23,* 239–253.

Coontz, S. (1992). *The way we never were.* New York: Basic Books.

Crawford, S. (1987). Lesbian families: Psychosocial stress and the family-building process. In Boston Lesbian Psychologies Collective (Eds.), New York: Plenum Press.

Crawford, S. (1988). Cultural context as a factor in the expansion of therapeutic conversation with lesbian families. *Journal of Strategic and Systemic Therapies, 7*(3), 2–10.

DeVine, J. L. (1984). A systemic inspection of affectional preference orientation and the family of origin. *Journal of Social Work and Human Sexuality, 2,* 9–17.

Faderman, L. (1984/1985). The new "gay" lesbians. *Journal of Homosexuality*, *10*(3/4), 85–95.

Faderman, L. (1991). *Odd girls and twilight lovers: A history of lesbian life in twentieth-century America*. New York: Columbia University Press.

Flaks, D. K., Ficher, I., Masterpasqua, F., & Joseph, G. (1994). Lesbians choosing motherhood: A comparative study of lesbian and heterosexual parents and their children. *Developmental Psychology, 31,* 105–114.

Forstein, M. (1986). Psychodynamic psychotherapy with gay male couples. In T. Stein & C. Cohen (Eds.), *Contemporary perspectives on psychotherapy with lesbians and gay men* (pp. 103–137). New York: Plenum Press.

Friedman, E. H. (1988). Systems and ceremonies: A family view of rites of passage. In B. Carter & M. McGoldrick (Eds.), *The changing family life cycle* (pp. 119–147). Boston: Allyn & Bacon.

Gergen, K. J. (1991). *The saturated self: Dilemmas of identity in contemporary life*. New York: Basic Books.

Goffman, E. (1963). *Stigma: Notes on the management of spoiled identity*. Englewood Cliffs, NJ: Prentice-Hall.

Goldner, V. (1985). Feminism and family therapy. *Family Process, 24,* 31–37.

Goldner, V. (1988). Generation and gender: Normative and covert hierarchies. *Family Process, 27,* 17–31.

Golombok, S., Spencer, A., & Rutter, M. (1983). Children in lesbian and single-parent households: Psychosexual and psychiatric appraisal. *Journal of Child Psychology and Psychiatry, 24,* 551–572.

Goodrich, T. J., Rampage, C., Ellman, B., & Halstead, K. (1988). *Feminist family therapy: A casebook*. New York: Norton.

Gottman, J., & Levenson, R. W. (1999). Dysfunctional marital conflict: Women are being unfairly blamed. *Journal of Divorce and Remarriage, 31*(3/4), 1–17.

Green, R.-J., Bettinger, M., & Zacks, E. (1996). Are lesbian couples fused and gay male couples disengaged?: Questioning gender straightjackets. In J. Laird & R.-J. Green (Eds.), *Lesbians and gays in couples and families: A handbook for therapists* (pp. 185–230). San Francisco: Jossey-Bass.

Green, R.-J., & Mitchell, V. (2002). Gay and lesbian couples in therapy: Homophobia, relational ambiguity, and social support. In A. S. Gurman & N. S. Jacobson (Eds.), *Clinical handbook of couple therapy* (3rd ed.). New York: Guilford Press.

Greene, B., & Boyd-Franklin, N. (1996). African American lesbians: Issues in couples therapy. In J. Laird & R.-J. Green (Eds.), *Lesbians and gays in couples and families: A handbook for therapists* (pp. 251–271). San Francisco: Jossey-Bass.

Hall Carpenter Archives, Lesbian Oral History Group. (1989a). *Inventing ourselves: Lesbian life stories*. London: Routledge.

Hall Carpenter Archives, Gay Men's Oral History Group. (1989b). *Walking after midnight: Gay men's life stories*. London: Routledge.

Hare-Mustin, R. (1978). A feminist approach to family therapy. *Family Process, 17*(4), 181–194.

Hare-Mustin, R. (1987). The problem of gender in family therapy theory. *Family Process, 26,* 15–33.

Harry, J. (1984). *Gay couples*. New York: Praeger.

Hartman, A., & Laird, J. (1983). *Family-centered social work practice*. New York: Free Press.

Herdt, G. (1992a). *Gay culture in America: Essays from the field*. Boston: Beacon Press.

Herdt, G. (1992b). Introduction: Culture, history, and life course of gay men. In G. Herdt (Ed.), *Gay culture in America: Essays from the field* (pp. 1–28). Boston: Beacon Press.

Herdt, G., & Koff, B. (2000). *Something to tell you: The road families travel when a child is gay.* New York: Columbia University Press.

Imber, Black, E. (1989). Rituals of stabilization and change in women's lives. In M. McGoldrick, C. M. Anderson, & F. Walsh (Eds.), *Women in families: A framework for family therapy.* New York: Norton.

Karpel, M. (1976). Individuation: From fusion to dialogue. *Family Process, 15,* 65–82.

Kirkpatrick, M., Smith, C., & Roy, R. (1981). Lesbian mothers and their children: A comparative survey. *American Journal of Orthopsychiatry, 5,* 545–551.

Kitzinger, C., & Wilkinson, S. (1997). Transitions from heterosexuality to lesbianism: The discursive production of lesbian identities. In M. R. Walsh (Ed.), *Women, men, and gender: Ongoing debates* (pp. 188–203). New Haven: Yale University Press.

Krestan, J. (1988). Lesbian daughters and lesbian mothers: The crisis of disclosure from a family systems perspective. *Journal of Psychotherapy and the Family, 3*(4), 113–130.

Krestan, J., & Bepko, C. S. (1980). The problem of fusion in the lesbian relationship. *Family Process, 19*(3), 277–289.

Krieger, S. (1982). Lesbian identity and community: Recent social science literature. *Signs, 8*(1), 91–108.

Kurdek, L. A. (1988). Perceived social support in gays and lesbians in cohabiting relationships. *Journal of Personality and Social Psychology, 54*(3), 504–509.

Kurdek, L. A., & Schmitt, J. P. (1985). Relationship quality of gay men in closed or open relationships. *Journal of Homosexuality, 12*(2), 85–99.

Kurdek, L. A., & Schmitt, J. P. (1987). Perceived emotional support from family and friends in members of homosexual, married, and heterosexual cohabiting couples. *Journal of Homosexuality, 14*(3/4), 57–68.

Laird, J. (1988). Women and ritual. In E. Imber-Black, J. Roberts, & R. Whiting (Eds.), *Rituals in families and family therapy* (pp. 331–362). New York: Norton.

Laird, J. (1989). Women and stories: Restorying women's self-constructions. In M. McGoldrick, C. M. Anderson, & F. Walsh (Eds.), *Women in families: A framework for family therapy* (pp. 427–450). New York: Norton.

Laird, J. (1993a). Lesbian and gay families. In F. Walsh (Ed.), *Normal family processes* (2nd. ed., pp. 282–328). New York: Guilford Press.

Laird, J. (1993b). Women's secrets—women's silences. In E. Imber-Black (Ed.), *Secrets in families and family therapy* (pp. 331–362). New York: Norton.

Laird, J. (1996). Invisible ties: Lesbians and their families of origin. In J. Laird & R.-J. Green (Eds.), *Lesbians and gays in couple relationships* (pp. 89–122). San Francisco: Jossey-Bass.

Laird, J. (1998). Theorizing culture: Narrative ideas and practice principles. In M. McGoldrick (Ed.), *Revisioning family therapy: Race, class, and gender in clinical practice* (pp. 20–36). New York: Guilford Press.

Laird, J. (1999). Gender in lesbian relationships: Cultural, feminist and constructionist reflections. *Journal of Marital and Family Therapy, 26*(4), 455–467.

Lerner, H. G. (1988). *Women in therapy.* Northvale, NJ: Jason Aronson.

Levy, E. (1989). Lesbian motherhood: Identity and social support. *Affilia, 4*(4), 40–53.

Lewin, E. (1993). *Lesbian mothers: Accounts of gender in American culture*. Ithaca, NY: Cornell University Press.

Liu, P., & Chan, C. S. (1996). Lesbian, gay, and bisexual Asian Americans and their families. In J. Laird & R.-J. Green (Eds.), *Lesbians and gays in couples and families: A handbook for therapists* (pp. 137–152). San Francisco: Jossey-Bass.

Luepnitz, D. A. (1988). *The family interpreted: Feminist theory in clinical practice*. New York: Basic Books.

Lukes, C. A., & Land, H. (1990). Biculturality and homosexuality. *Social Work, 35,* 155–161.

Lynch, F. R. (1992). Nonghetto gays: An ethnography of suburban homosexuals. In G. Herdt (Ed.), *Gay culture in America: Essays from the field* (pp. 165–201). Boston: Beacon Press.

McGoldrick, M., Anderson, C. M., & Walsh, F. (1989). *Women in families: A framework for family therapy*. New York: Norton.

McWhirter, D. P., & Mattison, A. M. (1984). *The male couple: How relationships develop*. Englewood Cliffs, NJ: Prentice-Hall.

Mencher, J. (1990). Intimacy in lesbian relationships: A critical re-examination of fusion. *Stone Center Work in Progress Series, No. 42,* pp. 1–12. Wellesley, MA: Wellesley College.

Miller, N. (1989). *In search of gay America*. New York: Harper & Row.

Minton, H. L., & McDonald, G. J. (1983/1984). Homosexual identity formation as a developmental process. *Journal of Homosexuality, 9*(2/3), 65–77.

Morales, E. (1996). Gender roles among Latino gay and bisexual men: Implications for family and couple relationships. In J. Laird & R.-J. Green (Eds.), *Lesbians and gays in couples and families* (pp. 272–297). San Francisco: Jossey-Bass.

Morningstar, B. (1999). Lesbian parents: Understanding developmental pathways. In J. Laird (Ed.), *Lesbians and lesbian families*. New York: Columbia University Press.

Patterson, C. J. (1991). Children of the lesbian baby boom: Behavioral adjustment, self-concepts, and sex-role identity. In B. Greene & G. Herek (Eds.), *Lesbian and gay psychology: Theory and clinical applications* (pp. 156–175). Thousand Oaks, CA: Sage.

Patterson, C. J. (1992). Children of lesbian and gay parents. *Child Development, 63,* 1025–1042.

Patterson, C. J. (1996). Lesbian mothers and their children: Findings from the Bay Area families study. In J. Laird & R.-J. Green (Eds.), *Lesbians and gays in couples and families: A handbook for therapists* (pp. 420–437). San Francisco: Jossey-Bass.

Peplau, L. A., & Cochrane, S. (1981). Value orientations in the intimate relationships of gay men. *Journal of Homosexuality, 6*(3), 1–19.

Peterson, J. L. (1992). Black men and their same-sex desires and behaviors. In G. Herdt (Ed.), *Gay culture in America: Essays from the field* (pp. 147–164). Boston: Beacon Press.

Ponse, B. (1978). *Identities in the lesbian world: The social construction of self*. Westport, CT: Greenwood.

Richmond, M. (1930). *The long view*. New York: Russell Sage Foundation.

Ricketts, W., & Achtenberg, R. (1989). Adoption and foster parenting for lesbians and gay men: Creating new traditions. *Marriage and Family Review, 14*(3/4), 83–118.

Roth, S. (1989). Psychotherapy with lesbian couples: Individual issues, female socialization, and the social context. In M. McGoldrick, C. Anderson, & F. Walsh (Eds.), *Women in families* (pp. 286–307). New York: Norton.

Roth, S., & Murphy, B. C. (1986). Therapeutic work with lesbian clients: A systemic therapy view. In M. Ault-Riche & J. C. Hansen (Eds.), *Women and family therapy* (pp. 78–89). Rockville, MD: Aspen.

Saghir, M. T., & Robins, E. (1973). *Male and female homosexuality: A comprehensive investigation.* Baltimore: Williams & Wilkins.

Sanders, G. (1993). The love that dares not speak its name: From secrecy to openness in gay and lesbian affiliations. In E. Imber-Black (Ed.), *Secrets in families and family therapy.* New York: Norton.

Savin-Williams, R. C. (1989). Parental influences on the self-esteem of gay and lesbian youths: A reflected appraisals model. *Journal of Homosexuality, 15,* 93–109.

Savin-Williams, R. (1996). Self-labeling and disclosure among gay, lesbian, and bisexual youths. In J. Laird & R.-J. Green (Eds.), *Lesbians and gays in couples and families: A handbook for therapists.* San Francisco: Jossey-Bass.

Savin-Williams, R. (2001). *Mom, dad. I'm gay: How families negotiate coming out.* Washington, DC: American Psychological Association.

Slater, S., & Mencher, J. (1991). The lesbian family life cycle: A contextual approach. *American Journal of Orthopsychiatry, 61,* 372–382.

Sophie, J. (1985/1986). A critical examination of stage theories of lesbian identity development. *Journal of Homosexuality, 12*(2), 39–51.

Stacey, J. (1996). *In the name of the family: Rethinking family values in the postmodern age.* Boston: Beacon Press.

Stacey, J., & Biblarz, T. J. (2001). (How) does the sexual orientation of parents matter? *American Sociological Review, 66*(2), 159–183.

Sullivan, A. (1997). *Same-sex marriage: Pro and con: A reader.* New York: Vintage Books.

Tanner, L. (2002). Pediatrics panel Oks gay adoption. Associated Press. Retrieved from http://www.contemporaryfamilies.org/.

Tasker, F. L., & Golombok, S. (1997). *Growing up in a lesbian family.* New York: Guilford.

Tiefer, L. (1995). *Sex is not a natural act and other essays.* Boulder, CO: Westview Press.

Walters, M., Carter, B., Papp, P., & Silverstein, O. (1988). *The invisible web: Gender patterns in family relationships.* New York: Guilford Press.

Walters, S. D. (2001). *All the rage: The story of gay visibility in America.* Chicago: University of Chicago Press.

Wardle, L. D. (1997). The potential impact of homosexual parenting on children. *University of Illinois Law Review,* 833–919.

Weston, K. (1991). *Families we choose: Lesbians, gays, kinship.* New York: Columbia University Press.

Weston, K. (1996). *Render me, gender me: Lesbians talk sex, class, color, nations, studmuffins.* New York: Columbia University Press.

Zacks, E., Green, R-J., & Marrow, J. (1988). Comparing lesbian and heterosexual couples on the Circumplex model. *Family Process, 24,* 487–507.

CHAPTER 8

ADOPTIVE FAMILIES

Cheryl Rampage
Marina Eovaldi
Cassandra Ma
Catherine Weigel-Foy

Adoption begins with a decision to parent a child not born or conceived of one's own body. Adoptive families are thus intentional families, bound together by belief, will, practice, and most of all love. Taken as a whole, adoption is a highly successful solution to the problem of providing permanent care and family relationships to children whose biological parents are unavailable (Brodzinsky, Lang, & Smith, 1995).

All families face numerous challenges as they move through their life course. Adoptive families face almost all of the challenges of nonadoptive families and several more that exist as a function of the unique circumstances of adoption, including the fact that every adopted child has two families. These circumstances make adopted families complex. There remain biases in society that view this complexity as deficiency. Language referring to "natural" or "real" parents is but one way this bias is revealed. The premise of this chapter, however, is that adoptive families are an expression of the diverse forms that human relations can take and are eminently capable of meeting children's needs for family and parents. Although historically, formal adoptive parenthood in the United States was almost entirely limited to heterosexual married couples, changes in law and custom over the past few decades have resulted in a considerable number of single people, as well as lesbian and gay couples, forming their families through adoption.

CURRENT ADOPTION PRACTICES
IN THE UNITED STATES

"Open adoption" has today become more the norm than the exception in domestic adoptions. Openness describes a continuum; it may mean a one-time exchange of pictures and letters between birth parents and adoptive parents, a series of letters and picture exchanges over the years, or a face-to-face, ongoing relationship in which the birthparent is incorporated into the adoptive family on a permanent basis.

The trend toward openness has been met with ambivalence by many adoptive parents, who worry about whether their child will feel divided loyalty between the birth family and the adoptive family. Most birth mothers, however, feel much more satisfied with the experience of making an adoption plan when they have more information about the adoptive family and at least the opportunity for ongoing contact of some sort (Brodzinsky & Schecter, 1990). The first large cohort of children to experience open adoption is just entering young adulthood, so it will be some time before the long-term effects of openness can be clearly assessed. However, anecdotal evidence suggests that adoptees value openness, and that it may actually facilitate the development of a fully integrated and coherent sense of self.

Another trend impacting contemporary adoption practices is the increasing number of children being adopted from abroad. As the number of healthy domestic infants available for adoption plummeted during the decade after abortion became legal, parents and adoption agencies looked to various parts of the world, where social upheaval or dire economic circumstances made governments receptive to the idea of foreign adoption as an alternative to institutional care for their orphaned or abandoned children.

The process of adopting from a foreign country creates several layers of complexity for American parents. First, the adequacy of care varies considerably from country to country, and even from one orphanage to another within the same country. Records vary in completeness and even accuracy. The amount of paperwork and bureaucracy results in the children being older at the time of placement than is the case in most domestic adoption, which means that there is a higher risk of a disrupted attachment, or no attachment at all. Particularly if the child is from a different ethnic or racial group than the parents, the physical dissimilarity among family members means that the fact of the adoption will always be public, open to comment and interpretation from strangers as well as friends.

Another social trend affecting current adoption practice is a preference for adoption over long-term foster care placement for children whose parents are alive, but whose function is compromised by addiction, criminal activity, mental illness, or some other disability. Increasingly, during the past two decades, child welfare departments of state governments have pressed for either speedy reunification of birth parents and children, or else prompt termination of parental rights, followed by placement in a permanent adoptive home. This policy, relatively new in most states, has created a pool of especially challenging adoption situations. Most of the children in this group are older; most have suffered some degree of neglect, and many have been abused. Many of the children have had multiple placements, and have thus experienced multiple losses. Some of them have severe attachment disorders. Child welfare agencies are attempting to help families cope with the variety of challenges that parenting such children creates (Smith & Howard, 1999).

The Decision to Adopt

Although many couples think positively about adoption as a method of family formation, most only seriously pursue adoption if they are unable to conceive or carry a pregnancy to term. Indeed, most adoption agencies require proof of infertility as a prerequisite to beginning the adoption process, unless the parents are willing to adopt an older or "special needs" child. Thus, loss is an issue from the very beginning of adoption. Most adoption professionals believe it is important that the prospective adoptive parents resolve the loss that infertility has created before entering the adoption process (Brinich, 1990). Resolving this loss means, in part, letting go of the idealized child that was hoped for, mourning that loss, and coming to accept it. Support groups such as RESOLVE attempt to assist couples in this process.

An alternative route to adoption is based on social or religious beliefs. In such cases, adoption is seen as the fulfillment of an obligation to do good and to care for those less fortunate than oneself. Parents who come to adoption in this manner often express an interest in adopting an older child or a child, with a significant disability.

Yet another path to adoption may begin with the decision of a single person, or a gay or lesbian couple, to raise a child, and to choose adoption over various reproductive technologies as a way to become parents. Some adoption agencies will work with single parents; few are yet willing to accept applications by lesbian and gay couples.

The Adoption Process

When parents decide to adopt, they face the considerable challenge of determining whether to adopt through an agency or privately (usually facilitated by an attorney), whether to adopt domestically or internationally, and whether to accept an older child (in the adoption field, this generally means a child 2 years or older), a child with identified problems, or a biracial child.

Because the vast majority of potential adoptive parents are white and their number greatly exceeds the number of healthy, white infants available for adoption, agencies have established stringent criteria for adoptive parents seeking to adopt these children. These criteria include maximum ages for parents (often 40 or 45 for a first child), a minimum number of years married (3–5), proof of infertility, and, in some cases, religious affiliation. Couples who meet agency requirements then undergo a "home study," in which complete medical and social histories are collected. Many agencies also ask potential parents to participate in preparatory seminars and/or support groups. Once parents have been approved and are licensed as foster parents, they begin the waiting process. This is a period of indeterminate length, sometimes as much as 2 years, during which prospective parents live with the stress of knowing that they may get a call telling them that they will receive their baby in 2 or 3 days. When the placement has been made, there is a waiting period of 6 months to 1 year before the family can go to court and finalize the adoption.

This process applies only to the domestic adoption of healthy, white infants, the only category of adoptable children in short supply. The entire approval process is expedited if parents are interested in adopting an older child, a mixed-race child, or a child with some significant disability. Similarly, African American couples who wish to adopt are liable to have their approval process expedited, because there are far fewer of them than there are African American children waiting to be adopted (Smith & Howard, 1999).

If their ages, marital status, gender orientation, mixed religious affiliations, or any other factors prevent couples from seeking the help of an agency in adopting, they may choose to adopt privately. Private adoptions, generally conducted with the assistance of an attorney, may involve the adoptive parents' direct solicitations through newspaper advertisements, letters to physicians, and requests of family and friends to seek a birth mother who is considering an adoption plan for her child. There is little regulation of this type of adoption. Parents must contract with an agency to do a home study, but the amount of psychological preparation or counseling is minimal.

NORMAL PROCESSES IN ADOPTIVE FAMILIES

Attachment

Attachment, a process of relationship formation, is central to the social development of human beings (Ainsworth, 1969, 1985, 1989; Bowlby, 1960, 1973, 1980). It is an affectionate bond that develops through positive, needs-satisfying, and pleasurable interaction. Attachment grows slowly, first between parents and child, eventually becoming the template for all future emotional relationships. The failure to develop a secure attachment, or the interruption of an established parent–child attachment, poses significant risks. Children placed for adoption within the first 12 months of life tend not to differ from nonadopted infants in developing secure attachment relationships (Singer, Brodzinsky, Ramsay, Stern, & Water, 1985). The important task of attachment formation in adoptive families may be more complicated if the child has suffered disrupted attachments from earlier caregivers, if the parents are unusually anxious, or if there is a poor match between parental expectations and the child's characteristics and behavior. Children placed after 12 months may be at risk for attachment problems and developmental difficulties (Bowlby, 1973; Yarrow & Goodwin, 1973; Yarrow, Goodwin, Manheimer, & Milowe, 1973). These children are likely to experience acute separation distress as a result of the severing of previous attachment relationships. Furthermore, in cases in which children have experienced multiple placements or suffered early maltreatment, the formation of secure attachments in the adoptive family may be compromised.

Children adopted after infancy may lose relationships with birth parent, siblings, and extended family members. They may suffer secondary losses of friends, pets, toys, foods, customs, and familiar surroundings. These children may also lose access to information about themselves. Adoptive parents may also experience secondary losses, such as the loss of an earlier relationship with a birth or hoped-for birth child. They may have experienced loss of status in the eyes of some people and loss of biological continuity. These losses may constrain both parents and child in their willingness to risk developing subsequent attachments.

Research confirms that children placed in adoptive homes soon after birth develop attachments to caregivers in the same way birth children do and, subsequently, do not perceive the loss connected to adoption until around age 8 (Brodzinsky & Brodzinsky, 1992). Cognitive development that occurs between ages 8 and 11 enables them to have a deeper understanding of adoption. The normal process of adaptive grieving by adopted children usually begins during this period (Brodzinsky, Radice, Hoffman, & Merkler, 1987).

The implications of attachment theory for the study of adoption are profound. Many adoption professionals believe that learning to cope with the inevitable losses associated with adoption is critical for the development of healthy attachments in the adoptive family. Yet, for many adoptive parents, the existence of previous attachment figures, such as birth parents or foster parents, is often experienced as a threat. Consequently, the parents may tend to minimize the importance of these figures in their child's life and provide little opportunity for the youngster to discuss feelings about these individuals. In such cases, the chances of coping effectively with adoption-related loss is compromised, leading to increased risk for problems in the adoptive family (Brodzinsky, et al., 1987; Brodzinsky & Brodzinsky, 1992; Nickman, 1985; Reitz & Watson, 1992).

Attachment is an interactional process influenced by aspects of both the child's and the parents' experiences. Difficulties sometimes arise even in the attachment of birth children to their biological parents because of temperament differences or a mismatch in personality styles. For a child entering the family at age 5 or 8, with a lot of emotional baggage and unmet needs, developing an attachment is even more complex. And just as the effect of past losses is a consideration for the child, resolution of past losses is also a challenge for adoptive parents. Some families adopt a child the same age as a child of theirs who died. Others grieve for the "normal" child their adopted child might have been if he or she had not suffered so many blows before coming into their lives. They grieve the damage done to their child and the pain the child is still experiencing.

Entitlement and claiming also affect parents' development of attachments to adopted children. The sense of being entitled to be parents of the child may be compromised by having to answer to agency workers or to policies, such as having to get permission to take a child out of state. Claiming a child as one's own is a feeling and a commitment. Parents may need encouragement and support that underscore their unique role as adoptive parents in order to make this commitment. In addition to being claimed by parents, adopted children need to be claimed as family by extended family members.

An added dimension of attachment formation in a family adopting an older child is the sibling connection. Some of the strongest, most positive attachments that children coming through the child welfare system have experienced are to siblings. Siblings in maltreating families often nurture each other and form strong bonds of dependence and loyalty. For many years after adoption, children may sustain feelings of responsibility or longing for siblings. Policies protecting children's rights to visit siblings while they are in foster care have been strengthened; however, other means are needed to support children's relationships with siblings after adoption (Smith & Howard, 1999).

Siblings already in the adoptive family are also affected by the arrival of an adopted child. Biological children of the adoptive parents may feel both an internal sense of privilege and unconscious guilt in the face of their entitlement. Biological or previously adopted children in the family, when they learn about the adoption of a new sibling, may begin to wonder about the circumstances of that sibling's birth, and then develop uncertainty or questions about their own origins.

Developing a Livable, Coherent Family Story

All families develop stories to describe events and convey the meaning of those events to others. Because adoptive families are built differently than biological families, this activity takes on greater significance. The family story has been called by various names, including the "life story" or the "adoption story." As family therapists, we prefer to refer to it as the "family story," because it is inclusive of individual development and places emphasis on the story as a vehicle for family development.

The family members' story about how their child came to live with them can provide a concrete link to the child's past and support his or her growing curiosity about origins. How the story is told is key. When told while the child, curled up on a parent's lap, basks in the concentrated attention from that parent, the message received is likely to encourage further exploration about adoption issues. This kind of telling contributes to the development of an environment ripe for reinforcing positive views about self and one's heritage. If, on the other hand, no story is developed, the child is likely to sense the barrier being set between the biological and adoptive families, and open exploration of adoption issues is constrained.

With the development of the child's cognitive skills at about age 8 comes the dawning awareness that the family came together out of experiences of loss. Smith and Howard refer to this as the knowledge that "somebody loves you and somebody doesn't" (1999, p. 90). Depending on how the context around telling the family story has developed, as well as on other child- and parent-specific variables (e.g., temperament and personality characteristics), the family story can become a vehicle through which loss can be addressed. Children's developing cognitive ability allows them to comprehend more details regarding birth parents and their decision to make an adoption plan, as well as what led the adoptive parents to adopt. In this way, the family story becomes richer and more nuanced, and can be returned to again and again to understand life in a meaningful way. By developing a satisfactory account for the cause of the losses, the child is helped to make sense of the loss and thus recover from it (Melina, 1989). Even if the child does not talk about adoption, it is important to assume that he or she is thinking about it. As with any story, there is always the public or official family story. But just as significant is the private version that each family member holds and often does not share.

Most adoption professionals endorse an "early telling" theory about when to begin to talk with children about adoption. Through telling the family story when their child is very young, parents encourage openness about discussing adoption. It also gives them more time to practice the telling. Even when the child is too young to grasp the meaning of adoption, the "early telling" sets the stage for an honest, fuller exchange at a later time (Melina, 1986). Although parents should decide when and what to tell their child about adoption, it can become problematic if the child first learns about his or her adoption from another family member. Clinical wisdom supports telling the story even before the child can really comprehend its significance, in order to avoid even a semblance of secrecy or shame about the issue of adoption.

What to tell children about their past is dependent on their age and developmental stage. In general, sharing accurate facts about the child's history is a good starting place. Of particular importance is information about transitions (i.e., where he or she was born, how he or she got to the adoptive home). With maturity, the child needs to hear about the interpretations of these facts. Telling the child that his or her birthparents probably did not consider the possibility of a pregnancy helps the child to begin to struggle to see the complexity of human behavior rather than just label the birthparents as irresponsible or uncaring people. With difficult information, it is particularly important to be sensitive to the child's developmental stage, to strive for a balance between honoring the birthparent and acknowledging hardships and limitations (Melina, 1989). Sometimes the most painful details are the very things that give coherence to the story. If there are knowledge gaps in what is known, acknowledging this is a first step. Suggesting what might have been the case can also be helpful. For example, if the birth mother's age is not known, the parent can suggest that she might have been in her twenties, because most mothers who place their children are that age. Some children press for more information about their identity, especially as they reach adolescence; helping them to contact the attorney or agency that arranged the adoption can resolve their questions. Others will extend the search to seek medical information about their birth family, or even have actual contact with birth family members. With the current milieu supporting more openness in the adoption process, some adopted children learn to deal with the presence of the biological family in their lives from an early age.

Telling the family's adoption story to the extended family and community requires parents to be prepared to meet the larger society's biases about adoption. Comments about how fortunate the child is or how wonderful the adoptive parents are for taking in another's child can bespeak an underlying belief that adoption is a less desirable way to create a family. In sharing their decision to adopt with extended family members, adoptive parents prepare the way for the arrival and welcoming of the child into the family. It is important to allow extended family members to give voice to their thoughts as they struggle with their own understanding of adoption, as well as with their own sense of loss of a biological grandchild, niece, nephew, or cousin. However, the decision to talk about a child's adoptive status with people outside the immediate social circle of the family might best be done on a "need to know" basis. It makes sense to inform the child's teacher, because some school projects will undoubtedly include identifying family roots. But a parent responding to a stranger's comment about whom the child looks like might not include information about the child's adoptive status. The process need not become an exercise in converting the world to a better understanding of adoption; working with one's own family, close friends, and professionals that touch a child's life is likely to be enough.

THE ADOPTIVE FAMILY LIFE CYCLE

Raising an adopted child to adulthood is both similar to and different from raising a biological child. All children require nurturance and discipline to reach maturity. The crucial variant in the pattern for adoptive parents is that they must make a definite decision to pursue adoption. They cannot drift into parenthood or accidentally adopt a child. Adoptive parents arrive at the decision to adopt for a variety of reasons. Most often, for couples, it is made following the acknowledgment of infertility. Almost always (except where parental rights are involuntarily terminated), the biological mother affirmatively decides to make an adoption plan for her child and proceeds through the process of legal termination of her parental rights. Biological fathers, if known or identifiable, must also give up their parental rights in order for a child to be available for adoption. The laws surrounding fathers' rights are newer and vary somewhat from state to state. Thus, loss is the very foundation of the adoptive family, necessitating additional parenting tasks. While tending to their own feelings regarding the loss of having a biological child, adoptive parents must also address the child's loss or abandonment by biological parents, possible loss of birthplace and cultural heritage, and the loss of security in knowing that he or she is and always was wanted. No matter how resolved these losses seem to be, they will reemerge at various points over the life cycle of both parent and child.

Other tasks follow on the heels of the adoption. Adoptive parents, as well as adoptees, must deal with the birth family either in reality, through an open adoption, or in fantasy. In open adoption, contact with the biological family can vary and requires sensitivity to the needs of all three parties involved: adoptee, biological family, and adoptive family. Where there is limited or no contact between biological and adoptive families, the fantasy about the birth family can affect the adoptive parents' perception and subsequent treatment of the child. The child's fantasies about the birth family can influence subsequent relations with the adoptive family. The importance of the adoptive parents' ability to create an environment where these fantasies and feelings can be dealt with cannot be overstated and is discussed further, later in the chapter.

Some adoptive families have the additional task of addressing the issues in becoming a multiracial family. Others face the tasks of integrating adopted children with biological children. Each of these realities presents extra challenges in parenting across the life cycle.

Parenting the Preschool Child

Two parenting issues emerge during the preschool years. The first depends on when the child is adopted. If adoption occurred during or after the second year of the child's life, parents may find it challenging to establish a secure parent–child attachment. The second issue to address during this stage deals with disclosure. Attachment between parent and child is significant, because it appears to be the best single predictor of behavioral and emotional adjustment among preschool children (Brodzinsky, Schecter, & Hening, 1992). Children who feel securely attached to their caregivers seem better able to weather the stresses of childhood. A child born abroad and adopted during toddlerhood or preschool years brings memories of prior relationships into the new family experience. Ending a meaningful caregiving relationship can push the child into grief for months. The lack of an early, adequate caregiving relationship can create withdrawal and failure-to-thrive responses in the adoptee. Children may also lose contact with the ethnic heritage and language they had begun to acquire. If they are allowed to talk about their past and do not worry that either biological or adoptive parent will feel betrayed by this, adjustment to the adoptive home is eased. Adoptive parents need to gather any information about the child's prior home and the names of important people, before the trail to this past disappears. Also, information about the child's habits, preferences, and vocabulary when in that home contribute to a smoother transition to the adoptive home.

Disclosing to a child that he or she is adopted is a trade-off between trust and comprehension (Rosenberg, 1992). Parents need to use their understanding and intuition of their child in determining how and when to talk about adoption. Although most parents wish they did not have to tell such news, they usually find that their fear of not being loved as a parent is unfounded. Disclosure during the preschool years is the beginning of a new task, the negotiation of meaning of the parent–child bond. This task continues for a lifetime.

Parenting the Elementary School Child

Parenting tasks during this period continue to center on disclosure issues. With entry into school, the child's and the family's world expands, necessitating further parental decisions regarding disclosure of the child's adoptive status. Also, the child's ability to comprehend adoption grows along with the struggle to integrate this new understanding in a meaningful way. These added tasks at this developmental period require parents to be thoughtful and sensitive to both their child and to the issues that get stirred up in them as a result, including parental anxiety about being perceived as "second best" by their child.

When the adoptee realizes that he or she has two sets of parents, the stage is set for seeking understanding of how and why this happened. Children may seek to know who is at fault for these circumstances and become more derogatory about both adoptive and birth parents as they question their own adequacy. Whether children know little or a great deal about the birth family, they may be prone to fantasize about which are the "better" parents. This may occur especially when children experience anger or sadness over reasonable limits set by the adoptive parents. Although the family romance is a coping mechanism typical of this age group, an obvious and profound difference between the adopted and nonadopted child is that the fantasized family exists in reality for both child and family.

On the coattails of the question of "Where do I belong?" comes the awareness and fear of impermanency in relationships. Testing limits during this time may be an expression of the child's wish or fear of being returned or given up. A child's misbehavior can trigger parents' questions about their own adequacy and cause them to wonder whether the child really has accepted them as parents.

Successfully traversing this developmental phase is facilitated by an adequate understanding of adoption issues for child, parent, and family. Parents who can anticipate, attend to, and acknowledge the often unspoken questions and fears of their child during this period prepare the way for the identity struggles of adolescence.

Parenting the Adolescent

Adolescence involves the complex interplay of normal developmental tasks and adoption issues. All adolescents press to rework the parent–child relationship as they grapple with independence, identity and individuation issues. For the adoptive family, this "reworking" is loaded with meaning. If attachment has been a difficult issue on which the family has worked, then the child's individuation efforts might be experienced as a threat to family cohesion. For some parents, adolescents' attempts at independence feel like abandonment. For adoptees with a secure sense of belonging in their adoptive family, developing a strong sense of self seems to follow readily. In these circumstances, Kaye (1990) suggests that adoptees who appear to minimize the identity struggle ought to be accepted as being truthful in their denial of difficulty. Not all adoptees experience particular difficulty during adolescence.

During this period, the adoptee's task is to integrate an identity that combines both genetic and psychological bonds. Adoptees may shift identities back and forth between the person they were raised to be and the person they believe they were born to become. This process of trying on identities requires parents to understand the struggle, yet set limits as needed to ensure safety. Another parental role in this process is to withstand criticism and comments about the adequacy of their parenting, including taking in the dreaded epithet, "You're not my real parents." If they respond defensively to such provocation, adoptive parents are at risk of recasting the adoption as a "mistake," and can get caught in fantasies about how their biological child would not have behaved in this way. Thus, the viability of the parent–child bond can be challenged. Through this struggle, adoptive parents and their children rework their connections with one another, and, if successful, arrive at acceptance of the complex but viable nature of their family system, which will always include adoptee, adoptive family, and biological family.

Essential to the reworking of the family relationships during adolescence is a full disclosure of the facts the adoptive parents have about the birth family. This disclosure (or redisclosure, if the parents have been very open about sharing information with their child) may prompt the adoptee to pursue further information about, or contact with, the birth family. Parents can be helpful guides to acquiring this information. For many adoptees with a closed or semi-open adoption contract, coming into possession of all the facts known to their parents about their birth family is often sufficient to satisfy the need to know about their biological roots, at least during this developmental phase (Brodzinsky, Smith, & Brodzinsky, 1998). Some adoptees resume the search during young adulthood, actually seeking contact with their birth parents. For adolescent adoptees in completely open adoptions, the reworking of family relationships in this stage includes defining the kind and amount of contact they want to have with the birth family.

Relationships in Adulthood

During young adulthood, adoptees continue the process of individuation, with further refinement of their identity and connectedness to their dual families. How well parent and child resolved the independence and abandonment issues during adolescence can be a good predictor of how smoothly the transition to young adulthood will progress (Rosenberg, 1992). The tasks in young adulthood involve establishing oneself in work and in relationships outside the family (see McGoldrick & Carter, Chapter 14, this volume).

With the diminished parental contact that is typical during this period, adoptees' struggles can become internal. As they establish an independent adult life, adoptees in closed and semi-open adoptions may be particularly aware of how dissimilar they feel to their adoptive family. Some adoptees, not satisfied with the information they have about their birth family, may institute an intensive search for their birth parents in order to address these issues. Life events, such as marriage, birth of a child, or death of the adoptive parent, can also trigger a search. One study found that searchers are primarily married females, averaging 29 years of age, employed in middle-income jobs (Schooler, 1993). Those who are supported by their parents in their search efforts will struggle less to integrate the new information into their identity as a young person. If parents have reservations regarding the search, they would do well to share these with the adoptee. Maintaining openness in communication during the search can provide opportunities for parents' concerns and fears to be allayed. Sharing in the discovery process offers both adoptee and adoptive parent a possibility to draw closer together. If parents are willing to be more active in the search (i.e., attend how-to workshops, search through telephone directories, etc.), communicating this to their child can also enhance their bond.

During and following the search, adoptive parents can expect the reemergence of their own issues regarding abandonment and fantasies about a "perfect" biological child. On the one hand, denying or acting out these issues can impair or even disrupt the parent–child relationship. On the other hand, if parents can collaborate with their child on the project of consolidating a sense of self that honors and integrates both biological and social influences, then the search experience itself can deepen and strengthen the parent–child attachment.

"SPECIAL NEEDS" ADOPTION

The federal government uses the term "special needs" to describe adoptable children who are either over the age of 5; from a minority background; physically, emotionally, or developmentally disabled; or part of a sibling group, all of whom are eligible for adoption (Public Law 96–172). Individual states can expand their definition of the term to include other children, such as those in foster care or children younger than age 5 (Glidden, 1990; Brodzinsky et al., 1998). States can regulate who can adopt "special needs" children, although, in practice, most states impose no particular restrictions (Glidden, 1990). In general, it is presumed that children falling into this category will be more difficult to place into adoptive homes.

The past two decades have seen a notable rise in the number of "special needs" adoptions (Smith & Howard, 1999). Previously unavailable for adoption, these children frequently remained in institutional settings or were repeatedly transferred within the foster care system. With the onset of legislation on *permanency planning*, articulated in the Adoption Assistance and Child Welfare Act of 1980 (Public Law 96-272), adoption agencies were pressed either to move children in the child welfare system back into their homes or to permanently place them with adoptive families (Glidden, 1990; Smith & Howard, 1999; Brodzinsky et al., 1995).

Parents of adopted children with *physical* disabilities generally report feeling pleased with their decision to adopt, and disruption rates of such adoptions are quite low (Rosenthal, Grozy, & Aguilar, 1991), perhaps because the parents clearly understand and accept the limitations and demands created by their child's physical disability. However, "special needs" adoptions involving children who are older, particularly if they have suffered multiple placement failures, emotional disturbance, or attachment problems, are very vulnerable to disruption and generally require extensive preparation and support to be successful (Smith & Howard, 1999).

Children with Physical Disabilities

Statistics regarding the numbers of adopted children with physical disabilities vary across studies and states because of differences in how the term is defined. In two prominent studies on children with special needs, physically disabling conditions were found in 33% of the children in one study and up to 38% in another (Groze, 1996; Barth & Berry, 1988). Adoptive parents are usually aware of any physical disabilities their child has prior to placement. This can be advantageous, because it allows for preparations of the child's arrival, such as changes to the physical environment. Whereas a birth parent will require a period of psychological adjustment following the birth of a disabled child, adoptive parents do not carry the burden of perceived responsibility for the child's disability (Melina, 1989). The majority of parents of children with physical disabilities report high levels of satisfaction with the adoption (Marx, 1990; Rosenthal, Groze, & Aguilar, 1991). Despite these positive aspects of parenting a physically disabled child, these families face several important challenges.

Developing realistic expectations for the child, as well as understanding the impact of having a child with physical disability, is important to overall adjustment for families (Smith & Howard, 1999; Melina, 1989). Children with disabilities require supportive services, oftentimes on a weekly basis. Family schedules require greater flexibility. Oftentimes, parents have to learn to be advocates for their children in school systems to acquire the resources needed for them to thrive. With the multiple adjustments and requirements on parents, families need to find a balance between serving the needs of the child and attending to the functioning of the family as a whole, so that disability is merely a part of everyday life and not the central characteristic.

Psychologically or Emotionally Abused Children

"Special needs" children frequently spend years in the foster care system. Many in the child welfare system have suffered some form of abuse and multiple transitions (Brodzinsky et al., 1998). The effect of emotional abuse can be profound, impacting the most fundamental elements of development, particularly in children's perceptions of the nature and value of interpersonal relationships. As a result, they almost always bring to their adoptive families an adaptive wariness.

Abuse and neglect impact identity development in several ways. The secrecy that frequently accompanies abuse communicates messages of shame to the child. Powerlessness or lack of self-efficacy results from repeated experiences of abuse over which the child has no control. Children who have been abused commonly manifest anger, depression, and other behavioral problems. Families adopting children who have had traumatic experiences need to understand the relationship between the way in which the child experienced the abuse and the behaviors he or she is manifesting. Children exposed to traumatic circumstances develop hypervigilance to their environment and difficulty with emotional and behavioral regulation (Smith & Howard, 1999). Adoptive families, therefore, may need to provide greater consistency and structure to aid children in learning self-regulation.

Factors Affecting Disruption of Adoption

When an adoption fails, and the child is returned to the custody of the state or agency, the adoption is said to be disrupted. In a review of literature on "special needs" adoption, Brodzinsky and colleagues (1995) found that between 10 and 20% of such adoptions disrupt. Child behavioral problems and older child adoptions are the primary reasons indicated for disruption of adoptions (Smith & Howard, 1999; Okun, 1996; Rosenthal, 1993). Researchers have suggested that there is likely a significant overlap between these two groups, in that older adopted children tend also to have a higher rate of histories with abuse, which commonly underlie behavioral problems (Brodzinsky et al., 1998). A past history of sexual abuse particularly is highly correlated with disruption (Smith & Howard, 1994, 1999).

INTERNATIONAL ADOPTION

International adoptions began after World War II, when families in the United States adopted children orphaned by the war (Simon & Altstein, 2000; Brodzinsky et al., 1998). Currently, most foreign-born adoptees are from China, Korea, and Russia (Simon & Alstein, 2000). In many ways, families adopting internationally are no different than other families that adopt. They desire a loving family, they have overcome many obstacles to create their family, and they have hopes and dreams for the future. International adoption does, however, involve issues not always confronted in domestic adoption.

Risks and Challenges

In general, children from other countries are at greater risk for malnutrition and communicable diseases that are better controlled in the United States. Malnutrition is a concern for children from Third World countries (Simon & Alstein, 2000). Most health risks, however, can be identified prior to adoption and immigration, and few are untreatable or have long-term consequences for children once treated (Brodzinsky et al., 1998).

The loss of the familiar accompanies any child who is adopted. Those adopted from abroad, however, lose not only the familiarity of their immediate caregivers but also the cultural context in which they were born. Depending upon the age of the child at the time of immigration, changes in language, food preferences, and culturally specific behaviors, such as the amount of physical touching, may be differences that require adjustment (Melina, 1989). In addition to language differences between parents and their children, racial differences and dissimilarities in appearance create another layer of complexity that families face.

Transracial Adoptions

Most international adoptions are transracial adoptions, because adoptive parents are predominantly Caucasian and the children available for adoption are predominantly from non-Caucasian countries (Simon & Alstein, 2000). Within the United States, there has been much debate over the importance of similarity in race between parents and children. In the 1970s transracial adoptions declined following condemnations by the National Association for Black Social Workers and the Native American community, who asserted that the placement of African American and Native American children with Caucasian parents was destructive to their identity and well-being (Simon & Alstein, 2000; Brodzinsky et al., 1995). This practice has gradually changed, based on the view that it is not in the best interest of children to be denied adoption in favor of waiting for a family of the same race given the long waiting period that such criteria create. Nonetheless, families who adopt a child from a different racial or ethnic group must be prepared to address issues that inevitably stem from that difference, including the complexity of being a bicultural family and the potential for insensitive, intrusive comments from strangers about the child's physical dissimilarity to the rest of the family. The best outcomes in such families are, in large part, a function of the parents' willingness to embrace their child's original culture and facilitate the child's ability to identify with it (J. Stigger, personal communication, September, 2001).

Acknowledging the physical differences while building a base of common experience and values is an important adaptive task for families who adopt children of different races (Friedlander, 1999; Melina, 1989; Benson, Sharma, & Roeehlkepartain, 1994). Research on adjustment of minority children suggests that being surrounded by other, culturally similar children is important in the development of positive self-esteem (Friedlander, 1999; Okun, 1996). Exposure of adoptive children to positive role models who are ethnically similar is important for development of healthy self-esteem and identity development (Friedlander, 1999).

Implications for Search Issues

Rules regarding how children are adopted, who can adopt, and follow-up procedures are vastly different depending upon the country from which a child is adopted. Despite the trend toward greater openness in domestic adoptions, laws abroad differ in terms of the amount of preadoption information available to adoptive parents. Records regarding birth parents are oftentimes no longer available by the time adoptees decide to search. For example, due to the one-child policy in China, daughters, who are less valued, are frequently abandoned by birth parents or relinquished to state-run orphanages. Little information regarding the birth mother or birth family is generally available to adoptive families, complicating later searches for birth parents.

Little is known about the impact of international adoption on the search process. In studies spanning two decades, beginning in 1971, Simon and Alstein (2000) found that most international adoptees living in five Midwest cities did not pursue the search for birth parents. Those who did search and find their birth parents were satisfied with their decision to do so and felt that the outcome drew them closer to their adoptive families. Overall, families with internationally adopted children reported feeling positive about the adoption, and the overwhelming majority of parents who adopted transracially expressed satisfaction with their choice to adopt a child of a different race (Simon & Alstein, 2000).

CLINICAL ISSUES

Over the past four decades, many adoptive families have received services through the Family Institute. In the past 3 years, we have developed an integrated program to serve the needs of these families, focusing specifically on how adoption impacts both individual and family development and functioning. We tried to discover what information might help adoptive families as they struggle to facilitate individual development and family cohesiveness, and what needed resources were not already available. Interviewing agencies, therapists, and academic researchers led us to develop a program that has three components. The first component focuses on education, for adults deciding to adopt or having already adopted, for therapists working with adoptive families, and for school personnel who relate to adoptive families. The second component is support groups for both adoptive children and adoptive parents. The third is providing family therapy.

Working with Individuals and Couples Considering Adoption

Professionals who work with adoptive families need to acquire specific information about the process and consequences of adoption, including the fact that the path to adoption often is strewn with disappointments, uncertain timetables, unremitting stress, and unfulfilled expectations. Many couples choose the path of adoption primarily due to infertility. This in itself can create problems, as discussed earlier. The excitement of finally creating a family through adoption can create high expectations for both the child and the parent–child relationship, even when the parents know that the child's state of health is compromised. Unrealized expectations can then produce stress on the family system and inhibit the growth and development of healthy attachment relationships. Our position is that parents beginning the process of adoption who understand and acknowledge the difficulties they may face will be far better equipped to enhance their child's ultimate emotional and physical health. Therefore, our therapy/ consultation with individuals and couples who consider adopting includes both an educational component and grief work.

We have come to think that working with individuals and couples considering adoption requires (1) knowledge about current legal and social trends in adoption, so as to be able to provide information regarding options; (2) awareness of the various resources in the area (i.e., lawyers, agencies, and parent networks); (3) familiarity with the educational programs that various agencies offer; (4) access to readings or places to observe children to facilitate learning about their various developmental stages; and (5) awareness of the issues that adopted children may experience more acutely, including separation, loss, anger, grief, and identity difficulties. Some of these issues are obvious in all stages of development; others surface at specific times.

Family Therapy

Family therapists who plan to work with adoptive families must understand the issues they are likely to encounter. In our work with adoptive families, we have identified a variety of themes imbedded in the problems that families report having. The recognition of these themes has stimulated us to design educational programs to help parents prepare for the challenges.

The literature supports our focus on the following issues or themes: acknowledgment or rejection of differences; anger or blaming; confusion between reality and fantasy; and relations complicated by fear of loss (Kaye, 1990; Kirk, 1964; Stein & Hoopes, 1985; Smith & Howard, 1999). The challenges to parents include relating to their child in terms of (1) attachment, (2) introduction of the concepts of sameness and differences, (3) repeated reference to the process of adoption and facilitation of the development of its meanings, (4) reinforcment of curiosity about origins, (5) awareness of the need to help mourn losses, (6) expectation of ambivalence and confusion, and (7) facilitation of a sense of self and the pursuit of information about birth parents. To complicate matters, while attempting all these tasks, parents must also deal with their own feelings, which often include a sense of powerlessness, guilt about their inadequacies or ambivalences, and fears of not being good-enough parents. Parents may also be constrained by unfinished business regarding their losses; marital difficulties; individual issues (that might have escalated as a result of loss or anxiety); or pressures from extended family, community, or job.

Adoptive families that come to therapy have a variety of perspectives. Some consider adoption as a possible source of their family's problem. They may focus on the child's history prior to adoption, their own ambivalence (regarding adoption, informing the child about adoption or birth parents, connecting with birth parents), or what they view as a poor fit between the child and family. Other families seek treatment without mentioning adoption. Some minimize it as a variable. Others deny the possibility that it is a variable (Hartman & Laird, 1990). In our experience, the latter families frequently have not considered being open with their child about differences, or have not encouraged grieving for losses.

Some families seek therapy only for the child they have identified as having problems. Much of the research on the adjustment of adopted children has focused on a clinical population of children who manifest adjustment difficulties generally characterized by externalizing symptomatology, including increased aggression, oppositional and defiant behaviors, lying, stealing, running away, substance abuse, and other antisocial tendencies (Cohen, Coyne, & Duvall, 1993; Fullerton, Goodrich, & Berman, 1986; Schechter, Carlson, Simmons, & Work, 1964). Most research has focused on characteristics of the children, leaving unanswered whether the families of these youngsters differ in any significant way from the families of nonadopted children with similar adjustment problems. Our approach attends to the entire family system, as well as to the individual child.

The Family Institute's model for therapy with adoptive families aims to assess children, parents, and families, and to develop short-term goals for all three. Our strategies and interventions often include offering an educational series or a support group to supplement the individual, couple, or family therapy. Our work with families with young children has included helping families develop life books, pictorial time lines, and rituals. With adolescents, within an activity or support group structure, our work has focused on journal writing, art projects, role playing, and reading other teens' stories about the search for their identity and the process of searching for a birth parent.

We have begun to explore the issues related to attachment problems and loss. Of course, the attachments of adopted as well as nonadopted children fall along a continuum from securely attached to unattached. The Illinois Adoption Preservation Project explored the association between separation and attachment issues of adopted children, and attachment problems in parent–child relationships (Smith & Howard, 1995). This study found that difficulties seem related to an adoptee's failure to come to terms with past loss, move through the grief process, and then emotionally engage with adoptive parents. It reported that children's support groups can elicit the expression of conflicts and fears that have not previously been verbalized to parents. For this reason, we recommend such groups as complements to family therapy. In addition, we work with parents, separately and in groups, to help them develop strategies for building attachment, including (1) trying to meet the child's needs, particularly during periods of high arousal; (2) repeatedly initiating positive interactions; (3) developing realistic expectations for their children; and (4) helping their children identify and express needs.

Experts specializing in work with maltreated children with attachment problems emphasize the need for strategies beyond traditional therapeutic approaches to "jump start" the child's frozen emotional development and to change his or her cognitive map of the world. We recommend networking with therapists who specialize in this work to obtain family referrals.

We operate with the idea that parenting success requires good preparation, realistic expectations, effective parenting skills, and adequate supports. Parenting adopted children is a different experience than rearing a biological child (Kirk, 1964). Acknowledging the inherent challenges of adoptive family life, creating a rearing environment that is conducive to open and supportive dialogue about these issues, and supporting the child's search for self and biological family of origin are critical tasks faced by adoptive parents (Brodzinsky & Brodzinsky, 1992; Schechter & Bertocci, 1990). Helping adoptive parents meet these challenges is the goal of our program.

A positive conclusion to therapy involves a ceremony acknowledging the circumstances that have brought parents to us for help and celebrating the changes they have made. Such a ceremony recognizes the unique circumstances that create membership in adoptive families. The process of family building and the emotions associated with each addition are reviewed; the ceremony concludes with affirmation of family attachments (Reitz & Watson, 1992).

CONCLUSIONS

Families formed by adoption are necessarily complex. Their stories always include loss, intervention by legal and social service professionals, and an awareness of their differences from most other families. When this complexity is accepted, when the losses are acknowledged and resolved, when parents and their children feel satisfied with adoption as a legitimate route to becoming a family, and when the community of family, friends and professionals who surround them is affirming, then the outcomes for adoptive families are very positive.

REFERENCES

Ainsworth, M. D. S. (1969). Object relations, dependency and attachment: A theoretical review of the infant–mother relationship. *Child Development, 40,* 969–1025.

Ainsworth, M. D. S. (1985). Attachment across the life span. *Bulletin of the New York Academy of Medicine, 61*(9), 792–812.

Ainsworth, M. D. S. (1989). Attachment beyond infancy. *American Psychologist, 44*(4), 709–716.

Barth, R. P. & Berry, M. (1988). *Adoption disruption: Rates, risks, and responses.* New York: Aldine de Gruyter.

Benson, P. L., Sharma, A. R., & Roeehlkepartain, E. C. (1994). *Growing up adopted: A portrait of adolescents and their families.* Minneapolis, MN: Search Institute.

Bowlby, J. (1960). Grief and mourning in infancy and early childhood. *Psychological Study of the Child, 15,* 9–52.

Bowlby, J. (1973). *Attachment and loss: Separation.* New York: Basic Books.

Bowlby, J. (1980). *Attachment and loss: Loss, sadness and dependency.* New York: Basic Books.

Brinich, P. (1990). Adoption from the inside out: A psychoanalytic perspective. In D. Brodzinsky & M. Schecter (Eds.) *The psychology of adoption* (pp. 42–61). New York: Oxford University Press.

Brodzinsky, D., & Brodzinsky, A. B. (1992). The impact of family structure on the adjustment of adopted children. *Child Welfare, 71,* 69–75.

Brodzinsky, D. M., Lang, R., & Smith, D. W. (1995). Parenting adopted children. In M. Bornstein (Ed.), *Handbook of parenting: Vol. 3. Status and social conditions of parenting* (pp. 209–232). Mahwah, NJ: Erlbaum.

Brodzinsky, S. M., Radice, C., Hoffman, L., & Merkler, K. (1987). Prevalence of clinical significant symptomatolgy in a non-clinical sample of adopted and nonadopted children. *Journal of Clinical Child Psychology, 16*(4), 350–356.

Brodzinsky, D. M., & Schecter, M. D. (1990). *The psychology of adoption.* New York: Oxford University Press.

Brodzinsky, D. M., Schecter, M. D., & Hening R. M. (1992). *Being adopted: The lifelong search for self.* New York: Doubleday.

Brodzinsky, D., Smith, D. W., & Brodzinsky, A. (1998). *Children's adjustment to adoption: Developmental and clinical issues.* Thousand Oaks, CA: Sage.

Cohen, N. J., Coyne, J., & Duvall, J. (1993). Adopted and biological children in the clinic: Families', parents', and children's' characteristics. *Journal of Child Psychology and Psychiatry, 34,* 545–562.

Friedlander, M. L. (1999). Ethnic identity development of internationally adopted children and adolescents: Implications for family therapists. *Journal of Marital and Family Therapy, 25*(1), 43–60.

Fullerton, C. S., Goodrich, W., & Berman, L. B. (1986). Adoption predicts psychological treatment resistances in hospitalized adolescents. *Journal of the American Academy of Child and Adolescent Psychiatry, 25,* 542–555.

Glidden, L. M. (Ed.). (1990). *Formed families: Adoption of children with handicaps.* Binghamton, NY: Haworth Press.

Groze, V. (1996). *Successful adoptive families: A longitudinal study of special needs adoption.* Westport, CT: Praeger.

Hartman, A., & Laird, J. (1990). Family treatment after adoption: Common themes. In D. Brodzinsky & M. Schecter (Eds.), *The psychology of adoption* (pp. 221–239). New York: Oxford University Press.

Howe, D., & Feast, J. (2000). *Adoption, search and reunion.* London: The Children's Society.

Kaye, K. (1990). Acknowledgement or rejection of differences? In D. Brodzinsky & M. Schecter (Eds.), *The psychology of adoption* (pp. 121–143). New York: Oxford University Press.

Kirk, H. D. (1964). *Shared fate.* New York: Free Press.

Marx, J. (1990). Better me than somebody else: Families reflect on their adoption of children with developmental disabilities. In L. M. Glidden (Ed.), *Formed families: Adoption of children with handicaps* (pp. 141–174). Binghamton, NY: Haworth Press.

Melina, L. (1986). *Raising adopted children: A manual for adoptive parents.* New York: Harper & Row.

Melina, L. (1989). *Making sense of adoption.* New York: Harper Perennial.

Nickman, S. L. (1985). Losses in adoption: The need for dialogue. *Psychological Study of the Child, 40,* 365–398.

Okun, B. F. (1996). *Understanding diverse families.* New York: Guilford Press.

Reitz, M., & Watson, K. W. (1992). *Adoption and the family system.* New York: Guilford Press.

Rosenberg, E. (1992). *The adoption life cycle: The children and their families through the years.* New York: Free Press.

Rosenthal, J. A. (1993). Outcomes of adoption of children with special needs. *The Future of Children, 3,* 77–88.

Rosenthal, J. A., Groze, V. K., & Aguilar, G. D. (1991). Adoption outcomes for children with handicaps. *Child Welfare, 70*(6), 623–636.

Schechter, M. D., & Bertocci, D. (1990). The meaning of the search. In D. Brodzinsky & M. D. Schechter (Eds.), *The psychology of adoption* (pp. 62–92). New York: Oxford University Press.

Schechter, M. D., Carlson, P., Simmons, S., & Work, H. (1964). Emotional problems in the adoptee. *Archives of General Psychiatry, 10,* 37–46.

Schooler, J. (1993). *The whole life adoption book.* Colorado Springs: Pinon Press.

Simon, R. J., & Alstein, H. (2000). *Adoption across borders.* New York: Rowman & Littlefield.

Singer, L. M., Brodzinsky, D. M., Ramsay, D., Stern, M., & Water, E. (1985). Mother–infant attachment in adoptive families. *Child Development, 56,* 1543–1551.

Smith, S. L., & Howard, J. A. (1994). The impact of previous sexual abuse on children's adjustment in adoptive placement. *Social Work, 39*(5), 491–501.

Smith, S. L., & Howard, J. A. (1995). *Adoption preservation in Illinois: Results of a four year study.* Springfield, IL: Department of Children and Family Services.

Smith, S. L., & Howard, J. A. (1999). *Promoting successful adoptions: Practice with troubled families.* Thousand Oaks, CA: Sage.

Stein, L. M., & Hoopes, J. L. (1985). *Identity formation in the adopted adolescent.* New York: Child Welfare League of America.

Watkins, M., & Fisher, S. (1993). *Talking with young children about adoption.* New Haven, CT: Yale University Press.

Yarrow, L. J., & Goodwin M. S. (1973). The immediate impact of separation: Reactions of infants to change in mother figure. In L. J. Stone, H. T. Smith, & L. T. Murphy (Eds.), *The competent infant* (pp. 1032–1040). New York: Basic Books.

Yarrow, L. J., Goodwin, M. S., Manheimer, H., & Milowe, I. E. (1973). Infant experiences and cognitive and personality development at 10 years. In L. J. Stone, H. T. Smith, & L. T. Murphy (Eds.), *The competent infant* (pp. 1273–1281). New York: Basic Books.

PART III

Cultural Dimensions in Family Functioning

CHAPTER 9

CULTURE
A Challenge to Concepts of Normality

Monica McGoldrick

In recent years, awareness of cultural diversity in our society and world has changed profoundly. We have witnessed some devastating and amazing transformations in ethnic group relationships in South Africa, Europe, the Middle East, the former Soviet Union, and elsewhere, while the United States is being transformed by rapidly changing demographics. We are experiencing the greatest rise in immigration in 100 years. More than 1 million legal and undocumented immigrants are arriving annually, most from Asia and Latin and South America. With streams of new immigrants imparting their unique cultures, American society has become characterized by unparalleled diversity.

The impact on geographic regions varies. In the Pacific region, for example, one fifth of Americans are foreign born, although in the Midwestern Farm Belt, this is true of only one person in 50. But overall, the percentages of African Americans, Latinos, and Asians have increased dramatically in recent decades.

For many decades, large cities were the main places where many different faces of Americans were visible. Today, however, America's suburbs, smaller cities, and even small towns are hardly as homogenous as they once were. Mental health professionals everywhere are being challenged to develop treatment models and services that are more responsive to a broad spectrum of ethnic, racial, and religious identities. As clinicians, our work requires us to clarify the various facets of their identity to increase their flexibility to adapt in this multicultural society. Our work entails helping clients negotiate the complex web of connections with their families and come to terms with the larger society, and with their history, while they create their future—all of which are cultural tasks.

Ethnicity refers to a group's common ancestry through which its individuals have evolved shared values and customs. It is deeply tied to the family, through which it is transmitted over generations, and it is reinforced—and at times invalidated—by the surrounding community. It is a powerful influence in determining identity. A sense of belonging and of historical continuity are basic psychological needs. We may ignore our ethnicity or deny it by changing our names and rejecting our families and social backgrounds, under the pressure to "pass" for the dominant group. Many immigrants have been forced to assimilate and to give up their names, their language, and their cultural connections in order to survive. What they lose is sense of their historical and cultural continuity and identity.

Our clients' personal contexts are largely shaped by the ethnic cultures in which they live and from which their ancestors have come. As Paolo Friere (1994) has described:

> No one goes anywhere alone, least of all into exile—not even those who arrive physically alone, unaccompanied by family, spouse, children, parents, or siblings. No one leaves his or her world without having been transfixed by its roots, or with a vacuum for a soul. We carry with us the memory of many fabrics, a self soaked in our history, our culture; a memory, sometimes scattered, sometimes sharp and clear, of the streets of our childhood. (p. 32)

Our sense of heritage and cultural belonging is vital to our identity. At the same time, the profound differences among us in our multicultural society must also be acknowledged. We need to balance between validating our connections with our own cultural heritage and negotiating and bridging the differences among us, and appreciating the common forces of our humanity.

Most of us are somewhat ambivalent about our ethnic identification. Even those who appear indifferent to their ethnic background would be proud to be identified with their group in some situations and embarrassed or defensive in others. Individuals most exposed to prejudice and discrimination are the most likely to internalize negative feelings about their ethnic identity. Often, ethnicity becomes such a toxic issue that people's response is not even to mention it, for fear of sounding prejudiced, although it may be a major factor in their response to each other.

The subject of ethnicity evokes deep feelings, and discussion frequently becomes polarized or judgmental, because of the pressure within our society to conform to the dominant cultural norms. Those of us born white, who conform to the dominant societal norms, probably grew up believing that "ethnicity" referred to others who were different. We were "regular." As Tataki (1993) has pointed out, we have always tended to view Americans as European in ancestry. At times, exclusion of outsiders becomes primary to group identity, which then becomes a negative, dysfunctional force defining group identity by its exclusion of others. And those in the group may become systematically unaware of their cultural biases and prejudice.

In *Nobody Knows My Name,* James Baldwin's comment on discovering what it means to be an American still holds a deep truth:

> Even the most incorrigible maverick has to be born somewhere. He may leave the group that produced him—he may be forced to—but nothing will efface his origins, the marks of which he carries with him everywhere. I think it is important to know this and even find it a matter of rejoicing, as the strongest people do, regardless of their station. . . . The time has come, God knows, for us to examine ourselves, but we can only do this if we are willing to free ourselves of the myth of America and try to find out what is really happening here. (1993, pp. 10–11)

Many in our country are left with a sense of cultural homelessness because their heritage is not acknowledged within our society. We must incorporate cultural acknowledgment into our theories and therapies, so that clients will not have to feel lost, displaced, or mystified, as James Baldwin did.

CULTURAL CLASHES: NEW AND GLARING ONES AND THOSE HIDDEN IN HISTORY

Ann Fadiman's (1998) account of the experience of a Hmong family with the health care system in California may serve as one of the most relevant documents on the concept of normality and the importance of cultural understanding for all family therapists and health care professionals. Fadiman shows how an understanding of culture must challenge all our assumptions, beginning with our decisions on how far back in history we go to assess presenting problems:

> If I were Hmong, I might feel that what happened when Lia Lee and her family encountered the American health care system could be understood fully only by beginning with the first beginning of the world. But since I am not Hmong, I will go back only a few hundred generations to the time when the Hmong were living in the river plains of north-central China. . . . Over and over again, the Hmong have responded to persecution and to pressures to assimilate by either fighting or migrating—a pattern that has been repeated so many times . . . that it begins to seem almost a genetic trait, as inevitable in its recurrence as their straight hair or their short, sturdy stature. . . . The Chinese viewed

the Hmong as fearless, uncouth, and recalcitrant. . . . The Hmong never had any interest in ruling over the Chinese or anyone else; they wanted merely to be left alone, which, as their later history was also to illustrate, may be the most difficult request any minority can make of a majority culture. (pp. 13–14)

The Lee family experienced repeated violations by well-meaning but ethnocentric health care personnel, who saw this loving family as uncaring, abusive, negligent, and ignorant, only because the yardstick they used to measure the family's values and relationships was that of the dominant U.S. psychological theories about individual and family behavior. The health care system's unwitting imposition of its own dominant values on this family shows how limited our perspectives are, unless we add a cultural lens to our psychological assessments.

As Sukey Waller, one of the few clinicians who managed to connect with the Lee family put it: "Psychological problems do not exist for the Hmong, because they do not distinguish between mental and physical illness. Everything is a spiritual problem" (quoted in Fadiman, 1998, p. 95). Waller shows an amazing natural creativity as a culture broker who must maneuver in relation to profoundly different concepts of normality. She says:

> I've made a million errors. When I came here everyone said you can't touch people on the head, you can't talk to a man, you can't do this, you can't do that, and I finally said, this is crazy! I can't be restricted like that! So I just threw it all out. Now I have only one rule. Before I do anything I ask, Is it okay? Because I'm an American woman and they don't expect me to act like a Hmong anyway, they usually give me plenty of leeway. (quoted in Fadiman, 1998, p. 95)

Hmong and other recent immigrant groups from distant cultures represent one extreme of the cultural difference we are presented with on a daily basis in various health care settings in our increasingly diverse society.

At the opposite end of the continuum of cultural experience, but still highly relevant for our clinical practice, are families many generations beyond immigration, whose ancestors have tried to assimilate into the so-called melting pot of our country's ethnic mix. It is our profound belief that cultural meanings may hold for many generations after migration and many generations after people have ceased to be aware of their heritage. Indeed, the suppression of the history of many cultural groups may lead to cultural patterns that they themselves fail to understand or appreciate. They may perceive their behavior as resulting purely from intrapsychic or familial factors, when, in fact, it derives from hidden cultural history. Tom Hayden, a fourth-generation Irish American who became a committed spokesman for the power of the hidden cultural identity, discusses the experience of so many in our country who have had to live with their deepest history denied:

> What price do we pay when those who pull the curtains of history allow us to know our history only dimly or with shame. [Ours is a] . . . story . . . of identity forever blurred by the winds of silence and the sands of amnesia. It is also a universal story of being rooted in uprootedness. . . . Themes of personal identity being threatened first with destruction and later by assimilation appear throughout our literature. . . . Themes that reverberate in each story are those of near destruction and survival, shame and guilt, the long fuse of unresolved anger, the recovery of pride and identity. (1998, pp. 8–9)

Hayden grew up experiencing himself as Catholic but not as Irish, thinking that he was "post-ethnic in an ethnic world," only to realize years later that this was a lie, and that he carried his suppressed ethnicity within:

> I had no historic rationale for why I was rebelling against my parents' achievement of respectability and middle-class comfort. There was no one teaching the Irish dimension of my radical discontent, in contrast to Jews and blacks who were instilled with values of their ancestors. . . . The Irish tradition . . . seemed more past than present, more sentimental than serious, more Catholic than political. (2001, pp. 68–69)

Hayden grew up mystified about his identity. His father, too, was mystified about what made Tom do what he had done, saying, "I don't know what influenced him when he went away, but it's not the way he was raised" (2001, p. 269). It was years before Hayden realized that his family's assimilation had made them seek "respectability" and conservatism as a way of "passing" for the dominant group, and had required his family, and indeed his whole cultural group, to appear to assimilate into the melting pot, but it had cost them their sense of who they were. Feeling himself an outsider in young adulthood, he joined the Civil Rights movement. His first task was to bring food to black sharecroppers who had been evicted from their lands in Tennessee. "Was it only coincidental that I responded to a crisis reminiscent of my evicted, starving Irish ancestors? So effective was the assimilation process that my parents couldn't comprehend why I would risk a career to prevent hunger, eviction and prejudice. I was Irish on the inside, though I couldn't name it at the time" (2001, p. 68).

Hayden's example illustrates the mystification that attempts to deny or ignore cultural history have on people's sense of their own identity. Cultural competence requires not a cookbook approach to cultural differences but an appreciation for the often hidden cultural aspects of our psychological, spiritual, and physical selves, a profound respect for the limitations of our own cultural perspective and an ability to deal respectfully with those whose values differ from our own.

IDENTITY IN CULTURAL CONTEXT

Cultural identity has a profound impact on our sense of well-being within society, and on our mental and physical health. Culture refers to the ongoing social context within which our lives have evolved. It is also a story of our evolving group identities as families migrate, organize, and reorganize themselves within community and social contexts to meet changing historical and geographic circumstances. Culture patterns our thinking, feeling, and behavior in both obvious and subtle ways, although we are not generally aware of it. It plays a major role in determining how we live our lives—how and what we eat; how we work, love, and celebrate; and, in the end, of course, how we die.

Our cultural background, as I use the term, refers to our ethnicity, but it is profoundly influenced also by social class, religion, migration, geography, gender oppression, and racism, as well as by family dynamics. All these factors influence how family members relate to their cultural heritage, to others of their cultural group, and to preserving cultural traditions. Furthermore, we live in a society in which our high rates of cultural intermarriage mean that citizens of the United States increasingly reflect multiple cultural backgrounds. Nevertheless, because of political, economic, and racial dynamics, our society is still highly segregated; that is, we tend to live in culturally and class-segregated communities, which also have a profound influence on our sense of our cultural identity.

Our very definitions of human development are ethnoculturally based. Eastern cultures, for example, tend to define the person as a social being and categorize development by the growth in the human capacity for empathy and connection. Many Western cultures, by contrast, begin by positing the individual as a psychological being and defining development as growth in the capacity for autonomous functioning. Even the definitions "Eastern" and "Western," as well as our world maps (Kaiser, 2001), reflect an ethnocentric view of the universe with Britain and the United States as the center of the universe.

African Americans (Boyd-Franklin, 1989; Hines & Boyd-Franklin, 1996) have a very different foundation for their sense of identity, expressed as a communal sense of "We are, therefore I am," contrasting starkly with the individualistic European ideal: "I think, therefore I am." In the United States, the dominant cultural assumptions have generally been derived from a few European cultures, primarily German, Dutch, and, above all, British assumptions that are taken to be the universal standard. The values of these few European groups have tended to be viewed as "normal," and values derived from other cultures have tended to be viewed as "ethnic." These other values have tended to be marginalized, even though they reflect the traditional values of the majority of the population.

Throughout the mental health field, therapeutic models have generally been presented as if they were free of cultural biases, rather than reflections of the social assumptions out of which they arise. For example, although human behavior results from an interplay of intrapsychic, interpersonal, familial, socioeconomic, and cultural forces, the mental health field has paid greatest attention to the first of these—the personality factors that shape life experiences and behavior. Family therapists have recognized that individual behavior is mediated through family rules and patterns, but we have not sufficiently appreciated how deeply these rules are rooted in cultural norms. The study of cultural influences on human emotional functioning has been left primarily to cultural anthropologists. And even they have more often explored these influences in distant non-European cultures rather than study the tremendous ethnic diversity within our own society. Only recently have some clinicians and researchers begun to consider the cultural assumptions underlying all our therapeutic models. But, generally, even mental health professionals who considered culture have tended to focus on marginalized, non-European groups, particularly African, Latino, and Asian, describing these cultures as to how they differ from the so-called norm.

When discussion of ethnicity has occurred, it has often focused on groups' "otherness" in ways that emphasize their deficits rather than their adaptive strengths or their place in the larger society. The emphasis has also been on how so-called "minorities" relate to the "dominant" societal values of "normality." In *Ethnicity and Family Therapy*, first published in 1982, my colleagues and I described the patterns of 20 different cultural groups, including many of European origin, summarizing issues of clinical relevance for each group. That work, expanded in 1996 to incorporate descriptions of more than 40 different ethnic groups, was meant to make clear that ethnicity pertains to and influences everyone's values. It is relevant to our thinking about every case—not just for marginalized or non-European families (McGoldrick, Giordano, & Pearce, 1996; McGoldrick, 1998). Thus everyone's assumptions must be investigated, not just those kept at the periphery of society. Working toward multicultural frameworks in our theories, research, and clinical practice requires that we challenge our society's dominant universalist assumptions, as we must do in our other societal institutions for democracy to survive (Dilworth-Anderson, Burton, & Johnson, 1993; Hitchcock, 2001).

STEREOTYPES

Although generalizing about groups has often been used to reinforce prejudices, one cannot discuss ethnic cultures without generalizing. In fact, we perpetuate covert negative stereotyping by failure to address culture explicitly in our everyday work. Yet many have eschewed the value of discussing ethnicity per se, considering socioeconomic, political, and religious influences more important (Falicov, 1995). Others avoid discussion of group characteristics altogether, in favor of individual family patterns, maintaining, "I prefer to think of each family as unique," or "I prefer to think of family members as human beings rather than pidgeonholing them in categories." Of course, we all prefer to be treated as unique and as human beings, but such assumptions prevent us from acknowledging the influence of cultural and group history on values and beliefs. The values, position, status, and privileges of families in our society are also profoundly influenced by their sociocultural location, which is deeply embedded in cultural as well as their class backgrounds, making these issues essential to our clinical assessment and intervention. In this sense, discussing cultural generalizations or stereotypes is the same as discussing "normal" families as a way to clarify the parameters of healthy family behavior through the lifecycle. Without some concept of norms, which are always cultural norms, we would have no compass in our clinical work at all.

Our underlying openness to making a space for those who are culturally different is the key to expanding our cultural understanding. We primarily learn about culture not by learning the "facts" of another's culture, but rather by changing our own attitudes about cultural difference (Fadiman, 1998). Cultural paradigms are useful to the extent that they help us challenge our long-held beliefs about "the way things are." But we cannot learn about culture cookbook fashion, through memorizing recipes for relating to other ethnic groups. Information we learn about cultural differences will, I hope, expand our understanding, particularly in respect to curiosity and humility about cultural differences. The best cultural training for family therapists might be to experience what it is like not to be part of the dominant culture—to gain the humility necessary for respectful cultural interactions based on more than a one-way hierarchy of normality, truth, and wisdom.

OUR EVOLVING ETHNICITIES

The concept of a group's "peoplehood" is based on a combination of geography, religion, and cultural history, and is retained whether or not members realize their commonalities with one another. The consciousness of ethnic identity varies greatly within and between groups. In groups that have experienced prejudice and discrimination, such as Jews and African Americans, family members may absorb the larger society's prejudice and become conflicted about their own identity. They may even turn against each other, with some trying to "pass" and others resenting them for doing so. Those who are close enough in appearance to the dominant group's characteristics may experience a sense of choice about which group to identify with, whereas others have no choice because of their skin color or other physical characteristics. Examples of internalized ethnic or racial prejudice include some group members' attempts to change their appearance through plastic surgery or other means to obtain "valued" characteristics. Families not part of the dominant culture are always under pressure to give up their values and conform to the norms of the more powerful, dominant group. Intrafamilial conflicts over the level of accomodation should be viewed not only as family conflicts but also as reflecting explicit or implicit pressure from the dominant culture as to which characteristics are to be more highly valued.

Individuals should not have to suppress parts of themselves in order to "pass" for normal according to someone else's standards. Being "at home" is about people having a sense of peace with who they really are, not fitting into rigidly defined group identities that strain people's basic loyalties. As family therapists, we believe in helping clients understand their ethnicity as a fluid, ever-changing aspect of who they are, not as something to be defined for them by others. The character Vivian Twostar in Erdrich and Dorris's *The Crown of Columbus* (1991), describes the complexity that this cultural self-definition always entails:

> I belong to the lost tribe of mixed bloods, that hodgepodge amalgam of hue and cry that defies easy placement. When the DNA of my various ancestors—Irish and Coeur d'Alene and Spanish and Navajo and God knows what else—combined to form me, the result was not some genteel indecipherable puree that comes from a Cuisinart. You know what they say on the side of the Bisquick box, under instructions for pancakes? Mix with fork. Leave lumps. That was me. There are advantages to not being this or that. You have a million stories, one for every occasion, and in a way they're all lies and in another way they're all true. When Indians say to me, "What are you? I know exactly what they're asking and answer Coeur d'Alene. I don't add, "Between a quarter and a half," because that's information they don't require, first off—though it may come later if I screw up and they're looking for reasons why. If one of my Dartmouth colleagues wonders, "Where did you study?" I pick the best place, the hardest one to get into, in order to establish that I belong. If a stranger on the street questions where [my daughter] gets her light brown hair and dark skin, I say the Olde Sodde and let them figure it out. There are times when I control who I'll be, and times when I let other people decide. I'm not all anything, but I'm a little bit of a lot. My roots spread in every direction, and if I water one set of them more often than others, it's because they need it more. . . . I've read anthropological papers written about people like me. We're called marginal, as if we exist anywhere but on the center of the page. We're parked on the bleachers looking into the arena, never the main players, but there are bonuses to peripheral vision. Out beyond the normal bounds, you at least know where you're not. You escape the claustrophobia of belonging, and what you lack in security you gain by realizing—as those insiders never do—that security is an illusion. . . . "Caught between two worlds," is the way we're often characterized, but I'd put it differently. We are the catch. (pp. 166–167)

This brilliant expression of a multifaceted cultural identity comprised of complex heritages illustrates also the impact of social location on the need to highlight one or another aspect of one's cultural background in a given context, in response to others' projections. The illustration also highlights what those who belong have to learn from those who are marginalized.

If we look carefully enough, everyone is a "hodgepodge." Developing "cultural competence" requires us to question the dominant values and explore the complexities of cultural identity. All of us are migrants moving between our ancestors' traditions, the worlds we inhabit, and the world we will leave to those who come after us. Our clinical work of healing may often entail helping clients locate themselves culturally, so they can overcome the sense of mystification, invalidation, or alienation that comes from not being able to feel culturally at home in their society.

For most of us, finding out who we are means putting together a unique internal combination of cultural identities. Maya Angelou (1986), an African American, naturally found it hard to feel culturally at home in the United States and for a period went to live in Africa, hoping in some way to find a sense of home for which she longed. She found that who she was could not be encompassed even by connecting with that important part of her heritage:

> If the heart of Africa still remained elusive, my search for it had brought me closer to understanding myself and other human beings. The ache for home lives in all of us, the safe place where we can go as we are and not be questioned. It impels mighty ambitions and dangerous capers. . . . We shout in Baptist churches, wear yarmulkes and wigs and argue even the tiniest points in the Torah, or worship the sun and refuse to kill cows for the starving. Hoping that by doing these things, home will find us acceptable or that barring that, we will forget our awful yearning for it. (p. 196)

Those who try to assimilate at the price of forgetting their connections to their heritage are likely to have more problems than those who maintain a positive sense of connection with their heritage (see Falicov, Chapter 11, this volume).

For these reasons we view "cultural genograms" as axiomatic for all work with clients or trainees (McGoldrick, Gerson, & Shellenberger, 1998; Hardy & Laszloffy, 1995; Congress, 1994). Genograms should help us contextualize our kinship network in terms of culture, class, race, gender, religion, and migration history. When we ask people to identify themselves ethnically, we are asking them to highlight themes of cultural continuity and identity to make them more apparent.

The definition of culture itself is highly complex. To define one's identity as belonging to a single ethnic group (e.g., Irish, Anglo, African

American) always oversimplifies matters, because we all reflect such cultural mixing, and no cultural process ever stands still, even for those from a single cultural background. We are always evolving ethnically. All of us have multiple cultural roots and are in the process of transforming our ethnic identity throughout our lives, influenced by the changing contexts in which we live.

We need to develop an open, flexible social system with flexible boundaries, so that people can define themselves by the groupings that relate to their heritages and practices and go beyond labels such as "minorities," "blacks," "Latinos," or "Americans." Our very language reflects the biases embedded in our society's dominant beliefs. The term "Latino," for example, refers simultaneously to Native Americans of hundreds of different groups throughout Latin and South America, as well as to immigrants from numerous other cultures, including Cubans of Spanish origin, Chinese who settled in Puerto Rico, families from Africa whose ancestors were brought to Latin and South America as slaves, and Argentinean Jews, whose ancestors lived in Europe for over 1,000 years, until the 1930s or 1940s (Falicov, 1996a, 1996b; Garcia-Preto, 1996a, 1996b; Bernal, 1996). The term "minority" peripheralizes groups whose heritage is different from that of the dominant groups. The term "black" obliterates the ancestral heritage of Americans of African heritage altogether and defines people only by their color. And the fact that there is no term to describe people of the United States—but only the inaccurate term "American," which makes invisible Canadians, Mexicans, and other Americans—is a serious handicap even to discussing these issues.

Ethnicity is indeed a complex concept. Jewish ethnicity, for example, is a meaningful term to millions of people (Rosen & Weltman, 1996). Yet it refers to people who have no single country of origin, and no single language of origin, and no single set of religious practices. Jews in the United States may come from Argentina, Russia, Greece, and Japan, and may have Ashkenazi roots. Or they may be Sephardic Jews from North Africa or Spain, with very different cultural traditions and migration patterns. Similar difficulty applies to definitions of Arabs (Abudabbeh, 1996), who may be Eastern Orthodox Syrians, Roman Catholic Lebanese, or Jordanian or Egyptian Muslims. Yet there is some sense of cultural connection among these groups. And the shared culture of the ethnic history of families of these backgrounds is not irrelevant to their adaptation in the United States.

We are all always in the process of ongoing cultural evolution. Our ethnic identity is ever-changing—incorporating ancestral influences, while forging new and emerging group identities. Group identities emerge in a complex interplay of members' relationships with each other (insiders) and with outsiders. We may feel negative, proud, and appreciative of our cultural heritage, or we may be unaware of the cultural groups to which we even belong. But our relationship to our cultural heritage will influence our well-being, as will our sense of our relationship to the dominant culture. Are we members of it? Are we "passing" as members? Do we feel like marginalized outsiders? Or are we outsiders who have so absorbed the dominant culture's norms and values that we do not even recognize that our internalized values reflect their prejudices and attempts to suppress cultural difference?

Our society's dominant definitions of cultural groups have shifted over time. In the 1700s only those of British and German ancestry were thought to be "white." As Ben Franklin put it:

> All Africa is black or tawny. Asia chiefly tawny. America (exclusive of the new Comers) wholly so. And in Europe the Spaniards, Italians, French, Russians and Swedes are generally of what we call a swarthy Complexion; as are the Germans also, the Saxons only excepted, who with the English make up the principal body of White People on the face of the Earth. I could only wish their numbers were increased. (quoted in Hitchcock, 2001, p. 18)

Over the centuries, we have greatly expanded the category of "white" cultures to include Europeans previously considered "ethnic" such as Poles, Italians, Irish, and Jews. People of mixed heritage are often pressed to identify with a single cultural group rather than being able to claim the true complexity of their cultural heritage (Root, 1992, 1996). The 2000 census was the first that allowed people to acknowledge any level of mixed heritage. Many have feared that it is only because the United States needs further expansion of the category "white," which will otherwise soon become a minority of the population.

The U.S. Census (2000), which has enormous power to determine the dominant cultural definitions of race and ethnicity, has severe limitations in its cultural categorizations. A glaring illustration is the definition of "white," which includes all those who have origins in Europe, the Middle East, and North Africa. The term "Asian" includes groups from Hmong to Pakistani. The obvious limitations of such categorizations are perhaps more evident since September 11, 2001. Cultural groups from Middle East countries such as Afganistan or Iraq are much more closely related to cultural groups in Pakistan that we have labeled "Asian," making one wonder whose interests it serves to use the categorization "white" at all. The only ethnicity that the latest census explored at all was "Hispanic." This very problematic category (Garcia-Preto, 1996a), which many consider a racist term developed by colonial powers, it is so general that it is about as relevant as using the term "American" to describe people of so many heritages. Furthermore, this categorization by the U.S. Census Bureau forced Brazilians to label themselves as "white" rather than "Hispanic, because of Portuguese settlement and language, although the cultural history of Puerto Ricans, Cubans, Dominicans, Argentinians, and other groups in

Latin and South America undoubtedly have much more in common with Brazilian cultures than with "white," North American cultures. The Census has been a conservative force within our society for 200 years, defining people in categories that oversimplify their heritage and cultural connections to each other and to their ancestors. People have been pressed into racial categories that have basically no meaning except to stratify people by their differences in skin color. These categorizations have been developed, rather, to affirm spurious racial categories that promote white supremacy in our society (Malcomson, 2000).

FACTORS INFLUENCING ETHNICITY

Essential to understanding culture is appreciating the interaction between ethnicity, gender, sexual orientation, class, race, religion, geography, migration, and politics, and how they have together influenced families in adapting to American life (Falicov, 1995). All these components are influenced also by the length of time since migration, a group's specific historical experience, and the degree of discrimination experienced in this society. Generally, people move closer to the dominant value system the longer they remain in the United States and the more they rise in social class. Families that remain within an ethnic neighborhood, who work and socialize with members of their group, and those whose religion reinforces ethnic values, will probably maintain their ethnicity longer than those who live in heterogeneous settings. And those who are systematically excluded from the dominant group by racism, anti-Semitism, sexism, homophobia, or other institutionalized bias, will continue to show the effects of this exclusion in their psychological and social makeup.

The family's migration experience may have a major influence on its cultural values. It matters to know why each family migrated—what they were seeking (e.g., survival, adventure, wealth) and what they were leaving behind (e.g., religious or political persecution, poverty). A family's dreams and fears when immigrating become part of its heritage. Parents' attitudes toward what came before and what lies ahead will have a profound impact on the expressed or tacit messages they transmit to their children. Families that have migrated tend to adapt more easily, such as Jews who migrated first to South America and later to the United States. Their previous migration probably taught them something about flexibility. Those who come as refugees, fleeing political persecution or the trauma of war, and who have no possibility of returning to their homeland, may have very different adaptations to American life than those who come seeking economic advancement, with the idea of returning to their homeland to retire. The political history surrounding migration may intensify cultural traits for a particular group, as illustrated, for example, in Fusco's account of the particular problems of Cuban immigrants over the past decades:

Americans often ask me why Cubans, exiled or at home, are so passionate about Cuba, why our discussions are so polarized, and why our emotions are so raw after thirty-three years. My answer is that we are always
fighting with the people we love the most. Our intensity is the result of
the tremendous repression and forced separation that affects all people
who are ethnically Cuban, wherever they reside. Official policies on both
sides collude to make exchange practically impossible. (1995, p. 3)

Adaptation is also affected by whether one family member migrated
alone or a large portion of the family, community, or nation came together. Families that migrate alone usually have a greater need to adapt to the
new situation, and their losses are often more hidden. Frequently, educated immigrants who come for professional opportunities move to places
where there is no one with whom they can speak their native language or
share family customs and rituals. When a number of families migrate together, as happened with the Scandinavians who settled in the Midwest,
they are often able to preserve much of their traditional heritage.

When a large part of the population or nation comes together, as
happened in the waves of Irish, Polish, Italian, and Jewish migration, discrimination against the group may be especially intense. The newest immigrants always pose a threat to those who came just before, who fear losing
their tenuous economic security and their rung on the ladder of social status.

Family members vary in how quickly they adapt, how much of their
heritage they retain, and the rate at which they learn English. The language of the country of origin serves to preserve its culture. It is important
to learn what language(s) were spoken while the children in the family
were growing up.

The East and West coasts, the entry points for most immigrants, are
likely to have greater ethnic diversity and ethnic neighborhoods, and people in these areas are more often aware of ethnic differences. The ethnic
neighborhood provides a temporary cushion against the stresses of migration, which are likely to surface in the second generation. Those immigrant families who moved to an area where the population was relatively
stable, for example, the South, generally had more trouble adjusting or
were forced to assimilate very rapidly.

When family members move away from an ethnic enclave, the stresses
of adaptation are likely to be severe even several generations after immigration. The therapist should learn about the community's ethnic network
and encourage the rebuilding of social and informal connections through
family visits, letters, or creating new networks.

Therapists need to be as attuned to migration stresses and ethnic
identity conflicts as they are to other stresses in a family's history (Hernandez & McGoldrick, 1999). Assessing such factors is crucial in determining
whether a family's dysfunction is a "normal" reaction to a high degree of

cultural stress, or whether it goes beyond the bounds of transitional stress and requires expert intervention.

All Americans have experienced complex stresses of migration; they may be "buried" or forgotten, and the cultural heritage before migration may have been suppressed or forgotten, but they influence the family's outlook, if sometimes subtly, as they try to accommodate to new situations. Many immigrant groups have been forced to abandon much of their ethnic heritage and have thus lost a part of their identity. Families are more vulnerable the more they have repressed their past. The effects of this hidden history may be all the more powerful for being hidden.

Families that have experienced trauma and devastation within their own society before even beginning the process of immigration will have a monumentally more difficult time adjusting to a new life than those who migrated for adventure or economic betterment. And the hidden effects of this history, especially when it goes unacknowledged, may linger for many generations, as illustrated by the history of the Irish (Hayden, 2001; McGoldrick, 1996), Armenians (Dagirmanjian, 1996), African Americans (Hines & Boyd-Franklin, 1996; Mahmoud, 1998), Latinos (Garcia-Preto, 1996a), and Jews (Cowan, 1982; Rosen & Weltman, 1996), among others.

The degree of ethnic intermarriage in the family also plays a role in the evolution of cultural patterns (McGoldrick & Garcia-Preto, 1984; Crohn, 1995; Petsonk & Remsen, 1988; Root, 2001). Although, as a nation, we have a long history of intercultural relationships, until 1967, our society explicitly forbade racial intermarriage and discouraged cultural intermarriage as well, because they challenged white supremacy. But traditional ethnic and racial categories are now increasingly being challenged by the cultural and racial mixing that has been a long-submerged part of our history. Maria Root (1992, 1996, 2001), one of the prime researchers in this area, has defined a special bill of rights for people of mixed race, asserting their right to define themselves for themselves, and not be limited by society's racial and ethnic stereotypes and caricatures.

Each generational cohort also has a different "culture," as do different geographic regions, urban and rural areas, socioeconomic contexts, and religious affiliations. In addition, we are all increasingly influenced by "popular culture," especially by television, which is unfortunately replacing family and community relationships for more and more people. Some families hold on to their ethnic identification, becoming clannish or prejudiced in response to a perceived threat to their integrity. Others use ethnic identification to push for family loyalty. For other groups, such an emotional demand for ethnic loyalty would probably not hold much weight.

The history of our country is at its core one of cultural loss created by immigration, persecution, poverty, slavery, and/or genocide. At the same time, our country has been largely defined by those seeking change from their ancestors' cultures. As Tataki (1993) states:

Indians were already here, while blacks were forcibly transported to America, and Mexicans were initially enclosed by America's expanding border. The other groups came here as immigrants: for them, America represented liminality—a new world where they could pursue extravagant urges to do things they had thought beyond their capabilities. Like the land itself, they found themselves "betwixt and between all fixed points of classification." No longer fastened as fiercely to their old countries, they felt a stirring to become new people in a society still being defined and formed. (p. 6)

The fluidity of cultural identity has always been an American trait. But a conservative backlash against multiculturalism has also waxed and waned, depending on the economics and politics of the moment. Anti-Arab and anti-Muslim feelings escalated to an extreme degree in the wake of the September 11, 2001 disaster, and white extremist skinheads and neo-Nazi groups at times escalate their fostering of racial and ethnic hatred, while we experience periodic increases of anti-immigrant reactions, depending on the labor needs of the country.

RACE AND RACISM

Race, unlike culture, is not an internal issue but rather a political issue operating to privilege certain people at the expense of others. Unlike culture, which operates from the inside out, influencing us because it represents values that have been passed down to us through generations of our ancestors, race is a construct that imposes judgment on us from the outside in, based on nothing more than our color or physical features. Many who come to the United States are deeply troubled when they experience racism here for the first time. Over time, reactions to our society's system of judgments about "race," and racism as a category to stratify people by skin color, tend to be internalized. Expectations of privilege and entitlement or invalidation tend to become internalized assumptions in response to this social force. All therapists must work actively to undo racism to eradicate this pernicious force in our society. The judgments about self or family that reflect these false categorizations are almost impossible to avoid making in therapy (see Boyd-Franklin, Chapter 10, this volume). Race is an issue of political oppression, not a cultural or genetic issue. As Ignatiev (1995) puts it: "No biologist has ever been able to provide a satisfactory definition of 'race'—that is, a definition that includes all members of a given race and excludes all others" (p. 19). Categorizing people by race serves to justify reducing all members of one group into an undifferentiated social status beneath that of all members of another group. Racism operates like sexism, a similar system of privilege and oppression, justified within the dominant society as a biological or cultural phenomenon that functions systematically to the advantage of certain members of society at the expense of others (Katz, 1978; Hardy & Laszloffy, 1992; Mahmoud, 1998; Hitchcock, 2001).

Although racism may be more subtle and covert today, the politics of race continue to be complex and divisive, and, unfortunately, whites remain generally unaware of the problems society creates for people of color. In a similar way that patriarchy, class hierarchies, and heterosexist ideologies have been invisible structural definers of all European groups' ethnicity, race and racism have also been invisible definers of their cultural values. The invisible knapsack of privilege (McIntosh, 1998) of all white Americans, just by virtue of the color of their skin, is something that most white ethnics do not acknowledge. Although there is a rapidly increasing rate of intermarriage among European groups and of whites with people of color, the percentages are still small. And the level of segregation in the United States between European Americans and people of color, especially African Americans, remains a profound problem in our society, and one that most whites do not notice. Racism and poverty have always dominated the lives of ethnic minorities in the United States. Race has always been a major cultural definer and divider in our society, because those whose skin color marked them as different have always suffered more discrimination than others. They could not "pass," as other immigrants might, leaving them with an "obligatory" ethnic and racial identification.

Racial bigotry and discrimination continue to be a terrible fact of American life, from college campuses to corporate boardrooms. Although conditions have improved since the 1950s, when blacks were not permitted to drink from the same water fountains as whites or to attend integrated schools, we still live in an essentially segregated society. The racial divide continues to be a painful chasm creating profoundly different consciousness for people of color than for whites. People find it even more difficult to talk to each other about racism than to talk about ethnicity. Each new racial incident ignites feelings and expressions of anger and rage, helplessness and frustration. Exploring our own ethnicity is vital to overcoming our prejudices and expanding our understanding of ourselves in context, but we must also take care in our pursuit of multicultural understanding not to diminish our efforts to overcome racism (Katz, 1978).

NOT ROMANTICIZING CULTURE

Just because a culture espouses certain values or beliefs does not make those values and beliefs sacrosanct. All cultural practices are not ethical. Mistreatment of women or children through disrespect, as well as physical or sexual abuse, is a human rights issue, no matter the cultural context in which it occurs. Every intervention is value laden. We must not use notions of neutrality or "deconstruction" to shy away from committing ourselves to core values upholding the respect, dignity, and worth of all human beings.

We must have the courage of our convictions, even while realizing that we can never be too certain that our perspective is the "correct" one. It means we must learn to tolerate ambiguities and continue to question our stance in relation to the position and values of our clients. And we must be especially careful about the power differential if we are part of the dominant group, because the voices of those who are marginalized are harder to hear. The disenfranchised need more support to have their position heard than do those who feel they are entitled because theirs are the dominant values.

In addressing racism, we must also deal with the oppression of women of color. This cannot be blamed solely on white society, for patriarchy is deeply embedded in African, Asian, and South American cultures. We must work for the right of every person to a voice and a sense of safety and belonging. We must challenge those who argue that cultural groups should be allowed to "speak for themselves." This ignores the issue of who speaks for the group, which is usually determined largely by patriarchal and class factors. Helping families define what is normal (healthy) may require supporting marginalized voices within the cultural groups that express liberating possibilities for family adaptation.

FAMILY THERAPY ISSUES

It is almost impossible to understand the meaning of behavior unless one knows something of the cultural values of a family. Even the definition of "family" differs greatly from group to group (McGoldrick et al., 1996). The dominant American (Anglo) definition focuses on the intact nuclear family, whereas African American families focus on a much wider network of kin and community. For Italians, there is no such thing as the "nuclear" family. To them, family means a strong, tightly knit three- or four-generational family that also includes godparents and old friends. The Chinese include as "family" all their ancestors, going all the way back in history, and all their descendants, or at least their male ancestors and descendents. Their definition of family also reflects a profoundly different sense of time than is held in the West.

Another obvious and essential variable is the family's attitude toward therapy. The dominant assumption is that talk is good and can heal a person. Therapy has even been referred to as "the talking cure." Talking to the therapist or to other family members is seen as the path to healing. Clients may not talk openly in therapy for many different reasons related to their cultural background or values. Consider the different value that cultures place on talk.

• African American clients may be uncommunicative, not because they cannot deal with their feelings, but because the context involves a representative of a traditional "white" institution, which they have never had reason to trust.

- In Jewish culture, analyzing and discussing one's experience may be as important as the experience itself for important historical reasons. Jews have long valued the clarifying and sharing of ideas and perceptions in examination of meaning in life. Given the anti-Semitic societies in which Jews have lived over centuries, with their rights and experiences often obliterated, one can understand how they have come to place great importance on analyzing, understanding, and acknowledging what has happened.

- In families of English descent, words tend to be used primarily to accomplish one's goals. They are valued mainly as utilitarian tools. As the son says about his brother's death, in the film *Ordinary People*: "What's the point of talking about it? It doesn't change anything."

- In Chinese culture, families may tend to avoid the dominant American idea of "laying your cards out on the table" verbally. They have many other symbolic ways of communicating, such as with food, rather than with words, so the talking cure as we know it would be a very foreign concept.

- Italians often use words primarily for drama, to convey the emotional intensity of an experience. They may be mystified when others, who take verbal expression at face value, hold them to their words, because for them, it is the interaction and the emotional relationship, not the words, that have the deepest meaning.

- An Irish client's failure to talk may have to do with embarrassment about admitting feelings to anyone, most especially to other family members. The Irish were forced by the British, who ruled them for centuries, to give up their language, which they found a cruel punishment. They are perhaps the world's greatest poets, using words to buffer experience—poetry and humor somehow make reality more tolerable. They use words not necessarily to tell the truth but perhaps to cover it up or embellish it. The Irish have raised poetry, mystification, double meanings, humorous indirection, and ambiguity to an art form in part, perhaps, because their history of oppression led them to realize that telling the truth could be dangerous.

- Norwegians might withhold verbal expression out of respect and politeness, which for them involves not openly stating their negative feelings about other family members. Such a custom may have nothing to do with guilt about "unacceptable" feelings or awkwardness in a therapy context, as it might for the Irish.

- In Sioux Indian culture, talking is actually proscribed in certain family relationships. A wife does not to talk directly to her father-in-law, for example, yet she may experience deep feelings of intimacy with him, a relationship that is almost inconceivable in our pragmatic world. The reduced emphasis on verbal expression seems to free Native American families for other kinds of experience of each other, of nature, and of the spiritual realm.

Cultural groups also vary greatly in the emphasis they place on various life transitions. Irish and African Americans have always considered death the most important life-cycle transition. The Irish place most emphasis on the wake, whereas African Americans spare no expense for a funeral. Italians, Asian Indians, and Poles tend to emphasize weddings, whereas Jews often pay particular attention to the bar or bas mitzvah, a transition from childhood that other groups hardly mark at all. Families' ways of celebrating these events differ also. The Irish tend to celebrate weddings (and every other occasion) by drinking, the Poles by dancing, the Italians by eating, and the Jews by eating, talking, and dancing.

Occupational choices, as well, reflect both personal necessity and group values. The Irish are overrepresented in politics and police work; Jews, in small businesses, medicine, law, and, above all, the mental health field; Germans, in engineering and science; immigrant Greeks and Chinese, in the restaurant business; and Koreans, in food stores.

Ethnic groups' distinctive problems are often the result of cultural traits that are conspicuous strengths in other contexts. For example, British American optimism leads to confidence and flexibility in taking initiative. But the same preference for upbeatness also blocks the ability to cope emotionally with tragedy or to engage in mourning. Historically, the British have perhaps had much reason to feel fortunate as a people. But optimism becomes a vulnerability when they must contend with major losses. They have few philosophical or expressive ways to deal with situations in which optimism, rationality, and belief in the efficacy of individuality are insufficient. Thus, they may feel lost when dependence on the group is the only way to ensure survival.

Concomitantly, groups vary in what they view as problematic behavior. The English may be concerned about dependency or emotionality; the Irish, about "making a scene"; Italians, about disloyalty to the family; Greeks, about any insult to their pride or *filotimo*; Chinese, about harmony; Jews, about their children not being "successful"; Puerto Ricans, about their children not showing respect; Arabs, about their daughters' virginity; and African Americans, about testimony or bearing witness.

Of course, groups also vary in how they respond to problems. The English see work, reason, and stoicism as the best response, whereas Jews often consult doctors and therapists to gain understanding and insight. Until recently, the Irish responded to problems by going to the priest for confession, "offering up" their suffering in prayers, or, especially for men, seeking solace through drink. Italians may prefer to rely on family support, eating, and expressing themselves. West Indians may see hard work, thrift, or consulting with their elders as the solution, and Norwegians might prefer fresh air or exercise. Asian Indians might focus on sacrifice or purity, and the Chinese, on food or prayer.

Groups also differ in attitudes toward seeking help. In general, Italians rely primarily on the family and turn to an outsider only as a last re-

sort. Black Americans have long mistrusted the help they receive from traditional institutions except the church, the only one that was "theirs."
Puerto Ricans and Chinese may somatize when under stress and seek medical rather than mental health services. Norwegians, too, often convert
emotional tensions into physical symptoms, which they consider more acceptable; thus, their preference of the doctor over the psychotherapist.
Likewise, Iranians may view medication and vitamins as a necessary part of
treating symptoms. Many potential patients experience their troubles so-
matically and strongly doubt the value of psychotherapy. And some groups
tend to see their problems as the result of their own (Irish, African Americans, Norwegians) or someone else's (Greeks, Iranians, Puerto Ricans)
sin, action, or inadequacy.

Cultures differ also in their attitudes about group boundaries. Puerto
Ricans, Italians, and Greeks all have similar rural, peasant backgrounds,
yet important ethnic differences exist among these groups. Puerto Ricans
tend to have flexible boundaries between the family and the surrounding
community, so that informal adoption is a common and accepted practice. Italians have much clearer boundaries within the family and draw
rigid boundaries between insiders and outsiders. Greeks have very definite
family boundaries, are disinclined to adopt children, and have deep feelings about the "bloodline." They are also strongly nationalistic, a value
that relates to a nostalgic vision of ancient Greece and to the country they
lost under hundreds of years of Ottoman oppression. By contrast, Italians
in the "old country" defined themselves first by family ties, second by their
village, and, third, if at all, by the region of Italy from which they came.
Only within a U.S. context did defining themselves by ethnicity became
relevant as they experienced discrimination by others. Puerto Ricans'
group identity has coalesced only within the past century, primarily in reaction to experiences with the United States. Each group's way of relating
to therapy will reflect its differing attitudes toward family, group identity,
and outsiders, although certain family characteristics, such as male dominance and role complementarity, are similar for all three groups.

Groups differ also in other patterns of social organization. African
Americans and Jewish families tend to be more democratic, with greater
role flexibility, whereas Greeks and Asian cultures tend to be structured in
a much more hierarchical fashion. All such differences significantly influence how a person might respond to meetings of the whole family together versus individual coaching or meeting with same-sex subgroups of family members. Therapists need to be aware of how their different methods
of intervention fit for clients of different backgrounds.

Appreciation of cultural variability leads to a radically new conceptual
model of clinical intervention. Helping a person achieve a stronger sense
of self may require resolving internalized negative cultural attitudes, cultural conflicts within the family or between the family and the community,
or in the wider context in which the family is embedded. A part of this

process involves identifying and consciously selecting ethnic values we wish to retain and carry on. Families may need coaching to distinguish deeply held convictions from values asserted for dysfunctional emotional reasons.

What is adaptive in a given situation? Answering this requires appreciation of the total context in which behavior occurs. For example, Puerto Ricans may see returning to the island as a solution to their problems. A child who misbehaves may be sent back to live with an extended family member. This solution may be viewed as dysfunctional if the therapist considers only that the child will be isolated from the immediate family, or that Puerto Rico may have fewer resources to meet the child's developmental needs. Rather than counter the parents' plan, the therapist may encourage them to strengthen their connectedness with family members in Puerto Rico with whom their child will be staying, for they will be using a culturally sanctioned network for support. The therapist's role in such situations may be that of a culture broker, helping family members to recognize their own ethnic values and to resolve the conflicts that evolve out of different perceptions and experiences.

There are many examples of such misunderstood behavior. Puerto Rican women are taught to lower their eyes and avoid eye contact, which American therapists are often taught to read as indicating an inability to relate interpersonally. Jewish patients may consider it essential to inquire about the therapist's credentials: Many other groups would perceive this as an affront, but for them, it is a needed reassurance. Iranian and Greek patient may ask for medication, give every indication of taking it, but then go home and not take it as prescribed. Irish families may not praise or show overt affection to their children for fear of giving them a "swelled head," which therapists may misread as lack of caring. Physical punishment, routinely used to keep children in line by many groups, including, until recently, the dominant groups in the United States, may be perceived as idiosyncratic pathological behavior rather than culturally accepted behavior, albeit a violation of human rights. This is not to justify child beatings, which have been widely accepted among many cultures. Rather, we must consider the cultural context in which a behavior evolves even as we try to shape it, when it does not reflect humanitarian or equitable values. The point is that therapists, especially those of dominant groups, who tend to take their own values as the norm must be extremely cautious in judging the meaning of behavior they observe, and in imposing their own methods and timetable of change.

CONCLUSIONS

Culturally respectful clinical work involves helping people clarify their cultural and self-identity in relation to their family, community, and history, while they also adapt to changing circimstances as they move through life. The following guidelines are meant to suggest the kind of inclusive thinking necessary for judging family problems and normal adaptation in cultural context:

- Assume that cultural, class, religious, and political background influences how families view their problems, until you have evidence to the contrary.
- Assume that a positive awareness of one's cultural heritage, just like a positive connection to one's family of origin, contributes to mental health and well being.
- Assume that a negative feeling or lack of awareness of one's cultural heritage is probably reflective of cutoffs, oppression, or traumatic experiences that have led to suppression of history.
- Assume that no one can ever fully understand another's culture, but that curiosity, humility, and awareness of one's own cultural values and history contribute to sensitve interviewing.
- Assume that clients from marginalized cultures have probably internalized society's prejudices about them, and those from dominant cultural groups have probably internalized assumptions about their own superiority and right to be privileged within our society.

REFERENCES

Abudabbeh, N. (1996). Arab families. In M. McGoldrick, J. Giordano, & J. K. Pearce (Eds.), *Ethnicity and family therapy* (2nd ed.). New York: Guilford Press.

Angelou, M. (1986). *All god's children need traveling shoes.* New York: Vintage.

Baldwin, J. (1993). *Nobody knows my name.* New York: Vintage.

Bernal, G. (1996). Cuban families. In M. McGoldrick, J. Giordano, & J. K. Pearce (Eds.), *Ethnicity and family therapy* (2nd ed.). New York: Guilford Press.

Boyd-Franklin, N. (1989). *Black families in therapy: A multisystems approach.* New York: Guilford Press.

Congress, E. P. (1994). The use of culturagrams to assess and empower culturally diverse families. *Families in Society, 75,* 531–540.

Cowan, P. (1982). *An orphan in history: Retrieving a Jewish legacy.* New York: Doubleday.

Crohn, J. (1995). *Mixed matches.* New York: Fawcett Columbine.

Dagirmanjgian, S. (1996). Armenian families. In M. McGoldrick, J. Giordano, & J. K. Pearce (Eds.), *Ethnicity and family therapy* (2nd ed.). New York: Guilford Press.

Dilworth-Anderson, P., Burton, L., & Johnson, L. (1993). Reframing theories for understanding race, ethnicity and families. In P. G. Boss, W. J. Doherty, R. LaRossa, W. R. Schumm, & S. K. Steinmetz (Eds.), *Sourcebook of family theories and methods: A contextual approach* New York: Plenum Press.

Erdrich, L., & Dorris, M. (1991). *The crown of Columbus.* New York: Harper.

Fadiman, A. (1998). *The spirit catches you and you fall down: A Hmong Child, her American doctors and the collision of two cultures.* New York: Farrar, Straus and Geroux.

Falicov, C. J. (1995). Training to think culturally: A multidimensional framework. *Family Process.*

Falicov, C. J. (1996a). *Latino families in therapy.* New York: Guilford Press.

Falicov, C. J. (1996b) Mexican families. In M. McGoldrick, J. Giordano, & J. K. Pearce (Eds.), *Ethnicity and family therapy* (2nd ed.). New York: Guilford Press.

Friere, P. (1994). *The pedagogy of hope.* New York: Continuum.

Fusco, C. (1995). *English is broken here: Notes on cultural fusion in the Americas.* New York: New Press.

Garcia-Preto, N. (1996a). Latino families: An overview. In M. McGoldrick, J. Giordano, & J. K. Pearce (Eds.), *Ethnicity and family therapy* (2nd ed.). New York: Guilford Press.

Garcia-Preto, N. (1996b). Puerto Rican families. In M. McGoldrick, J. Giordano, & J. K. Pearce (Eds.), *Ethnicity and family therapy* (2nd ed.). New York: Guilford Press.

Hardy, K. V., & Laszloffy, T. A. (1992). Training racially sensitive family therapists: Context, content and contact. *Families in Society, 73*(6). 363–370.

Hardy, K. V., & Laszloffy, T. A. (1995). The cultural genogram: Key to training culturally competent family therapists. *Journal of Marital and Family Therapy, 21*(3), 227–237.

Hayden, T. (Ed.). (1998). *Irish hunger.* Boulder, CO: Roberts Reinhart.

Hayden, T. (2001). *Irish on the inside: In search of the soul of Irish America.* New York: Verso.

Hernandez, M., & McGoldrick, M. (1999). Migration and the family life cycle. In B. Carter & M. McGoldrick (Eds.), *The expanded family life cycle.* Boston: Allyn & Bacon.

Hines, P. M. & Boyd-Franklin, N. (1996). African American families. In M. McGoldrick, J. Giordano, & J. K. Pearce (Eds.), *Ethnicity and family therapy* (2nd ed.). New York: Guilford Press.

Hitchcock, J. (2001). *Unraveling the white cocoon.* Dubuque: Kendall/Hunt.

Ignatiev, N. (1995). *How the Irish became white.* New York: Routledge.

Kaiser, W. L. (2001). *A new view of the world: Handbook to the Peters projection world map.* New York: Friendship Press.

Katz, J. H. (1978). *White awareness: Handbook for anti-racism training.* Norman: University of Oklahoma Press.

Mahmoud, V. (1998). The double bind dynamics of racism. In M. McGoldrick (Ed.), *Revisioning family therapy: Race, culture and gender in clinical practice.* New York: Guilford Press.

Malcomson, S. (2000). *One drop of blood: The American misadventure of race.* New York: Farrar, Straus & Giroux.

McGoldrick, M. (1996). Overview: Ethnicity and family therapy. In M. McGoldrick, J. Giordano, & J. K. Pearce (Eds.), *Ethnicity and family therapy* (2nd ed.). New York: Guilford Press.

McGoldrick, M. (Ed.). (1998). *Revisioning family therapy: Race, culture and gender in clinical practice.* New York: Guilford Press.

McGoldrick, M., & Garcia-Preto, N. (1984). Ethnic intermarriage. *Family Process, 23*(3), 347–362.

McGoldrick. M., Giordano, J., & Pearce, J. K. (1996). *Ethnicity and family therapy* (2nd ed.). New York: Guilford Press.

McGoldrick, M., Pearce, J. K., & Giordano, J. (1982). *Ethnicity and family therapy.* New York: Guilford Press.

McIntosh, P. (1998). White privilege: Unpacking the invisible knapsack. In M. Mc-Goldrick (Ed.), *Re-visioning family therapy from a multicultural perspective.* New York: Guilford Press.

Petsonk, J., & Remsen, J. (1988). *The intermarriage handbook: A guide for Jews and Christians.* New York: Morrow.

Root, M. P. P. (Ed.). (1992). *Racially mixed people in America.* Thousand Oaks, CA: Sage.

Root, M. P. P. (Ed). (1996). *The multiracial experience: Racial borders as the new frontier.* Thousand Oaks, CA: Sage.

Root, M. P. P. (2001). *Love's revolution: Interracial marriage.* Philadelphia: Temple University Press.

Rosen, E., & Weltman, S. (1996). Jewish families: An overview. In M. McGoldrick, J. Giordano, & J. K. Pearce (Eds.), *Ethnicity and family therapy* (2nd ed.). New York: Guilford Press.

Tataki, R. (1993). *A different mirror: A history of multicultural America.* Boston: Little, Brown.

U.S. Census Bureau. (2000). Racial and ethnic classifications used in Census 2000 and beyond: Population division. Retrieved on-line at www.census.gov/dmd.

CHAPTER 10

RACE, CLASS, AND POVERTY

Nancy Boyd-Franklin

In order to evaluate what is "normal" in the development of any family, clinicians and researchers must explore the larger social context in which the family lives. Race and class are two of the most complex and emotionally loaded issues. In the United States, for poor, inner-city, African American families, the day-to-day realities of racism, discrimination, classism, poverty, homelessness, violence, crime, and drugs create forces that continually threaten the family's survival. Many clinicians who have no framework with which to view these complicated interrelationships become overwhelmed. The purpose of this chapter is to provide a framework that will be helpful in understanding and working with these families. The first part of the chapter explores the complexity of these issues for African American families and the second, the issues that race, class, and poverty raise for family therapists.

Two cautions are in order. First, discussing race, class, and poverty in one chapter necessitates a less thorough treatment of each than is warranted. A second caveat is that race, class, and poverty are not monolithic constructs that apply unilaterally. Race, for example, has many different levels of meaning for African American individuals and families in the United States. Class as an issue is equally complex and not merely a socioeconomic distinction. For many African Americans, class or socioeconomic level does not foreordain value system: For example, a family classified as "poor" because of income may have "middle-class" values. Also, a "culture of poverty"—coping mechanisms necessary for survival "on the streets"—may exist in families. Finally, the societal realities of racism, oppression, and classism contribute to the challenges that many African American families experience (Hill, 1999).

RACISM AND OPPRESSION

It is important to explore the societal context of life for African American families. Historically, they share both a common African heritage and the degradation of slavery in the United States. In order for Americans of European ancestry to have justified slavery, persons of African American descent had to be viewed as subhuman. Thus, for African Americans, skin color became a "mark of oppression." The oppression of slavery—and later segregation and discrimination—contributed to a sense of rage that persists to this day in many African Americans.

Slavery created a legacy for white people as well. Grier and Cobbs (1968) and Hines and Boyd-Franklin (1996) have indicated that the consequences of slavery were as evident in the children of slavemasters as they were in the children of slaves. Race continues to be an extremely conflicted issue for many white Americans. For some, the issue elicits emotions of guilt, rage, or fear. The increasing numbers of bias-related incidents in this country reveal that these old wounds remain an indelible part of the American psyche (Jones, 1997).

THE ISSUE OF RACE

For African Americans, the concept of race has many levels of meaning. On one level, it identifies those persons of African ancestry and implies a shared origin. Often, it applies to shared physical characteristics such as skin color, hair texture, and appearance (Carter, 1995; Helms & Cook, 1999). However, African Americans as a race present in many different skin colors and appearances, because individuals may have various mixtures of ancestry, including Native American and European elements.

Jones (1997) and Pinderhughes (1989) have shown that "over time, race has acquired a social meaning . . . via the mechanism of stereotyping. . . . Status assignment based on skin color identity has evolved into complex social structures that promote a power differential between Whites and various people of color" (Pinderhughes, 1989, p. 71). Hopps (1982) has stated that "although many forms of exclusion and discrimination exist in this country, none is so deeply rooted, persistent or intractable as that based on color" (p. 3). For this reason, many African American families' perceptions of the world—including self-identity, racial pride, child rearing, educational and school-related experiences, job or employment opportunities, or lack of them, financial security or the lack of it, as well as treatment in interpersonal encounters and male–female relationships—are screened through the lens of the racial experience (Boyd-Franklin, 1989; Boyd-Franklin & Franklin, 1998; Grier & Cobbs, 1968; Taylor, Jackson, & Chatters, 1997).

IMPACT OF RACE ON CHILD REARING

Many African American parents, aware of the degrading messages their children receive from society, particularly through the school systems, make a conscious effort to instill a sense of racial pride and strong positive identity in their children (Franklin, Boyd-Franklin, & Draper, 2002; McAdoo, 2002). A further challenge in child rearing for African Americans is combating pervasive negative images, particularly in the media.

Thus, within such a context, "normal family development" requires many African American parents to educate their children to the realities of racism and discrimination, and to prepare them for the negative messages they may encounter. African American parents, interviewed for the book *Boys Into Men: Raising Our African American Teenage Sons* (Boyd-Franklin, Franklin, & Toussaint, 2000), frequently stated that they felt that they had to be more "vigilant" in order to raise an African American child today, particularly a male child. However, parents must walk a fine line between giving children the tools to understand racism, so that they do not internalize the process, and instilling in them a belief that they can achieve despite the odds and overcome racism, without becoming consumed with rage and bitterness. This is a complex task and a difficult developmental journey for a family or an individual to navigate (Boyd-Franklin et al., 2000).

RACISM, THE INVISIBILITY SYNDROME, AND GENDER ISSUES

There are many levels of complications of racism with which African Americans must contend in the process of "normal family development." The legacy of slavery and oppression has contributed to a fear in American society of African American males that begins at a very early age. Franklin (1992, 1999) has referred to an "invisibility factor," a paradoxical process by which the high skin-color visibility of African American men causes society to view them with fear and, as a consequence, to treat them as if they are "invisible."

African American male children, who may begin school being perceived as "cute" by teachers, at a very young age (7, 8, or 9) are viewed as a threat. Kunjufu (1985), in his book *Countering the Conspiracy to Destroy Black Boys*, discusses the "fourth-grade failure syndrome," in which teachers (and therapists) often become intimidated by African American male children and begin to label them as aggressive, hyperactive, and as failures (Boyd-Franklin et al., 2000).

African American families are thus in a double bind, particularly when rearing sons. Although racism clearly exists for both male and female African American children, society tends to be more punitive toward and restrictive of male children. The risk in raising sons to be assertive is that society will see them as aggressive. The consequences of this have many levels of impact, including labeling within the school system, high dropout and unemployment rates, overrepresentation in the prison system, and, most tragically, early death on the streets (Boyd-Franklin et al., 2000).

CLASS

Social class is extremely complicated in the United States, particularly when coupled with issues of race. Many African American families find that their experiences of class distinctions within their own communities are very different from the class categories applied in the broader American society (Hill, 1993; 1999). For example, on the one hand, many poor, working-class African American families are considered "middle class" within their own communities because of their values, aspirations, and expectations for their children. On the other hand, class status is very precarious for many African Americans. In times of economic recession, African Americans are particularly vulnerable to layoffs and often fall victim to "last hired, first fired" policies.

THE "CLASS NOT RACE" MYTH

There has long been a tendency in the social sciences, as well as in the mental health field, to minimize the importance of race and to focus more on class variables. A prominent sociologist, William Julius Wilson, in his book *The Declining Significance of Race* (1980), argued that whereas race and racism were factors in the past in creating the poverty of African Americans, the opportunities of the late 1960s and 1970s made middle-class status available to many African Americans. However, Wilson incorrectly concluded that because there now exists an African American middle class, class has replaced race as the salient distinction, with the vast numbers of African American families who are trapped in the vicious cycle of poverty constituting an "underclass." Although he modified his views in his more recent books (1987, 1996), Wilson's initial work had a major impact on public policy.

Wilson's original theory is far too simplistic in dismissing the complex interplay of variables such as race, class, and poverty. Thomas and Hughes (1986), Boyd-Franklin (1989), and Hill (1999) have argued that there is a continuing significance of race that must be explored in assessing the normal family processes of African Americans. It is important to acknowledge class and race together with oppressive poverty in working with inner-city families.

MIDDLE-CLASS AFRICAN AMERICAN FAMILIES

Although this chapter primarily focuses on the experience of African American families living in poverty, it is important here to explore briefly the growth of the black middle class and the unique issues facing these families. Within the last two decades, there has been an increase in the number of middle-class black families. Hill (1999) estimates this number at approximately 25% of the African American community. There is even a small percentage (5%) of upper-class African American families today. Hill (1999) cautions us to

> be careful not to exaggerate the growth of the middle and upper class among blacks because they are often not economically comparable with the white middle and upper classes. . . . First, as Oliver and Shapiro (1995) and Anderson (1994) observe, most middle and upper class black families attain their status through [two] incomes and occupations, while comparable whites achieve their status through wealth and assets, which are ten times greater than blacks. Second, several observers (Duncan, 1992; Reich, 1994) have noted the growth of the white middle class has slowed and the gap between them and the white upper class has been widening. There is similar evidence that the growth in the black middle class has also slowed in recent decades (Billingsley, 1992; Hill, 1993). . . . The steady decline in scholarships and grants for black college students is likely to slow the growth of the black middle class even further during the 21st century. (p. 77)

Middle-class, educated African Americans who encountered a "glass ceiling" when anticipating promotions in their professions were rudely reminded of the existence of an institutionalized racism in this country. Bias-related incidents in cities and on college campuses increased. Many African Americans began to experience a "white backlash" from those who felt their own opportunities threatened, and the "blaming the victim" philosophy of an earlier era has since returned.

Despite the economic gains by some African Americans, there has been an enduring yet more subtle quality to the racism that has emerged in the 21st century. Racism is often less overt and more covert, but just as painful (Jones, 1997). Ellis Cose (1993), in his book *The Rage of the Privileged Class,* describes the anger and rage felt by many middle- and upper-class blacks when they continue to encounter overt racial assaults and more subtle "microaggressions" despite their high educational and socioeconomic level (Pierce, 1988). Tokenism persists, with the hiring and promotion of relatively few African Americans to high-level positions.

POVERTY AND THE "VICTIM SYSTEM"

Although a number of African Americans have benefited from job and educational opportunities, many African American communities remain mired in multigenerational poverty (Hill, 1993, 1999). These families are faced with drug and alcohol abuse, gangs, crime, homelessness or increasingly dangerous public housing, violence and death, teenage pregnancy, high unemployment, high school dropout rates, poor educational systems, and ongoing issues with the police and the justice system (Boyd-Franklin et al., 2000). They see little in terms of options for their children, and many feel trapped, which leads to what Pinderhughes (1982; 1989) has termed as "the victim system":

> A victim system is a circular feedback process which . . . threatens self-esteem and reinforces problematic responses in communities, families and individuals. The feedback works as follows: Barriers to opportunity and education limit the chance for achievement, employment, and attainment of skills. This limitation can, in turn, lead to poverty or stress in relationships, which interferes with adequate performance of family roles. (1982, p. 109)

Many of these individuals feel trapped, disempowered, and a growing rage, as demonstrated by the Los Angeles riots in May 1992. Economic conditions for these families have worsened; many live in fear for themselves and their children.

As Boyd-Franklin et al. (2000) have shown, adolescence begins early within poor, inner-city communities when, at a very young age, children are faced with pressures related to sexuality, household responsibility, drugs, and alcohol use. Random violence, particularly drug-related violence, has become a major concern for poor, inner-city families. Parents struggle with helpless feelings about preventing "the streets" from taking over their children. This sense of futility and disempowerment is a potent issue for many poor African American families.

CHRONIC POSTTRAUMATIC STRESS DISORDER

Inner-city children and families commonly experience chronic trauma and stress. Children and adults living in housing projects or housing shelters often report intense fear in walking through darkened halls, or past deserted buildings and crack houses. It is not unusual for children to have to walk through a "needle park" to get to school, or to climb over crack vials and discarded syringes in the playground. Many are acquainted from an early age with violence in their homes in the form of child abuse, sexual abuse, drug overdose, and AIDS. Children often begin to exhibit behavior problems after witnessing traumatic events, such as violent deaths in their communities. In addition to acting-out behaviors manifested in oppositional or conduct disorders, these children often experience anxiety or depressive symptoms. However, the classic features of posttraumatic stress disorder—nightmares, flashbacks of the traumatic event, generalized fear and anxiety, and fears of entering areas where traumatic events occurred—are often overlooked by clinicians.

RACE AND POVERTY

Although there are significant numbers of poor families in this country who are not African American, and many have lived for generations in poverty, poor African Americans experience a dual oppression based on race and class (Hill, 1999). Whereas members of other ethnic groups have attained upward mobility within one or two generations of immigrating to the United States, chronic unemployment and high dropout rates for African American youth (particularly men aged 15–25) have affected many families' views of their options.

RACISM AND POVERTY, ANGER, AND RAGE

The combination of discrimination and oppression, augmented by racism and poverty, has produced a fierce anger in many African Americans (Cose, 1993; Jones, 1997). For African American families trapped in poverty and assaulted by unemployment, high dropout rates, drugs, violence, crime, and homelessness (at times, the result of urban gentrification), anger and rage have been growing for decades. Often, rage is turned on those living in the community, as can be seen in incidents of "black on black" crime. It can be acted out through conduct-disordered or delinquent behavior, or in the family, by stealing, child abuse, or domestic violence. Finally, rage can be internalized and manifested as depression, or self-destructive drug or alcohol abuse.

Both African American and white service providers must be aware that anger and rage may be directed against them. This anger and rage frequently paralyzes well-meaning clinicians who work in these communities. Training programs must address this issue and prepare clinicians for it by helping them learn not to personalize it, and by teaching them effective strategies for joining and building trust with these families (Boyd-Franklin, 1989; Boyd-Franklin & Bry, 2000).

ATTITUDES OF MENTAL HEALTH WORKERS TOWARD POOR AFRICAN AMERICAN FAMILIES

In the mental health field, poor African Americans have tended to be pathologized and labeled as "unmotivated" or "lazy," "disorganized," "deprived," or "disadvantaged," too often leading clinicians to "blame the victim" and dismiss these families as untreatable. Intervention models often offer a limited focus on "individuals" or "families," without considering their social context. Mental health workers who enter inner-city communities may thus be overwhelmed and ill-equipped to cope with the realities of poverty, for example, homelessness, teenage pregnancy, unemployment, crime, appalling living conditions, hunger, poor health care, and maltreatment of the poor by public agencies such as schools, police, and juvenile justice and court systems. As a consequence, mental health workers and family therapists may find themselves mirroring the lack of empowerment that these families feel.

RESPONSES OF POOR AFRICAN AMERICAN FAMILIES TO MENTAL HEALTH SERVICES

For many families, poverty has led to a greater likelihood of intrusion by outside agencies, especially the welfare department. Often, inner-city families live with the fear of removal of their children by child protective agencies. Many African Americans have a long memory for the policies of the past, such as the Aid to Dependent Children, which would often be withheld if a man was contributing to the support of a family. This policy set a disincentive for past generations of couples to marry when pregnancy occurred. Women, moreover, were often motivated to claim that they headed "single-parent" households and men remained peripheral to their families, a factor that contributed significantly to the "invisibility" of African American men (Franklin, 1992, 1999). Even though the laws have now changed, generations within African American communities were impacted by these policies.

This legacy of intrusion by social and child protective services, police, legal, and criminal justice systems into poor African American communities has resulted in a "healthy cultural paranoia" or suspicion (Boyd-Franklin, 1989; Grier & Cobbs, 1968). Although this pattern is evident in other poor families, it is far more intense with the added variable of racism. This "healthy cultural paranoia" extends toward "helping institu-

tions" and "helping professions" as well. Thus, schools and teachers, social
service agencies and social workers, mental health clinics and therapists of
all disciplines, hospitals, and medical, nursing, and other health care professionals are faced with families who are suspicious of their efforts. Service providers who are unaware of the legacy of racism and classism may
personalize this initial response and erroneously presume that these families do not want their services or cannot be treated.

Another complication is that many African American families, particularly those living in the inner city, are not self-referred and thus may feel
coerced to enter treatment. There is also a very widely held stigma in this
community that therapy is "for crazy, sick, or weak people," or for "white
folks." In addition, because of "healthy cultural paranoia," poor African
Americans may tell their children that family business is "nobody's business but our own," and may caution against "airing the dirty laundry outside the family." Therefore, mental health service providers may find it
necessary to address these issues first and establish trust with families before any intervention can take place (Boyd-Franklin, 1989).

STRENGTHS AND SURVIVAL SKILLS

Many social scientists and service providers have tended to focus on the
deficiencies in inner-city African American families. Viewing families
through a deficit lens blinds one to their inherent strengths and survival
skills. It is extremely important that public policy and clinical training programs focus on the strengths that must be mobilized to produce change.

The first strength is an extensive kinship network comprised of
"blood" and "nonblood" family members (Billingsley, 1968, 1992, 1994;
Boyd-Franklin, 1989; Hill, 1972, 1999; Logan, 2001; McAdoo, 1996, 2002;
Stack, 1974) who help these families survive by providing support, encouragement, and "reciprocity" in terms of sharing goods, money, and services.
This network might include older relatives such as great-grandparents,
grandmothers, grandfathers, aunts, uncles, cousins, and older brothers
and sisters, all of whom may participate in child rearing, as well as "nonblood relatives" such as godparents, babysitters, neighbors, friends,
church family members, ministers, ministers' wives, and so forth.

Because it is "normal" for African American families to be connected
to such a network, those families who come to the attention of mental
health services may have become isolated or disconnected from their traditional support network. Families may become disconnected as the key
"switchboard" family members of the older generation begin to die. These
are often the family members who kept the family together through
Thanksgiving and Christmas dinners, special holidays, family reunions,
and "family news" such as births, deaths, and marriages. Also, family members who engage in substance abuse may become "cutoff" from their fami-

ly network because their stealing from the family in order to support a drug habit has given rise to much anger. Additionally, a "cutoff" may occur when a family member becomes homeless as a result of being "burnt out" or evicted. In some inner-city areas, entire neighborhoods have been dispossessed through arson or efforts of gentrification.

Establishing trust is frequently difficult at first, particularly if the therapist is of a different race, class, or culture. However, once trust has been established after a number of contacts, families are often more willing to share vital information and their genograms, family trees, or "real family" networks.

The task for therapists is often to search for persons who represent "islands of strength" within the family (Billingsley, 1992; Logan, 2001). Unfortunately, these family members often do not come in to agencies or clinics. Therefore, in order to identify and/or meet the individuals who really hold the power in African American families, the worker may have to obtain the family's permission to visit the home.

It is not unusual for poor African American mothers to present at mental health centers as overwhelmed single parents with their children. In traditional clinical settings, the distress presented by such women has been overpathologized by locating the source of their problems in their own character disorders, and misapplication of diagnoses such as "borderline." It is crucial to appreciate the context of their sense of being overwhelmed or their disorganization and lack of resources to manage realistically overwhelming situations. Therapists should avoid making snap judgments on the basis of first impressions and instead broaden their lens and familiarize themselves with the formal and informal networks to which the family may be connected. For families who are "cut off" from these support systems, a part of the therapy must focus on helping them to resolve conflictual issues in order to reconnect with their families of origin or to form new support networks within their communities. Such an approach might prove particularly empowering for poor families who experience a sense of isolation and fear within their own communities.

RELIGION, SPIRITUALITY, AND OTHER SURVIVAL SKILLS

Many African American families have gained strength from their spiritual and/or religious orientation (Billingsley, 1994; Boyd-Franklin & Lockwood, 1999; Hill, 1993; Walsh, 1999). Particularly for the older generation, this translates into church membership and a feeling of community or connectedness with a "church family" (Billingsley, 1994; Boyd-Franklin, 1989). Many poor families have used this church family to provide role models and support with child rearing. For families who fight a constant battle to "save their children from the streets," churches often provide an alternative network for friends, and male and female adult role models who have achieved stature and distinction, including the minister, the minister's wife, deacons, deaconesses, elders, and trustee boards. These role models are very visible and active. The church community also provides activities such as junior choir, afterschool and summer activities, and babysitting during services.

Many younger African American families in inner-city areas either have rebelled against this support system or have become disconnected and dispirited (Aponte, 1994). It is essential that we learn from the functional, poor families in African American communities who identify these supports for themselves and their children. Service providers should be aware of the "church families" and be acquainted with the ministers in African American communities, who have a great deal of influence and can sometimes provide help and support for a family that is homeless, for a mother who is struggling to raise her children alone and searching for afterschool activities, or for a chronically mentally ill adult who has become "cut off" from his or her extended family after the death of the main caregiver.

It is also important to note a distinction between "spirituality" and "religious orientation" in African Americans (see Walsh & Pryce, Chapter 13, this volume.) Family members who may not have a "church home" or formal membership in a church community may still have a deep, abiding "spirituality." In the Afrocentric tradition and view of the world, the "psyche" and the "spirit" are one. Therefore, spirituality is often a strength and a survival mechanism for African American families that can be tapped, particularly in times of death and dying, illness, loss, and bereavement. Thus, family members may not go to church, but they may "pray to the Lord" when times are hard.

LOVE OF CHILDREN: ANOTHER LOOK AT EXTENDED FAMILY CHILD-REARING PRACTICES

Therapists working with African American, inner-city families may find themselves making judgments about values regarding child rearing. Because of the harshness of their lives and the skills necessary for survival in a racist society, many African American families have adopted the strict discipline known as "spare the rod, spoil the child" (Boyd-Franklin et al., 2000). It is important for clinicians to recognize that for these families this concept of discipline is often a "normal family value." Despite what may be seen by therapists as abusive treatment of children, this parenting practice is often rooted in feelings of love and concern in families who fear for their children's well-being, particularly that of their male children. Reframes with these families that focus on caring intentions, such as "You love him (or her) so much that you are trying to teach him right and protect him from harm," are very powerful. Once this respect has been given, parental family members will be more able to hear "But I have the sense that all of your efforts do not seem to be working."

Some families preach this "tough" philosophy but are very inconsistent in their parenting. Once the underlying love has been recognized, these parents can hear the need for consistency. Another variable related to consistency has to do with extended family involvement in child rearing. Researchers have documented the widespread pattern of "multiple mothering or fathering," in which parenting responsibilities are often shared by grandmothers, grandfathers, aunts, uncles, cousins, older brothers and sisters, and "nonblood relatives," such as ministers, church family members, neighbors, friends, and babysitters (Billingsley, 1968, 1992; Boyd-Franklin, 1989; Hill, 1972, 1999; Hines & Boyd-Franklin, 1996; Logan, 2001; McAdoo, 1996, 2002; Stack, 1974). These supports often provide aid and strength to overburdened parents; however, the negotiation of these relationships can be complex, and inconsistencies in parenting may develop because so many individuals are involved. In family assessments, practitioners need to look beyond the household to identify important kin. Alas, overvaluing the "nuclear family" in the dominant culture may blind workers to the rich, multigenerational ties. The clinician's task in working with such family networks is to open communication between the "parental" figures and reach consensus on boundaries, rules, and disciplinary practices.

SINGLE-PARENT FAMILIES

There is a tendency in the social science literature to treat single-parent families as if they represent a homogeneous group. In fact, there are many different kinds of single-parent families, whose circumstances vary according to family functioning, capabilities of the parent, socioeconomic and income level, employment, and degree of extended family support (see Anderson, Chapter 5, this volume).

In an earlier work (Boyd-Franklin, 1989), service workers were cautioned about the tendency to mislabel automatically all single-parent families as dysfunctional. *The fact of single parenthood does not automatically make a family "dysfunctional"* (Boyd-Franklin, 1989; McAdoo, 2002; Murray & Brody, 2002). Lindblad-Goldberg, Dukes, and Lasley (1988) compared functional and dysfunctional low-income, African American, single-parent families living in Philadelphia. The functional families predictably had clear boundaries and role responsibilities. They were not isolated but drew readily on the support of their extended family kinship network.

There are also differences in the ways in which families became single-parent entities. Increasing numbers of African American single parents become single through divorce, separation, or death (a trend that mirrors a similar pattern in American society as a whole) (Boyd-Franklin,

1989). Also, a number of women in their 30s and 40s become single parents by choice as they become older and are concerned about being childless. Although these trends are important, the largest number of African American single parents initially attain that status through unwed, teenage pregnancy.

TEENAGE PREGNANCY

One of the most complicated phenomena in African American communities is the issue of teenage pregnancy. There has been an ongoing tendency in social science literature to "blame the victim" and to label these young women as irresponsible (McAdoo, 1996; Tatum, Moseley, Boyd-Franklin, & Herzog, 1995). This phenomenon must be viewed within the context of poverty, unemployment, racism, and the general sense of hopelessness that frequently pervades inner-city urban communities. For many young women living in these conditions, having a child becomes a "rite of passage" to womanhood. Unemployment and lack of opportunity affect both young women and men in inner-city African American neighborhoods. Wilson (1987) has clearly shown that when men had jobs or believed they had prospects as breadwinner/provider, they were significantly more likely to marry. Unfortunately, the realities of a declining economy and the results of racism and discrimination leave them with few options. For some African American men who feel disenfranchised, having a child becomes a way to demonstrate manhood. Because they lack the sense of a future, immediate pleasure and the potency involved in creating a life become part of a more present-oriented way of life. Once a child is born, if the mother is too young to be employed, the child is placed on Aid to Dependent Children (welfare). This system further reinforces the exclusion or "invisibility" of the man by decreasing a family's financial support if he is present. Generally, because girls become pregnant as young as age 13, 14, or 15, older women in the family are usually actively involved in child care. This creates complex family and parenting dynamics.

MULTIGENERATIONAL ISSUES

For many of these young women, single parenthood and teenage pregnancy constitute multigenerational family patterns—both the mother and the grandmother in the family also became pregnant during their adolescent years. Often, as a daughter approaches puberty, there is increased anxiety within the family system (Tatum et al., 1995). Families react in a variety of ways, the most common of which are (1) to become overly rigid, restrictive, and punitive with the child in an attempt to protect her from pregnancy; or (2) to feel overwhelmed with this multigenerational family transmission process (Bowen, 1976) and to "throw up their hands," leaving the child with the responsibility of raising herself. These adolescents often appear very much out of control, and parents often feel helpless to make a difference. It is paradoxical that either of these extreme responses increase the risk that the girl will carry out the family script of multigenerational teenage pregnancy. Family treatment that explores these issues openly between the generations in a family can help to break this cycle.

EMPOWERMENT

In confronting the obstacles of racism, classism, poverty and the "victim system," many inner-city African American families feel disenfranchised and powerless. Therefore, a key factor in any treatment approach must focus on empowerment (Boyd-Franklin, 1989; Boyd-Franklin & Bry, 2000). This concept of empowerment is multifaceted, consisting of the empowerment of both the "executive" or parental system in the family (Minuchin, 1974) and the families to intervene in the multiple systems that impact and intrude on their lives.

Structural family therapy, which encourages clinicians to put parental figures in charge of their children, is a very powerful approach (Minuchin, 1974; Aponte, 1976, 1994). When these families feel that they are "losing their children to the streets," it is very empowering to pull extended family members together to fight and "take their children back from the streets" (Boyd-Franklin et al., 2000).

Empowerment through Multiple Family Groups

Social isolation (homelessness and lack of support networks) exacerbates mental health problems. One approach that is extremely empowering to family members, as well as to the clinicians who work with them, is the multiple family group therapy intervention. Families who lack support systems are brought together in a group with other families in their community that are struggling to overcome similar problems. Together they become a support system for each other and often form relationships that continue beyond the life of the group (Boyd-Franklin & Bry, 2000). This approach is especially valuable for single parents who face myriad challenges on their own.

African American families traditionally search out and create social supports when moving to a new community. However, because of the fear of violence, crime, and drugs, many inner-city African American families today find themselves isolated, virtually held hostage within their own homes and apartments. Therefore, it is truly empowering to introduce these families to one another and bring them together around their common concerns for their children, because the enhanced sense of community destigmatizes common dilemmas. It is both comforting and personally empowering to know that one is not alone and that there exists support for change. An example of such a support situation would be for families to be able to go together to discuss with the principal at their children's school their concerns related to drugs, crime, and so forth.

Empowerment through a Multisystems Model

Treatment must take into consideration the fact that, as discussed earlier, poor, inner-city African-American families cope with the intrusiveness of many organizations, such as agencies, schools, hospitals, police, courts, juvenile justice systems, welfare, child protective services, and housing and mental health services on a daily basis (Boyd-Franklin, 1989; Boyd-Franklin & Bry, 2000; Henggeler & Borduin, 1990; Henggeler & Santos, 1997). Empowerment within this context means identifying the various agencies or institutions that affect a family's life. An eco map (Boyd-Franklin, 1989; Hartman & Laird, 1983) can be helpful in diagramming these systems. The family members can then be empowered to intervene in these systems in the following ways: (1) calling meetings of various agencies that have the power to make decisions for their families; (2) writing letters, and getting letters from therapists, doctors, and so forth, in support of their families; (3) obtaining a therapist's support to be empowered to ask for conferences with supervisors of resistant workers. The key here is that clinicians must resist the urge to do all of the work themselves. Family members must be empowered to take charge of these issues.

Empowerment of Clinicians

Training programs in all disciplines in the mental health field have not been effective in adequately preparing clinicians for working with poor African American families. Well-meaning, eager clinicians may be unprepared for the racial tension, anger, and "healthy cultural paranoia" they encounter. They also may well be overwhelmed by the realities of poverty, or be unprepared to cope with the myriad multisystems levels and agencies that are factors in these families' lives. There are also difficulties in outreach, because families may not have phones, or they may live in dangerous neighborhoods. Practitioners may find it helpful to work through natural community bases in schools, churches, and health care clinics.

The process of training clinicians to work effectively with families who are dealing with racism, classism, and poverty is also one of empowerment. It is not surprising that this process must begin by helping therapists to look at themselves—at their own values, upbringing, and attitudes about race, class, and poverty. There are now a number of excellent training tools available. Pinderhughes's (1989) book, *Understanding Race, Ethnicity and Power*, describes in detail a training program designed to help therapists explore these issues. Aponte (1985, 1994) has long been a pioneer in helping therapists explore their own use of self with poor families. His training program at Hannemann Hospital in Philadelphia is a model of such an approach.

In *Black Families in Therapy: A Multisystems Approach* (Boyd-Franklin, 1989), a chapter is devoted to the therapist's use of self with relevant countertransference issues for African American patients and white clinicians. The last chapter explores the role of training and supervision in the process of empowering clinicians. The multisystems model (Boyd-Franklin, 1989; Boyd-Franklin & Bry, 2000) addresses and helps prepare clinicians to deal more effectively with the complex issues of race, culture, class, and poverty, and also to look at African American families within the context of their history and culture, and to recognize the strengths that can be utilized to produce empowerment.

Work with African American inner-city families requires a therapist who is prepared to be "active" and committed to activating families toward their own empowerment. It also requires supervisors who are committed to being "on the front lines" with their trainees and empowering them to look at the complex and difficult questions of race, class, poverty, and at their own values and responses to these issues. Beyond didactic teaching, this model produces empowerment by focusing on the process of supervision and training as an opportunity to develop the "person of the therapist" (Aponte, 1985, 1994). It is only through a very personal process that therapists can be trained to recognize the complex issues discussed in this chapter, to be true to themselves, and to allow their own humanity to be communicated to the families with whom they work.

Empowerment through Social Policy Intervention

Strong social policy programs must address this issue of empowerment of families and communities by incentives that encourage self-determination. These programs should provide housing to counteract homelessness, and better and more responsive educational systems and work incentives. Those in the mental health field, including family therapists, social workers, psychologists, and psychiatrists, must unite to put these key issues back on the national agenda.

In 1996, the Personal Responsibility and Work Opportunity Reconciliation Act was passed. Hill (1999) discussed the ways in which this "welfare reform" legislation ended federally guaranteed, long-term entitlements for poor families with dependent children and gave states the responsibility for administering welfare programs through "block grants." Hill has observed that

> one block grant, Block Grants to States for Temporary Assistance for Needy Families (TANF), is designed to help welfare recipients leave the

rolls within specified time limits: two years to obtain jobs, and a maximum of five years to receive welfare benefits. Although the second block grant is designed to provide subsidized child care for welfare recipients who are able to obtain jobs, many observers predict that the funds are inadequate for the large number of recipients who will need child care assistance. (p. 154)

Hill does not consider this legislation to be at all concerned with helping welfare recipients to find their way out of poverty and become self-sufficient. His critique of welfare reform focuses on six major weaknesses:

(1) It has fixed amounts that will not be responsive to economic downturns and periodic recessions; (2) it has inadequate resources for providing extended training and education to enhance the capabilities of "long-term" recipients with few marketable skills; (3) it will place most recipients into short-term, low-wage jobs with no health benefits; (4) it has inadequate funds to provide subsidized child care for the large numbers of recipients who are expected to find jobs; (5) it relies on churches and other nonprofit institutions to provide increased assistance to the poor with limited government resources; and (6) it is likely to increase the number of persons who are homeless, poor, and in foster care. (p. 155)

Another policy area that must be addressed is kinship care. Historically, African American families have "informally adopted" children into the homes of extended family members. Unfortunately, prior to 1980, many African American children were removed from their homes and placed in foster care, when viable kinship placements were available. In 1980, however, with the passage of the Adoption Assistance and Child Welfare Act (PL 96–272), a number of changes began to occur (Hill, 1999). This legislation strongly encouraged family preservation services. Many states began to implement procedures for locating viable extended family caregivers. Major discrepancies remain, however. Even though kinship care is more likely to be utilized for placement, kin caregivers are usually not given adequate funding to provide for these children (Hill, 1999). As a result, many of these caregivers, often elderly relatives, incur a large financial burden. There is a need for major federal and state legislation to provide funding to support viable kinship care for African American families.

CHANGE IN SOCIETAL ATTITUDES THAT FOSTER RACISM, CLASSISM, AND POVERTY

Ultimately, mental health providers must accept a personal sense of social responsibility for changing those attitudes that foster racism, classism, and poverty. The first step is honestly acknowledging the existence of these phenomena and learning about their complex interplay. On the microcosm level, we can begin with ourselves and the families with whom we work. Many mental health clinicians, however, like the families they serve, become overwhelmed when asked to move to a "macro" level. If these issues are ever to be resolved fully in any society, we must be willing to speak out for and advocate change in our own agencies and clinics, communities, and local, state, and national governments.

REFERENCES

Anderson, C. (1994). *Black labor, white wealth.* Edgewood, MD: Duncan & Duncan.

Aponte, H. (1976). Underorganization in the poor family. In P. J. Guerin (Ed.), *Family therapy: Theory and practice* (pp. 432–446). New York: Gardner Press.

Aponte, H. (1985). The negotiation of values in therapy. *Family Process, 24*(3), 323–338.

Aponte, H. (1994). *Bread and spirit: Therapy with the new poor.* New York: Morton Press.

Billingsley, A. (1968). *Black families in white America.* Englewood Cliffs, NJ: Prentice-Hall.

Billingsley, A. (1992). *Climbing Jacob's ladder: The enduring legacy of African-American families.* New York: Simon & Schuster.

Billingsley, A. (Ed.). (1994). The Black church. *National Journal of Sociology, 8*(1–2) (double edition).

Bowen, M. (1976). Theory in the practice of psychotherapy. In P. J. Guerin (Ed.), *Family therapy: Theory and practice* (pp. 42–90). New York: Gardner Press.

Boyd-Franklin, N. (1989). *Black families in therapy: A multisystems approach.* New York: Guilford Press.

Boyd-Franklin, N., & Bry, B. H. (2000). *Reaching out in family therapy: Home-based, school, and community interventions.* New York: Guilford Press.

Boyd-Franklin, N., & Franklin, A. J. (1998). African American couples in therapy. In M. McGoldrick (Ed.), *Revisioning family therapy: Race, culture, and gender in clinical practice* (pp. 268–281). New York: Guilford Press.

Boyd-Franklin, N., Franklin, A. J., & Toussaint, P. (2000). *Boys into men: Raising our African American teenage sons.* New York: Plume.

Boyd-Franklin, N., & Lockwood, T. W. (1999). Spirituality and religion: Implications for psychotherapy with African American clients and families. In F. Walsh (Ed.), *Spiritual resources in families and family therapy* (pp. 90–103). New York: Guilford Press.

Carter, R. T. (1995). *The influence of race and racial identity in psychotherapy: Toward a racially inclusive model.* New York: Wiley.

Cose, E. (1993). *The rage of the privileged class.* New York: HarperCollins.

Duncan, G. (1992, February 12). *The disappearing middle-class.* Testimony before the U.S. House of Representatives Select Committee on Children, Youth and Families, 102nd Cong., 2nd Sess., pp. 186–206. Washington, DC: U.S. Government Printing Office.

Franklin, A. J. (1992). Therapy with African-American men. *Families in Society: The Journal of Contemporary Human Services, 73*(6), 350–355.

Franklin, A. J. (1999). The invisibility syndrome and racial identity development in psychotherapy and counseling of African American men. *Counseling Psychologist, 27*(6), 761–693.

Franklin, A. J., Boyd-Franklin, N., & Draper, C. (2002). A psychological and educational perspective on Black parenting. In H. McAdoo (Ed.), *Black children: Social, educational and parental environments* (2nd ed., pp. 119–140). Thousand Oaks, CA: Sage.

Grier, W., & Cobbs, P. (1968). *Black rage.* New York: Basic Books.

Hartman, A., & Laird, J. (1983). *Family-centered social work practice.* New York: Free Press.

Helms, J., & Cook, D. (1999). *Using race and culture in counseling and psychotherapy.* Boston: Allyn & Bacon.

Henggeler, S. W., & Borduin, C. (1990). *Family therapy and beyond.* Pacific Grove, CA: Brooks/Cole.

Henggeler, S. W., & Santos, A. B. (1997). *Innovative approaches for difficult-to-treat populations.* Washington, DC: American Psychiatric Press.

Hill, R. (1972). *The strengths of black families.* New York: Emerson-Hall.

Hill, R. (Ed). (1993). *The research on the African-American family: A holistic perspective.* Westport, CT: Auburn House.

Hill, R. (1999). *The strengths of African American families: Twenty-five years later.* Lanham, MD: University Press of America.

Hines, P. M., & Boyd-Franklin, N. (1996). African American families. In M. McGoldrick, J. K. Pearce, & J. Giordano (Eds.), *Ethnicity and family therapy* (2nd ed., pp. 66–84). New York: Guilford Press.

Hopps, J. (1982). Oppression based on color [editorial]. *Social Work, 27*(1), 3–5.

Jones, J. (1997). *Prejudice and racism* (2nd ed.). New York: McGraw-Hill.

Kunjufu, J. (1985). *Countering the conspiracy to destroy black boys* (Vol. 1). Chicago: African-American Images.

Lindblad-Goldberg, M., Dukes, J., & Lasley, J. (1988). Stress in black, low-income, single-parent families: Normative and dysfunctional patterns. *American Journal of Orthopsychiatry, 58*(1), 104–120.

Logan, S. L. M. (Ed.). (2001). *The Black family: Strengths, self-help, and positive change* (2nd ed.). Boulder, CO: Westview Press.

McAdoo, H. (Ed.). (1996). *Black families* (3rd ed.). Thousand Oaks, CA: Sage.

McAdoo, H. (Ed) (2002). *Black children: Social, educational and parental environments* (2nd ed.). Thousand Oaks, CA: Sage.

Minuchin, S. (1974). *Families and family therapy.* Cambridge, MA: Harvard University Press.

Murray, V. M., & Brody, G. H. (2002). Racial socialization processes in single-mother families: Linking maternal racial identity, parenting, and racial socialization in rural, single-mother families with child self-worth and self-regulation. In H. McAdoo (Ed.), *Black children: Social, educational and parental environments* (2nd ed., pp. 97–118). Thousand Oaks, CA: Sage.

Oliver, M., & Shapiro, T. (1995). *Black wealth/white wealth.* New York: Routledge.

Pierce, C. (1988). Stress in the workplace. In A. F. Coner-Edwards & J. Spurlock (Eds.), *Black families in crisis: The middle class* (pp. 27–34). New York: Brunner/Mazel.

Pinderhughes, E. (1982). Afro-American families and the victim system. In M.

McGoldrick, J. K. Pearce, & J. Giordano (Eds.), *Ethnicity and family therapy* (pp. 108–122). New York: Guilford Press.

Pinderhughes, E. (1989). *Understanding race, ethnicity and power: The key to efficacy in clinical practice.* New York: Free Press.

Reich, R. (August 31, 1994). The fracturing of the middle class. *The New York Times,* p. A-19.

Solomon, B. (1976). *Black empowerment: Social work in oppressed communities.* New York: Columbia University Press.

Stack, C. (1974). *All our kin: Strategies for survival in a black community.* New York: Prentice-Hall.

Tatum, J., Moseley, S., Boyd-Franklin, N., & Herzog, E. (1995, February–March). A home based family systems approach to the treatment of African American teenage parents and their families. *Zero to Three: Journal of the National Center for Clinical Infant Programs, 15*(4), 18–25.

Taylor, R. J., Jackson, J. S., & Chatters, L. M. (1997). *Family life in Black America.* Thousand Oaks, CA: Sage.

Thomas, M., & Hughes, M. (1986). The continuing significance of race: A study of race, class and quality of life in America, 1972–1985. *American Sociological Review, 51,* 830–841.

Walsh, F. (Ed.). (1999). *Spiritual resources in family therapy.* New York: Guilford Press.

Wilson, W. J. (1980). *The declining significance of race* (2nd ed.). Chicago: University of Chicago Press.

Wilson, W. J. (1987). *The truly disadvantaged: The inner city, the underclass and public policy.* Chicago: University of Chicago Press.

Wilson, W. J. (1996). *When work disappears: The world of the new urban poor.* New York: Knopf.

CHAPTER 11

IMMIGRANT FAMILY PROCESSES

Celia Jaes Falicov

T he new century demands a new road map—one that reflects a search for communion and understanding in an increasingly global village. As we explore the superhighways and backroads of changing demographics, immigrant families appear at every turn. The adaptations that emerge from the changes imposed by migration on individual and family life deserve our careful study to better inform delivery of social, medical, and educational services attuned to the special needs of immigrants.

Concepts from family systems theory and family therapy, supplemented with concepts from studies on migration, can be used to deepen our understanding of the family transformations brought about by migration. Key constructs used in this chapter include migration loss, based on Pauline Boss's (1991, 1999) concept of ambiguous loss and a family sense of coherence (Antonovsky, 1987; Antonovsky & Sourani, 1988), which is a central component of relational or family resilience (Walsh, 1996, 1998).

This chapter expands on my earlier writings about the dilemmas of personal, family, and social transformation faced by immigrants and their capacity to find "both/and" solutions rather than forcing an "either/or" choice about incorporation of cultural change (Falicov, 1998a, 2002). This position differs from the common deficit-oriented description of immigrants living "*between* two worlds" and not fitting in either one. It is also different from classical acculturation theory, in which the immigrant gradually assimilates to mainstream culture. Rather, many families are able to live "*in* two worlds," alternating their everyday practices, rituals, and cultural codes depending on the context in which they find themselves, or finding new hybrid cultural mixes over the generations. I describe the emergence of a number of immigrant practices that may amount to *spontaneous rituals,* that encapsulate various family and social restitutive attempts following migration. Situations in which migration risks test families' capacity for blending continuity and change are also addressed.

VARIATIONS IN THE EXPERIENCE OF MIGRATION

In this chapter, generalizations emerge about the family and social experiences associated with the changes imposed by migration for many groups. However, it is important at all times to remember that each immigrant family participates in multiple contexts of insertion and exclusion, and acquires partial perspectives imparted by ethnicity, class, education, geography, climate, religion, nationality, and occupation that interact to form particular *ecological niches* (Falicov, 1995). Families derive their shared and individual meanings from their particular ecological niches and unique personal histories.

Notable variations are mediated by the degree of choice about migration, proximity and accessibility to country of origin, gender, age and generation, education, developmental stage of the family life cycle, family form, community social supports, and experiences of racial or economic discrimination in one's own country or in the country of adoption.

The experience may be altered significantly depending on whether migration is voluntary or involuntary. Those forced to leave beloved homelands for religious, political, or war-related reasons may have experienced trauma and feel intensely ambivalent about their longing to return and the necessity of departure. Such anguish may be ameliorated in those who left willingly in search of a more prosperous life.

Proximity between homeland and new land also mediates the intensity of the loss. The ability to make frequent visits or even reside in both countries—dubbed a "two-home," transnational, or binational arrangement—alleviates some of the immigrants' pain by maintaining a sense of belonging and participation, a much less feasible option for those whose homelands are far away and unreachable, or politically and economically unfeasible.

Gender and generation alter the migration experience as well. Migration is vastly different for women and men; infants, children, or adolescents; and young adults or aged persons. Developmental issues such as language acquisition, socialization, insertion in peer groups, acquisition of cultural codes, and a formed or unformed sense of national identity figure into the equation.

Whether members of the family unit migrate together or in sequential stages, the family composition before migration or the family form that evolves after migration—from extended three- and four-generation families to two-generation nuclear arrangements, to single-parent or intermarried couples, among others—may imply multiple family connections or disconnections that affect outcomes of coping with the stresses of adaptation.

Negative or ambivalent receptions, discrimination, and shortage of adequate economic and social opportunities because of race and/or class alter radically the ability to absorb the losses of migration. Community social supports also vary widely depending on the opportunities for reconstructing ruptured social networks and re-creating cultural spaces in ethnic neighborhoods or in work settings. Without such connections, isolation may contribute to a host of biopsychosocial consequences.

All of these factors make up specific configurations for each family and influence the resources and constraints, as well as the meaning of the migration experience. The local knowledge and experiences reflected in each individual description of the migration experience are always infinitely more complex, complete and nuanced than any attempts at generalization. At the same time, it is important that clinicians and researchers address common issues and challenges.

THE EXPERIENCE OF MIGRATION LOSS

Despite their myriad differences, immigrants in the United States encounter to one degree or another the loss, grief, and mourning that are characteristic of the migration experience (Alvarez, 1995; Shuval, 1982; Garza-Guerrero, 1974; Johnston, 1976; Warheit, Vega, Auth, & Meinhardt, 1985; Sluzki, 1979; Grinberg & Grinberg, 1989; Westermeyer, 1989; Rodriguez, 1992; Hoffman, 1989; Potocky-Tripodi, 2000). These losses have been compared with the processes of grief and mourning precipitated by the death of loved ones. Yet migration loss has special characteristics that distinguish it from other kinds of losses (Falicov, 2002). Compared with the inescapable fact of death, migration is both larger and smaller. It is larger because migration brings with it losses of all kinds. For the immigrants, gone are family members and friends who stay behind; gone is the familiar language, the customs and rituals, the food and music, the comforting identification with the land itself. The losses of migration touch the family back home and reach forward to shape future generations born in the new land.

Yet migration loss also is smaller than death, because despite the grief and mourning occasioned by physical, social, and cultural uprooting, the losses are not absolutely clear, complete, and irretrievable. All are still alive but just not immediately reachable or present. Unlike coping with the finality of death, after migration it is always possible to fantasize an eventual return or forthcoming reunion. Like Janus, one face is turned to the new shore, the other toward the familiar harbor. Furthermore, immigrants seldom migrate toward a social vacuum. A relative, friend, or acquaintance usually waits on the other side to help with work, housing, and guidelines for life in the new country. A social community and ethnic neighborhood reproduce in pockets of remembrance the sights, sounds, smells, and tastes of one's village or country (Falicov, 1998a). All of these elements create a remarkable mix of emotions: sadness and elation, losses and restitution, and absence and presence that make grieving incomplete, postponed, ambiguous.

Ambiguous Loss

The concept of ambiguous loss proposed by Pauline Boss (1991, 1999) describes situations in which loss is unclear, incomplete, or partial. Basing her thesis on stress theory, Boss describes two types of ambiguous loss. In one type, family members are physically absent but psychologically present (the family with a soldier missing in action, the dissapearance of a family member, as in Kosovo or Argentina; the noncustodial parent in divorce; the child gone off to college; and the migrating relative). In the second type, family members are physically present but psychologically absent (the family living with an Alzheimer's patient or chronically ill person; the parent or spouse who is emotionally unavailable due to stress or depression).

Migration represents what Boss (1999) calls a "crossover," in that it has elements of both types of ambiguous loss. Although beloved people and places are left behind, they remain keenly present in the psyche of the immigrant; at the same time, homesickness and the multiple stresses of adaptation may leave some family members emotionally unavailable to support and encourage others. The very decision to migrate has at its core two ambivalent poles. For many immigrants, frustrations with economic or political conditions compel the move and result in new opportunities and gains but love of family and surroundings pull in another direction.

Lack of Transitional Rituals

It is perhaps because of this ambiguous, inconclusive, impermanent quality that migration as a life transition is devoid of clear rituals or rites of passage at any point during its various stages of development. The preparations that precede the actual departure may bear some similarities to rituals, but practices such as packing symbolic, meaningful objects (e.g., photographs or other mementos, including a small cache of native soil) are random and idiosyncratic, and do not involve family members or friends. There is no formal structure, no designated place or time, no cultural collective celebration that allows people to come together to mark the transition, try to transcend it, and provide a container for the strong emotions everybody is feeling. Thus, migration is similar to other transitions that lack cultural rituals: An aborted or a stillborn child represents a future life that was cut off; a divorce leaves partners feeling that what could have been is no longer possible. Even the term "adopted country," like an adopted child not raised by its biological parents, suggests that there was a "homeland," map of a possible territory that could have been inhabited but is no longer accessible.

Uprooting of Meanings

In comparison with other ambiguous losses, what is distinctive and most dramatic about migration is the uprooting of entire systems of meanings: physical, social, and cultural. Peter Marris (1980), an urban ecologist, suggests that the closest human counterpart to the root structure that nourishes a plant is the systems of meaning that provide familiarity with a physical, social, and cultural reality. If we take the uprooting metaphor further, we can see that when a plant is plucked from the earth, some residue of soil always remains attached to the roots. Good gardeners know that when replanting in the new soil, they must not wash away this little bit of residue of the old soil, in order to minimize shock and ensure the success of the tranplantation.

Although immigrants no longer have the depth and expanse of the native soil to nourish their roots, the little bit of original native soil they bring with them is represented in the type of households they recreate, the traditions they pass on to their children, the language they speak, the foods they cook and the friendships they form, the connections they keep with their country of origin, and the family and social rituals that evolve over time. It seems plausible, therefore, that, as in the case of plants, families that deal with the uprooting of meanings and the ambiguous losses of migration by holding on to and re-creating parts of the old context while adapting to their new ecologies are able to develop firmer family and cultural foundations that, in turn, may contribute to the healthy growth of future generations.

DUAL VISIONS: CONTINUITY AND CHANGE

The migration experience disrupts family stability and in turn poses more intense struggles to regain continuity in the midst of new challenges and opportunities. From a family systems viewpoint, for a family to be both flexible and stable during crucial family transitions, the tendencies toward both change and continuity need to occur simultaneously. What is needed to cope with life challenges is an integration of the two processes, so that a sense of continuity, identity, and stability can be maintained while new patterns of behavior, interactions, or beliefs evolve (Hansen & Johnson, 1979; Melitto, 1985; Walsh, 1998; Falicov, 1993; Sluzki, 1983)

The flow of people and information between cultures, and the increasing globalization of the world lead immigrant families to develop new ways of finding connectedness—renewing contacts with their culture of origin, reinventing old family themes in this country, while opening up possibilities for carving out new lives. In the field of migration studies, new acculturation theories fit with this idea insofar as the concepts they offer reflect a dynamic balance of continuity and change. Terms such as "binationalism," "bilingualism," "biculturalism," and "cultural bifocality" describe dual visions, ways of maintaining contact with familiar cultural practices while making new spaces manageable. Unlike linear models of assimilation, new constructs of alternation, hybridization, segmented acculturation, or syncretism provide frameworks for describing continuous family connections along with discontinuous adaptations.

Among these, the alternation framework proposes that individuals can alternate or switch language and cultural codes according to the social context at hand (La Framboise, Coleman, & Gerton, 1993; Ogbu & Matute-Bianchi, 1986; Rouse, 1992). Those social contexts, so variable in our multicultural society, comprise "cultural borderlands" (Rosaldo, 1989; Anzaldúa, 1987) in which people move and live, and where behavior is readily, flexibly alternated according to the need at hand. The result is a sense of fit or partial belonging in more than one cultural and language context.

The theme of ambiguous loss and integration is not circumscribed to the first stages of migration. Choices about affirming cultural meaning systems or adapting to change are made throughout a family's initial transplantation and for other generations to come. There are compelling psychological reasons for retention of cultural and family identities, among them the family's attempt at preserving a *sense of family coherence* with its evolving story and the application of its practiced customs.

Sense of Coherence and Family Resilience

In a rapidly changing world, we search for recognizable patterns in the midst of discontinuities. Some of these reliable patterns, the prevailing cultural narratives of and about a group, may make the world understandable, but inevitably, they also "prune from experience those events that do not fit the dominant evolving story that we and others have about us" (White & Epston, 1990, p. 11). By selectively and purposefully maintaining some aspects of cultural narratives while pruning others, resilient immigrant families are able to restore a sense of continuity and coherence to their lives.

The concept, *sense of coherence,* was developed by Aaron Antonovsky (1987) as a model for understanding the spontaneous emergence of healthy as opposed to pathogenic responses to crisis situations. It assumes that our normal state is disorder and chaos, but that human beings also make continuous attempts to promote health and stability in the midst of disruption and change. A sense of coherence involves a global orientation to life as comprehensible, manageable, and meaningful, in spite of its many challenges. A family's sense of coherence (Antonovsky & Sourani,

1988) refers to the perceived coherence of family life in coping with specific crises. The concept addresses meaningfulness and purpose in life, and a larger and deeper existential confidence than is implied in concepts such as *mastery* or *locus of control*, which focus more narrowly on self-reliance and specific coping strategies. According to Walsh (1996, 1998), this sense of coherence (and hopefulness) is one of the key ingredients of *family or relational resilience*, those processes by which families surmount persistent stress.

In the next sections, I explore immigrant families' attempts to restore meaning and purpose in life by creating "both/and" balances that keep continuity alive while integrating change in several areas: family connectedness, awareness of anti-immigrant realities, and emergence of spontaneous rituals.

FAMILY TRANSFORMATIONS

Extended Families

In spite of national and class variations, many immigrants come from countries that favor collectivistic narratives involving three-generational and extended family lifestyles. A primary component of the collectivistic narrative of self and family is an internalized obligation to help extended family members throughout life, regardless of how good, or not so good, those relationships might be. At least in some large populations of immigrants, family obligations and supports seem to withstand migration and persist in some form for one. two. or more generations. Furthermore, the emphasis on family relationships appears to be an enduring psychosocial feature of family life and not just a marshaling of family forces in reaction to migration (Suárez Orozco & Suárez Orozco, 1995b). Nevertheless, the realities of migration frequently involve temporary or permanent separation or disconnection between the nuclear and the extended family.

The Psychological Presence of Extended Family

Many immigrants do not live in kin-based communities, and years may pass before face-to-face interactions with extended family members can take place. To deal with the stresses of these family losses and the movement toward family nuclearization, immigrants often construct a psychologically present family of origin and continue to express family connectedness through long-distance phone calls, remittances, concerns and preoccupations, and occasional visits. For example, studies show that as families of Mexican descent acculturate, they become increasingly involved and competent in dealing with the norms of outside social systems, but their basic internal family system allegiances remain unchanged (Rueschenberg & Buriel, 1989; Sabogal, Marín, Otero-Sabogal, Marí, & Perez-Stable, 1987). Acculturated adult Mexicans, and perhaps other Latinos, including those whose parents and own children are born in the United States and live in small nuclear family households, learn how to behave in a dominant culture that values assertiveness, independence, and achievement. But they do not tend to acquire mainstream internal patterns of family interaction, keeping instead the values and meanings of collectivistic families in terms of their cohesion, visiting patterns, interdependence or interpersonal controls. They live dual lives, functioning as mainstream Americans in the affairs of the community at large, but continuing their ethnically patterned lives within their own closed circle.

The Physical Presence of Extended Family

From a family systems viewpoint, a large and stable collectivistic group generates complexity, affectional attachments, options for fulfilling instrumental or expressive functions, and alternatives for resolving problems and modeling behaviors. In extended family settings, multiple caretakers may create various types of primary attachments, so processes of separation–individuation and marital differentiation may evolve differently and require other parameters of analyses than those applied to small nuclear families (Falicov, 1992, 1996, 1998a, 1988b). Because models of family life have been based almost exclusively on the prevailing cultural form in the United States, the nuclear family, as we attempt to understand the role of extended family members in immigrant families, we have few guidelines about the complexities of these family arrangements before and after migration.

Extended family members who are physically present play a significant role in shoring up the family as it struggles for continuity and copes with change. Their collectivistic sense drives a concern for one another's lives, a pulling together to weather crises, and sociocentric values that teach children to care about others (Harwood, Miller, & Irizarry, 1995). These patterns yield support among adult siblings by pooling of money and resources, or closeness between adult children and their parents. In the immigrant context, these patterns of mutual support may be a measure of relational resilience. They foster narrative coherence (Cohler, 1991) and continuity in the face of ruptured attachments and the disruptive experiences of relocation.

The presence of extended family members does not, however, guarantee that all is well for the immigrant family. The depiction of family closeness is sometimes taken to such extremes that images of picturesque family life dominate, while tensions and disconnections among extended family members simmer below, discounted or ignored. Indeed, not everything is good in extended families, and nobody knows it better than the people who live in them. Migration may exacerbate preexisting family problems. Large families generate different problems than small families. For examples, triangles involving husband, wife, and mother-in-law, or coalitions involving mother, grandmother, and child, may be more common in three- than in two-generational arrangements. Closely tied, richly joined networks may generate their own problematic patterns that need to be looked at both culturally and contextually (Falicov & Brudner-White, 1983; Falicov, 1998b).

The Children of Immigrants

Children of immigrants do not experience migration loss with the same poignancy as their parents, but they are often exposed to their parents' mixed perceptions and emotions about their many losses and present hardships. Parents may be psychologically absent because of these tensions. Furthermore, children and adolescents are central participants in the family's evolving cultural narratives and the homegrown cultural spaces that re-create a subjective, altered past in the present. Children help mix continuity with change in their language, values, and identities. Thus, they co-construct with the parents and with society the family's transformations.

Immigrant parents, as they re-create familiar patterns and perpetuate customs, may help instill a sense of cohesion and connectedness that binds together even distant generations. When immigrant parents ensure the psychological presence of absent relatives, they may expand the meaning of family to broader identifications with their country of origin for their children, a finding that suggests deep intergenerational roots in ethnic and national identifications (Troya & Rosenberg, 1999). Suárez-Orozco and Suárez-Orozco (1995a) research findings also point to the strong positive role that family connectedness and ethnic affiliation plays in the motivation to achieve in school of children and adolescents who identify with their immigrant parents' dreams and sacrifice.

Generational Conflicts

Depictions of immigrant parents' relationships with their preadolescent, adolescent, or adult children almost invariably include eruptions of conflicts. This conflict is said to be based on the fact that children, who learn to speak English and understand American ways much faster than their parents, become translators of the culture and the language. They often act as parents to their parents, and the hierarchical reversal that ensues strips authority from the parent. This pattern has been observed many times, yet new studies reveal a much greater variety of outcomes.

Suárez Orozco and Suárez Orozco (1995a) found much less

parent–child conflict in the stories told by Mexican and Mexican American adolescents than in those of white American adolescents. They tie these findings to the familistic tendencies of Mexicans, whose sense of self is deeply embedded in social others rather than being defined "against" others, as is more typical of individualistic cultures. This coincide with recent findings (Szapocznik & Santisteban, personal communication, 2000) that acculturation per se does not create conflict and loss of parental authority so long as a strong family orientation is maintained in the home. Only when parents and children do not share languages at all does the acculturation gap become so large that the family may not have the resources to resolve conflicts that appear.

Similarly, Rumbaut's (1999) work with several Asian and Latino groups demonstrates important differences in generational conflict between situations of *dissonant acculturation,* which separates children and parents along language and cultural lines, and *selective acculturation,* in which both parents and children are able to retain language and culture to some extent and in some areas of life. The latter is more common when a community of the same ethnicity and sufficient size and institutional diversity surrounds the family and helps to slow down the cultural shift. This selective style preserves parental authority and provides a strong bulwark against the deleterious effects of racial and ethnic discrimination. A third type of acculturation found in Rumbaut's study is *consonant acculturation,* whereby both parents and children abandon language and culture at about the same pace, a situation most often found when parents are professionals and quickly incorporated in mainstream institutional settings.

Taking into account the connections between nurturance and control in parenting behavior may be very useful when trying to understand the behavior of immigrant parents who may emphasize one over the other when raising their children without the supports of their own families, social networks, and cultural institutions. Family therapy research has shown that nurturant, emotionally supportive and positively involved parents are much more respected and have greater leadership with their children (Mackey, 1996). This important integration of the two dimensions of nurturance and control clarifies the differences between authoritarian and authoritative parenting, the latter containing many elements of support, empathy, and understanding, along with guidance, supervision, and discipline (Steinberg, Dornbusch, & Brown, 1992), a finding that may apply to clinical work with many immigrant populations.

Gender-Based Conflicts

Gender also enters into the equation of migration in complex ways. In search of a better economic or political future, historically, men took the lead on the migration journey. They left wife and children behind, sent remittances, and reunited with the family later, typically in the United

States. Sometimes, men acquired a second wife and children, thus having one family in each country. Increasingly, as women from developing countries take up the journey by themselves, they often leave their children with family caretakers, send remittances, and work to be reunited later. Sometimes, many years pass before reunification, and many family reorganizations may take place.

Both men and women experience emotional difficulties following individual or solo migration and use a variety of coping mechanisms that appear to follow their gender socialization, such as seeking help for depression or psychosomatic problems in women, and alcohol dependence or violent behaviors in men. Over time, the presence of community—particularly conational support—networks help to ameliorate the symptoms of isolation and disenfranchisement, especially in women (Vega, Kolody, Valle, & Weir, 1991). When men and women migrate together, sometimes polarizations take place that reflect the ambiguities about leaving and staying, with one supporting the decisions to return, while the other opposes it. Other times, the polarizations focus on one parent supporting language and cultural continuity, with the other sponsoring language and cultural change.

The positions that men and women assume in these polarizations seem to depend at least in part on the historical moment and the encounter of cultures that may create different ambiguities, gains, or losses, for the two genders in the country of adoption compared to the country of origin. Immigrant men from traditional patriarchal cultures and ecological niches often feel threatened and disempowered by the more Western, egalitarian values influencing their wives and children in American mainstream culture (Rouse, 1992). Whereas studies 20 years ago reported slower cultural and language adaptations in women than in men, more recent studies indicate that women adapt to the cultural changes faster than men and may be more at peace with the decision to settle, citing gains of greater economic and personal freedoms (Hondagneu-Sotelo, 1994; Troya & Rosenberg, 1999). These changes are likely to be tied to the increased participation of women in the workforce; thus, many immigrant women feel torn by the dual vision and double shift of maintaining ethnic traditional lifestyles within the home while becoming modernized in their outside work settings.

AWARENESS OF ANTI-IMMIGRANT RECEPTIONS

The adaptation to a life of uncertainty and ambivalent feelings depends to a large extent on the number and type of external contextual stresses families face in the new country. Striving for economic stability and psychological equilibrium in the new land is riddled with pressure to assimilate the dominant culture's negative judgment of dark-skinned, poor immigrants and deprives them of legal resources in the face of oppressive institutional treatment and derogatory stereotypes.

While the concept of "dual visions" characterizes the inner workings of many immigrant families, it also captures the nature of the family interactions with external, larger systems. The concept of "double consciousness," which Du Bois (1903) first used to describe the social situations of African Americans, is useful to understand the situation of many immigrants, because it encompasses a perception of who one really is as a person within one's own group, and in the attributions of the larger society's story regarding that group. Racial, ethnic, and economic discrimination shape the individual stories of most immigrants, particularly those from disadvantaged classes and poor countries, who are almost always perceived as the "other," not us. Choices to develop more empowering narratives are sorely limited by the larger culture's negative views of immigrants.

When immigrant children from various ethnic groups (Chinese, Haitian, Central American, Dominican, and Mexican) were asked what was most difficult about immigration, discrimination and racism were recurrent themes in the research data. Researchers Suárez-Orozco and Suárez-Orozco (2000), codirectors of this large-scale, longitudinal Harvard Immigration Project, observed that immigrant children develop a keen eye for their reception and incorporate these socially negative reflections in the image of themselves and their ethnic identity. Parents' positive mirroring often cannot compensate for the distorted reflections children encounter in daily life. The conceptual model is very useful in describing a number of ways in which immigrant children react to negative social mirroring and stresses that hope is essential for positive outcome. In fact, hope and confidence that social marginalization is a temporary rather than permanent price to pay, and a belief that the family will triumph over the odds, are elements that keep alive immigrants' dream of a better life for themselves and their children.

In the next section, I describe a number of practices that appear with regularity in the lives of immigrants that not only reflect a spirit of pride and respect for their language and cultural background but also demonstrate that awareness of social situation and flexibility to transform family life to the present requirements facilitate success and adaptation.

THE EMERGENCE OF SPONTANEOUS RITUALS

Immigrants deal with the massive uprooting of meanings and migration loss with attempts at physical, social, and cultural restitution through a number of practices that create makeshift physical, social, and cultural bridges across the absences. These actions have a number of characteristics that bear many similarities with *rituals*: They are catalysts for feeling, thinking, and action; they validate ties between past, present, and future;

and they contain both sides of the ambiguity—presence and absence, connection and disconnection, gain and loss, ideal and real. Such actions tend to be repetitive and incorporate continuity in the midst of change and familiarity in the midst of strangeness. In fact, immigrants find themselves almost magnetically drawn to the situations that follow, when nobody really instructs them to do so. It may be tempting to speculate that these rituals have psychological and social "functions." However, it seems preferable to assume simply that these activities have psychological cognitive and emotional *effects* in the way all rituals do.

Visits Home, Communications, and Money Remittances: Rituals of Connection

Longing for one's country makes visits home a priority. Visits close the gap between that which is psychologically present and physically absent. Trips to the country of origin serve to revive, renew, and reinforce personal and cultural connections rather than allow such connections to stagnate or wither away. Some immigrants make it a ritual to go home for special holidays or family reunions. The actual experience is rife with paradoxes, sweet interpersonal nourishment, and bitterness at what is no longer accessible. The return to the country of adoption may be full of regret but also relief at the newfound freedom or opportunity.

Historically, most voluntary immigrants, and even refugees, often managed to maintain connections through letters, messages, packages. Ease of transportation and telecommunications has increased the possibilities of immigrants staying in contact and have made modern-day migrations a transnational experience. Today, many immigrants from poor countries all over the world send money home as soon as they are able. These remittances contribute significantly to the economic sustenance of their families and even their countries, maintaining both their social continuity and long-distance presence.

The actions of visiting, communicating, and sending money home are filled with planning and caring that may be said to amount to carrying out *rituals of connection*, in that they may involve ritualized practices, such as contacting intermediaries at a specific time of the month, purchasing money orders, going to the post office, setting up joint transnational bank accounts, and getting an acknowledgment from the people receiving the remittance. These behaviors may have the same psychological effects as the Sunday visit to one's elderly parents nearby.

Re-creating Ethnic and Social Spaces: Re-creation Rituals

In most cities where immigrants live, one can find distinct ethnic neighborhoods. These urban landscapes reproduce in public environments the sights, smells, sounds, flavors, and tastes of the native country. Open markets and Sunday flea markets reproduce with uncanny fidelity the meeting places of the past. This collective cultural revival meeting may be thought as a psychological return, a representational form of "cultural mourning" (Ainslie, 1998). These makeshift, "as if" environments where cultural memories remain alive become *rituals of re-creation,* of "pretending" to be at home, which is clearly much better than not being home at all. These powerful actions not only help reestablish links with the lost land, but they also help transform the receiving cultures into more familiar places. No doubt, they reflect continuity. Yet the ethnic and social spaces have elements of difference, the dominant culture being ever-present through the money, the products, the mix of languages.

The vicissitudes of the disruption of lifelong networks, and the attempts at reconstructing them (Sluzki, 1989), attest to the immigrants' constructive attempts to make present the absent—ways of saying "hello again" in the midst of the many good-byes. Most immigrants seem to be able to reconstruct networks of conationals in the urban environments toward which they gravitate. Again, we can observe that these transformational phenomena synthesize both/and, the old and the new.

Reminiscing about the Past: Memory Rituals

In popular media depictions, immigrants are portrayed as telling stories about their countries, recounting the details of their migration saga, repeating old proverbs and pining away for the special foods or customs of their country. They are also known to make either idealized or denigrating judgments about the differences between their country of origin and the country of adoption. These practices have the effect of promoting personal and cultural continuity by building connections with those in the new land, mostly the immigrant's own children. It is a mistake to think of this storytelling as merely a quaintly nostalgic or sentimental self-indulgence. Much of it serves to create a coherent narrative past and to make meaning out of inevitable changes and transition into present circumstances, as well as hopes and dreams for the future.

The perpetual ambiguities of the migration story may create a powerful cognitive and emotional magnet within a family system. The migration story may become the family's dominant story—the way it makes sense of all other aspects of life, the magnet that provides meaning and narrative coherence (Cohler, 1991). Experiences of failure, success, sadness, resignation, heroism, marital conflict, the wife's newfound assertiveness, the ungrateful adult children, the nascent freedom to be oneself, all can be contained within an explanation: "This is happening to us because we came here."

The gap between physical absence and psychological presence may be particularly intense for immigrants who maintain the dream of permanent return. For them, ambiguous loss may translate into a frozen grief, like that of an individual after divorce, whose unrealistic reunion fantasies block the development of new attachments and commitments. A family may remain unable to mobilize their resources, make settlement decisions, or take full advantage of existing opportunities.

Preserving Culturally Patterned Rituals

Processes of continuity and change in an immigrant family's resilience to migration loss over the generations can be studied through the transmission of family and cultural rituals (Bennett, Wolin, & McAvity, 1988). Family systems theorists and practitioners have long known about the power of rituals (Imber-Black, Roberts, & Whiting, 1988) to restore continuities with a family's heritage and reaffirm a sense of cultural identity.

Nowhere is collectivism better reflected and reinforced than in the celebration of *cultural and religious family rituals*. Such extended family celebrations proclaim and reaffirm family pride, unity, and connection. From birth to death, life-cycle transitions are honored and celebrated in ways that are patterned in ethnic ways: Marriages, baptisms, graduations, and funerals are gatherings in which a sense of belonging is reaffirmed. Ritual celebrations offer an opportunity for collective contribution, and collaboration and reinforcement of ethnic gender and generation patterns.

The enactment of traditional rituals and celebrations may come to represent an immigrant family's balance between continuity and change. Even when original cultural contents have shifted or faded, rituals continue to have the inherent power to strengthen families by reinforcing old bonds and reaffirming blended social identities. Studies of immigrant families should include a close look at the persistence and evolving new shapes of cultural family rituals, from routine family interactions (dinners or prayers) to celebrations of birthdays, holidays, and rites of passage, as well as the old and new meanings family members associate with them.

An immigrant's *daily family rituals,* such as meal preparation, home decoration, forms of daily greeting, and dress may mimic the local customs of the original culture, but they also mix the new elements of language and customs of the adoptive culture that the children of immigrants bring home.

Even when immigrants cannot transport the physical and social landscapes, belief systems reflected in *religious* and *folk medicine rituals* have transportability. Perhaps the most transportable ritual is prayer. Indigeneous beliefs and rituals about health, illness, and cures also persist, along with the growing acceptance of current medical practices; for example, a family may consult an indigenous healer for a case of "fright," while also turning to a mainstream physician to deal with the same symptoms of nervousness (Falicov, 1999).

The emergence of spontaneous rituals of connection, re-creation of social and ethnic spaces, memory rituals, and the preservation of cultural rituals in the lives of immigrants illustrate the ambiguous, conflictual nature of immigrants' losses and attachments. Yet embedded in these spontaneous rituals are healthy "both/and" responses or "solutions," which demonstrate that people learn to live with the ambiguity of never resolving the losses of migration or achieving final closure in the experience. Work with immigrant families could greatly profit from an exploration of the place of rituals in their lives. It seems possible that the immigrants' abandonment of the rituals just described, or alternatively, their excessive reliance on the performance of these cultural and religious rituals at the expense of adaptations to the new culture, could point toward problematic adaptations.

IMMIGRANT FAMILIES' RISKS

Sometimes families' brave and complex attempts at integrating continuity and change, and restoring a sense of narrative coherence fail in the face of either intense loss or of irreparable ambiguity. Among several categories of disruptive outcomes, I discuss three types of situations to illustrate how the ambiguous losses in migration are compounded by a confusing family context, a lack of clarity as to who is in and who is out of the family system or subsystems. Pauline Boss (1991) labeled this phenomenon "boundary ambiguity." Situations that heighten the risks of boundary ambiguity include reluctant or unprepared migrations, separations and reunions in the nuclear family, and family life-cycle transitions.

Reluctant and Unprepared Migrations

In family migrations, not all family members have equal say over the decision to migrate. There may be subtle power lines and asymmetries that involve gender and generation. Among those coaxed into migration somewhat against their will are children and adolescents, wives who reluctantly follow their husbands, and older parents who are hastily convinced by their adult children to take on the journey, often after losing a spouse (Falicov, 1998a). In such situations, migration loss is further compounded by the lack of readiness to migrate and the constant ambivalence about the decision. The reluctant immigrant may feel torn by family loyalties, inconclusive good-byes, and lingering obligations to family members left behind, with difficulties in defining the important relationships in their lives. It is not surprising, therefore, that coaxed or reluctant individuals experience more ambivalence and difficulties of adaptation than those who actively elect to migrate, and that they may often present with clinical symptoms of depression, anxiety, or psychosomatic problems.

Separations and Reunions among Nuclear Family Members

When a father or a mother migrates first, leaving family or children behind to be reunited at a later time, the family membership confusion that ensues may be mild and temporary or prolonged and intense. Even when a parent remains connected through monetary remittances, if sufficient time passes, the family left behind may reorganize into a single-parent household or find internal or external substitutes to supplement the functions and feelings left vacant. At the time of reunion, boundaries and relationships need to change again to allow for reentry of the absent member into the family system. Meanwhile, confusion may reign as to whether an absent mother or father is truly a part of the system and could be reincorporated again.

Another common migratory pattern that may lead to boundary ambiguity occurs when immigrant parents leave one or more children behind with grandparents or other close relatives. Children are left so that their parents can face the dangers of illegal passage, the economic hardships, the instability of employment, and the lack of adequate caretaking in the new country without the added worry of having youngsters under wing. Sometimes a child may be left behind with a grandparent to assuage the immigrants' guilt about leaving and to symbolize that migration is provisional and experimental rather than permanent. However, these separations and subsequent reunions complicate the experiences of loss and reconnection, and raise issues of inclusion and exclusion for members of the three generations (Falicov, 1998a, 2002).

Although these stresses present significant risks, many families cope succesfully with separations and reunions, and are able to maintain healthy definitions of family life that may include multiple caretakers for the same child. Research is needed with different immigrant groups to understand the family and cultural meanings, and the contextual factors that may support or aggravate family separations and reunifications.

Life-Cycle Transitions

Like all families, immigrant families undergo life-cycle changes such as birth, leaving home, illness, and death. These transitions require reorganizations of the family that involve varying degrees of stress. When nonambiguous, irretrievable losses occur in the life of an immigrant family—perhaps the death of a relative back home—the uncertainty of old good-byes accentuates migration loss. The immigrant family may even experience the appearance of other ambiguous losses, such as a teenager leaving home or a spouse separating and divorcing, as more stressful than if they had occurred in a context that did not involved migrations.

Family transitions that involve members of the family who have stayed behind in the country of origin may be particularly stressful. Many immigrants postpone visiting an aging parent for lack of money or time; sometimes they avoid thinking about the topic, because they may feel overwhelmed by guilt at not being able to do as much as expected for their loved ones at a distance. And when a death occurs, they may feel overwhelmed by deep regret. Migration mourning that was proceeding toward acceptance, toward "living with it," suddenly becomes complicated by sadness and guilt at not having made the effort to see more frequently the parent, sibling, or friend who just died. There may be worry about not being present to help other family members with the loss and unbearable loneliness at not participating in communal grieving. Renewed questions about the wisdom of the decision to migrate and where one really belongs—with the family back home or the present one—further complicate the feelings of emptiness and despair.

CONCLUSIONS

Many immigrant families deal in flexible and creative ways with the ambiguous losses of migration. They are able to restore a sense of coherence to their lives by developing dual visions and lifestyles that preserve central themes of a cultural family life, while incorporating new ideas and skills. They are also able to make positive existential meaning out of the experience of migration, while being aware of obstacles and social injustices. The emergence of new rituals that re-create cultural and social spaces, rekindle the past, and maintain long-held spiritual beliefs and religious or health practices, actions that in the past had been regarded as deficits or rigidities, can be interpreted in a "both/and" frame as active attempts at restitution that bolster rather than constrain family adaptations.

Traditional imagery has regarded the immigrant's connection with the past as a wistful staring into the pages of a black-and-white photo album, or as listening teary eyed to the gramophone music of the old country. But a more apt metaphor for depicting contemporary immigrant family resilience is the richly ambiguous sound of fusion bands that mix ethnic sounds with new cultural beats. Indeed, many immigrants apply "both/and" perspectives as they blend hybrid mixtures of traditional themes with new tastes, values, and views.

ACKNOWLEDGMENT

Some of the concepts utilized in this chapter also appear in Falicov (2002).

REFERENCES

Ainslie, R. C. (1998). Cultural mourning, immigration, and engagement: Vignettes from the Mexican experience. In M. M. Suárez-Orozco (Ed.), *Crossings* (pp. 285–305). Cambridge, MA: Harvard University Press.

Alvarez, M. (1995). *The experience of migration: A relational approach in therapy* (Work in Progress, No. 71). Wellesley, MA: The Stone Center, Wellesley College.

Antonovsky, A. (1987). *Unraveling the mystery of health.* San Francisco: Jossey-Bass.

Antonovsky, A., & Sourani, T. (1988). Family sense of coherence and family adaptation. *Journal of Marriage and the Family, 50,* 79–92.

Anzaldúa, G. (1987). *Borderlands/la frontera: The new mestiza.* San Francisco: Spinster/Aunt Lute.

Bennett, L. A., Wolin, S. J., & McAvity, K. J. (1988). Family identity, ritual, and myth: A cultural perspective on life cycle transitions. In C. J. Falicov (Ed.), *Family transitions: Continuity and change over the life cycle* (pp. 211–234). New York: Guilford Press.

Boss, P. (1991). Ambiguous loss. In F. Walsh & M. McGoldrick (Eds.), *Living beyond loss: Death in the family.* New York: Norton.

Boss, P. (1999). *Ambiguous loss: Learning to live with unresolved grief.* Cambridge, MA: Harvard University Press.

Cohler, B. (1991). The life story and the study of resilience and response to adversity. *Journal of Narrative and Life History, 1,* 169–200.

Du Bois, W. E. B. (1903). *The souls of black folk.* Chicago: McClurg.

Falicov, C. J. (1992). Love and gender in the Latino marriage. *American Family Therapy Academy Newsletter, 48,* 30–36.

Falicov, C. J. (1993, Spring). Continuity and change: Lessons from immigrant families. *American Family Association Therapy Newsletter,* pp. 30–36.

Falicov, C. J. (1995). Training to think culturally: A multidimensional comparative framework. *Family Process, 34,* 373–388.

Falicov, C. J. (1996). Mexican families. In M. McGoldrick, J. Giordano, & J. Pierce (Eds.), *Ethnicity and family therapy* (2nd ed., pp. 169–182). New York: Guilford Press.

Falicov, C. J. (1998a). *Latino families in therapy: A guide to multicultural practice.* New York: Guilford Press.

Falicov, C. J. (1998b). The cultural meaning of family triangles. In M. McGoldrick (Ed.), *Re-visioning family therapy: Race, culture, and gender in clinical practice.* New York: Guilford Press.

Falicov, C. J. (1999). Religion and spiritual folk traditions in immigrant families: Therapeutic resources with Latinos. In F. Walsh (Ed.), *Spiritual resources in family therapy* (pp. 104–120). New York: Guilford Press.

Falicov, C. J. (2002). Ambiguous loss: Risk and resilience in Latino immigrant families. In M. Suárez-Orozco (Ed.), *Latinos: Remaking America* (pp. 274–288). Berkeley: University of California Press.

Falicov, C. J., & Brudner-White, L. (1983). The shifting family triangle: The issue of cultural and contextual relativity. In C. J. Falicov (Ed.), *Cultural perspectives in family therapy* (pp. 51–65). Rockville, MD: Aspen.

Garza-Guerrero, A. C. (1974). Culture shock: Its mourning and the vicissitudes of identity. *Journal of the American Psychoanalytic Association, 22,* 408–429.

Grinberg, L., & Grinberg, R. (1989). *Psychoanalytic perspectives on migration and exile.* New Haven, CT: Yale University Press.

Harwood, R. L., Miller, J. G., & Irizarry, N. L. (1995). *Culture and attachment: Perceptions of the child in context.* New York: Guilford Press.

Hoffman, E. (1989). *Lost in translation: A life in a new language.* New York: Penguin.

Hondagneu-Sotelo, P. (1994). *Gendered transitions.* Berkeley: University of California Press.

Imber-Black, E., Roberts, J., & Whiting, R. (Eds.). (1988). *Rituals in families and family therapy.* New York: Norton.

Johnston, R. (1976). The concept of the "marginal man": A refinement of the term. *Australian and New Zealand Journal of Science, 12,* 145–147.

LaFramboise, T., Coleman, H. L., & Gerton, J. (1993). Psychological impact of biculturalism: Evidence and theory. *Psychological Bulletin, 114*(3), 395–412.

Mackey, S. K. (1996). Nurturance: A neglected dimension in family therapy with adolescents. *Journal of Marital and Family Therapy, 22*(4), 489–508.

Marris, P. (1980). The uprooting of meaning. In G. V. Coelho & P. I. Ahmed (Eds.), *Uprooting and development: Dilemmas of coping with modernization* (pp. 101–116). New York: Plenum Press.

Melitto, R. (1985). Adaptation in family systems: A developmental perspective. *Family Process, 24*(1), 89–100.

Ogbu, J. U., & Matute-Bianchi, M. A. (1986). Understanding sociocultural factors: Knowledge, identity, and social adjustment. In California State Department of Education, Bilingual Edcation Office (Ed.), *Beyond language: Social and cultural factors in schooling* (pp. 73–142). Sacramento: California State University, Los Angeles Evaluation, Dissemination and Assessment Center.

Potocky-Tripodi, M. (2000). Where is my home?: A refugee journey. Writer's showcase presented by *Writer's Digest,* Lincoln, NE: Universe.

Rodriguez, R. (1992). *Days of obligation: An argument with my Mexican father.* New York: Viking.

Rosaldo, R. (1989). Culture and truth: The remaking of social analysis. Boston: Beacon Press.

Rouse, R. (1992). Making sense of settlement: Class transformation, cultural struggle and transnationalism among Mexican immigrants in the United States. In N. G. Schiller, L. Basch, & C. Blanc-Szanton (Eds.), *Towards a transnational perspective on migration.* New York: New York Academy of Sciences.

Rueschenberg, E., & Buriel, R. (1989). Mexican American family functioning and acculturation: A family systems perspective. *Hispanic Journal of Behavioral Sciences, 11*(3), 232–244.

Rumbaut, R. G. (November 12, 1999). *It takes a family (and a village): Patterns of incorporation among children of immigrants.* Presentation at the 61st National Concil on Family Relations Annual Conference: Borders, Boundaries, and Beacons: Diverse Families in Dynamic Societies, Irvine, CA.

Sabogal, F., Marín, G., Otero-Sabogal, R., Marín, B. V., & Perez-Stable, P. (1987). Hispanic familism and acculturation: What changes and what doesn't. *Hispanic Journal of Behavioral Sciences, 9*(4), 397–412.

Shuval, J. T. (1982). Migration and stress. In L. Goldberger & S. Breznitz (Eds.), *Handbook of stress: Theoretical and clinical aspects* (2nd ed., pp. 641–657). New York: Free Press.

Sluzki, C. E. (1979). Migration and family conflict. Family Process, 18(1), 379–392.

Sluzki, C. E. (1983). The sounds of silence. In C. J. Falicov (Ed.), *Cultural perspectives in family therapy* (pp. 68–77). Rockville, MD: Aspen.

Sluzki, C. E. (1989). Network disruption and network reconstruction in the process of migration/relocation. *Berkshire Medical Center Department of Psychiatry Bulletin, 2*(3), 2–4.

Steinberg, L., Dornbusch, S. M., & Brown, B. B. (1992). Ethnic differences in adolescent achievement. *American Psychologist, 47*(6), 723–729.

Suárez-Orozco, M. M., & Suárez-Orozco, C. E. (1995a). *Transformations: Immigration, family life and achievement motivation among Latino adolescents.* Stanford, CA: Stanford University Press.

Suárez-Orozco, C., & Suárez-Orozco, M. (1995b). Migration: Generational discontinuities and the making of Latino identities. In L. Romanucci-Ross & G. DeVos (Eds.), *Ethnic identity: Creation, conflict, and accommodation* (3rd ed.). Walnut Creek, CA: Altamira Press.

Suárez-Orozco, C., & Suárez-Orozco, M. (2000). *Children of immigration.* Cambridge, MA: Harvard University Press

Troya, E. & Rosenberg, F. (1999). "Nos fueron a Mexico": Que nos paso a los jovenes exiliados consureños? *Sistemas Familiares, 15*(3), 79–92.

Vega, W. A., Kolody, B., Valle, R., & Weir, J. (1991). Social networks, social support, and their relationship to depression among immigrant Mexican women. *Human Organization, 50,* 154–162.

Volkan, V. D., & Zintl, E. (1993). *Life after loss: The lessons of grief.* New York: Scribner's.

Walsh, F. (1996). The concept of family resilience: Crisis and challenge. *Family Process, 35*(3), 261–282.

Walsh, F. (1998). *Strengthening family resilience.* New York: Guilford Press.

Warheit, G., Vega, W., Auth, J., & Meinhardt, K. (1985). Mexican-American immigration and mental health: A comparative analysis of psychosocial stress and dysfunction. In W. Vega & M. Miranda (Eds.), *Stress and Hispanic mental health* (pp. 76–109). Rockville, MD: National Institute of Mental Health.

Westermeyer, J. (1989). *Psychiatric care of migrants: A clinical guide.* Washington, DC: American Psychiatric Press.

White, M., & Epston, D. (1990). *Narrative means to therapeutic ends.* New York: Random House.

CHAPTER 12

CHANGING GENDER NORMS

Transitional Dilemmas

Shelley A. Haddock
Toni Schindler Zimmerman
Kevin P. Lyness

Gender is a fundamental organizing principle of people's lives, family relationships, and society. Women and men have powerful expectations about gender and intimate relationships in contemporary society. "Traditional" societal gender expectations for how men and women should behave and what they should value continue to influence our lives and shape our family relationships. Yet these societal expectations are in transition, and many people today are striving to define themselves and their family relationships in new, less restrictive ways. They believe that traditional gender expectations often keep them from finding their own individually defined purpose and fulfillment. They are searching for ways to live and love free from the constraints of rigid, gender-based expectations and inequities.

In this chapter, we describe gender as a social construction and explain how it continues to organize our lives and relationships. We provide evidence that although gender norms are in transition in the United States, ideological and structural barriers continue to prevent many families from translating their egalitarian ideals into daily realities. We also illustrate that, despite these barriers, a growing number of families have been able to reject gender as an ideological justification for inequality in family life. Finally, we believe that therapists need to address gender and power dynamics proactively to assist clients in recognizing and overcoming gender-based constraints.

THE SOCIAL CONSTRUCTION OF GENDER

Until recently, gender was believed to derive naturally from one's biological sex. "Becoming a woman" or "becoming a man" was understood as a "natural" process, and perceived differences between men and women in personality and orientation were linked to biology (Ellman & Taggart, 1993). In recent decades, however, several theoretical traditions have evolved to better explain the role of gender in people's lives and relationships (see Risman, 1998). Despite differences in their conceptualizations of gender, contemporary gender theorists (e.g., Bem, 1993; Chodorow, 1989; Coltrane, 1998; Connell, 1987; Ferree, 1990; Gilligan, 1982; Hare-Mustin & Maracek, 1990; Lorber, 1994; Risman, 1998; West & Zimmerman, 1987) agree that whereas sex is based on relatively distinct biological factors, gender is a social construction. West and Zimmerman (1987) have argued that rather than being what we are, gender is something that we do. We are expected to "do gender"—to exhibit or enact those attributes or actions that are defined as masculine or feminine in a particular cultural context (Coltrane, 1998).

In this socially constructed gender system, the prescriptions for each gender are defined in relation to the other. Maleness and femaleness are cast as dichotomized and polarized categories; human capacities are divided up and relegated, as if they belong naturally to one gender and not the other (Ellman & Taggart, 1993). Traditionally, manhood is defined narrowly in instrumental terms—rationality, stoicism, independence, aggressiveness, and achievement orientation. Womanhood is defined in expressive terms—nurturance, emotionality, dependence, selflessness, and relationship orientation. Supposed differences between the genders are exaggerated, with similarities suppressed (Ferree, 1990; Hare-Mustin & Maracek, 1990). Individuals are judged positively if they comply with the social expectations for their gender and negatively if they do not (Ellman & Taggart, 1993). For instance, in contemporary U.S. culture, men or boys are commonly referred to as "wimps" or "fags" for showing supposedly feminine qualities, such as emotionality and vulnerability (Katz & Earp, 1999). Women are commonly perceived as "bitches" or "pushy" if they exhibit the "masculine" quality of assertiveness (Lerner, 1997).

The dichotomized categories of gender are granted unequal social value (Ferree, 1990). Male characteristics are regarded as the ideal standard for human behavior, and there is an implicit assumption that male attributes and experiences are somehow gender-neutral and normative (Katz & Earp, 1999). In their presumed difference from men, women's qualities and experiences are devalued and used to justify inequality (Hare-Mustin, 1989).

These constructed gender differences are used as a justification for sex stratification (Hare-Mustin & Maracek, 1990; Lorber, 1994). Gender is considered a reasonable and legitimate basis for the distribution of rights, resources, power, privilege, and responsibilities (Baber & Allen, 1992; Feree, 1990; Risman, 1998). On the basis of gender, men as a group have had more privilege and women have been oppressed in virtually every culture (Lorber, 1994).

Gender is intertwined with other dimensions of social expectations and power. Race, social class, sexual orientation, and religion also organize men's and women's lives and family relationships. "We exist in social contexts created by the intersections of systems of power (e.g., race, class, gender, and sexual orientation) and oppression (prejudice, class stratification, gender inequality, and heterosexist bias)" (Bograd, 1999, p. 276). Not all men are equally privileged in our society, nor are all women affected by multiple oppressions. Yet in every cultural group, men have more privilege and status than do their mothers or sisters (Risman, 1998). In understanding the gender-based nature of people's lives and relationships, it is important to consider them in the context of powerful cultural and religious beliefs, along with the socioeconomic conditions that influence family processes.

Men's privilege and women's oppression result from "a complex system of structures, processes, relations, and ideologies, not just from men's control over women" (Baber & Allen, 1992, p. 7). In some cultures, these systems of power function almost invisibly, and people enact them intentionally or unintentionally. Certainly, some women and children are mistreated by men who intentionally abuse their privilege (McGoldrick, Broken Nose, & Potenza, 1999), yet other women may not experience intentional oppression by any particular man or group of men. However, in a gender-based society, the influence of societal ideologies and institutions that grant men privilege and oppress women persist (Risman, 1998).

Feminist scholars share the common goal of eradicating inequality, yet there are disparities among feminist theorists as to why gender differences exist as well as in their proposed solutions. Scholars at the Wellesley College's Stone Center for Developmental Services and Studies (Belenky, Clinchy, Goldberger, & Tarule, 1986; Gilligan, 1982; Jordan, 1997; Jordan, Kaplan, Miller, Stiver, & Surrey, 1991; Miller, 1986) believe that biology and socialization interact to create some of the differences between women and men. In their view, the primary problem is that women's characteristics, values, and ways of knowing (or of making sense of the world) and relating have been devalued, whereas men's characteristics are held as the ideal. In this view, the solution to gender inequality lies less in eradicating gender difference and more in elevating the social value assigned to characteristics traditionally associated with women. Other theorists (e.g., Hare-Mustin & Marecek, 1990) emphasize the similarities between women and men, and contend that perceived gender differences are a result of centuries of socialization and unfair access to resources, opportunities, and experiences (Baber & Allen, 1992). In this view, the solution emphasized is one of changing the ideologies that exaggerate gender differences.

FAMILIES ARE ORGANIZED BY GENDER

Family and gender are so intertwined that it is impossible to understand one without reference to the other (Coltrane, 1998). Families are not merely influenced by gender; rather, families are *organized* by gender. Gender is as central to understanding families as is the concept of generation: Gender and generation are the two fundamental, organizing principles of family life (Goldner, 1989). The names of family roles (mother, son, sister, nephew, grandma, uncle) tell us both the gender and generational location of family members. Gender typically indicates as much about the expectations for, and status or power of, a person in a family as does generational location.

The influence of gender on family life must be understood at multiple levels; gender has consequences at the personal, relational, and societal levels (Risman, 1998). At the personal level, individuals respond to gender-based expectations for how they should feel and behave, what they should want and value, and how they should look. Gender shapes our identities, and the real and perceived life choices available to us. At a relational level, gender organizes the social processes of everyday life, particularly in our family or intimate relationships. For instance, in most heterosexual couples, men are still viewed as the primary breadwinner even if the female partner is employed full-time (Friedman & Greenhaus, 2000), and employed women continue to shoulder the majority of household and child care obligations (Hochschild, 1997).

Gender also operates at the societal level. Societal ideologies and institutions related to the gender-based nature of family roles change in response to economic and cultural circumstances. Contemporary gender expectations are best understood in a historical context. In the late 19th century, industrialization and urbanization brought a redefinition of gender roles in families (Coontz, 1992). In the transition from the farm to the factory, paid work in the labor force became separate from nonpaid work at home. This "separate sphere ideology" included three assumptions that continue to have significant implications for the gender-based nature of family relationships (Williams, 2000). First, men were viewed as "naturally" suited for employment; being a good husband and father was reductively equated with being a good economic provider. Second, women were seen as naturally suited for caretaking and homemaking, and motherhood was viewed as an all-encompassing responsibility and sole source of identity and fulfillment for women (Braverman, 1989). Third, workplace norms and practices were based on an expectation that workers (i.e., men) did not have caregiving responsibilities (which were handled by wives), and therefore could devote themselves to professional pursuits without "interference" from family responsibilities.

The separate sphere ideology spawned cultural assumptions that the organization of family roles according to traditional gender expectations and gender-based power was essential to *normal family processes* and healthy child development (Boss & Thorne, 1989). The breadwinner–homemaker family became reified as the "normal" and "ideal" family. The influential theories of Parsons and Bales (1955) granted academic credibility to these ideas, making the faulty assumption that this family pattern—unique to a particular time and place—was the universally ideal family type (Walsh, 1998). By doing so, they helped to construct gender-based expectations and power differentials that continue to be viewed as "normal" today.

The separate sphere ideal has been more of a cultural symbol than an actual reality (Coontz, 1992; Skolnick, 1991). Even at its peak during the 1950s, the breadwinner–homemaker family was a reality primarily for upper- and middle-class white families. In marginalized ethnic and lower socioeconomic-level families, men have had relatively few opportunities for advancement in the public world, and women typically have worked outside the home for pay (Coltrane, 1998). Still today, when only a small minority of families include a breadwinner father and homemaker mother (Barnett & Rivers, 1996), the separate sphere ideal contributes to belief systems and practices that encourage gender-based expectations and inequality at the relational level of family life by placing women at a disadvantage in the workplace and discouraging men from doing family work.

Gender inequality is manifested in intimate relationships in many ways but often reflects assumptions about which person's needs and desires are given top priority (Knudson-Martin & Mahoney, 1998). Reviews of the relevant research (e.g., Williams, 2000) reveal that men typically hold the bulk of the power in heterosexual families of all racial backgrounds. Gender-based power differentials can manifest in both partners' prioritizing the man's career and personal interests; expecting less responsibility from him in household coordination, chores, and parenting; granting him greater influence in important family decisions; prioritizing his leisure time and allowing him more discretionary spending; and expecting from him less emotional investment in family relationships (McGoldrick, Anderson, & Walsh, 1989; Rabin, 1996; Zvonkovic, Greaves, Schmeige, & Hall, 1996). These gender-based power differentials also can influence both partners to assume that the female partner should be primarily responsible for parenting and housework, and—from a position of restricted power—for maintaining effective family functioning, and that she should limit outside activities, including paid employment and leisure, so that these activities do not pose a threat to the family (McGoldrick et al., 1989; Rabin, 1996). Although many gay and lesbian couples also structure their relationships according to power differentials (Carrington, 1999; Renzetti, 1997), several scholars (e.g., McWhirter, Sanders, & Reinisch, 1990) have found that the relationships of same-sex couples tend to be characterized by more egalitarianism than heterosexual relationships.

Gender also influences parenting behavior. As a primary and influential socializing agent of children (Coltrane, 1998), parents teach what is "appropriate" and "inappropriate" behavior for each gender, and how the genders should interact with one another. From a very young age, parents model or openly express their ideas about how gender should be done. For instance, children learn that performing a disproportionate amount of the housework and child care is part of being a woman and doing gender appropriately (West & Zimmerman, 1987). Until children can *do gender* themselves, adults perform this function for them.

Parents often begin the process of gender socialization before the birth of a child. They often want to know the sex of their unborn child in order to choose gender-appropriate names and clothing (Grieshaber, 1998). During preschool years, parents tend to give their children gender-stereotyped toys: Boys receive more vehicles, sports equipment, and military toys, and girls receive more dolls and domestic toys (Etaugh & Liss, 1992). Parents also interact differently with their children depending on their gender (Lindsey, Mize, & Pettit, 1997; Sandnabba & Ahlberg, 1999), rewarding gender-typical play and punishing atypical play (Lytton & Romney, 1991). Chores also are often assigned in a gender stereotypical fashion (McHale, Bartko, Crouter, & Perry-Jenkins, 1990). Additionally, Crouter, McHale, and Bartko (1993) found that in families in which the father is the sole breadwinner, fathers spend three times more time in dyadic activities with sons than with daughters; in dual-earner families, fathers spend similar amounts of time with sons and daughters.

Consequences of Gender-Based Family Life

Although the gendering of family life has historically been considered normal and desirable—and continues to be considered as such by some political and religious groups (Faludi, 1991), scholars and practitioners have highlighted the many negative consequences that can result from compliance with rigid gender expectations and the resulting power differentials in intimate relationships. Gender constraints at the personal level restrict freedom for both women and men (Goldner, 1989), discouraging the development of their full human capacities. For instance, when men enact traditional expectations to be stoic and autonomous breadwinners, they often fail to develop more meaningful relationships with children and become isolated from partners, friends, and their own inner experience (Rosen, 1999; Silverstein, 1996). When women enact expectations to prioritize the needs of others at the expense of their own, they often become lonely (Schwartz, 1994) and depressed (Papp, 2000), and sacrifice personal goals (McGoldrick, 1999).

The gendering of family life sets up inequitable skews between most marital or intimate partners (Walsh, 1989). A significant body of empirical research has established that gender-based power differentials are corrosive to family relationships. In her review of the literature, Bernard (1982) concluded that two marriages exist—*his* and *hers*. His is more satisfying than hers. McGoldrick (1989) reviewed numerous studies that found that married women's sense of well-being is lower than that of married men's. Although inequality is clearly detrimental to women, it also negatively influences men by compromising the quality of their family relationships, which are generally as central to men's happiness and well-being as they are to women's (Barnett & Rivers, 1996). Inequity in marital or intimate partnerships has been consistently shown to have negative effects on relationship satisfaction, regardless of whether partners are under- or over-benefiting (DeMaris & Longmore, 1996; Feeney, Peterson, & Noller, 1994; Peterson, 1990; VanYperen & Buunk, 1994), although underbenefiting is more harmful than overbenefiting (VanYperen & Buunk, 1994).

Several scholars (Rabin, 1996; Schwartz, 1994; Steil, 1997) contend that deep friendship and sustained intimacy are unattainable in a relationship based on power differentials. When a relationship is structured primarily around the needs and desires of one person, it leads to relationship "failures" of empathy, interest, respect, and authenticity, and a resulting dehumanizing of the woman, which preclude the possibility of friendship and intimacy (Schwartz, 1994). Beavers (1985) found that the greater the power differential between partners, the more dysfunctional and unsatisfying the marriage. Gottman's longitudinal research on married couples found that "when a man is not willing to share power with his partner, there is an 81 percent chance that his marriage will self-destruct" (Gottman & Silver, 1999, p. 100).

Tragically, in a large number of couples, these power differentials are characterized by intrafamilial abuse, resulting in potentially dire consequences, including psychological trauma, physical injury, and death of the victim, who is typically female (Bograd, 1999; McGoldrick et al., 1999; Renzetti, 1997). Although estimates of prevalence rates differ, scholars agree that the problem is at epidemic proportions. For example, in 1998, women experienced about 900,000 violent offenses at the hands of an intimate partner; the rate of intimate partner violence for women is 7.7 per 1,000, while that for men is 1.5 per 1,000; nearly three out of four victims of murder by an intimate partner are women, and women are victims of 85% of violent nonlethal crime (Rennison & Welchans, 2000). Although violence also exists among gay and lesbian couples (Renzetti, 1997), much family violence is linked to traditional gender ideologies and the abuse of male privilege (see Haddock, 2002; McGoldrick et al., 1999). Graham-Bermann and Brescoll (2000) found that the amount of physical violence and emotional abuse experienced by mothers is positively related to how much children believe in the inherent superiority and privilege of men in the family. This finding reveals the damaging transmission of destructive gender attitudes across generations.

Children are negatively influenced by gender norms in other ways.

For instance, Pipher (1994) argued that increasing numbers of American girls suffer from depression, eating disorders, addictions, and suicide attempts, because girls try to conform to rigid gender expectations. By focusing on their appearance or acting less intelligent so as not to intimidate boys, for instance, they stifle their creative spirit and damage their self-esteem. Muuss (1999) noted that one likely cause of eating disorders lies in social attitudes; positive personality attributes are associated with thinness. Kindlon and Thompson (1999) linked emotional illiteracy in boys, which can result from adherence to traditional gender norms for boys, to depression, substance abuse and addiction, anger and violence, and difficulties in forming later relationships and in expressing emotional vulnerability.

GENDER AND FAMILY NORMS IN TRANSITION

In the past 40 years, key economic and social conditions, particularly women's increased employment and the Women's Movement, have challenged traditional conceptualizations of gender, fueling dramatic shifts in the structure of family life. Some segments of society perceive these changes negatively, bemoaning the "breakdown of the family," and arguing that the maintenance of the separate sphere ideology is the best route to an ideal society and family life (Faludi, 1991). However, many women and men in the United States do not embrace the "Father Knows Best" days of segregated gender roles and gender-based power differentials (Coontz, 1992). Instead, men increasingly want to forge more intimate relationships with their children and partners, and many women want to develop interests and identities in addition to those of intimate partner and mother (Rosen, 1999; Walsh, 1998). Increasing numbers of women and men are choosing to forge full identities and lives that may not include marriage, intimate partnership, or parenthood (Coltrane, 1998).

These progressive attitudes and beliefs about gender are reflected in a new cultural ideal for intimate partnerships; an ideal that many family scholars agree is more companionate and egalitarian (Coltrane, 1998). There is increasing empirical evidence that more women and men endorse equality as an important element of intimate relationships than in past decades. For example, Ferber and Young (1997) found that in an undergraduate sample, men and women expected to do nearly equal amounts of housework, felt that such a division of work was fair, and had expectations that both spouses would work, compared to statistics they cited from 1976, in which "no more than 2% of either men or women thought that husbands and wives should be equally responsible for housework" (p. 69). Recent data show consistently high levels of egalitarian expectations for marriage in college-age women, with 82–94% endorsing egalitarian responses in various domains of married life (Botkin, Weeks, & Morris, 2000). These shifting attitudes are especially prevalent among younger individuals, urban residents, and those in higher socioeconomic-level groups (Fleming, 1988; Keith & Schafer, 1991). In a recent study of middle-class, dual-earner couples, most women and men rated marital equality as "very important" in their own marriages (Rosenbluth, Steil, & Whitcomb, 1998). Additionally, several scholars (e.g., Carrington, 1999) have found that egalitarianism is considered ideal in most gay and lesbian relationships.

Scholars (Coltrane, 1996; Deutsch, 1999; O'Connell, 1993; Schwartz, 1994) also have documented that some families are moving toward shared parenting and more liberal gender socialization for children. Cowan and Cowan (2000) found that fathers in the United States are more involved with rearing children than previous generations, helping their wives more in pregnancy and taking on more responsibilities for early childhood tasks. Researchers (e.g., Coltrane, 1996; Parke, 1996; Risman, 1986) also have noted that the more involved fathers are, the more they tend to encourage sons and daughters equally, and use similar interaction and play styles for both.

Despite these significant attitude changes, the actual dynamics of heterosexual relationships have changed very little. Initially, many researchers assumed that women's increased employment would result in less conformity to gender expectations and more egalitarian intimate relationships (e.g., Hardill, Green, Dudleston, & Owen, 1997). Despite the widespread goal of lessening the influence of gender expectations on individual lives and relationships, only a slow trend in this direction is evident (Risman & Johnson Summerford, 1998). Across many recent studies, contemporary marriages are consistently structured by gender-based power differentials (Rosenbluth et al., 1998; also see Steil, 1997). Even women who are employed shoulder nearly 80% of the "second shift" of household chores and child care (Hochschild & Machung, 1989; Williams, 2000). In a recent study of 860 business professionals, employed mothers spent more than three times the number of hours per week on child care activities than did men (Friedman & Greenhaus, 2000). Women are the primary caretakers of ill and elderly family members (McGoldrick, 1999; Walsh, 1999) and are primarily responsible for the emotional and organizational labor of the family (Zimmerman, Haddock, Ziemba, & Rust, 2001; McGoldrick, 1999). Men's needs are prioritized in other areas, such as marital decisions (Zvonkovic et al., 1996), career (Friedman & Greenhaus, 2000), and finances (Steil & Weltman, 1991).

The desire to free one's family relationships from gender-based inequities does not translate easily to its achievement (Blaisure & Allen, 1995; Hochschild & Machung, 1989; Knudson-Martin & Mahoney, 1998). According to recent research, many couple relationships are marked by incongruence between an ideological commitment to equality and inequitable interactional patterns (Carrington, 1999; Deutsch, 1999; Rabin, 1996). Rosenbluth et al. (1998) found that despite their participants' endorsement of equality as ideal and very important in their marriages, fewer than 28% equally shared household tasks. Carrington (1999) found a similar pattern among some gay and lesbian couples, who held a strong commitment to equality, yet did not translate this principle into daily divisions of family work. This incongruence can appear in parenting practices as well; parents may verbally express beliefs about gender equality to children, then—often unwittingly—behave in ways that contradict these beliefs (Walsh, 1998). For instance, parents may model gender inequities if the mother typically responds to a child's needs because the father is "busy," or if they expect a daughter to help more with household chores than her brother.

Many contemporary couples deal with the incongruence between their egalitarian ideals and unequal interactional patterns by developing *gender myths,* which are intended to veil the inequities in the relationship and support the illusion of equality (Carrington, 1999; Hochschild & Machung, 1989). An example of myth making can be seen in couples' explanations that women provide a disproportionate share of child care because it is their individual choice or a need for control, or because of their "superior parenting" (Deutsch, 1999, p. 48). Another common myth involves the role of fathers and the high quality of their parenting. Men tend to compare their own parenting with their fathers and their peers (rather than their female partner), which leads them to assess themselves favorably, without realizing that they are doing less than their wives (Deutsch, 1999). As Rosen (1999) argues, "Since the model for high-quality fathering is so abysmally lacking in our society, their boasts about the quality of their own involvement is hard to assail" (p. 135).

Other studies (e.g., Hochschild & Machung, 1989) reveal myths related to household labor in heterosexual couples. Although many women define inequitable division of labor as unfair (VanYperen & Buunk, 1994), other women—who are responsible for the majority of household chores—describe their relationships as fair and themselves as satisfied (DeMaris & Longmore, 1996). Deutsch refers to this as the "myth of women's power at home" (p. 48). DeMaris and Longmore (1996) found that among dual-earner couples (drawn from the National Survey of Families and Households) who define housework as an unfair burden *on the husband,* he was doing only 36–39% as much of the routine housework as the woman, and in "fair" relationships, men did only 19% as much routine housework as women. In those families in which housework was seen as unfair to the wife, the men did 13–14% as much routine housework as women.

BARRIERS TO EQUALITY IN FAMILIES

How can the typical pattern of continued inequality in families be explained despite many people's desires to form egalitarian relationships?

Gender so thoroughly organizes our lives at the personal, relational, and societal levels that even those who ideologically reject gender inequality are often compelled to "choose" options that undermine their egalitarian principles (Baber & Allen, 1992; Risman, 1998); societal structures and ideologies often make the gender-based choice the seemingly logical one (Risman, 1998). Although women and men maintain free will in making decisions, their agency is limited by social institutions and ideologies that link non-gender-based choices with personal hardship (Risman, 1998), such as loss of male privilege and power, gender identity tensions, fears about harming family relationships, and societal censure.

Below, we briefly provide examples of societal ideologies and structures that directly reinforce gender inequities in families [for more information on societal barriers, see Barnett & Rivers, 1996; Carrington, 1999; Coltrane, 1998; Deutsch, 1999; Dusky, 1996; Galinsky, 1999; Hare-Mustin & Marecek, 1990; Holcomb, 1998; McGoldrick, et al., 1989; Risman, 1998; Schwartz, 1994; Williams, 2000]. The assumptions that underlie the separate sphere ideology continue to operate powerfully in society, serving as constraints to gender equality in family life. Social ideologies continue to cast men and women as radically different and gender-based inequities in families as normative or even desirable. In addition, economic structures that assume that employees do not have family responsibilities, and ideologies related to motherhood, have detrimental effects on family life.

Gender Ideologies in Popular Media

Traditional ideologies about how men and women should express gender remain dominant in popular culture (Hare-Mustin & Maracek, 1990; Holtzman, 2000). Katz and Earp (1999) and Kilbourne (2000) demonstrate the pervasiveness of these ideologies in the mass media (e.g., television, movies, and magazines). Studies of the best-selling self-help literature on relationships in the 1990s (Zimmerman, Haddock, & McGeorge, 2001; Zimmerman, Holm, & Haddock, 2001) show that many self-help books, particularly the most popular, recommend traditional gender behaviors and continued inequality (e.g., *Men Are from Mars, Women Are from Venus* [Gray, 1992]; and *The Rules* [Fein & Schnieder, 1995]). These books endorse acceptance of gender stereotypes as "normal" and immutable; for instance, many implicitly and explicitly suggest that men are naturally unemotional, aggressive, and disengaged from or uninterested in family life, and that women are manipulative, submissive, overly responsible for family life, and overly concerned with attractiveness. These books encourage men and women to form intimate relationships based on power differentials, encouraging women, for instance, to adapt to men's needs and placate men. Self-help books have become a constant and integral part of contemporary society; many readers turn to these books for supposedly expert advice on how to improve their intimate relationships. Unfortunately, in many of these books, they receive advice that is potentially detrimental to the quality of their relationships. As is noted in each study, however, other leading self-help books (e.g., *Dance of Anger* [Lerner, 1997]) do promote empowerment and gender equality.

The Gender-Based Economic System

Despite an increasingly diverse workforce, the economic system continues to revolve around several implicit, gender-based assumptions: that the ideal worker is a (white) male who is employed full time; that his (female) partner is either not employed or is a secondary wage earner, and that she bears primary responsibility for housework, child care, and elder care (Friedman & Greenhaus, 2000). Such an economic system creates a foundation for societal and familial inequality, leading to numerous negative consequences for the majority of workers whose lives and families do not fit this "ideal" model.

The assumption of natural differences in women's and men's aptitudes, orientations, and obligations continues to keep women's pay low, to exclude them from certain professions (i.e., science and business), and to block their access to career advancement (i.e., the glass ceiling) (see Coltrane, 1998; Friedman & Greenhaus, 2000; Williams, 2000). For instance, women in general make 73% of men's annual earnings (U.S. Bureau of the Census, 2001). These inequities in the economic system contribute to many men's sense of entitlement to their female partners' unpaid domestic labor and to greater influence in decision-making power than their partner (Coltrane, 1998). These sexist economic practices also contribute to the disproportionately high rates of poverty among single-mother families (Williams, 2000), especially among families headed by mothers who also face racial discrimination.

Economic structures are stratified not only by gender but also by race (Almeida, Woods, Messineo, Font, & Heer, 1994). In relation to white men's earnings, African American men earn 78%, and African American women earn 64%; Hispanic men earn 63%, and Hispanic women earn 52% (U.S. Bureau of the Census, 2001). For men of color, the societal expectation that men ideally provide the sole source of income for their families collides with racial discrimination. Almeida et al. (1994) suggested that some men of color may respond to exclusions from economic sources of power by trying to exert control over female partners out of a desire to prove their "manhood." Other scholars have explained the higher levels of egalitarianism in African American families compared to white families, for instance, as a reflection of the relatively common practice of dual earning in these families that has resulted from discrimination against black men in the paid labor force (Benokraitis, 1999).

These inaccurate economic assumptions create difficulties for those who balance employment with family responsibilities. These gender-based assumptions fuel the common practice of expecting unrealistic commitments of time and energy from employees. In fact, people in the United States work more hours per week than in any other industrialized country, and these hours have been increasing over the past 20 years, particularly among men (Galinsky, 1999). These workplace practices, in combination with social expectations to perform as breadwinner, have kept many men peripherally involved in family life and have prevented them from participating in household management and from forming intimate, daily connections with their partners and children (Walsh, 1989). These assumptions also justify the failure of many workplaces to implement family-friendly alternatives, such as flexibility in scheduling hours and on-site child care programs.

Balancing family and work is even more difficult for women. In anticipation of conflicts, some women believe that they must make the life-defining "choice" between an active and satisfying career or a fulfilling family life (Holcomb, 1998). Other women believe they must limit their career "choices" to those that allow more flexibility and time for family—decisions that often are associated with lower pay and prestige (Friedman & Greenhaus, 2000). In families with sufficient economic means, some women "choose" to stop working or work part-time for an extended period following the birth of children—a decision that can have long-term implications for not only for their own economic well-being but also that of their children, especially in situations of divorce or death of a spouse (Williams, 2000). Men rarely face these real and perceived life choices. Whereas men feel that they are fulfilling their family commitments by working, women have to justify why working does not make them bad mothers (Coltrane, 1998).

Recent analyses of pay differentials between men and women in various family situations further illustrate the bias in the economic system against workers who maintain family responsibilities. Researchers have found that women without children earn more than mothers (Friedman & Greenhaus, 2000). Although parenthood is associated with pay loss for women, it is an asset for men. Fathers earn more than men without children. To understand this difference in pay, Friedman and Greenhaus found only one factor that accounts for the difference: Fatherhood is associated with more authority on the job. However, the economic system even discriminates against fathers who have more family responsibilities. Friedman and Greenhaus found that single-earner men earn more than dual-earner men, and they could find no factors (e.g., psychological involvement, number of hours worked, job performance) to account for this discrepancy. Similarly, 1999 survey data of nearly 2,700 men shows that married men who have a stay-at-home wife make considerably more per hour than men married to women with full-time jobs (Chun & Lee, 2001). These researchers conclude that having a wife who handles family responsibilities is an advantage for men at work. These inequities in the workplace will likely end only when the economic system is based on the reality that virtually all paid workers are also family workers (Risman, 1998).

Ideologies about Motherhood

Although the view of motherhood as an all-encompassing occupation is a modern invention, it has become a widely accepted cultural assumption (Risman, 1998) that contributes to beliefs that mothers cannot simultaneously be loving and effective parents while also engaging in paid employment, self-care activities, or other pursuits. It is important to note that societal expectations related to motherhood differ based on social class; often, the same political groups in American society that encourage (white, middle-class) mothers to "stay home" for the sake of their children also argue that mothers on welfare should find gainful employment (Eitzen & Zinn, 2000).

Today, most two-earner families need both incomes for economic viability (Galinsky, 1999), and virtually all single parents must work for pay. Despite the reality that the vast majority of mothers must or prefer to work, societal ideologies continue to support the notion that it is best that they do not. Working mothers often are depicted in the media as lacking time for their children, their families, and their employers. Their children are frequently portrayed as desperate for parental love and attention while being "raised" by child care providers (Holcomb, 1998). The media are replete with alarming and inaccurate information about the outcomes for children of employed mothers (Holcomb, 1998; Galinsky, 1999). These media portrayals are not harmless; rather, they have become embedded in contemporary culture, shape Americans' collective psyches (Barnett & Rivers, 1996), and result in women's overresponsibility for parenting, their tendency to curtail other pursuits to live up to unrealistic motherhood ideals, and their common experiences of unwarranted guilt for out-of-home employment to ensure the economic viability of their family or to fulfill personal goals (Deutsch, 1999). This view of motherhood also reduces fathers to peripheral roles in family life, primarily valued for their paychecks but viewed as caregivers inferior to mothers.

It is important to recognize that these persisting cultural myths have been debunked by decades of empirical research. In her review of the relevant research, Galinsky (1999) noted that studies have found either no impact or a positive impact from maternal employment. Maternal employment in and of itself does not affect the mother–child relationship, does not diminish the influence of parents on children, and does not influence children's assessment of the quality of their mothers' parenting. Few, if any, differences in children's intellectual ability or achievement are related to maternal employment. Despite common beliefs that children do not have enough time with their employed mothers, empirical evidence shows that children have more time with their parents now than they did 20 years ago, and it is with fathers—not mothers—that children report having too little time (Galinsky, 1999). Moreover, children of employed mothers are no more likely to feel that they have too little time with their mothers than are children of stay-at-home mothers.

Many unrecognized benefits for families derive from women's employment. The most obvious benefit is increased income. Maternal employment has the most positive effect on children's development in low-income families, particularly when children receive warm and responsive care at home and from child care providers (Galinsky, 1999). Economic resources allow families to enhance the quality of their children's physical environment and provide high-quality medical care and more educational opportunities and resources. Maternal employment also has consistently been associated with better physical and emotional health for women (Barnett & Rivers, 1996). There is some evidence that maternal employment is associated with increased independence and self-competence in children (Crosby, 1991). Additionally, Hoffman (1989) found that girls of working mothers score better on social adjustment tests, do better in school, and have more professional accomplishments than children whose mothers are not employed. Given sexist practices in the workplace, a noteworthy finding is that the positive outcomes of maternal employment for women and their children are particularly strong when women have a high degree of control or authority at work, and are highly invested in and satisfied with their jobs (Friedman & Greenhaus, 2000). Many men are still reluctant to accept their wives as equal providers a reluctance that is less common among working-class men than other men (Coltrane, 1998); however, women's employment has been found to relieve pressures on men to be the sole breadwinner, which may create more psychological space and time for them to engage actively in family life (Schwartz, 1994). Moreover, women's employment allows them greater ability to negotiate for fairness in the marital relationship (Lennon & Rosenfeld, 1994).

The gender-based economic system and myths of motherhood may explain why, for most couples, inequality becomes even more pronounced with parenthood (e.g., Carter, 1999; Cowan & Cowan, 2000). Deutsch (1999) argued that "children create an inequality of crisis proportions" (p. 5) for several reasons. First, overall workload increases greatly with children, and the workplace is often inflexible in offering family-friendly work hours or options (Carter, 1999). Second, because women are more likely to stop working for a period of time or reduce their hours to part-time, the presence of children often coincides with a reduction in women's earning potential (Williams, 2000) and a resultant decline in their relational power (Rabin, 1996). Moreover, beliefs that women are ideally and instinctively suited for parenting lead many couples to centralize the mother's child care role.

DESPITE BARRIERS, SOME FAMILIES REJECT GENDER AS A JUSTIFICATION FOR INEQUALITY IN FAMILY LIFE

Although it is important to recognize that societal ideologies and structures constrain women and men, it is equally important to recognize that individuals maintain personal agency within these constraints. As people individually and collectively struggle and experiment with new ways to live, the social ideologies and practices evolve (Risman, 1998). Unfortunately, transformations in social norms occur slowly and lag behind change in individuals and families (Baber & Allen, 1992). However, in their review of research on egalitarian families, Risman and Johnson-Summerford (1998) noted that by the early 1990s, structural and ideological constraints had changed enough to allow equity-oriented men and women to negotiate egalitarian relationships. They found that, although still rare, the number of these families has grown steadily.

In their study of "fair families," Risman and Johnson-Summerford (1998) noted that these families "rejected gender as an ideological justification for inequality or even difference in the negotiation of their marital relationship. . . . The interactions of these couples appeared to be guided by rules of fairness and sharing within egalitarian friendships" (1998, pp. 38–39). Similarly, Schwartz (1994) found that the equal couples in her study could be distinguished by their dedication to fairness and collaboration in housework, parenting, and decision making. She noted as particularly striking that this equality was not emphasized by the couple for its own sake, but in the service of developing an intense companionship. In a cross-cultural study of egalitarian couples, instead of organizing relationships around power, egalitarian couples structured "empowerment" into the foundation of their relationship (Rabin, 1996). In this model, partners stand together, unlike the traditional model in heterosexual relationships, in which the woman "stands behind her man." This model fits Goodrich's (1991) description of relational empowerment as power shared with one's partner rather than power over the other.

The most salient finding common to many studies of egalitarian relationships (e.g., Haddock et al., 2001; Rabin, 1996; Schwartz, 1994) is that these partners spontaneously describe each other as their best friend. Schwartz found that equal couples prioritize their relationship above all else; they share a profound degree of intimacy, communicate often, enjoy a great deal of time together, and understand one another well. They are highly committed to each other, viewing their relationship as unique and one another as irreplaceable. A growing body of research finds that equal marital or intimate partnerships are more intimate and satisfying (e.g., DeMaris & Longmore, 1996; Feeney et al., 1994; Gottman, 1999; Keith & Schafer, 1998; Peterson, 1990; Steil, 1997; VanYperen & Buunk, 1994). Gottman found that the happiest and most stable long-term marriages were ones in which the partners shared power and mutually accepted influence from one another (see Walsh, Chapter 2, this volume). Beavers and Hampson (1990) found that optimally functioning families show less gender stereotyping, both in couple relationships and in parenting (see Greene et al., Chapter 4, this volume).

Research reveals that it is not just intimate partnerships that benefit when women and men resist compliance with gender norms. Friedman and Greenhaus (2000) conclude that satisfaction with personal growth for both genders tends to be enhanced when engaging in an aspect of life that has been undervalued in traditional gender roles: for men, investment in family; for women, investment in both career and personal interests. For instance, Gottman and Silver (1999) found that men who share power with their wives lead more fulfilling lives:

> This new type of husband and father leads a meaningful and rich life. Having a happy family base makes it possible for him to create and work effectively. Because he is so connected to his wife, she will come to him not only when she is troubled but when she is delighted. When the city awakens to a beautiful fresh snowstorm, his children will come running for him to see it. The people who matter most to him will care about him when he lives and mourn him when he dies. (p. 110)

Gottman (1997) found that these "emotionally intelligent" men also tend to be outstanding fathers. More specifically, the children of these men benefit from their father's emotional awareness and ability to model a wide range of emotions, evidenced by the children's significantly better performance in school and in relationships with others. In contrast, "an emotionally distant dad—one who is harsh, critical, or dismissive of his children's emotions—can have a deeply negative impact. His kids are more likely to do poorly in school, fight more with friends, and have poor health" (p. 26). Reviews of the literature (Coltrane, 1998; Engle, 1997) reveal that fathers who have a warm and responsive involvement with their children contribute greatly to their children's intellectual, social, and emotional development. Boys of these fathers also hold less stereotyped gender attitudes as adolescents and young adults (Hardesty, Wenk, & Morgan, 1995).

Women also benefit from equality in relationships; empirical research has found that women in equal relationships have better physical health, higher self-esteem, and more autonomy than women in unequal relationships (McGoldrick, 1989). Women suffer from less depression when they perceive household labor as shared fairly with their partner (Bird & Rogers, 1998). Additionally, the more voice women have in decision making, the less dysphoria they experience and the greater their well-being (Steil, 1997). Researchers in many countries have found that children also benefit when women have more authority in the family; women tend to spend more money on items (e.g., clothing, food) and experiences (e.g., schooling) that benefit children (Cagatay, Elson, & Grown, 1995).

ATTENDING TO GENDER IN FAMILY THERAPY

Feminist Critique of Family Therapy

Gender and power issues are at the heart of many couple and family problems, yet they have been too often ignored in clinical theories and practice (Walsh & Scheinkman, 1989). In the past 25 years, feminist scholars (e.g., Avis, 1986; Bograd, 1986; Chaney & Piercy, 1988; Goldner, 1985, 1989; Goodrich, Rampage, Ellman, & Halstead, 1988; Zimmerman & Haddock, 2001; Hare-Mustin, 1978, 1989; Luepnitz, 1988; McGoldrick et al., 1989; Prouty, 2001; Walters, Carter, Papp, & Silverstein, 1988) have challenged the field of family therapy to attend to the critical influences of gender and power in its theories, practice, and training.

Feminists have highlighted many problematic aspects of family therapy models (see Goldner, 1985; Hare-Mustin, 1978; Taggart, 1989; Walsh & Scheinkman, 1989). A primary criticism has been that family therapy models encourage neutrality or reinforcement of power differentials between men and women. These models are based on an assumption that each member of the system has equal power and influence in both the cause of problems and the development of solutions (Taggart, 1989). However, because women and men do not occupy equal positions of power in society, it is often not possible for them to influence change equally, as the notion of circular causality implies. Therapists' failure to recognize power differentials can lead to blaming the victim, as in the classic example of partner abuse: Circular causality would imply that the perpetrator and victim are equally responsible for the perpetrator's abusive behavior. Such a notion is unethical and potentially lethal (see special section on domestic violence in Volume 25 of the *Journal of Marital and Family Therapy*).

Feminists also have argued that a bias against women is evident in the field. For example, until only recently, mother blaming was prevalent throughout the mental health field, as in the assumption that schizophrenia was caused by a "schizophrenogenic mother," and that most individual difficulties in childhood or adulthood were rooted in early deficiencies in the mother–child relationship (McGoldrick et al., 1989). Early family therapy models widened the lens beyond early childhood dyadic relationships to ongoing family transactional patterns. Yet they persisted in viewing mothers negatively.

The concerns of feminist scholars have been validated by recent empirical research. Haddock and Bowling (2001) analyzed a national sample of family therapists who responded to a vignette. The dual-earner couple in the vignette was experiencing difficulties with inequitable division of labor and concerns about the effects of maternal employment on the children. Less than one-third of therapists addressed division of labor between the couple in their treatment plan. In their conceptualizations of the problem, 40% of the sample pathologized the female client (compared to 3% for the male client). In relation to the clients' concerns about maternal employment, almost 80% of the sample either failed to recognize the influence of societal myths about maternal employment or actively reinforced these myths (e.g., 10% of the sample indicated that if the couple asked them the drawbacks of dual earning for children, they would have mentioned that these children *typically* feel unloved and neglected). Also of concern was that 20% of the sample recommended that the *female* client consider changes to her work schedule as a possible solution to the couple's difficulties.

In analyses of the American Association for Marriage and Family Therapy Master Series training tapes over a 10-year period, Haddock, MacPhee, and Zimmerman (2001) and Haddock and Lyness (2001) found that even eminent therapists often reinforce traditional gender-based expectations and power differentials in therapy. A finding of particular concern in these studies was the disrespectful manner in which female clients were treated by several of the male founders of the field of marriage and family therapy. In several interactions, these therapists made inappropriate comments about women's appearance and negatively labeled their emotions. Werner-Wilson, Price, Zimmerman, and Murphy (1997) also found evidence of gender bias in the practice of therapy; they found that therapists interrupt female clients three times more frequently than they interrupt male clients, even when controlling for the amount of time each gender talks in therapy.

Gender-Aware Therapy in Practice

Clients often fail to recognize gender and power as central to their presenting problems. Yet therapists have an ethical responsibility to highlight and respectfully question how individual and relationship difficulties may be related to gender. It is therapists' responsibility to develop a framework that allows them to use a *gender lens* in conceptualizing and addressing all presenting problems, including relationship dissatisfaction, sexual dysfunction, depression, substance abuse, and eating disorders. Attention to power differentials is particularly important in situations of domestic violence; therapists must interrupt cycles of emotional and physical abuse, and confront the disrespectful and demeaning treatment of women by abusive partners (see Haddock, 2002).

As a tool to help therapists focus their attention on gender and power in family therapy, Haddock, Zimmerman, and MacPhee (2000) developed the Power Equity Guide (Appendix 12.1). Also see Haddock and Zimmerman (2001) for a handout based on the Guide, to be used with clients. The purpose of the Guide is to delineate major goals and themes that characterize a feminist-informed approach to therapy. The

Guide does not provide a set of techniques or strategies; rather, it provides therapists with a framework for organizing the therapy process, a method for translating feminist principles into specific behaviors in therapy, and a tool for tracking their progress in incorporating these principles. The Guide delineates three central goals in the practice of gender-informed therapy: (1) to empower clients to honor and integrate all aspects of themselves, especially those not supported by dominant culture; (2) to eliminate or reduce power differentials between partners; and (3) to manage the power differentials between therapist and clients.

Critical to the success of gender-aware therapy is respect for clients' values and beliefs (e.g., religion, culture), which may influence therapeutic goals related to gender and equality (Lyness, Haddock, & Zimmerman, in press). Feminist-informed practice does not prescribe a new "norm" that all couples and families should adopt; rather, it encourages flexibility and choice for each family to develop its own relationships with mutual respect and reciprocity in accord with personal and family values. Rather than imposing particular ideas about gender, it is important for therapists to take a stance of respectful curiosity, asking clients questions about their values, how these values were formed, which values they want to reinforce, and which they want to change. Such an approach by therapists avoids prescribing a "one size fits all" approach to gender and equality.

CONCLUSIONS

Gender is a powerful organizing force in families, and gender norms continue to be in transition. There are many barriers to achieving gender equality in our society, and in couples and family life. Increasingly, we are recognizing that gender-based stereotypes and inequality are damaging to family members and their relationships, and that there are clear benefits to equality in families. Therapists can serve as a bridge to equality; however, they may need first to overcome their own gender bias and consciously attend to gender and power in their work with families. As a primary goal, feminist-informed therapists must help their clients reduce the constraints of rigid gender expectations and expand the possibilities for their own growth.

REFERENCES

Almeida, R., Woods, R., Messineo, T., Font, R. J., & Heer, C. (1994). Violence in the lives of the racially and sexually different: A public and private dilemma. *Journal of Feminist Family Therapy, 5*(3/4), 99–126.

Avis, J. M. (1986). Feminist issues in family therapy. In F. Piercy & D. Sprenkle (Eds.), *Family therapy sourcebook* (pp. 213–242). New York: Guilford Press.

Baber, K. M., & Allen, K. R. (1992). *Women and families: Feminist reconstructions.* New York: Guildford Press.

Barnett, R. C., & Rivers, C. (1996). *She works, he works: How two-income families are happy, healthy, and thriving.* Cambridge, MA: Harvard University Press.

Beavers, W. R. (1985). *Successful marriage: A family systems approach to couples therapy.* New York: Norton.

Beavers, W. R., & Hampson, R. B. (1990). *Successful families: Assessment and intervention.* New York: Norton.

Belenky, M. F., Clinchy, B. M., Goldberger, N. R., & Tarule, J. M. (1986). *Women's ways of knowing: The development of self, voice, and mind.* New York: Basic Books.

Bem, S. L. (1993). *The lenses of gender: Transforming the debate on sexual inequality.* New Haven, CT: Yale University Press.

Benokraitis, N. V. (1999). *Marriages and families: Changes, choices, and constraints* (3rd ed.). Upper Saddle River, NJ: Prentice-Hall.

Bernard, J. (1982). *The future of marriage.* New Haven, CT: Yale University Press.

Bird, C. E., & Rogers, M. L. (1998). *Parenting and depression: The impact of the division of labor within couples and perceptions of equity,* PSTC Working Paper No. 98-109. Providence, RI: Brown University Population Studies and Training Center.

Blaisure, K. R., & Allen, K. R. (1995). Feminists and the ideology and practice of marital equality. *Journal of Marriage and the Family, 57,* 5–19.

Bograd, M. (1986). A feminist examination of family therapy: What is women's place? *Women and Therapy, 5,* 95–106.

Bograd, M. (1999). Strengthening domestic violence theories: Intersections of race, class, sexual orientation, and gender. *Journal of Marital and Family Therapy, 25,* 275–290.

Boss, P., & Thorne, B. (1989). Family sociology and family therapy: A feminist linkage. In M. McGoldrick, C. M. Anderson, & F. Walsh (Eds.), *Women in families: A framework for family therapy* (pp. 78–96). New York: Norton.

Botkin, D. R., Weeks, M. O., & Morris, J. E. (2000). Changing marriage role expectations: 1961–1996. *Sex Roles, 42,* 933–942.

Braverman, L. (1989). Beyond the myth of motherhood. In M. McGoldrick, C. M. Anderson, & F. Walsh (Eds.), *Women in families: A framework for family therapy* (pp. 227–243). New York: Norton.

Cagatay, N., Elson, D., & Grown, C. (1995). Gender, adjustment, and macroeconomics. *World Development, 23,* 1830–1845.

Carrington, C. (1999). *No place like home: Relationships and family life among lesbians and gay men.* Chicago: University of Chicago Press.

Carter, B. (1999). Becoming parents: The family with young children. In B. Carter & M. McGoldrick (Eds.), *The expanded family life cycle: Individual, family, and social perspectives* (3rd ed., pp. 249–273). Boston: Allyn & Bacon.

Chaney, S. E., & Piercy, F. P. (1988). A feminist family therapy behavior checklist. *American Journal of Family Therapy, 16,* 305–318.

Chodorow, N. (1989). *Feminism and psychoanalytic theory.* New Haven, CT: Yale University Press.

Chun, H., & Lee, I. (2001). Why do married men earn more: Productivity or marriage selection. *Economic Inquiry, 39,* 307–319.

Coltrane, S. (1996). *Family man: Fatherhood, housework, and gender equity.* Oxford, UK: Oxford University Press.

Coltrane, S. (1998). *Gender and families.* Thousand Oaks, CA: Pine Forge Press.

Connell, R. W. (1987). *Gender and power: Society, the person, and sexual politics.* Stanford, CA: Stanford University Press.

Coontz, S. (1992). *The way we never were: American families and the nostalgia trap.* New York: Basic Books.

Cowan, C. P., & Cowan, P. A. (2000). *When partners become parents: The big life change for couples.* Mahwah, NJ: Erlbaum.

Crosby, F. J. (1991). *Juggling: The unexpected advantages of balancing career and home for women and their families.* New York: Free Press.

Crouter, A. C., McHale, S. M., & Bartko, W. T. (1993). Gender as an organizing feature in parent–child relationships. *Journal of Social Issues, 49*(3), 161–174.

DeMaris, A., & Longmore, M. A. (1996). Ideology, power, and equity: Testing competing explanations for the perception of fairness in household labor. *Social Forces, 74,* 1043–1071.

Deutsch, F. M. (1999). *Halving it all: How equally shared parenting works.* Cambridge, MA: Harvard University Press.

Dusky, L. (1996). *Still unequal: The shameful truth about women and justice in America.* New York: Crown.

Eitzen, D. S., & Zinn, M. B. (2000). The missing safety net and families: A progressive critique of the new welfare legislation. *Journal of Sociology and Social Welfare, 27,* 53–72.

Ellman, B., & Taggart, M. (1993). Changing gender norms. In F. Walsh (Ed.), *Normal family processes* (pp. 377–404). New York: Guilford Press.

Engle, P. L. (1997). The role of men in families: Achieving gender equity and supporting children. *Gender and Development, 5*(2), 31–40.

Etaugh, C., & Liss, M. (1992). Home, school, playroom: Training grounds for adult gender roles. *Sex Roles, 26,* 129–147.

Faludi, S. (1991). *Backlash: The undeclared war against American women.* New York: Crown.

Feeney, J., Peterson, C., & Noller, P. (1994). Equity and marital satisfaction over the family life cycle. *Personal Relationships, 1,* 83–99.

Fein, E., & Schneider, S. (1995). *The rules: Time-tested secrets for capturing the heart of Mr. Right.* New York: Warner Books.

Ferber, M. A., & Young, L. (1997). Student attitudes toward roles of women and men: Is the egalitarian household imminent? *Feminist Economics, 3,* 65–83.

Ferree, M. M. (1990). Beyond separate spheres: Feminism and family research. *Journal of Marriage and the Family, 52,* 866–884.

Fleming, J. (1988). Public opinion on change in women's rights and roles. In S. Dornbusch & M. Stobber (Eds.), *Feminism, children, and the new families* (pp. 47–66). New York: Guilford Press.

Friedman, S. D., & Greehaus, J. H. (2000). *Work and family—allies or enemies?* New York: Oxford University Press.

Galinsky, E. (1999). *Ask the children: What America's children really think about working parents.* New York: Morrow.

Gilligan, C. (1982). *In a different voice: Psychological theory and women's development.* Cambridge, MA: Harvard University Press.

Goldner, V. (1985). Feminism and family therapy. *Family Process, 24,* 31–47.

Goldner, V. (1989). Generation and gender: Normative and covert hierarchies. In M. McGoldrick, C. M. Anderson, & F. Walsh (Eds.), *Women in families: A framework for family therapy* (pp. 42–60). New York: Norton.

Goodrich, T. J., Rampage, C., Ellman, B., & Halstead, K. (1988). *Feminist family therapy: A casebook.* New York: Norton.

Goodrich, T. J. (1991). *Women and power: Perspectives for family therapy.* New York: Norton.

Gottman, J. M. (1997). *Raising an emotionally intelligent child: The heart of parenting.* New York: Simon & Schuster.

Gottman, J. M. (1999). *The marriage clinic: A scientifically-based marital therapy.* New York: Norton.

Gottman, J. M., & Silver, N. (1999). *The seven principles for making marriage work.* New York: Random House.

Graham-Bermann, S., & Brescoll, V. (2000). Gender, power, and violence: Assessing the family stereotypes of the children of batterers. *Journal of Family Psychology, 14,* 600–612.

Gray, J. (1992). *Men are from Mars, women are from Venus: A practical guide for improving communication and getting what you want in your relationships.* New York: HarperCollins.

Grieshaber, S. (1998). Constructing the gender-based infant. In N. Yelland (Ed.), *Gender in early childhood* (pp. 15–35). New York: Routledge.

Haddock, S. A., & Bowling, S. (2001). Therapists' approaches to the normative challenges of dual-earner couples: Negotiating outdated societal ideologies. *Journal of Feminist Family Therapy, 13*(2/3), 91–120.

Haddock, S. A. (2002). Training family therapists to assess for and intervene in partner abuse: A curriculum for graduate courses, professional workshops, and self-study. *Journal of Marital and Family Therapy, 28,* 193–202.

Haddock, S. A., & Lyness, K. P. (2001). Three aspects of the therapeutic conversation in couple's therapy: Does gender make a difference? *Journal of Couple and Relationship Therapy, 1*(1), 3–17.

Haddock, S. A., MacPhee, D., & Zimmerman, T. S. (2001). AAMFT Master Series Tapes: An analysis of the inclusion of feminist principles into family therapy practice. *Journal of Marital and Family Therapy, 27,* 487–500.

Haddock, S. A., & Zimmerman, T. S. (2001). The Power Equity Guide: An activity to assist couples in negotiating a fair and equitable relationship. *Journal of Activities in Psychotherapy Practice, 1,* 1–16.

Haddock, S. A., Zimmerman, T. S., & MacPhee, D. (2000). The power equity guide: Attending to gender in family therapy. *Journal of Marital and Family Therapy, 26,* 153–170.

Haddock, S. A., Zimmerman, T. S., Ziemba, S., & Current, L. (2001). Ten adaptive strategies for work and family balance: Advice from successful dual earners. *Journal of Marital and Family Therapy, 27,* 445–458.

Hardesty, C., Wenk, D., & Morgan, C. S. (1995). Parental involvement and the development of gender expectations in sons and daughters. *Youth and Society, 26,* 283–297.

Hardill, I., Green, A. E., Dudleston, A. C., & Owen, D. W. (1997). Who decides what?: Decision making in dual-career households. *Work, Employment, and Society, 11,* 313–326.

Hare-Mustin, R. (1978). A feminist approach to family therapy. *Family Process, 17,* 181–194.

Hare-Mustin, R. (1989). The problem of gender in family therapy theory. In M. McGoldrick, C. M. Anderson, & F. Walsh (Eds.), *Women in families: A framework for family therapy* (pp. 61–77). New York: Norton.

Hare-Mustin, R., & Marecek, J. (1990). *Making a difference: Psychology and the construction of gender.* New Haven, CT: Yale University Press.

Hochschild, A., & Machung, A. (1989). *The second shift: Working parents and the revolution at home.* New York: Viking.

Hochschild, A. R. (1997). *The time bind.* New York: Henry Holt.

Hoffman, L. W. (1989). Effects of maternal employment in the two-parent family. *American Psychologist, 44,* 283–292.

Holcomb, B. (1998). *Not guilty: The good news about working mothers.* New York: Scribner.

Holtzman, L. (2000). *Media messages: What film, television, and popular music teach us about race, class, gender, and sexual orientation.* Armonk, NY: Sharpe.

Jordan, J. V. (Ed.). (1997). *Women's growth in diversity: More writings from the Stone Center.* New York: Guilford Press.

Jordan, J. V., Kaplan, A. G., Miller, J. B., Stiver, I. P., & Surrey, J. L. (1991). *Women's growth in connection: Writings from the Stone Center.* New York: Guilford Press.

Katz, J., & Earp, J. (1999). *Tough guise: Violence, media, and the crisis in masculinity* [VHS]. Northampton, MA: Media Education Foundation.

Keith, P. & Schafer, R. (1991). *Relationships and well-being over the life stages.* New York: Praeger.

Keith, P. M., & Schafer, R. B. (1998). Marital types and quality of life: A reexamination of a typology. *Marriage and Family Review, 27,* 19–35.

Kilbourne (2000). *Still killing us softly III.* Cambridge, MA: Cambridge Documentary Films.

Kindlon, D., & Thompson, M. (1999). *Raising Cain: Protecting the emotional life of boys.* New York: Ballentine.

Knudson-Martin, C., & Mahoney, A. R. (1998). Language and processes in the construction of equality in new marriages. *Family Relations, 47,* 81–91.

Lennon, M. C., & Rosenfeld, S. (1994). Relative fairness and the division of housework: The importance of options. *American Journal of Sociology, 100,* 506–531.

Lerner, H. (1997). *The dance of anger: A woman's guide to changing the patterns of intimate relationships.* New York: HarperCollins. (Original published in 1985)

Lindsey, E. W., Mize, J., & Pettit, G. S. (1997). Differential play patterns of mothers and fathers of sons and daughters: Implications for children's gender-role development. *Sex Roles, 37,* 643–661.

Lorber, J. (1994). *Paradoxes of gender.* New Haven, CT: Yale University Press.

Luepnitz, D. A. (1988). *The family interpreted: Feminist theory in clinical practice.* New York: Basic Books.

Lyness, K. P., Haddock, S. A., & Zimmerman, T. S. (in press). Contextual issues in marriage and family therapy: Gender, culture, and spirituality. In L. Hecker & J. Wetchler (Eds.), *An introduction to marriage and family therapy.* Binghamton, NY: Haworth.

Lytton, H., & Romney, D. M. (1991). Parents' differential socialization of boys and girls: A meta-analysis. *Psychological Bulletin, 109,* 267–296.

McGoldrick, M. (1989). Women through the family life cycle. In M. McGoldrick,

C. M. Anderson, & F. Walsh (Eds.), *Women in families: A framework for family therapy* (pp. 200–226). New York: Norton.

McGoldrick, M. (1999). Women and the family life cycle. In B. Carter & M. Mc-Goldrick (Eds.), *The expanded family life cycle: Individual, family, and social perspectives* (3rd ed., pp. 106–123). Boston: Allyn & Bacon.

McGoldrick, M., Anderson, C. M., & Walsh, F. (1989). *Women in families: A framework for family therapy.* New York: Norton.

McGoldrick, M., Broken Nose, M. A., & Potenza, M. (1999). Violence and the family life cycle. In B. Carter & M. McGoldrick (Eds.), *The expanded family life cycle: Individual, family, and social perspectives* (3rd ed., pp. 470–491). Boston: Allyn & Bacon.

McHale, S. M., Bartko, W. T., Crouter, A. C., & Perry-Jenkins, M. (1990). Children's housework and psychosocial functioning: The mediating effects of parents' sex-role behaviors and attitudes. *Child Development, 61,* 1413–1426.

McWhirter, D., Sanders, S., & Reinisch, J. M. (Eds.). (1990). *Homosexuality/heterosexuality: Concepts of sexual orientation.* New York: Oxford University Press.

Miller, J. B. (1986). *Toward a new psychology of women* (2nd ed.). Boston: Beacon Press.

Muuss, R. E. (1999). Eating disorders: Anorexia nervosa and bulimia. In R. E. Muuss & H. D. Porton (Eds.), *Adolescent behavior and society: A book of readings* (pp. 396–408). Boston, MA: McGraw-Hill.

O'Connell, M. (1993). *Where's Papa: Fathers' role in child care.* (Population Trends and Public Policy No. 20). Washington, DC: Population Reference Bureau.

Papp, P. (2000). Gender differences in depression: His or her depression. In P. Papp (Ed.), *Couples on the fault line: New directions for therapists* (pp. 132–153). New York: Guilford Press.

Parke, R. D. (1996). *Fatherhood.* Cambridge, MA: Harvard University Press.

Parsons, T., & Bales, R. (1955). *Family socialization and interaction process.* Glencoe, IL: Free Press.

Peterson, C. C. (1990). Husbands' and wives' perceptions of marital fairness across the family life cycle. *International Journal of Aging and Human Development, 31,* 179–188.

Pipher, M. (1994). *Reviving Ophelia: Saving the selves of adolescent girls.* New York: Ballantine.

Prouty, A. (2001). Experiencing feminist family therapy supervision. *Journal of Feminist Family Therapy, 12*(4), 171–204.

Rabin, C. (1996). *Equal partners, good friends: Empowering couples through therapy.* London: Routledge.

Rennison, C. M., & Welchans, S. (2000, May). *Intimate partner violence.* Bureau of Justice Statistics Special Report. Washington, DC: U.S. Department of Justice, Office of Justice Programs.

Renzetti, C. M. (1997). Violence and abuse among same-sex couples. In A. Cascarelli (Ed.), *Violence between intimate partners: Patterns, causes, and effects* (pp. 70–89). Boston: Allyn & Bacon.

Risman, B. J. (1986). Can men "mother"?: Life as a single father. *Family Relations, 35,* 95–102.

Risman, B. J. (1998). *Gender vertigo: American families in transition.* New Haven, CT: Yale University Press.

Risman, B. J., & Johnson-Summerford, D. (1998). Doing it fairly: A study of post-gender marriages. *Journal of Marriage and the Family, 60,* 23–40.

Rosen, E. J. (1999). Men in transition: The "new man. " In B. Carter & M. Mc-Goldrick (Eds.), *The expanded family life cycle: Individual, family, and social perspectives* (3rd ed., pp. 124–140). Boston: Allyn & Bacon.

Rosenbluth, S. C., Steil, J. M., & Whitcomb, J. H. (1998). Marital equality: What does it mean? *Journal of Family Issues, 19*(3), 227–244.

Sandnabba, N. K., & Ahlberg, C. (1999). Parents' attitudes and expectations about children's cross-gender behavior. *Sex Roles, 40,* 249–263.

Schwartz, P. (1994). *Love between equals: How peer marriage really works.* New York: Free Press.

Silverstein, L. (1996). Fathering is a feminist issue. *Psychology of Women Quarterly, 20,* 3–37.

Skolnick, A. (1991). *Embattled paradise.* New York: Basic Books.

Steil, J. M. (1997). *Marital equality: Its relationship to well-being of husbands and wives.* Thousand Oaks, CA: Sage.

Steil, J. M., & Weltman, K. (1991). Marital inequality: The importance of resources, personal attributes, and social norms on career valuing and domestic influence. *Sex Roles, 24,* 161–179.

Taggart, M. (1989). Epistemological equality as the fulfillment of family therapy. In M. McGoldrick, C. M. Anderson, & F. Walsh (Eds.), *Women in families: A framework for family therapy* (pp. 97–116). New York: Norton.

U.S. Bureau of the Census. (2001). *Little progress on closing wage gap in 2000* (Current Population Survey). Washington, DC: U.S. Government Printing Office.

VanYperen, N. W., & Buunk, B. P. (1994). Social comparison and social exchange in marital relationships. In M. J. Lerner & G. Mikula (Eds.), *Entitlement and the affectional bond: Justice in close relationships* (pp. 89–115). New York: Plenum Press.

Walsh, F. (1989). Reconsidering gender in the marital quid pro quo. In M. McGoldrick, & C. M. Anderson (Eds.), *Women in families: A framework for family therapy* (pp. 267–285). New York: Norton.

Walsh, F. (1998). *Strengthening family resilience.* New York: Guilford Press.

Walsh, F. (1999). Families in later life: Challenges and opportunities. In B. Carter & M. McGoldrick (Eds.), *The expanded family life cycle: Individual, family, and social perspectives* (3rd ed., pp. 307–326). Boston: Allyn & Bacon.

Walsh, F., & Scheinkman, M. (1989). (Fe)male: The hidden gender dimension in models of family therapy. In M. McGoldrick, & C. M. Anderson (Eds.), *Women in families: A framework for family therapy* (pp. 479–520). New York: Norton.

Walters, M., Carter, B., Papp, P., & Silverstein, O. (1988). *The invisible web: Gender patterns in family relationships.* New York: Guilford Press.

Werner-Wilson, R., Price, S., Zimmerman, T. S., & Murphy, M. (1997). Client gender as a process variable in marriage and family therapy: Are women clients interrupted more than men clients? *Journal of Family Psychology, 11,* 373–377.

West, C., & Zimmerman, D. (1987). Doing gender. *Gender and Society, 1,* 125–151.

Williams, J. (2000). *Unbending gender: Why family and work conflict and what to do about it.* New York: Oxford University Press.

Zimmerman, T. S., & Haddock, S. A. (2000). The weave of gender and culture in the tapestry of a MFT training program: Promoting social justice in the practice of family therapy. *Journal of Feminist Family Therapy, 12*(2/3), 1–32. Reprinted in T. S. Zimmerman (Ed.), *Integrating Gender and Culture in Family Therapy Training* (pp. 1–32). Binghamton, NY: Haworth Press.

Zimmerman, T. S., Haddock, S. A., & McGeorge, C. (2001). Mars and Venus: Unequal planets. *Journal of Marital and Family Therapy, 27,* 55–68.

Zimmerman, T. S., Haddock, S. A., Ziemba, S., & Rust, A. (2001). Family organizational labor: Who's calling the plays? *Journal of Feminist Family Therapy, 13*(2/3), 65–90.

Zimmerman, T. S., Holm, K., & Haddock, S. A. (2001). A decade of advice for women and men in the best-selling self-help literature. *Family Relations, 50,* 122–133.

Zvonkovic, A., Greaves, K., Schmeige, C., & Hall, L. (1996). The marital construction of gender through work and family decisions. *Journal of Marriage and the Family, 58,* 91–100.

APPENDIX 12.1
THE POWER EQUITY GUIDE: ATTENDING
TO GENDER IN FAMILY THERAPY

Feminist-Informed Family Therapy

Feminist-informed family therapy is based on several principles, including the following:

* Gender, as an organizing principle of society, has been and continues to be the basis for:
    * the inequality and oppression of women,
    * power differentials between men and women,
    * assignment of certain traits and expectations (i.e., gender identity formation).
* Interpersonal and family interactions should be conceptualized in this larger societal context, and therefore gender is also understood as an organizing principle of family life.
* Gender intersects with other primary dimensions of social life, including race, class, and sexual orientation that influence interpersonal and family interactions.
* Interactions and identity formations emerging from this societal context are often detrimental to individual, relationship, and family well-being;
* The goal of therapy involves assisting clients to:
    * understand, critically examine, and effectively negotiate gender-based constraints and other oppressions, thereby increasing their sense of options and personal agency, and
    * develop egalitarian relationships characterized by mutuality, reciprocity, intimacy, and interdependency.

Uses of the Power Equity Guide

The Guide reminds the user of the many areas in which the above principles are relevant to family life. It is a training, therapy, and research tool that can be used in the following ways.

Summarizing: The Guide summarizes key goals and themes that characterize a gender-informed approach to therapy. Its straightforward design makes this therapeutic approach more understandable and manageable, and provides a common language to facilitate discussion.

Treatment Planning: The Guide assists therapists in generating specific interventions that are consistent with a feminist approach. It is useful for therapists at all developmental levels who wish to incorporate feminist principles into their practice. It can also be used in therapy to facilitate conversations with clients and set personal and relationship goals.

Evaluating: The Guide provides supervisors and researchers with an effective means for evaluating the practice of gender-informed family therapy.

Directions for Specific Uses
- **For training:** The Guide can be used to introduce the basic principles of gender-informed family therapy. Further, students can use the Guide to brainstorm various interventions; to examine power and gender dynamics in their families, relationships, or society; or to analyze live or video therapy sessions.
- **For therapy:** The Guide can be used for treatment planning and to track progress in incorporating these principles into the therapeutic process. In the spaces provided, therapists can write specific strategies for assessing and intervening in each relevant area to accomplish the respective goal. Upon termination of the case, therapists can assess their success in incorporating relevant feminist principles. Therapists can use the Guide with clients to facilitate conversation, assess relationship dynamics, and set goals.
- **For supervision:** Supervisors can use the Guide to assist supervisees with treatment planning, offering specific strategies for assessing and intervening in relevant areas to accomplish the respective goals. During live or video supervision, supervisors can use the Guide to organize and present feedback to supervisees regarding their effectiveness in incorporating feminist principles.
- **For research:** Researchers can use the Guide to further develop an empirical base for feminist-informed family therapy. For instance, the Guide can be used to conduct outcome or process research, and to measure the effectiveness of various training methods.

Important Note
In the practice of gender-informed family therapy, therapists are proactive in addressing feminist principles. When therapists remain neutral or silent about power differentials or inequality, they are communicating support of such arrangements. However, it is also important for therapists to respect clients' choices and values with regard to gender, tailoring therapy to their needs, personal and cultural values, and goals. Additionally, it is not necessary or realistic to address all areas highlighted by the Guide in any one therapy session, or even one case. Rather, we recommend a systematic, thoughtful approach to addressing client concerns from a feminist standpoint, using the principles as a guide. And, finally, as each couple is unique, it is not the expectation that a couple would necessarily achieve equality in each area. For instance, one partner may take more responsibility for child care and another for household labor.

With sensitivity to the influence of the societal context on individuals and relationships, attempt to understand, accomplish, or evaluate the following gender-informed family therapy goals as they are addressed throughout the therapeutic process.

	Inattentive to Gender/ Power	Attentive to Gender/ Power

Goal 1: Eliminate or reduce power differentials between clients and their partners.

Decision-making: Encourage shared decision-making power between partners regarding various aspects of life (e.g., entertainment, vacations, living environment).
Comments:

1 2 3 4 5 N/A

Communication and Conflict Resolution: Encourage respectful and collaborative communication and conflict resolution between partners.
Comments:

1 2 3 4 5 N/A

Work, Life Goals, and/or Activities: Encourage partners to grant equal value to other's career, work, life goals, and/or activities.
Comments:

1 2 3 4 5 N/A

Housework: Encourage an equitable distribution of labor within the context of the couple's work/family arrangement (e.g., dual-income or breadwinner/homemaker).
Comments:

1 2 3 4 5 N/A

Finances: Encourage shared knowledge of financial information and decision-making power.
Comments:

1 2 3 4 5 N/A

Sex: Encourage a mutual, consensual sexual relationship based on intimacy.
Comments:

1 2 3 4 5 N/A

	Inattentive to Gender/ Power		Attentive to Gender/ Power			

Relationship Maintenance: Encourage both partners to take responsibility for the quality of their relationships with one another, children, family, and friends.
Comments:

Rating: 1 2 3 4 5 N/A

Relationship Characteristics: With attention to both larger relationship patterns and the ways these patterns are reflected in the intricacies of daily interaction,

(a) Promote relationships characterized by mutuality, reciprocity, and interdependence, and by a balance between intimacy and autonomy.
Comments:

Rating: 1 2 3 4 5 N/A

(b) Take a strong stance against behaviors intended to control (e.g., through intimidation, manipulation, or coercion) another's actions, time, and relationships.
Comments:

Rating: 1 2 3 4 5 N/A

Abuse and Violence: Proactively assess for and take a strong stance against violent or abusive behaviors. Attend to safety issues.
Comments:

Rating: 1 2 3 4 5 N/A

Relationship Separation or Divorce:

(a) Communicate that personal well-being need not be jeopardized by an intimate relationship. When deemed appropriate, encourage clients to consider the option of ending a relationship.
Comments:

Rating: 1 2 3 4 5 N/A

(b) Attend to ways that separation/divorce often differentially affect women; support equitable financial arrangements between and continued parental involvement by both partners.
Comments:

Rating: 1 2 3 4 5 N/A

	Inattentive to Gender/ Power			Attentive to Gender/ Power		
Parental Responsibility: Encourage both parents to share responsibility for and equally participate in parenting with consideration to the couple's work/family arrangement. Avoid mother-blaming. **Comments:**	1	2	3	4	5	N/A

Parenting style: Assist parents to:

(a) Manage their power effectively by incorporating feminist principles into their parenting style (e.g., listen to children's ideas, give children choices, involve children in decision making as appropriate). **Comments:**	1	2	3	4	5	N/A
(b) Eliminate power differentials between siblings (e.g., divide household chores equitably and in a gender-neutral fashion, intervene in sibling rivalry). **Comments:**	1	2	3	4	5	N/A

Goal 2: Empower clients to honor and integrate all aspects of themselves, including those not supported by dominant culture.

Female Clients: Encourage female clients to:

(a) Cultivate their capacity to be more attentive to self-care; to be more assertive and independent; to pursue personal time, space, and interests; to pursue their own goals and desires; and to develop a social support system **Comments:**	1	2	3	4	5	N/A
(b) Explore nontraditional life/career choices and resist societal pressures to conform to or value themselves according to gender-based expectations (i.e., defining self only in terms of wife and mother, choosing service-oriented professions, valuing themselves according to their appearance) while supporting and encouraging choices they consciously make that are traditional. **Comments:**	1	2	3	4	5	N/A

	Inattentive to Gender/ Power			Attentive to Gender/ Power		

(c) Explore and respond to the influence of oppression on themselves and their relationships and negotiate and manage problematic situations due to sexism.

1 2 3 4 5 N/A

Comments:

Male Clients: Encourage male clients to:

(a) Cultivate their capacity to be more attentive to relationship maintenance; to be more emotionally expressive and available; to be more vulnerable with their partner, children, and appropriate others; and to develop a support system that ideally includes men.

1 2 3 4 5 N/A

Comments:

(b) Explore nontraditional life/career choices and resist societal pressures to conform to or value themselves according to gender-based expectations (i.e., defining self only in terms of career, valuing themselves according to their earning potential).

1 2 3 4 5 N/A

Comments:

(c) Encourage male clients to become aware of their privileged social position and assist them in exploring how this privileged status may influence them and their relationships.

1 2 3 4 5 N/A

Comments:

Children:

(a) Empower (and help parents empower) children to resist constricting gender-based expectations (i.e., boys don't cry, girls only play with dolls, etc.)

1 2 3 4 5 N/A

Comments:

	Inattentive to Gender/ Power	Attentive to Gender/ Power

(b) Be conscious of (and help parents be conscious of) messages given to children regarding the social constructions of gender, race, class, sexual orientation, and disability. Encourage (and help parents encourage) children to think critically about these social constructions (e.g., why women and other marginalized groups are under-represented, such as in government positions, as main characters in books, and in some historical accounts).　　　**1　2　3　4　5　N/A**
Comments:

Marginalized Clients: Encourage clients of marginalized status to explore and respond to the influence of oppression on themselves, their lives, their relationships, and the presenting problem. Assist them to negotiate and manage problematic situations due to racism, classism, homophobia, and other oppressions.　　　**1　2　3　4　5　N/A**
Comments:

Majority Clients: Encourage clients of majority status to become aware of their privileged social position, assisting them in exploring how this privileged status may influence them, their relationships, and the presenting problem.　　　**1　2　3　4　5　N/A**
Comments:

Goal 3: Manage the power differential between therapist and client.

Goal-setting: Collaboratively set goals and attend to the goals of all clients.　　　**1　2　3　4　5　N/A**
Comments:

Stance: Maintain a collaborative versus an expert stance.　　　**1　2　3　4　5　N/A**
Comments:

	Inattentive to Gender/ Power		Attentive to Gender/ Power			

Disclosure of gender-based values: Disclose own   1   2   3   4   5   N/A
gender-based values and beliefs (i.e., inform clients of
your belief that it is important to understand problems
in social context).
Comments:

Disclosure of other relevant values: When relevant,   1   2   3   4   5   N/A
disclose personal values related to controversial topics,
relationships, or decisions (i.e., abortion, homosexuality,
divorce, etc.) and refer when personal values may
impede the therapeutic process.
Comments:

Inclusion of all family members, including children: 1   2   3   4   5   N/A
Appropriately balance time and attention to all clients.
Include children in sessions in developmentally
appropriate ways.
Comments:

Self of the therapist: Demonstrate comfort with   1   2   3   4   5   N/A
instrumental and expressive behaviors, role modeling
a person who has loosened gender-socialized constraints
(i.e., display competence and authority as well as
empathy and nurturance).
Comments:

**Attention to stereotypes, prejudices, and socially based
power differentials:** Be aware of:
  (a) Power differentials in the therapeutic relationship 1   2   3   4   5   N/A
       based on gender, race, class and/or sexual
       orientation (i.e., differences in race and class of
       therapist and client);
       Comments:

  (b) Stereotypes and assumptions that may lead to   1   2   3   4   5   N/A
       negative judgments based on gender, race, class,
       sexual orientation, or disability.
       Comments:

	Inattentive to Gender/ Power			Attentive to Gender/ Power		
Demonstrate acceptance of various family forms: Affirm the "normalcy" and strengths of various family forms (e.g., single-parent, gay or lesbian, dual-earner, breadwinner/homemaker, and step-families). **Comments:**	1	2	3	4	5	N/A
Evaluation process: Implement evaluation process of therapist, encourage client feedback, and accept and address feedback with a non-defensive stance. **Comments:**	1	2	3	4	5	N/A
Communicate respect: Avoid labeling, pathologizing, and/or interrupting clients, etc. **Comments:**	1	2	3	4	5	N/A
Boundaries: Communicate care and commitment while maintaining clear and appropriate boundaries. **Comments:**	1	2	3	4	5	N/A

CHAPTER 13

THE SPIRITUAL DIMENSION OF FAMILY LIFE

Froma Walsh
Julia Pryce

O ver the centuries and across cultures, spiritual beliefs and practices have anchored and nourished families and their communities. Families have lit candles, prayed together, meditated, and quietly turned to faith for solace, strength, and connectedness in their lives. At times of crisis and adversity, spiritual beliefs and practices have fostered recovery from trauma, loss, and suffering. Today, the vast majority of families adopt some form of expression for their spirituality. Yet mental health professionals and social scientists have tended to neglect this vital dimension in their understanding of family functioning and in the treatment of distress. This chapter briefly examines the growing importance and diversity of religion and spirituality for families and considers their influence in family coping and resilience.

Spirituality is not simply a special topic, although some families may have particular spiritual concerns. Rather, like culture and ethnicity, it involves streams of experience that flow through all aspects of life, from family heritage to personal belief systems, rituals and practices, and shared faith communities. Spiritual beliefs influence ways of dealing with adversity, the experience of pain and suffering, and the meaning of symptoms. They also influence how people communicate about their pain; their beliefs about its causes and future course, their attitudes toward helpers—clergy, physicians, therapists, faith healers, the treatments they seek, and

Revised from Chapters 1 and 2 in Froma Walsh (Ed.). (1999). *Spiritual resources in family therapy*. New York: Guilford Press.

their preferred pathways to recovery. Many who seek help for physical, emotional, or interpersonal problems are also in spiritual distress. It is therefore important for clinicians and researchers to attend to the spiritual practices and beliefs of families as a source of understanding, as well as a potential contribution to family healing and growth.

RELIGION AND SPIRITUALITY IN A CHANGING WORLD

At the dawn of the 21st century there has been a resurging interest in religion and spirituality as people have sought greater meaning, harmony, and connection in their lives. Over recent decades, families worldwide have experienced tumultuous social and economic dislocations, generating widespread spiritual malaise (Lerner, 1994). As the world changes at an accelerated pace, daily lives may seem on the brink of chaos. Harried, fragmented schedules undermine a sense of identity, well-being, and purpose (Hochschild, 1997). Poverty and lack of hope for future possibilities can generate despair—literally, loss of spirit (Aponte, 1994). Among the affluent, the accumulation of material goods fails to provide fulfillment. The saturation of media images of sex and violence leaves a hunger for substance and moral integrity. Besieged parents are unsure how to raise their children well in a hazardous world, and how to counter destructive pressures of popular culture (Pipher, 1997). The ethos of the "rugged individual" and decades of self-orientation contribute to the breakdown of communities and the fraying of our social fabric, accompanied by a widespread sense of isolation, powerlessness, and despair (Bellah, Madsen, Sullivan, Swidler, & Tipton, 1985). Many feel adrift on their own fragile life rafts in a turbulent sea (Lifton, 1993).

Amid such changes, marriage and family life have become more challenging over recent decades. With the growing diversity of family forms and cultural values, changing gender roles, and varied life-cycle course, no single model fits all. Instead, families need to reinvent themselves, many times over, to fit the demands of our times (Walsh, 1998a; see Chapter 1, this volume). Disruption and confusion accompany changes in the structure of family relationships as members redefine their values, practices, and living arrangements.

As baby boomers age and grapple with their own mortality and the death of loved ones, there is a growing impetus to explore the meaning of life and the mystery of a spiritual afterlife. The AIDS epidemic heightened consciousness of life and death issues. The rise of terrorism has shattered American illusions of invulnerability. With the attacks of 9/11 many were jolted into awareness of the precariousness of life and the interconnections of all people on our planet. In the aftermath, people turned, above all else, to their loved ones and to their faith for meaning, support, and strength in facing an uncertain future.

It may be an illusion that life was ever more secure in earlier times as seen through the rose-colored lens of nostalgia (Walsh & McGoldrick, 1991). Yet many are alarmed by a seeming collapse of universal moral values in the relativism of our postmodern era (Browning, Miller-McLemore, Couture, Lyon, & Franklin, 2001). The rise in religious fundamentalism in many parts of the world can be seen as one expression of a need to return to traditions that provide clear structure, pure values, and absolute certainties in the face of rapid social change. Buffeted by societal and global forces seemingly beyond control or comprehension, many feel a yearning for inner peace, for a sense of wholeness and coherence in fragmented lives, and for more meaningful connection with others beyond the self.

DEFINING RELIGION AND SPIRITUALITY

As we consider the concepts of religion and spirituality in contemporary families, it is important to clarify our understanding of these terms, which are often used interchangeably. Wright, Watson, and Bell (1996) offer some useful distinctions between religion, as extrinsic, organized systems, and spirituality, as more intrinsic personal beliefs and practices.

Religion: Organized Belief System and Affiliation

"Religion" can be defined as an organized belief system that includes shared, and usually institutionalized, moral values, beliefs about God or a Higher Power, and involvement in a faith community. Religions provide standards and prescriptions for individual virtue and family life grounded in core beliefs. Particular ideas and practices are often unquestioned, accepted as right or true. Congregational affiliation provides social and health benefits, as well as support in times of crisis.

Rituals and ceremonies offer participants a sense of collective self. In all religions, the family is central in rites that mark the birth of a new member, entry into the adult community, marriage vows, and the death of a loved one. For instance, the practice of Judaism is centered on the family observance of rituals, from weekly Shabbat candle lighting to the major holidays in the Jewish calendar year and rites of passage across the life cycle. Each ritual is significant, connecting family members with their larger community and its history, their covenant with God, and their survival over adversity.

Spirituality: Transcendent Beliefs and Practices

Spirituality, an overarching construct, refers more generally to transcendent beliefs and practices. Spirituality can be experienced either within or outside formal religious structures and is both broader and more personal. A simple, yet profound definition of spirituality is "that which connects one to all there is" (Griffith & Griffith, 2001). Spirituality involves an active investment in an internal set of values and fosters a sense of meaning, wholeness, harmony, and connection with others (Stander, Piercy, Mackinnon, & Helmeke, 1994). One's spirituality may involve belief in a supreme being, a striving toward an ultimate human condition, or a unity with all life, nature, and the universe (Wright et al., 1996). Spiritual resources might range from secular humanistic principles to congregational affiliations to personal practices of meditation or traditional faith-healing rituals. It may include numinous experiences that are holy or mystical. Spiritual and religious belief systems provide faith explanations of past history and present experiences; for many, they predict the future and offer pathways toward understanding the ultimate meanings of life and existence (Campbell & Moyers, 1988).

Spirituality invites an expansion of consciousness, along with personal responsibility for and beyond oneself, from local to global concerns. A child's growing moral awareness evolves out of spiritual belief systems (Coles, 1990, 1997). Morality involves the activity of informed conscience: judging right and wrong based on principles of fairness, decency, and compassion (Doherty, 1995, 1999). Moral or ethical values spur actions beyond repair to improve conditions, to respond to the suffering of others, to dedicate efforts to help others, and to alleviate injustice (Perry & Rolland, 1999). At their best, ethical values promote humanity.

Universally, the spirit is seen as our vital essence, the source of life and power. In many languages the word for "spirit" and "breath" are the same: in Greek, *pneuma;* in Hebrew, *reach;* in Latin, *spiritus* (Weil, 1994). Similarly, the soul has been seen over the ages as the source of human genuineness, depth, joy, sorrow, and mystery. Herbert Anderson (1994; 1999), a leading theological educator on marriage and the family, defines the "soul" as something like the visualizing center of life, the quality of living with ourselves and others. We can only glimpse it in part and cannot penetrate its essence. Taking a double view, Anderson describes soul as everywhere but nowhere, in every cell of the body and also capable of self-transcendence. Thus, we are both soul-filled bodies and embodied souls. As Thomas Moore (1992) affirms, "It takes a broad vision to know that a piece of sky and a chunk of the earth lie lodged in the heart of every human being, and if we are to care for that heart we will have to know the sky and earth as well as human behavior" (p. 20). Such perspectives are strikingly akin to Native American spirituality (Deloria, 1994).

Some regard the "loss of soul" as a primary source of the maladies of our times, afflicting individuals and society. Moore (1992) asserts: "When soul is neglected . . . it appears symptomatically in obsessions, addictions, violence, and loss of meaning" (p. xi). The temptation is to isolate these symptoms or try to eradicate them one by one; but the root problem is the loss of wisdom about the soul, resulting in a deficit of human spirit. Someone in despair is referred to as a "lost soul," lacking purpose or community, struggling to survive. Much of the suffering that is given pathological labels in therapeutic settings may also be understood as maladies of the soul, yearnings for meaning and connection.

Tending to the soul involves purposeful activity and restful replenishing. When lost in a multitude of activities and petty concerns, the soul is endangered. Soul also involves vulnerability and uncertainty; as humans, all are susceptible to being wounded. The soul is nourished by living without pretense or armor, approaching all experience with openness, courage, and compassion.

SPIRITUAL BELIEFS AND PRACTICES: GROWING IMPORTANCE AND DIVERSITY

The United States is one of the most religious nations in the industrialized world in the level of attested spiritual beliefs and practices. Since 1939, Gallup surveys have been polling Americans about their spiritual/religious beliefs and affiliations.[1] Religious interest and church attendance surged after World War II, through the 1950s, with televised evangelists reaching into family homes. Religious involvement declined somewhat from the late 1960s through the 1980s, but found renewed vitality in the 1990s, in an expanding landscape of faiths. Today, 85% of all adults say religion is important in their lives; nearly 60% consider it very important, and one-third view it as the most important part of their lives (Princeton Religion Research Center; Gallup, 1996; Gallup & Lindsey, 1999).

Intertwining of Spirituality and Family Functioning

Spirituality and family life are deeply intertwined (Burton, 1992; D'Antonio, Newman, & Wright, 1982). Family process research has found that transcendent spiritual beliefs and practices are key ingredients in healthy family functioning (Beavers & Hampson, 1990, Chapter 20, this volume; Stinnett & DeFrain, 1985). A system of values and shared beliefs that transcend the limits of their experience and knowledge enables family members to better accept the inevitable risks and losses in living and loving fully. Gallup surveys (Gallup & Lindsey, 1999) consistently support these findings: Nearly 75% report that their family relationships have been strengthened by religion in the home. Over 80% say that religion was important in their family of origin, when they were growing up. Notably, these people were also significantly more likely to report that religion greatly strengthens current family relationships.

Family Values

Family values have become a hotly debated topic in political discourse. Some conservatives have asserted that the changing family forms and gender roles over recent decades have led to the demise of the family and the decay of "family values." In an era of growing family diversity and a rich variety of kinship patterns, it is crucial to move beyond the myth that one model of the family is the paragon of virtue for all to emulate and that others are inherently damaging (Stacey, 1996; see Walsh, Chapter 1, this volume). Family form has been confused with family substance: Family processes and community connections that strengthen the quality of relationships are most crucial for families and their members to thrive (Walsh, 1998a).

All families have values—even those who have difficulty in their consistent practice. Some contemporary family values break with cultural and religious traditions, as in the conviction that men and women should be equal partners in marriage and family life (see Haddock, Zimmerman, & Lyness, Ch. 12, this volume). Yet most families uphold values that maintain continuity with the past in terms of commitment, personal responsibility, and the strong desire to raise children to be healthy and have a good life (Doherty, 1999). In recent surveys (Gallup, 1996), "family ties, loyalty, and traditions" were ranked as the main factors thought to strengthen the family. Next, were "moral and spiritual values based on the Bible," which far outranked "family counseling," "parent training classes," and "government laws and policies."

Spirituality across the Family Life Cycle

Spirituality involves dynamic processes that ebb and flow, and change in meaning over the life course and across the generations (Worthington, 1989). In the family life cycle, marriage often brings religious considerations to the fore. Conflict may arise over the wedding itself, such as whether to have a religious or civil ceremony. Even partners of the same faith may differ in their particular sect or degree of observance and preferences for clergy and marital vows. Families of origin may exert pressures for wedding plans in line with their own convictions, often fueling intergenerational conflict and in-law triangles that can reverberate over the years. The desire for a religious commitment ceremony by gay and lesbian couples may be met with family or congregational disapproval (see Laird, Chapter 7, this volume).

Interfaith marriage can complicate the issues couples ordinarily bring to any relationship (Falicov, 1995; see McGoldrick, Chapter 9, this volume). Under stress, tolerance for differences can erode, particularly if one way is believed to be right and morally superior, with the other viewed as wrong or even immoral. It can matter a great deal whether both families of origin approve of the marriage and attend the wedding. In some cases, the choice of a spouse from a different religious background may express rebellion against parental values and authority (Friedman, 1985). Family acceptance or disapproval can have long-lasting ramifications for the success or failure of the marriage and for intergenerational relations.

Remarriage can also pose unexpected dilemmas. For orthodox Jews, a woman wishing to remarry after divorce must obtain a "get," or written permission from her ex-spouse, although a man wanting to remarry is not expected to do so (Rosen & Weltman, 1996). The Catholic Church allows divorce but only sanctions remarriage in cases of annulment. This strict ruling has led many Catholics to leave the church at remarriage. Other couples may decide to live together without legal remarriage or religious rites. Desire to remarry has also led a growing number of Catholics to petition the church for annulment of a former marriage. Such annulments are commonly granted, especially to influential men, even after a long marriage and over objections of a wife and children, who may be deeply wounded that an annulment invalidates their prior family life and legitimacy. It is crucial to explore such potentially painful and conflict-laden religious issues in working clinically with separated, divorced, and remarried families, and with co-habiting couples.

The vast majority of parents want their children to have religious training (Gallup & Lindsey, 1999). In interfaith marriages, differences that initially attracted partners may over time become contentious in raising children. Couples who may have viewed religion as unimportant in their lives may later find that one or both partners care deeply about the religious upbringing of their children. Conflicts may arise over decisions about rituals such as christening, baptism, or bar/bat mitzvah. Here again, the older generation, now as grandparents, may make their religious preferences strongly known. Previous acceptance of their children's choice of a nontraditional wedding or an interfaith marriage may shift when they consider the moral development and religious identification of their grandchildren. This is an especially agonizing issue in the Jewish community, with high rates of interfaith marriage in recent decades. Studies suggest that if the gentile partner converts to Judaism, children are more likely to grow up with a Jewish identity and practice the faith.

Most teenagers say it is important for parents and younger children to attend services together (Gallup, 1996). Sometimes it is the children who draw parents back to religious roots. It may surprise some that 95% of teenagers report that they believe in God, and nearly 50% claim they went to church or synagogue in the past week. Three in four say they pray when alone. Over 60% report a great deal of interest in discussing the existence of God; over 50% express interest in discussing life's meaning and how to make moral decisions (Gallup, 1996). Like their parents, over 80% of teenagers follow Judeo-Christian faiths. Only 9% state no religious preference.

Young adults, particularly those in college, often distance from their religious upbringing (Elkind, 1971). Of note, 15% of college freshmen report no religious preference (Gallup, 1996). Some young adults simply become less involved and lose faith, whereas others more actively question their religion or cut off altogether from their family's traditions. Many explore other religions or nontraditional ways of experiencing spirituality. A family member who chooses to convert or "marry out" may be seeking to rebalance the family's ethnic or religious orientation, moving away from some values and toward others. In some cases, this may express an attempt to separate and differentiate from one's family of origin (Friedman, 1985). Parents may experience such a choice as a rejection of them. Indeed, some young adults may wish to cut off from religious or parental upbringing that was experienced as oppressive. More often, though, it is simply a natural attraction between two individuals of diverse backgrounds in an increasingly multicultural society.

Middle to later life is a time of growing saliency of spiritual values as family members grapple with questions about the meaning of life, deal with the deaths of parents and other loved ones, and begin to face their own mortality (Erikson, Erikson, & Kivnick, 1986). Over half of all adults expect religion to become increasingly important to them as they age. Surveys find that active congregational participation and prayer tend to increase over adulthood. Whereas only 35% of young adults aged 18–29 attend their place of worship weekly, 41% of persons aged 30–49, 46% of those aged 50–64, and 56% of those over 65 attend weekly. The wisdom of elders is surely deepened by their growing spirituality (Walsh, 1998c).

Growing Religious Pluralism

The principle of respect and tolerance for religious differences was a core value in the founding of the United States (Gaustad, 1966). Although predominantly Christian through the mid- 20th century (Greeley, 1969), the population has grown increasingly diverse in spiritual beliefs and practices in recent decades. The religious landscape has changed dramatically as people seek spiritual expression and connection in varied ways.

Over 90% of Americans identify with a specific religion. The country remains primarily Christian (84%), and largely Protestant (58%), although membership has been shifting from mainline to Baptist and other evangelical denominations (Gallup & Lindsey, 1999). Twenty-six percent of Americans are Roman Catholic. Additionally, 1% are Mormon (Church of the Latter-Day Saints), and 1% are Eastern Orthodox (such as Greek or Russian).

Many denominations are hard to distinguish; terms such as "fundamentalist," "evangelical," and "charismatic" are blurred, overlapping, and in flux. Nearly 20% of adults think of themselves as belonging to the religious Right (Gallup, 1996), with the highest identification for women,

Southerners, blacks, seniors, and those who did not attend college. This is actually a heterogeneous group. For some, the "Christian Right" is a broad based interracial, interfaith coalition combining fundamentalist visions of religion with politically and socially conservative agendas. Yet among those who consider themselves "born again" or evangelical Christians (18%), only one-third hold conservative social and political ideologies and identify with the religious Right. Therefore, it is important to clarify each family's beliefs without making assumptions.

The non-Christian proportion of the U.S. population has been rising rapidly: from 3.6% in 1900, to 9.9% in 1970, to 14.6% by 1995 (Gallup, 1996). Two percent of Americans identify as Jewish (down from 5% in the1950s but stable since 1972). Five percent follow other religions— Islam, Hinduism, and Buddhism, each currently at 1%, are growing rapidly. (Worldwide, Muslims will soon outnumber Christians.) Still others identify with such faiths as Sikh, Bahaii, Shintoism, and Taoism. A strong revival of Native American spiritual heritage has occurred. Some are drawn to mysticism from varying religious traditions. The New Age movement blends a range of approaches for people whose spiritual needs have not been met by conventional religions.

Some are drawn to religious cults, cutting off from their families and communities to live communally and follow the ideology of a charismatic leader, who may be seen as a prophet (Galanter, 1989). Anguished families may seek help to recover and "deprogram" a family member lost to such groups. The turn of the millennium saw an upsurge in apocalyptic prophecies of the end of the world, "doomsday cults," and survivalist communes. Religious extremist groups, although small in number, have posed a growing threat of violence. Although Muslim fundamentalist terrorists view themselves as adherents of Islam, the Koran does not condone the killing of innocent people or suicide, and the vast majority of Muslims abhor such acts. In the United States, violence has also been sparked by members of right-wing white militia movements, many associated with extremist Christian groups that espouse creeds of racism and religious intolerance. Imposition of the dogmatic belief that there is only one "true religion" has led to catastrophic consequences throughout human times, as in holy wars to convert, subjugate, or annihilate nonbelievers.

Religious Congregations

With organized religion flourishing in many forms, there are currently over 2,000 denominations plus countless independent churches and faith communities (Gallup, 1996; Lindner, 1998). There are nearly 500,000 churches, temples, and other places of worship, from small storefront congregations to huge amphitheaters drawing thousands of worshipers. Membership in a church, synagogue, or other religious body has been consistently high—nearly 7 in 10 persons—over the past 50 years. Nearly 6 in 10 persons report that they attend services monthly; 4 in 10 attend weekly (including 50% of all women compared to 37% of men).

Most religious congregations encourage active participation through choir and prayer groups, suppers and social gatherings, as well as service and charity work. Religious support groups help members find strength in helping one another. Congregants view the clergy as dealing well with the needs of their parishioners and the problems of their communities. Religious leaders are generally held in high esteem: Clergy are ranked second to pharmacists as the profession most respected in terms of honesty and ethical standards—slightly ahead of doctors, dentists, engineers, and college professors (Gallup, 1996). (Ranked lowest are members of Congress and car salesmen!)

Religion and Multicultural Influences

Religion and culture are interwoven in all aspects of spiritual experience. Frank McCourt (1998) describes the image of God he formed in his Irish Catholic upbringing:

> We didn't hear much about a loving God. We were told God is good and that was supposed to be enough. Otherwise the Irish Catholic God of my memory is one the tribes of Israel would have recognized, an angry God, a vengeful God, a God who'd let you have it upside your head if you strayed, transgressed, coveted. . . . He had His priests preaching hellfire and damnation from the pulpit and scaring us to death. We were told that the Roman Catholic Church was the One True Church, that outside the Church there was no salvation. (p. 64)

McCourt developed two different versions of God in his head—Irish and Italian:

> Our faith was mean, scrimped, life-denying. We were told this was a vale of tears, transitory, that we'd get our reward in heaven, if, that is, we'd stop asking those dumb questions. . . . Statues and pictures of the Virgin Mary in the Irish churches seemed disembodied and she seemed to be saying, "Who is this kid?" In contrast Italian art portrayed a voluptuous, maternal Mary with a happy infant Jesus at her bosom. (p. 64)

McCourt wondered: "Was it the weather? Did God change His aspect as He moved from the chilly north to the vineyards of Italy?" (p. 64). He thought that, all in all, he'd prefer the Italian expression of Catholicism to the Irish one.

Religious adherence and more personal spiritual beliefs and practices vary greatly across and within cultures. For instance, U.S. Muslims include African Americans and immigrants from South Asia, the Middle East, north and sub-Saharan Africa, Pakistan, and Indonesia. All Muslims perform the same daily prayers and share a common set of precepts from the

Holy Koran that guide daily life. Yet each family places a distinct cultural stamp on its practices (Mahmoud, 1996). Within cultures, differences are also found between families from rural, traditional backgrounds and those from urban settings, with more education and middle-class values. Religion is further intertwined with influences such as race, recent immigration, and the degree of fit vis-à-vis the dominant culture or local community. Religious prejudice or outright discrimination leads some to suppress their religious identification or expression.

Ethnicity influences religious preference, yet it is crucial not to reflexively link religion with ethnicity. Although Hispanics are commonly assumed to be Catholic, in fact, just 60% are Catholic, whereas 25% are Protestant. Contrary to popular belief, only one-third of Arab Americans are Muslim; many are Christian. Although most Irish are Catholic, those from Northern Ireland may well be Protestant. Streams of recent immigrants from Southeast Asia may be Christian or bring Eastern religious traditions. Some come, as immigrants did historically, fleeing religious persecution in their country of origin, such as Russian Jews. Refugees from the former Yugoslavia are not only Serbian, Croatian, or Bosnian, but also Orthodox Christian, Catholic, or Muslim—differences that carry heavy historical meaning (i.e., the imposition of Islam by invading Turks) and have fueled hatred and bloodshed across generations.

Among African Americans, 73% are Protestant, 10% are Catholic, and a growing number are Muslim (Gallup, 1996). Blacks of all faiths are far more likely than others to consider religion important: Religious experience starts young and continues throughout their lives. Most African Americans participate actively in their local church congregation. They take religion seriously, practice it fervently, and look to it for strength in dealing with adversity (Billingsley, 1992; Boyd-Franklin & Lockwood, 1999; see Chapter 10, this volume).

The wide spectrum of faiths today has been called a "supermarket" of religions. However, in a predominantly Christian nation of European origins, we must be cautious not to superimpose the template of western European values on other belief systems and practices that may not be understood in Christian terms. It is crucial not to judge diverse faith traditions, particularly those of tribal peoples, as inferior when they differ from Euro-Christian standards, such as African healing traditions (Some, 1994). Early Euro-American conquerors viewed Native Americans as primitive heathens and regarded their spiritual beliefs and practices as pagan witchcraft. Such attitudes led the government and religious missionary programs to educate and acculturate Indians in Christianity and Western ways, eradicating their own tribal language, religion, and customs. Children, taken from their families and isolated in boarding schools, were stripped of their cultural identity and religious heritage. Today, native youth are returning in large numbers to the spiritual roots of their ancestors, seeking identity and worth in their spiritual community (Deloria, 1994).

Common Spiritual Beliefs and Practices

It may surprise many secular therapists and social scientists that 96% of Americans believe in God or a universal spirit, although these conceptions vary widely. Only 3% are atheists, not believing in the existence of God, and 1% are agnostic, uncertain about whether God exists (Gallup, 1996; God in America, 1998). Some think of God as a "force" that maintains a balance in nature, but most people believe in a personal God who watches over and judges people. Eight persons in 10 feel that God has helped them to make decisions. Most believe that God performs miracles today. Many say they have felt the presence of God at various points in their lifetime and believe that God has a plan for their lives. The closer people feel to God, the better they feel about themselves and others. Most people believe that they will be called before God on Judgment Day to answer for their sins (Gallup, 1996). Eighty percent of Americans believe in an afterlife; 72% believe in heaven, and most believe in angels. Fifty-six percent believe in Hell, and 50% believe in the devil. Seventy-five percent rate their own chances of going to heaven as excellent or good (even though a few are not sure of its existence)!

The vast majority of Americans are Christian or Jewish, who believe the Bible was either the literal or inspired word of God and regard the Ten Commandments as valid rules for living. For Muslims, the Koran builds on those foundations and provides specific guidelines and prohibitions for individual, family, and community life (Almeida, 1996). Every religion has a precept akin to "Treat others as you would want them to treat you."

Religious beliefs profoundly influence character development. Eight people in 10 say that their religious convictions help them to respect themselves and other people, and to assist those in need. Six in 10 report that religion answers their questions and helps them to solve their problems. Furthermore, most say their beliefs keep them from doing things they know they should not do. One-third report a profound spiritual experience, either sudden or gradual, that dramatically altered their lives. Those who say religion is the most important influence in their lives, and those who receive a great deal of comfort from their faith, are far more likely to feel close to their families, to find their jobs fulfilling, and to be hopeful about the future (Chamberlain & Zika, 1992).

Prayer and Meditation

Prayer has strong meaning for Americans: 90% say they pray in some fashion at least weekly; 75% pray daily (Gallup, 1996). For most, prayer originates in the family and is centered in the home. Prayer at bedtime and saying Grace or giving thanks to God before meals are common practices. Most people report that they pray whenever they feel the need. Almost all (98%) pray for their family's health and happiness. Few (5%) pray for bad tidings for others. Prayer generates feelings of hope and peace. Most who pray (86%) believe it makes them better persons. Nearly all report that their prayers have been heard and answered. Most (62%) say they got what they hoped for, and most (62%) have received divine inspiration or a feeling of being led by God. Twenty-five percent report a voice or vision as a result of prayer. Some (30%) have stopped praying for long periods of time, mostly because they got out of the habit. Few (10%) stopped because they had lost their faith, were angry with God or the church, or felt their prayers had not been answered.

Every religion values some form of prayer or meditation. It may involve chanting, reading scriptures, or rituals such as lighting candles or incense, reciting a rosary, or, for Muslims, observing the call to prayer five times daily. Most pray to a Supreme Being, such as God, Allah, Jehovah, or to Jesus Christ. Very few report that they pray to a transcendent or cosmic force, or to "the god within." One reason to pray is to express praise and gratitude for life itself. A deeper reason is to keep life in perspective, which is considered the most difficult lesson people must learn.

Meditation offers a way for the mind to seek clarity and the heart to find tranquility (Bell, 1998). Meditation can empty the mind of "noise" and ease tension, pain, and suffering. Becoming mindful in still and focused concentration, as in Buddhist practice, can lead to more deliberate action (Nhat Hanh, 1991). A contemplative atmosphere can be found in communion with nature or appreciation of art; quietly listening to music, whether sacred or secular, can be deeply spiritual. Shared meditative experiences foster genuine and empathic communication, reduce defensive reactivity, and deepen couple and family bonds (Bell, 1998).

Rites and Rituals

In every culture, sacred ceremonies and rituals serve invaluable functions in connecting individuals with their families and communities, as well as guiding them through life passage and times of adversity (Imber-Black & Roberts, 1992). Rituals can celebrate family holidays, traditions, achievements, and reunions. They can ease difficult transitions or unfamiliar situations and summon courage through the darkest hours. In times of crisis and profound sorrow, they can script family actions and responses, as in funeral rites or memorial services. Rituals also connect a particular celebration or tragedy with all human experience, and a birth or a death and loss with others.

Patriarchy, Sexism, and Heterosexism

Patriarchy, a cultural pattern embedded in most religious traditions, has been a dominant force and powerful legacy. At its worst, it has sanctioned the subordination and abuse of women and children (Bottoms, Shaver,

Goodman, & Qin, 1995; Bridges & Spilka, 1992). In Genesis (3:16) Eve was admonished, "In pain you shall bring forth children; yet your desire shall be for your husband, and he shall rule over you." The traditional daily prayers of Orthodox Jewish men, as well as Muslims, have included thankfulness to God (Allah) for not having been born a woman. In Islamic law, the failure of a wife to produce a male offspring is grounds for divorce (Brook, 1995). Christianity, as well, has preached a doctrine of separate and unequal sexes. St Paul told women: "You must lean and adapt yourselves to your husbands. The husband is the head of the wife." Timothy (2:11–15) pronounced, "Let a woman learn in silence with all submissiveness. I permit no woman to teach or to have authority over men; she is to keep silent." The Hindu Code of Manu (ca. 100 A.D.) declared "In childhood a woman must be subject to her father; in youth to her husband; and when her husband is dead, to her sons. A woman must never be free of subjugation." In China, Confucius (551–479 B.C.) boldly proclaimed, "One hundred women are not worth a single testicle!"(Bowman, 1983). Over the centuries, prevalent cultural norms have supported religious dogma and institutions in rigidifying more patriarchal gender roles. A legacy of this devaluation is the still-common practice of infanticide and abandonment of daughters; in many parts of Asia, abortion of a female fetus is sanctioned.

The denigration of women has alienated many from their religious roots. Some have turned to the Bahai faith (Huddleston, 1999) and to reform movements within many religions, which promote the equality of men and women in family life and society. Others have found new sources of meaning and esteem through nontraditional expressions of spirituality and interest in ancient, goddess-centered or wicca traditions. Carol Gilligan's (1982) seminal research challenged androcentric standards of moral development. Feminist scholars have sought to reinterpret and claim their rightful place in religious traditions.

Religious beliefs may underlie sexist patterns in couple and family relationships. A wife's depression or wish to leave a marriage may result from her husband's controlling and demeaning behavior, which is grounded in fundamentalist religious tenets that a wife should be submissive. One fundamentalist Christian woman reported that her husband was right to beat her because she had challenged his authority. Her husband concurred that this was her problem. As family therapists, we have an ethical responsibility to challenge beliefs that are harmful to any member, whether based in family, ethnic, or religious traditions. Above all, every religion upholds the core principles of respect for others, and the dignity and worth of all human beings.

The condemnation of homosexuality in religious doctrine has been a source of deep anguish for gay men and lesbians, who have felt exiled from most traditional faith communities (Fortunato, 1982). Some denominations preach an abhorrence for homosexual practice alongside a loving acceptance of homosexual persons as human beings created by God. Such a dualistic attitude nevertheless perpetuates stigma and shame, pathologizing "unnatural" sexual behavior as deviating from the proper norm (Laird & Green, 1996; see Laird, Chapter 11, this volume). It is important to explore religious roots of rejection of gay offspring by a family of origin.

Gay men and lesbians have increasingly been forging their own spiritual pathways (O'Neill & Ritter, 1992). Long-standing religious opposition to same-sex unions is currently being challenged by a growing number of clergy. With deep schisms over these issues in many Christian denominations in recent years, most parishioners are far more tolerant than official church doctrine.

Interfaith Boundaries, Tolerance, and Marriage

Through the mid–20th century, there were sharp divisions between different religious faiths and denominations, especially along social class and ethnic lines (Browning, Miller-McLemore, Couture, Lyon, & Franklin, 1977; Gallup, 1996). In recent years, 25% of adults have changed faiths or denominations from the one in which they were raised, mostly because they preferred another orientation or because of interfaith marriage.

Traditionally, many religions prohibited interfaith marriage, strongly discouraging young people from even dating someone of another denomination. Currently 32% of Catholics, 52% of Jews, and 57% of Buddhists marry outside their faith. As noted earlier, the high rate of intermarriage by Jews is of deep concern to their community (Forster & Tabachnik, 1993). Although blacks are only half as likely as whites to oppose interracial marriages, they are more opposed than whites to interfaith marriages (Gallup, 1996). Yet, in general, acceptance has grown with the support of ecumenical and interfaith movements, and the blurring of racial and ethnic barriers. Most parents and children show increasing religious tolerance and favor public school courses to provide nondevotional instruction about various world religions. Most think that all religions are essentially good, and that people can be ethical even if they don't believe in God.

Discontinuities and New Connections

Congruence between religious/spiritual beliefs and practices yields a general sense of well-being and wholeness, whereas a dissonance can induce shame, guilt, or spiritual malaise. Discontinuities often exist between religious teachings and personal spiritual beliefs and practices. Many eschew formal institutionalized religion yet lead deeply spiritual lives. Others adhere to religious rituals without finding spiritual meaning in them. Even with the reported importance of religion, it does not necessarily change people's lives. There is often a gap between their faith and knowledge of the religion, its core tenets, and family religious roots. Many revere their holy scriptures but few read or study them. One survey found that although 93% of homes contain a Bible, 58% of respondents couldn't name five of the Ten Commandments; 10% thought Joan of Arc was Noah's wife (Shorto, 1997).

There is another gap between beliefs and practices. Many are strong believers but do not actively participate in congregational life. Most view their faith as a matter between themselves and God. Whereas Orthodox Jews center their lives on observance of traditional laws and practices, 62% of American Jews believe they can be "religious" without being "particularly observant" (Jewish Theological Seminary, New York, cited by Shorto, 1997).

It is important to distinguish between surface religion, such as attending church for social reasons, and deep, transforming faith that is lived out in daily life, relationships, and service to others. It is the level of spiritual commitment that makes a significant difference in personal well-being and concern for others. Those with a deeply integrated and lived-out faith gain strength from their religious convictions and often spend significant time helping those in need. They are more likely to be tolerant of other faiths and are more giving and forgiving in their personal relationships.

Most Americans are highly independent in their spiritual lives. For instance, Catholics are among the most devout worshipers, yet 64% agree that one can be a good Catholic without going to Mass, and 82% say that using birth control is "entirely up to the individual" (Gallup, 1996). The vast majority (78%) disagree with the Church's refusal to sanction remarriage after divorce. Sixty-two percent believe that those who have abortions are still good Catholics, and 58% believe the Church should relax its standards prohibiting abortions. Personal attitudes about abortion, euthanasia, and the death penalty are strongly polarized within and across religions. Younger people tend to be more liberal in these beliefs than their elders, often arousing intergenerational tensions within families.

Religion and spirituality are expected to grow in significance over the coming decades, shaped less by institutions and more by the people who seek meaning and connection. In our rapidly changing world, religion is less often a given that people are born into and accept unquestioningly. Instead, individuals, couples, and families commonly pick and choose among beliefs and practices to fit their lives. Canadian sociologist Reginald Bibby calls this trend "religion à la carte" (cited in Gallup, 1996, p. 8); for Deloria (1994), combining elements of varied faiths is like a platter of "religious linguini." As religious diversity within families increases, many are creating their own recipes, blending Christianity and Native American spirituality, Judaism and Zen Buddhism. Most are taking a broader ecumenical view. As McGoldrick and Giordano (1996, p. 8) observe, "We are all migrants, moving between our ancestors' traditions, the worlds we inhabit, and the world we will leave to those who come after us."

SPIRITUALITY AND CONNECTEDNESS

Faith is inherently relational from our earliest years, when fundamental convictions about life are shaped within caretaking relationships. Intimate bonds with authentic communication ("I and Thou") are expressions of spirituality and offer pathways for spiritual growth (Buber, 1921/1970; Fishbane, 1998). Deep connections are experienced with "kindred spirits" and "soul mates." Caring relationships with partners, family members, and close friends nourish spiritual well-being; in turn spirituality deepens and expands connections with others. It can be spiritually enriching to care for an infant or a frail elder, to befriend strangers, or to receive the loving kindness of others. For many, belief in a personal relationship with God strengthens them through their darkest hours (Becvar, 1996; Griffith, 1999).

Faith, intimacy, and resilience are intertwined (Higgins, 1994). Love sustains lives and infuses them with meaning. Victor Frankl (1946/1984), in recounting his experiences in Nazi prison camps, came to the realization that salvation is found through love. As he visualized the image of his wife, a thought occurred: "I didn't even know if she were still alive. I knew only one thing—which I have learned well by now: Love goes very far beyond the physical person of the beloved. It finds its deepest meaning in his spiritual being, his inner self."

The transcendent sense of family and community is forged through shared values, commitment, and mutual support through adversity. Banning together in activism for such concerns as environmental protection or social justice can be a powerful expression of spirituality (Perry & Rolland, 1999). In contrast to the highly individualized concept of human autonomy centered on the "self" in Western societies, most cultures in the world consider the person as embedded within the family and larger community. The African theologian John Mbiti (1970) describes this sociocentric view of human experience with the dictum, "I am because we are."

Spiritual connection and renewal can be found in nature and in great works of art, literature, and music that communicate our common humanity. Music offers a powerful transcending experience. African-American gospel "spirituals," blues, jazz, and "soul" music were creative expressions forged out of the cauldron of slavery, racism, and impoverished conditions, transcending those scarring experiences through the resilience of the human spirit.

Often, people who have had negative experiences of religion in childhood, find such ways of expressing their spirituality. The author Alice Walker found hers through communion with nature, creative writing, and activism. In a collection of essays, Walker (1997) wrote about her life as an activist and her faith in the human heart. She described her beloved mother, who was devoted to her rural church, as someone who took action, took children in need into her home, and looked out for the welfare of others in her struggling, isolated community. She notes that her mother would not have thought of herself as an activist but would have called it just being a person.

Walker's own spiritual journey began in a childhood subjected to "white orthodox Christianity," which her parents followed. She dropped out at age 13, feeling that the preacher and the church structure reinforced the gender inequality she saw elsewhere. She found that instead of church attendance, nature nourished her through long country walks, being out in the rain, or running with the wind. She became what she calls a "born-again pagan," experiencing spirituality through the land as a country dweller, a peasant. Her activist spirit found powerful expression in her writing and her work in movements for social justice. Her deep spirituality nourished her conviction that if you just accept conditions and do nothing, nothing changes, and you shut down; instead, activism transforms; it's impossible to stay depressed about anything if you act to change it (Walker, 1997).

IMPLICATIONS FOR CLINICAL PRACTICE

Most people who come for therapeutic help today are seeking more than symptom reduction, problem-solving, or communication skills; they are seeking deeper meaning and connections in their lives. For many, spiritual distress is at the core of physical, emotional, and relational problems. Clinicians are only beginning to develop ways to integrate this vital dimension in therapeutic work and to encourage spiritual connections in family and community life.

Moreover, psychotherapy itself, long considered a healing art, can be a profoundly spiritual experience for both clients and therapists, yet this has been a hidden aspect of clinical work (Walsh, 1999b). The very essence of the therapeutic relationship and meaningful change is ultimately spiritual in nature, fostering personal transformation, wholeness, and relational connection with others.

Throughout the mental health field, until only recently, spirituality has been purposefully left out of clinical training and practice, regarded as a taboo subject to be checked at the office door by both client and therapist. Therapists have been reluctant to raise the subject and uncomfortable in dealing with it when it does arise. When clients sense that spirituality doesn't belong in the clinical context, they censor themselves from bringing this dimension of their lives into the therapeutic conversation.

Currently, there is a growing surge of interest in spirituality by mental health professionals. Yet most feel ill-equipped in their training, constrained from broaching the subject with clients, and unsure how to approach the spiritual dimension of their therapeutic practice. Clinicians are encouraged to move beyond these barriers and find ways to incorporate spirituality in clinical assessment and intervention, in an effort to understand spiritual sources of distress and tap resources in healing, recovery, and resilience.

Overcoming Barriers

Several influences have contributed to the long-standing lack of attention to spirituality in clinical practice and family research (Prest & Keller, 1993).

Sacred and Secular

One assumption has been that religion is not the proper domain of mental health professionals. Like the larger society's founding principle of separation of the religious from the secular, rigid boundaries separated spiritual concerns as "off limits" from psychotherapy. Therapists were trained not to intrude into clients' "private" spiritual matters or impose their own religious views. Spiritual distress was seen to exist in a separate realm from physical and psychosocial distress, restricted to the domain of clergy or pastoral counselors. Likewise, spiritual healing practices were deemed outside the province of mental health and health care.

Power and Influence

A related barrier involves the potential in the therapeutic relationship for vulnerable clients, in distress, to adopt their therapist's spiritual orientation. Concerns about therapists' persuasion and clients' susceptibility stem from recognition of the power of the therapist and the dependent position of clients. Therefore, professionals were trained to remain objective and unbiased. To protect clients, they were advised to be cautious not to reveal their own values or practices. However, there has been growing recognition that therapists cannot be neutral or value-free. Inescapably, therapy involves the interaction of therapists' and clients' value systems. Just as other aspects of culture (e.g., ethnicity, social class, and gender) influence client and therapist constructions of norms, problems, and solutions, so too does the spiritual dimension of experience. What we ask and pursue—or do not—influences the therapeutic relationship, course, and outcome.

We best respect clients not by avoiding discussion of spirituality altogether, but by demonstrating active interest in exploring and understanding *their* values and practices. In doing so, it is important to affirm and encourage those that foster well-being. At times, certain beliefs or practices may be challenged if they contribute to distress or are harmful to others, such as when violence is rationalized by citing fundamentalist religious precepts. To be both self-aware and sensitive to clients, is important for therapists to examine and come to understand their own orientation to religion and spirituality. It is best to recognize spiritual influences and work collaboratively in ways that foster resilience and empowerment in clients, their family relationships, and their communities (Walsh, 1998b).

Science and Faith

Historically, the psychological and the spiritual were one and the same. In fact, *psyche* is the Greek word for spirit. Some problems are still seen and treated as possession by spirits in many traditional cultures (Comas-Diaz, 1981; Falicov, 1999). Over the centuries, faith healers and clergy have held influential roles as counselors in their communities, tending to emotional suffering and marital/family relational problems.

Despite psychotherapy's roots in spiritual healing traditions, 20th century developments in the mental health field produced a schism: The scientific paradigm emerged as the dominant epistemology, along with skepticism toward faith-based approaches. Although many marriage and family therapists came out of pastoral counseling traditions, most mental health professionals have been trained to uphold firm boundaries between the "helping professions" and faith-based healing. Professional disciplines have sought to gain scientific credibility and status through empirically based practice, distancing from aspects of client experience and therapeutic processes that presumably could not be observed and measured.

Increasingly, possibilities for integration of science and spirituality are being pursued. Qualitative studies are gaining credence as methods to explore the meaning of experiences, yielding more knowledge about the role of faith beliefs and practices in problem construction and solution (Wright et al., 1996). Quantitative studies have begun to find empirical support for spiritual influences in mental health (Gartner, Larson, & Allen, 1991; Hood, Spilka, Hunsberger, & Gorsuch, 1996) and physical well-being (Koenig et al., 1998), and for the healing power of prayer (Dossey, 1993). Studies of meditation document its influence in reducing stress and blood pressure, improving sleep and mental alertness, managing chronic pain, and raising self-esteem and lowering reactivity in relationships. Over the past decade, the mental health disciplines have brought greater attention to religion and spirituality in research and practice (e.g., Shafranske, 1996; Steere, 1997; Woolfolk, 1998).

Healing and Treatment

Family therapists have approached healing in terms of a therapeutic relationship that encourages clients' own inherent healing potential. This collaborative approach is at the core of strength-based and resilience-oriented models of practice (Walsh, 1998b). Distinct from curing, healing is seen as a natural process in response to injury or trauma. Sometimes people heal physically but do not heal emotionally, mentally, or spiritually; badly strained relationships remain unhealed. Some may recover from an illness but not regain a spirit to live and love fully. Yet we can heal psychosocially even when we do not heal physically, or when a traumatic event cannot be reversed. The literal meaning of healing is becoming whole, and when necessary, adapting and compensating for losses of structure or function (Weil, 1994). Our faith in each family's desire to be healthy and its potential for healing and growth can encourage family members' best efforts (see Walsh, Chapter 15, this volume).

Healing and treatment are quite different concepts. Healing involves a gathering of resources within the person, the family, and the community, and is fostered through the therapeutic relationship; treatment is externally administered by experts. Western scientific medicine has focused on identifying external agents of disease and developing technological weapons to defeat them. An unbalanced focus on pathology rather than health contributes to despair (Weil, 1994). In contrast, medicine grounded in Eastern religious and philosophical traditions is based on a set of beliefs about healing processes and the importance of mind–body interactions. Healing is a functional system, not an assemblage of structures. Chinese medicine, for instance, explores ways of increasing internal resilience as resistance to disease, so that people can remain healthy regardless of the harmful influences to which they are exposed. This belief in strengthening protective processes assumes that the body has a natural ability to heal and grow stronger. A number of recently developed "alternative" approaches to medicine and psychotherapy draw on these beliefs to decrease pain and foster greater well-being (e.g., Kabat-Zinn, 1990).

Resources for diagnosis, self-repair, and regeneration exist in all of us and can be activated as need arises. Strengths-based approaches to practice encourage a family's own healing resources and reduce vulnerability. Emphasis has shifted from earlier focus on therapist techniques to see the fundamental power for change as residing within the family, and to encourage clinicians to tap into the family's own healing forces (Minuchin, 1992). In strengthening resilience, we inspire people to believe in their own possibilities for regeneration. Therapy best fosters this resilience in two ways: through a healing therapeutic relationship that is a collaborative partnership with clients, and by activating relationship networks as a healing environment for the relief of suffering and renewal of life passage. Our faith in each family's desire to be healthy and its potential for healing and growth can encourage best efforts.

The general public has indicated a need for mental health and health care professionals to attend to the spiritual dimension in their practice. Recent surveys found that 81% of respondents prefer to have their own spiritual practices and beliefs integrated into any counseling process; 75% want physicians and therapists to address spiritual issues as part of their care. Half of elderly people say they want their doctors to pray with them as they face death (Gallup, 1996). In general, clients are less interested in their therapists' spiritual orientation and more interested in sharing their own spiritual concerns. When therapists neglect the potential relevance of clients' spiritual beliefs and practices, and when clients hold back spiritual concerns, therapy can leave them feeling fragmented (Bergin, 1991).

Among the early pioneers in family therapy, Gregory Bateson (1979) was visionary in seeing the unity of mind and nature in all experience. Virginia Satir stood out in embracing a broad spirituality in her practice approach (1977/1988). More recently, a number of family therapists have been breaking down barriers to explore ways to bring spirituality into therapeutic work (e.g., Anderson & Worthen, 1997; Becvar, 1996, 1998; Griffith & Griffith, 2001; Kramer, 1995; Prest & Keller, 1993; Stander et al., 1994; Walsh, 1999c). Weaver, Koenig, and Larson (1997) have called for greater collaboration with clergy in family therapy training, practice, and research. Some therapists offer special approaches with very religious families (Butler & Harper, 1994; Griffith, 1986; Nakhaima & Dicks, 1995; Rotz, Russell, & Wright, 1993; Stewart & Gale, 1994). Others address issues such as violence in fundamentalist marriages (Whipple, 1987) or the painful spiritual challenges of gay men and lesbians (Markowitz, 1998; O'Neill & Ritter, 1992). Doherty (1995, 1999) criticized psychotherapy's overemphasis on self-interest and called for greater sensitivity in therapy to the moral responsibilities in loving relationships and community. His message resonates with pioneer family therapist Ivan Boszormenyi-Nagy's (1987) emphasis on the ethical dimension of intergenerational relationships (Fishbane, 1999).

Incorporating Spirituality in Family Assessment

Just as family therapists have recognized the importance of inquiring about ethnicity and other aspects of culture, assessment should routinely explore the spiritual dimension of clients' lives. Therapists should note religions orientations on family genograms, (McGoldrick, Gerson, & Shellenberger, 1998) and also explore their significance for clients. It is important to clarify, for example, whether identifying as Christian is based in deeply held convictions or a family background that has not been followed meaningfully. Is religion associated with a loving Christ or with sin and punishment? With congregational support or rigid hierarchy and doctrine? Can a broader or more personal approach to spirituality open up potential resources in everyday life?

Table 13.1 suggests some fruitful lines of inquiry in exploring the spiritual dimension of individual, couple, and family experience. Particular attention should be focused on exploring ways that religious beliefs or experiences may contribute to current distress. It is also important to consider how past, current, or potential spiritual resources can be identified and drawn on to ease distress, strengthen resilience in dealing with adversity,

TABLE 13.1. Inquiry into the Spiritual Dimension of Clients' Individual and Family Experience to Explore Sources of Distress and Potential Therapeutic Resources

- How important is religion or a more personal spirituality in current lives? In the family of origin? What are clients' desires for future spirituality?

- To what extent do individuals, couples and families identify with a particular religion? How observant are they in practices and congregational involvement?

- How are religious differences within a couple or family handled and accepted? How do they contribute to conflict or estrangement?

- With intermarriage and/or conversion, how was the decision made? Has it been supported by families of origin? Has it been regretted?

- What are clients' concepts of the "ideal" marriage and family of their faith? Roles of wife/mother; husband/father; sons and daughters? How do they view themselves and their own family by comparison?

- How has adversity or trauma wounded the spirit?

- How have religious/spiritual beliefs or practices contributed to problems or blocked healing and growth?

- Have religious precepts (e.g., sexist or heterosexist) contributed to client suffering or abuse?

- Has a spiritual void or cutoff from religious roots exacerbated suffering or alienation?

- How might clients' past, current, or potential spiritual resources be drawn on for healing, change, and growth?
    Personal and shared faith for comfort, strength, and mutual support
    Spiritual practices (e.g., prayer, meditation, ritual)
    Congregational affiliation and support
    Spiritual guidance and counsel by clergy

or help clients accept what cannot be changed in order to foster healing, change, and growth.

In therapeutic work, it is important to learn how each family, from its own distinct sociocultural background, blends the core principles of faith with varied aspects of family members' lives. For some, traditional religious beliefs and practices can be a positive stabilizing resource in weathering crisis. For others, they have become outmoded and fail to serve as a foundation for psychosocial and spiritual well-being. Family members who feel oppressed by religious dogma may find alternate constructions and practices consonant with larger spiritual beliefs, without rejecting spirituality altogether.

Even when presenting problems do not ostensibly involve spirituality, a spiritual source of distress may emerge. One woman was referred for therapy by her mother-in-law, who was concerned about her daughter-in-law's continued inconsolable grief, many months after the stillbirth of her second child. Exploration with the therapist revealed the daughter-in-law's profound sense of guilt. Raised in a devout Catholic family, she fell in love with a Jewish man; they married in a civil ceremony, because religion did not seem very important to them at that time in their lives. When their first child, a son, was born, they agreed to handle their differences by not bringing him up in either faith. With the stillbirth of the second child, the woman believed that God was punishing her for not having baptized her son. Reluctant to reveal this to her Jewish husband and his family, she had withdrawn from them and kept her concerns to herself. Individual and couple sessions were combined to involve both partners for mutual support, open communication, and decision making. Consultation with a priest and rabbi was also helpful to them.

Tapping into Spiritual Resources for Healing, Recovery, and Resilience

Suffering, and often the injustice or senselessness of it, are ultimately spiritual issues (Wright et al., 1996). Adversity and suffering have vastly different meanings in various religious traditions (Smith, 1991), and each faith in its own way calls forth resilience (Wolin, Muller, Taylor, & Wolin, 1999), the capacity to rebound from adversity strengthened and more resourceful (Walsh, 1998b; see Chapter 15, this volume). Resilience is an active process of endurance, self-righting, and growth out of crisis or persistent life challenges. Family resilience involves key transactional processes that enable the family system to rally in times of crisis, buffering stress, reducing the risk of dysfunction, and supporting optimal adaptation for all members. Family belief systems are a powerful influence in making meaning of adversity and suffering; they can facilitate—or constrain—growthful change (Dallos, 1991; Wright et al., 1996). When relationships have been hurtful, family members can be helped to seek compassion, reconciliation, and forgiveness, which are central to the teachings of all major religions (Hargrave, 1994).

The paradox of resilience is that the worst of times can also bring out the best. A crisis can lead to transformation and growth in unforeseen directions. It can spark a reordering of life priorities for more meaningful connections. In the midst of suffering, the hardship endured can lead to spiritual growth. In turn, spiritual beliefs and practices strengthen the ability to withstand and transcend adversity. Keys to resilience, such as meaning making, hope, courage, perseverance, and connectedness are all enhanced by spirituality (Walsh, 1998b). Faith supports the belief that adversity can be overcome. Studies suggest that beyond simply being religious what matters most is being able to give meaning to a precarious situation, having faith that there is some greater purpose or force at work, and finding solace and strength in these outlooks (see Walsh, 1998b).

In their longitudinal study of resilience in poor multiethnic families in Hawaii, Werner and Smith (1992) found that religion is an important protective factor from childhood through adulthood. Religious faith and affiliation—including Buddhist, Catholic, Mormon, Jehovah's Witness, and others—strengthened individuals and their families through times of adversity by providing a sense of hope, mission, and salvation. Many credited highly structured religious groups for their resilience. One woman described her deep church involvement since adolescence and her abiding faith in God: "When I felt like life wasn't worth living, there was a God who loved me and would help me come through." Follow-up studies found that resilience could be forged, transforming lives throughout the life cycle. A crisis could become an epiphany, opening lives to a spiritual dimension previously untapped.

Spiritual distress, an inability to invest life with meaning, impedes coping and mastery in the face of life challenges. Religious ideas or experiences may contribute to guilt, shame, or worthlessness. From sources in family history, culture, and spirituality, we can help clients invest in traditions, rituals, or spiritual communities that link them in more positive ways. For many, new spiritual wellsprings can be tapped to offer a larger vision of humanity and connection that inspires their best.

Health Benefits of Faith

Beliefs are powerful influences in health and illness (Antonovsky, 1987). Medical studies find that faith, prayer, and spiritual rituals can strengthen health and healing by triggering emotions that influence physiological systems (Ellison & Levin, 1998). Older persons with strong religious beliefs are more likely to be satisfied with their lives and to have lower blood pressure, reducing the risk of heart disease (Koenig et al., 1998). Among elderly persons, both depression and alcohol abuse are reduced by prayer (Ayele, 1998). Those who find strength and comfort in religious outlooks survive surgery at a far higher rate than those who lack faith (Oxman, Freeman, & Manheimer, 1995). The solace and hopefulness of strong faith appear even more important than frequency of participation in religious services or activities. A review of medical studies on the efficacy of prayer (Dossey, 1993) similarly found that prayer triggers emotions that in turn positively impact the immune and cardiovascular systems, thereby improving health. At the same time, caution is advised not to attribute failure to recover to a lack of personal spiritual piety.

Facing Death; Recovering from Loss

Facing death and the loss of a loved one are the most painful of all family challenges. Western Christian belief systems heighten the dilemma of acceptance in their emphasis on mastery and control over destiny. The end of life is approached in terms of loss of control and the failure of treatments—or of will. In contrast, Eastern and indigenous tribal spiritual traditions approach death as a natural part of the human life cycle. Buddhism teaches that in accepting death, we discover life. Indian tribal religions approach death within the larger context: viewing human beings as an integral part of the natural world (Deloria, 1994). In death, as the soul enters the spirit world, the body is contributed and becomes the dust that nourishes the plants and animals that in turn feed people during their lifetime. Because the family and tribal community are seen as a continuing unity, death, although saddening, is simply a transitional event in a much larger human life cycle.

People of many faiths believe that the spirit lives on after the death of the body. Some believe the soul resides in a spirit world for all eternity; many believe they can be in contact or receive visits from spirits, particularly in times of need, to offer reassurance to the bereft, or when a serious wrong has not been addressed. For believers, the spirits of the deceased live on in the minds, hearts, and stories of loved ones. They can haunt as ghosts or become guardian angels and guiding spirits, inspiring best efforts and actions.

Religious beliefs can impede family response to loss (Bohannon, 1991), especially with complicated deaths, such as suicide, that may be morally condemned (Domino & Miller, 1992). They can also facilitate family adaptation (Gilbert, 1992). The end of life offers gifts to those who face it openly with courage and compassion, reaching out to loved ones. More than any other human experience, death and loss can teach us about the meaning of life and put us in touch with what most matters in our lives; thus, the experience can be transforming. Therapists can help families face death and loss by encouraging members' full presence and participation in the dying process, drawing on their spiritual beliefs and practices to assist them.

Some devastating losses can turn people away from faith. A deeply religious couple was referred for counseling after the death of their only child. When asked if they were able to find solace in their faith, the husband shouted, "I'm angry at God!" As the therapist explored the meaning of the loss for him, he sobbed, "I believe that when something happens, there's always a reason. And I just can't fathom what the reason is here. We did everything right, by the book. God took our son. And it's not fair. He never had a chance at life." Therapists trained to help families solve problems may feel helpless and uneasy at such times; we are powerless to stop death or bring back a loved one. Often, consultation with clergy can help people find their spiritual moorings.

Recovery from Substance Abuse and Addictions

Researchers and clinicians have often overlooked the role of spiritual beliefs and practices in preventing substance abuse and relapse (Gorsuch, 1995). An emphasis on spirituality has been a key component in 12-step programs of recovery from addictions, such as Alcoholics Anonymous

(Minnick, 1997), which can be a valuable adjunct to couple or family therapy (Berenson, 1990). In addition to offering fellowship and group support, these programs address spiritual issues concerning identity, integrity, inner life, and interdependence (Peteet, 1993). The steps are designed to promote a spiritual awakening that prepares individuals and family members to practice the principles of abstinence and greater well-being in all aspects of their lives. The connection with a Higher Power through prayer and meditation also facilitates reflection that sustains them through times of trouble. Often, this spiritual awakening sparks life-altering transformations.

Overcoming Barriers of Racism and Poverty

Religious faith and congregational support help families to survive and transcend impoverished conditions, barriers of racism, and other adversity (Billingsley, 1992; Boyd-Franklin & Lockwood, 1999; see Boyd-Franklin, Chapter 10, this volume). In *Bread and Spirit,* Harry Aponte (1994) urges therapists to attend to spiritual as well as practical needs of poor families that have lost hope and faith in their chances for a better life. At the core, they suffer a poverty of despair, a wounding of the soul in a pervasive sense of injustice, helplessness, and rage at the inequalities surrounding them. Aponte encourages therapists to go beyond theory and technique to reach for meaning and purpose in people's lives:

> Therapy can be an enemy or a friend to spirit. The technology of therapy has attempted to replace tradition, ritual, and customs. . . . However, just as medication can only succeed when it cooperates with the healing powers of the body, therapy only works when it joins with the indigenous forces of culture and faith in people's lives. (p. 8)

In the midst of despair, a spirit of love, courage, and hope can be rekindled. Aponte (1999) believes that therapists can make a difference by recognizing that potential and joining in a revitalization of family and community spirit.

Reconnecting with Family Religious Roots

Therapists trained to look to family-of-origin history for problems and conflicts need to rebalance their focus to search for strengths. Faith is often a powerful source of resilience in weathering losses and adaptive challenges. Discovering such connections and the strength of religious roots can be a valuable part of therapeutic work, especially where experiences of oppression or forced migration have shattered a coherent sense of identity and severed linkages with ancestors. For instance, many African American descendants of Muslims brought from west Africa as slaves may be unaware of this heritage, because the practice of African religions was suppressed.

Islam was often practiced in secret and passed down surreptitiously in oral history or by "strange" customs. Mahmoud (1996) has found that in doing genograms with African Americans in clinical practice, a story might surface of a distant relative who prayed facing east, refused to eat pork, or gave children non-Christian names. Restoring vital bonds with a family's religious heritage can be healing and empowering.

Use of Meditation and Rituals

Meditation is becoming widely used to enhance the work of therapy in various ways. Therapists' own practice of meditation outside therapy can increase therapeutic rapport, focus, and effectiveness with greater ease and success as the process flows more naturally (Rosenthal, 1990). In therapy, contemplative questions can facilitate reflection or respectfully challenge constraining or harmful beliefs. Therapists can encourage clients to practice meditation in a variety of forms, either in or between sessions, according to their spiritual beliefs, preferences, and comfort. Contrary to concerns that fragile clients might experience dissociation, meditation supports integration and wholeness: a clearer knowledge and acceptance of oneself and a deeper connection with others (Bell, 1998). Deep breathing exercises connect mind, body, and spirit (Nhat Hanh, 1991). At the same time therapists are cautioned to proceed slowly and prepare clients for whom painful memories and feelings may emerge, such as survivors of trauma, helping them to hold such experiences in a safe, bounded, and centered way (Barrett, 1999). A therapist might have a client visualize and describe a caring person and interaction from childhood, such as the secure and comforting feeling of being cradled in the arms of a grandmother.

   Therapists can also ask about and encourage spiritual rituals that have been meaningful in a family's past (Imber-Black & Roberts, 1992). They can help clients transform empty rituals into meaningful ones, create new ceremonies, or bridge formal religious differences in an expression of spirituality that is both more personal and transcendent. Including children and elders in rites of passage, especially around loss and disruptive transition, is especially important in their adaptation.

Encouraging Faith-Based Activism

The Reverend Martin Luther King, a guiding spirit to so many oppressed people throughout the world, maintained an abiding faith that social justice will prevail. Yet his was not a passive faith, waiting for a better world to happen. Rather, it was a rallying call of individual and collective action to bring about change. Studies have found that people gain resilience in overcoming adversity and heal from trauma through collaborative efforts to right a wrong or to bring about needed change in larger systems

(Walsh, 1998b). Following her daughter's brutal murder, one mother, consumed by rage and helplessness, did not want to go on living. At her therapist's encouragement, she visited her daughter's grave to seek inspiration for the path ahead. That night, she slept deeply for the first time and awoke "knowing" that her daughter's spirit would want her to forge a larger purpose and benefit to others out of the tragedy. She turned self-destructive feelings into concerted action with other families and community leaders to reduce neighborhood violence. Perry and Rolland (1999) bring this vital dimension of faith-based activism into clinical practice.

Responsiveness to Spiritual Diversity

As societies become increasingly diverse, clinicians have more contact with different faiths and the need to develop a spiritual pluralism with knowledge and respect for varied beliefs and practices. Therapeutic approaches and services need to be sensitive and responsive to this spiritual diversity. Clinicians, especially those from dominant cultural groups, must be cautious not to take their own values as the norm, or be judgmental toward faith differences. Instead, they should seek to understand the meaning and function of faith for each family and its members.

Cultural traditions and spiritual beliefs must be understood and integrated in a holistic approach to mental health and health care (see McGoldrick, Chapter 9; Falicov, Chapter 11, this volume). When one Hmong family from southeast Asia brought a young daughter to a hospital emergency room with a seizure, a cross-cultural crisis ensued (Fadiman, 1997) The family members wanted the daughter's distress alleviated, but they did not want to stop her seizures, which they believed to be sacred trance states signifying positive connection with the spiritual world. As they put it, "The spirit catches you and you fall down." The well-intentioned medical staff obtained a court-ordered removal of the girl from her parents in order to treat her seizures. However, this only heightened her distress and alienated the family, which refused further treatment after the girl's return home, resulting in tragedy. If the health care professionals had tried to understand and work with the spiritual beliefs of the family, instead of taking an adversarial approach, the tragedy might well have been averted.

With growing religious diversity *within* families, therapists may need to take a role somewhat like that of a culture broker (McGoldrick & Giordano, 1996). Where there is conflict or estrangement, therapists can help partners, parents, or extended family members to better understand and respect one another's beliefs and practices. To resolve conflicts, therapists can help members avoid polarization or shift from a stance of "moral superiority" to an acceptance of different spiritual pathways. If a therapist is of the same religion as clients, it can be easier to form a natural rapport. However, one can easily overidentify with them or be hesitant to question beliefs assumed to be fundamental.

Clinical training can encourage therapists to explore their own family religious traditions and reflect on their own spiritual journeys (Roberts, 1999). Therapists may not be knowledgeable about the many, varied religious orientations of clients and are not trained to offer religious counseling. Yet clinical practice can be informed by the emerging literature on common beliefs and practices in families of various faith traditions (see, e.g., Almeida, 1996, on Hindu families; Butler & Harper, 1994, on religious Christian couples; Comas-Diaz, 1981, on Puerto Rican Espiritismo; Cornwall & Thomas, 1990, on Mormon families and communities; Daneshpour, 1998, on Muslim families). McGoldrick (see Chapter 9, this volume) stresses that culturally sensitive practice begins with awareness of the profound influence of core beliefs and an openness to learn from clients. As with other cultural matters, therapists need to openheartedly listen and explore spiritual concerns and beliefs that have profound implications for healing and growth.

NOTE

1. Nearly all reported statistics on religious beliefs and affiliations, in reference works such as *Encyclopedia Brittanica* and *World Almanac,* are obtained from a single source, Gallup Surveys, conducted by the Princeton Religion Research Center, headed by George Gallup, Jr. Quarterly newletters reporting recent polls on paticular topics can be obtained by contacting the Center at 1–609–921–8112.

   Actual membership data reported by Christian church denominations throughout North America are gathered by the National Council of Churches of Christ and are presented in the *Yearbook of American and Canadian Churches 1998,* edited by Eileen Lindner.

REFERENCES

Almeida, R. (1996). Hindu, Christian, and Muslim families. In M. McGoldrick, J. Giordano, & J. Pearce (Eds.), *Ethnicity and family therapy* (2nd ed., pp. 395–423). New York: Guilford Press.

Anderson, H. (1994). The recovery of the soul. In B. Childs & D. Waanders (Eds.), *The treasure in earthen vessels: Explorations in theological anthropology* (pp. 208–223). Louisville, KY: Westminster/John Knox Press.

Anderson, H. (1999). Feet planted firmly in midair: A spirituality for family living. In F. Walsh (Ed.), *Spiritual resources in family therapy* (pp. 157–178). New York: Guilford Press.

Anderson, D. A., & Worthen, D. (1997). Exploring a fourth dimension: Spirituality as a resource for the couple therapist. *Journal of Marital and Family Therapy, 23,* 2–12.

Antonovsky, A. (1987). *Unraveling the mystery of health.* San Francisco: Jossey-Bass.

Aponte, H. (1994). *Bread and spirit: Therapy with the new poor.* New York: Norton.

Aponte, H. (1999). The stresses of poverty and the comfort of spirituality. In F.

Walsh (Ed.), *Spiritual resources in family therapy* (pp. 76–89). New York: Guilford Press.

Ayele, H. (1998, May). Faith and prayer linked to better quality of life. *Proceedings of the American Geriatric Society Annual Meeting.* Seattle, WA.

Barrett, M. J. (1999). Healing from trauma: The quest for spirituality. In F. Walsh (Ed.), *Spiritual resources in family therapy* (pp. 157–178). New York: Guilford Press.

Bateson, G. (1979). *Mind and nature: A necessary unity.* New York: Dutton.

Beavers, W. R., & Hampson, R. B. (1990). *Successful families: Assessment and intervention.* New York: Norton.

Becvar, D. (1996). *Soul Healing: A spiritual orientation in counseling and therapy.* New York: Basic Books.

Becvar, D. (1998) (Ed.). *The family, spirituality, and social work.* Binghamton, NY: Haworth.

Bell, L. G. (1998). Start with meditation. In T. Nelson & T. Trepper (Eds.), *101 interventions in family therapy* (Vol. 2). New York: Haworth.

Bellah, R. N., Madsen, R., Sullivan, W., Swidler, A., & Tipton, S. (1985). *Habits of the heart.* Berkeley: University of California Press.

Berenson, D. (1990). A systemic view of spirituality: God and twelve step programs as resources in family therapy. *Journal of Strategic and Systemic Therapies.*

Bergin, A. E. (1991). Values and religious issues in psychotherapy and mental health. *American Psychologist, 46,* 394–403.

Billingsley, A. (1992). *Climbing Jacob's ladder: The enduring legacy of African-American families.* New York: Simon & Schuster.

Bohannon, J. R. (1991). Religiosity related to grief levels of bereaved mothers and fathers. *Omega, 23,* 153–159.

Boszormenyi-Nagy, I. (1987). *Foundations of contextual family therapy.* New York: Brunner/Mazel.

Bottoms, B. L., Shaver, P. R., Goodman, G. S., & Qin, J. (1995). In the name of God: A profile of religion-related child abuse. *Journal of Social Issues, 51,* 85–111.

Bowman, M. (1983, November/December). Why we burn: Sexism exorcised. *The Humanist,* 28–29.

Boyd-Franklin, N., & Lockwood, T. W. (1999). Spirituality and religion: Implications for psychotherapy with African American clients and families. In F. Walsh (Ed.), *Spiritual resources in family therapy* (pp. 90–103). New York: Guilford Press.

Bridges, R. A., & Spilka, B. (1992). Religion and the mental health of women. In J. F. Schumaker (Ed.), *Religion and mental health* (pp. 43–53). New York: Oxford University Press.

Brook, G. (1995). *Nine parts of desire: The hidden world of Islamic women.* New York: Anchor Books.

Browning, D. S., Miller-McLemore, B., Couture, P., Lyon, K., & Franklin, R. (1977). *From culture wars to common ground: Religion and the American family.* Louisville, KY: Westminster Press/John Knox Press.

Browning, D. S., Miller-McLemore, B., Couture, P., Lyon, K., & Franklin, R. (2001). *From culture wars to common ground: Religion and the American family* (2nd ed.). Louisville, KY: Westminster Press/John Knox Press.

Buber, M. (1970). *I and thou.* New York: Charles Scribner's Sons. (Original published in 1921)

Burton, L. A. (1992). *Religion and the family: When God helps.* New York: Haworth Press.

Butler, M. H., & Harper, J. M. (1994). The divine triangle: God in the marital system of religious couples. *Family Process, 33,* 277–286.

Campbell, J., & Moyers, B. (1988). *The power of myth.* New York: Doubleday.

Chamberlain, K., & Zika, S. (1992). Religiosity, meaning in life, and psychological well-being. In J. F. Schumaker (Ed.), *Religion and mental health* (pp. 138–148). New York: Oxford University Press.

Coles, R. (1990). *The spiritual life of children.* Boston: Houghton Mifflin.

Coles, R. (1997). *The moral intelligence of children.* New York: Random House.

Comas-Diaz, L. (1981). Puerto Rican Espiritismo and psychotherapy. *American Journal of Orthopsychiatry, 51,* 636–645.

Cornwall, M., & Thomas, D. L. (1990). Family, religion, and personal communities: Examples from Mormonism. *Marriage and Family Review, 15,* 229–252.

Dallos, R. (1991). *Family belief systems, therapy, and change.* Philadelphia: Open University Press.

Daneshpour, M. (1998). Muslim families and family therapy. *Journal of Marital and Family Therapy, 24,* 355–368.

D'Antonio, W. V., Newman, W. M., & Wright, S. A. (1982). Religion and family life: How social scientists view the relationship. *Journal for the Scientific Study of Religion, 21,* 218–225.

Deloria, V., Jr. (1994). *God is red: A native view of religion* (2nd. ed.). Golden, CO: Fulcrum.

Doherty, W. J. (1995). *Soul searching: Why psychotherapy must promote moral responsibility.* New York: Basic Books.

Doherty, W. J. (1999). Morality and spirituality in therapy. In F. Walsh (Ed.), *Spiritual resources in family therapy* (pp. 179–192). New York: Guilford Press.

Domino, G., & Miller, K. (1992). Religiosity and attitudes toward suicide. *Omega, 25,* 271–282.

Dossey, L. (1993). *Healing words: The power of prayer and the practice of medicine.* San Francisco: Harper.

Elkind, D. (1971). The development of religious understanding in children and adolescents. In M. P. Strommen (Ed.), *Research of religious development* (pp. 655–685), New York: Hawthorn Books.

Ellison, C. G., & Levin, J. S. (1998). The religion-health connection: Evidence, theory, and future directions. *Health Education and Behavior, 25,* 700–720.

Erikson, E. H., Erikson, J. M., & Kivnick, H. Q. (1986). *Vital involvement in old age.* New York: Norton.

Fadiman, A. (1997). *The spirit catches you and you fall down.* San Francisco: Ferrer.

Falicov, C. (1995). Cross-cultural marriages. In N. Jacobson & A. Gurman (Eds.), *Clinical handbook of couple therapy* (Vol. 3, pp. 231–246). New York: Guilford Press.

Falicov, C. (1999). Religion and spiritual folk traditions in immigrant families: Therapeutic resources with Latinos. In F. Walsh (Ed.), *Spiritual resources in family therapy* (pp. 104–120). New York: Guilford Press.

Fishbane, M. (1998). I, thou, and we: A dialogical approach to couple's therapy. *Journal of Marital and Family Therapy, 24,* 41–58.

Fishbane, M. D. (1999). Honor thy father and thy mother. In F. Walsh (Ed.), *Spiritual resources in family therapy* (pp. 136–156). New York: Guilford Press.

Forster, B., & Tabachnik, J. (1993). Jews-by-choice: Conversion factors and outcomes. In M. Lynn & D. Moberg (Eds.), *Research in the social scientific study of religion* (Vol. 5, pp. 123–155). Greenwich, CT: JAI Press.

Fortunato, J. (1982). *Embracing the exile: Healing journeys of gay Christians*. San Francisco: HarperCollins.

Frankl, V. (1984). *Man's search for meaning*. New York: Simon & Schuster. (Original published in 1946)

Friedman, E. H. (1985). *Generation to generation: Family process in church and synagogue*. New York: Guilford Press.

Galanter, M. (1989). *Cults and new religious movements*. Washington, DC: American Psychological Association.

Gallup, Jr., G. (Ed.). (1996). *Religion in America: 1996 report*. Princeton, NJ: Princeton Religion Research Center.

Gallup, G., Jr., & Lindsey, D. M. (1999). *Surveying the religious landscape: Trends in U. S. beliefs*. Harrisburg, PA: Morehouse.

Gartner, J., Larson, D. B., & Allen, G. D. (1991). Religious commitment and mental health: A review of the empirical literature. *Journal of Psychology and Theology, 19*, 6–25.

Gaustad, E. S. (1966). *A religious history of America* (rev. ed.). San Francisco: Harper & Row.

Gilbert, K. (1992). Religion as a resource for bereaved parents. *Journal of Religion and Health, 31*, 19–30.

Gilligan, C. (1982). *In a different voice: Psychological theory and women's development*. Cambridge, MA: Harvard University Press.

God in America [Special issue]. (1998). *Life, 21*(13).

Gorsuch, R. L. (1995). Religious aspects of substance abuse and recovery. *Journal of Social Issues, 51*, 65–83.

Greeley, A. (1969). *Why can't they be all like us?* New York: American Jewish Committee.

Griffith, J. L. (1986). Employing the God–family relationship with religious families. *Family Process, 25*, 609–618.

Griffith, J. L., & Griffith, M. E. (2001). *Encountering the sacred in psychotherapy: How to talk with people about their spiritual lives*. New York: Guilford Press.

Griffith, M. E. (1999). Opening therapy to conversations with a personal God. In F. Walsh (Ed.), *Spiritual resources in family therapy* (pp. 209–222). New York: Guilford Press.

Hargrave, T. (1994). *Families and forgiveness*. New York: Brunner/Mazel.

Higgins, G. O. (1994). *Resilient adults: Overcoming a cruel past*. San Francisco: Jossey-Bass.

Hochschild, A. (1997). *Time bind*. New York: Holt.

Hood, R. W., Spilka, B., Hunsberger, B., & Gorsuch, R. (1996). *The psychology of religion: An empirical approach* (2nd. ed.). New York: Guilford Press.

Huddleston, J. (1999). *The earth is but one country* (4th ed.) New Delhi: Baha'i Publishing Trust.

Imber-Black, E., & Roberts, J. (1992). *Rituals for our times: Celebrating, healing, and changing our lives and our relationships*. New York: HarperCollins.

Kabat-Zinn, J. (1990). *Full catastrophe living: Using the wisdom of your mind and body to face stress, pain, and illness*. New York: Dell.

Kramer, S. Z. (1995). *Transforming the inner and outer family: Humanistic and spiritual approaches to mind–body systems therapy*. New York: Haworth.

Koenig, H., George, L., Hays, J. Larson, D., Cohen, H., & Blazer, D. (1998). The relationship between religious activities and blood pressure in older adults. *International Journal of Psychiatry, 28,* 189–213.

Laird, J., & Green, R. -J. (Eds.). (1996). *Lesbians and gays in families and family therapy.* San Francisco: Jossey-Bass.

Lerner, M. (1994). *Jewish renewal: A path to healing and transformation.* New York: Putnam.

Lifton, R. J. (1993). *The protean self: Human resilience in an age of fragmentation.* New York: Basic Books.

Lindner, E. W. (1998). *Yearbook of American and Canadian churches 1998* (66th ed.). Nashville: Abingdon Press.

Mahmoud, V. (1996). African American Muslim families. In M. McGoldrick, J. Giordano, & J. Pearce (Eds.), *Ethnicity and family therapy* (pp. 112–128). New York: Guilford Press.

Markowitz, L. (1998). Essential conversations: Raising the sacred in therapy. *In the family, 3*(3), 7–13.

Mbiti, J. S. (1970). *African religions and philosophy.* Garden City, NY: Anchor Books.

McCourt, F. (1998, December). God in America: When you think of God, what do you see? *Life, 21*(13), 60–74.

McGoldrick, M., Gerson, R., & Shellenberger, S. (1998). *Genograms: Assessment and intervention* (2nd. ed.). New York: Norton.

McGoldrick, M. & Giordano, J. (1996). Overview. In M. McGoldrick, J. Giordano, & J. K. Pearce (Eds.), *Ethnicity and family therapy* (pp. 1–28). New York: Guilford Press.

Minnick, A. M. (1997). *Twelve step programs: Contemporary American quest for meaning and spiritual renewal.* New York: Praeger.

Minuchin, S. (1992). *Family healing: Strategies for hope and understanding.* New York: MacMillan.

Moore, T. (1992). *Care of the soul: A guide for cultivating depth and sacredness in everyday life.* New York: HarperCollins.

Nakhaima, J. M., & Dicks, B. H. (1995). Social work practice with religious families. *Families in Society: Journal of Contemporary Human Services, 76,* 360–368.

Nhat Hahn, T. (1991). *Peace is every step: The path of mindfulness in everyday life.* New York: Bantam Books.

O'Neil, C., & Ritter, K. (1992). *Coming out within: Stages of spiritual awakening for lesbians and gay men.* New York: HarperCollins.

Oxman, T. E., Freeman, D. H., & Manheimer, E. D. (1995). Lack of social participation or religious strength and comfort as risk factors for death after cardiac surgery in the elderly. *Psychosomatic Medicine, 57,* 5–15.

Perry, A. D. V., & Rolland, J. S. (1999). Spirituality expressed in community action and social justice: A therapeutic means to liberation and hope. In F. Walsh (Ed.), *Spiritual resources in family therapy* (pp. 272–292). New York: Guilford Press.

Peteet, J. R. (1993). A closer look at a spiritual approach in addictions treatment. *Journal of Substance Abuse Treatment, 10,* 263–267.

Pipher, M. (1997). *The shelter of each other: Rebuilding our families.* New York: Ballantine.

Prest, L. A., & Keller, J. F. (1993). Spirituality and family therapy: Spiritual beliefs, myths, and metaphors. *Journal of Marital and Family Therapy, 19,* 137–148.

Roberts, J. (1999). Heart and soul: Spirituality, religion, and rituals in family therapy training. In F. Walsh (Ed.), *Spiritual resources in family therapy* (pp. 256–271). New York: Guilford Press.

Rosen, E. J., & Weltman, S. F. (1996). Jewish families: An overview. In M. McGoldrick, J. Giordano, & J. Pearce (Eds.), *Ethnicity and family therapy* (pp. 611–630). New York: Guilford Press.

Rosenthal, J. (1990). The meditative therapist. *Family Therapy Networker, 14,* 38–41, 70–71.

Rotz, E., Russell, C. S., & Wright, D. W. (1993). The therapist who is perceived as "spiritually" correct: Strategies for avoiding collusion with the "spiritually one-up" spouse. *Journal of Marital and Family Therapy, 19,* 369–375.

Satir, V. (1988). *Peoplemaking.* Palo Alto, CA: Science and Behavior Books. (Original published in 1977)

Shafranske, E. P. (Ed.). (1996). *Religion in the clinical practice of psychology.* Washington, DC: American Psychological Association Press.

Shorto, (December 7, 1997). *The New York Times Magazine,* p. 61.

Smith, H. (1991). *The world's religions: Our great wisdom traditions* (rev. ed.) New York: HarperCollins.

Some, M. P. (1994). *The healing wisdom of Africa.* New York: Tarcher/Putnam.

Stacey, J. (1996). *In the name of the family: Rethinking family values in the postmodern age.* Boston: Beacon Press.

Stander, V., Piercy, F. P., MacKinnon, D., & Helmeke, K. (1994). Spirituality, religion, and family therapy: Competing or complementary worlds? *American Journal of Family Therapy, 22,* 27–41.

Steere, D. A. (1997). *Spiritual practice in psychotherapy: A guide for caregivers.* New York: Brunner/Mazel.

Stewart, S. P., & Gale, J. E. (1994). On hallowed ground: Marital therapy with couples on the religious right. *Journal of Systemic Therapies, 13,* 16–25.

Stinnett, N., & DeFrain, J. (1985). *Secrets of strong families.* Boston: Little, Brown.

Walker, A. (1997). *Anything we love can be saved: A writer's activism.* New York: Random House.

Walsh, F. (1998a). Beliefs, spirituality, and transcendence: Keys to family resilience. In M. McGoldrick (Ed.), *Re-visioning family therapy* (pp. 62–77). New York: Guilford Press.

Walsh, F. (1998b). *Strengthening family resilience.* New York: Guilford Press.

Walsh, F. (1998c). Families in later life: Challenges and opportunities. In B. Carter & M. McGoldrick (Eds.), *The expanded family life cycle* (3rd. ed., pp. 307–326). Needham Heights, MA: Allyn & Bacon.

Walsh, F. (1999a). Religion and spirituality: Wellsprings for healing and resilience. In F. Walsh (Ed.), *Spiritual resources in family therapy* (pp. 3–27). New York: Guilford Press.

Walsh, F. (1999b). Opening family therapy to spirituality. In F. Walsh (Ed.), *Spiritual resources in family therapy* (pp. 28–58). New York: Guilford Press.

Walsh, F. (Ed.). (1999c). *Spiritual resources in family therapy.* New York: Guilford Press.

Walsh, F., & McGoldrick, M. (1991). *Living beyond loss: Death in the family.* New York: Norton.

Weaver, A. J., Koenig, H. G., & Larsen, D. B. (1997). Marriage and family therapists and the clergy: A need for clinical collaboration, training, and research. *Journal of Marital and Family Therapy, 23,* 13–25.

Weil, A. (1994). *Spontaneous healing.* New York: Knopf.

Werner, E. E., & Smith, R. S. (1992). *Overcoming the odds: High risk children from birth to adulthood.* Ithaca, NY: Cornell University Press.

Whipple, V. (1987). Counseling battered women from fundamentalist churches. *Journal of Marital and Family Therapy, 13,* 251–258.

Wolin, S. J., Muller, W., Taylor, F., & Wolin, S. (1999). Three spiritual perspectives on resilience: Buddhism, Christianity, and Judaism. In F. Walsh (Ed.), *Spiritual resources in family therapy* (pp. 121–135). New York: Guilford Press.

Woolfolk, R. (1998). *The cure of souls: Science, values, and psychotherapy.* San Francisco: Jossey-Bass.

Worthington, E. L., Jr. (1989). Religious faith across the lifespan: Implications for counseling and research. *Counseling Psychologist, 17,* 555–612.

Wright, L., Watson, W. L., & Bell, J. M. (1996). *Beliefs: The heart of healing in families and illness.* New York: Basic Books.

PART IV

Developmental Perspectives on Family Functioning

CHAPTER 14

THE FAMILY
LIFE CYCLE

Monica McGoldrick
Betty Carter

W e are born into families. We develop, grow, and hopefully die in the context of our families. Our problems are framed by the formative course of our family's past, the present tasks it is trying to master, and the future to which it aspires. Embedded within the larger sociopolitical culture, the family life cycle is the natural context within which to frame individual identity and development, and to account for the effects of the social system (Carter & McGoldrick, 1999a; McGoldrick & Carter, 1999a).

Until recently, therapists and researchers have paid little attention to the family life cycle and its impact on human development (Carter & McGoldrick, 1999b). Even now, most psychological theories relate at most to the nuclear family, ignoring the multigenerational context of family connections that pattern our lives over time. But our dramatically changing family patterns, which can assume many varied configurations over the lifespan, are forcing us to take a broader view of both development and normalcy. It is becoming increasingly difficult to determine what family life-cycle patterns are "normal," which causes great stress for family members, who have few consensually validated models to guide the passages they must negotiate. Furthermore, in our rapidly changing world, we are having to recognize that life-cycle definitions and norms are relative, depending on the sociocultural context (Hines, 1999; Hines, Garcia-Preto, McGoldrick, Almeida, & Weltman, 1999; Falicov, 1999; Kliman & Madsen, 1999; Johnson & Colucci, 1999)

Just as the texture of life has become a more complicated fabric, so too must research and therapeutic models change to reflect this complexity, appreciating both the context around the individual as a shaping environment and the evolutionary effect of time on human development. From a family life-cycle perspective, symptoms and dysfunction are examined within a systemic context and in relation to what the culture considers "normal" functioning over time. From this perspective, therapeutic interventions aim at helping to reestablish the family's developmental momentum, so that it can proceed forward to foster each member's development.

THE FAMILY AS A SYSTEM MOVING THROUGH TIME

Families comprise persons who have a shared history and a shared future. They encompass the entire emotional system of at least three and frequently four or even five generations, held together by blood, legal, and/or historical ties. Relationships with parents, siblings, and other family members go through transitions as they move along the life cycle. Boundaries shift, psychological distance among members changes, and roles within and between subsystems are constantly being redefined. It is extremely difficult, however, to think of the family as a whole because of the complexity involved. As a system moving through time, the family has basically different properties from all other systems. Unlike all other organizations, families incorporate new members only by birth, adoption, commitment, or marriage, and members can leave only by death, if then. No other system is subject to these constraints. A business organization can fire members it views as dysfunctional, or, conversely, members can resign if the structure and values of the organization are not to their liking. In families, however, the pressures of membership with no exit available can, in the extreme, lead to psychosis. In nonfamily systems, the roles and functions of the system are carried out in a more or less stable way by replacement of those who leave for any reason, and people move on into other organizations. Although families also have roles and functions, the main value in families is the relationships, which are irreplaceable. If a parent leaves or dies, another person can be brought in to fill a parenting function, but this person can never replace the parent in his or her personal emotional aspects. Even in situations such as a divorcing couple without children, the bonds linger, so that it is difficult to hear of an ex-spouse's death without being shaken.

In our times, people often act as if they can choose membership and responsibility in a family. In fact, there is very little choice about whom we are related to in the complex web of family ties. Children, for example, have no choice about being born into a system, nor do parents have a choice, once children are born, adopted, or fostered, as to the existence of the responsibilities of parenthood, even if they neglect these responsibilities. In fact, no family relationships except marriage or committed partnerships are entered into by choice. Even in those cases, the freedom to choose whomever one wishes is a rather recent option, and the decision to marry is probably much less freely made than people usually recognize at the time (McGoldrick, 1999a). Although partners can choose not to continue a marriage relationship, they remain coparents of their children, and the former marriage continues to be acknowledged with the designation "ex-spouse." People cannot alter whom they are related to in the complex web of family ties over all the generations. Obviously, family members frequently act as if this were not so—they cut each other off because of conflicts, or they claim to have "nothing in common"—but when family members act as if family relationships are optional, they do so to the detriment of their own sense of identity and the richness of their emotional and social context.

Despite the current dominant American pattern of nuclear families living on their own and often at great geographical distance from extended family members, they are still emotional subsystems that react to past, present, and anticipated future relationships within the larger multigenerational family system. The many options and decisions to be made can be confusing: whether or whom to marry, where to live, how many children to have, if any, how to conduct relationships within the immediate and extended family, and how to allocate family tasks. As Hess and Waring (1984) observed:

> As we moved from the family of obligatory ties to one of voluntary bonds, relationships outside the nuclear unit (as well as those inside it) . . . lost whatever normative certainty or consistency governed them at earlier times. For example, sibling relationships today are almost completely voluntary, subject to disruption through occupational and geographic mobility, as indeed might be said of marriage itself. (p. 303)

Spiritual and cultural factors also play a major role in how families go through the life cycle (Walsh, 1999; Hines, Garcia-Preto, McGoldrick, Almeida, & Weltman, 1999). Not only do cultural groups vary greatly in their breakdown of family life-cycle stages and definitions of the tasks at each stage, but also it is clear that even several generations after immigration, the family life-cycle patterns of groups differ markedly (Hernandez & McGoldrick, 1999; McGoldrick, Giordano, & Pearce, 1996). Furthermore, families' motion through the life cycle is profoundly influenced by the historical era in which they are living (Elder, 1992; Neugarten, 1979). Family members' worldviews, including their attitudes toward life-cycle transitions, are profoundly influenced by the time in history in which they have grown up. People who lived through the Great Depression, who came of age during the Vietnam War, who experienced the black migration to the north in the 1940s, who grew up in the 1950s "baby boomer" generation—all these cohorts have profoundly different orientations to the meaning of life, influenced by the eras in which they lived (Elder, 1986).

We must also pay close attention to the enormous anxiety generated by the chronic, unremitting stresses of poverty and discrimination, especially as the economic and racial divide in our society widens. At the millennium, as the conservative crusade for so-called "family values" intensified, it became necessary to evaluate the stress for families, especially women, caused by the relentless criticism of working mothers (Crittenden, 2001), the attacks on abortion rights, and the stigmatization of divorced, gay and lesbian families, and unmarried mothers and their children. The era of the traditional, stable multigenerational extended family of yore should not be romanticized as a time when mutual respect and satisfaction existed between the generations. It was supported by sexism, classism, racism, and heterosexism. In this traditional patriarchal family structure, respect for parents and obligations to care for elders were based on control of the resources, reinforced by religious and secular sanctions against those who did not conform to the normative standards of the dominant group. Now, with the increasing ability of younger family members to determine their own fate in marriage, work, and economic security, the power of elders to demand filial piety is reduced. As women are now demanding lives of their own, whereas before, their roles were limited primarily to the caretaking of others, our social institutions are being pressed to fit with these changing needs. But these institutions lag far behind.

In different cultures and classes, the ages of multigenerational transitions differ markedly. Indeed, the stages of the life cycle are rather arbitrary breakdowns. The notion of childhood has been described as the invention of 18th-century Western society, and adolescence as the invention of the 19th century (Aries, 1962), related to the cultural, economic, and political contexts of those eras. The notion of young adulthood as a separate phase appears to be an invention of the 20th century, and that of women as individuals, of the late 20th century. The lengthy phases of the empty nest and older age are also primarily developments of the 20th century, brought about by the smaller number of children and the longer lifespan in our era. Given the current changes in the family, the 21st century may become known for developing the norms of serial marriage and unmarried parenthood as part of the life cycle process. In all other contemporary cultures, and during virtually all other historical eras, the breakdown of life-cycle stages has differed from our current definitions. To add to this complexity, cohorts born and living through various periods differ in fertility, mortality, acceptable gender roles, migration patterns, education, needs and resources, and attitudes toward family and aging.

Families characteristically lack time perspective when they are having problems. They tend generally to magnify the present moment, overwhelmed and immobilized by their immediate feelings, or they become fixed on a moment in the future that they dread or desire. They lose the awareness that life means continual motion from the past and into the future, with a continual transformation of familial relationships. As the sense of motion becomes lost or distorted, therapy involves restoring a sense of life as process and movement from one state toward another.

UNDERSTANDING THE LIFE CYCLE: THE INDIVIDUAL, THE FAMILY, THE CULTURE

To understand how people evolve, we must examine their lives within the context of both the family and larger cultural contexts, which change over time. Because "the family" is no longer organized solely around a married heterosexual couple raising their children, but rather many various structures with different organizing principles, our job of identifying family stages and emotional tasks of the life cycle is much more complex. But even within the diversity of family forms, we have used some unifying principles that define stages and tasks, such as the emotional disequilibrium generated by adding and losing family members during life's many transitions (Hadley, Jacob, Milliones, Caplan, & Spitz, 1974; Ahrons & Rodgers, 1987; Ahrons, 1999; McGoldrick & Carter, 1999b).

Each system (individual, family, and cultural) can be represented schematically (see Figure 14.1) along two time dimensions: one is historical (the vertical axis), and the other is developmental and unfolding (the

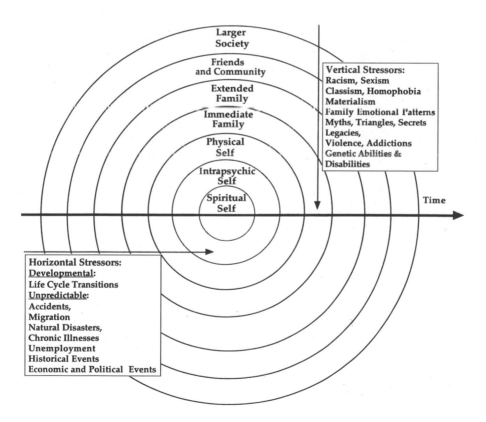

FIGURE 14.1. The context for assessing problems.

horizontal axis). For the individual, the vertical axis includes the biological heritage and intricate programming of behaviors with one's given temperament, possible congenital disabilities, and genetic makeup. The horizontal axis relates to the individual's emotional, cognitive, interpersonal, and physical development over the lifespan within a specific sociohistorical context. Over time, the individual's inherent qualities can either become crystallized into rigid behaviors or elaborated into broader and more flexible repertoires (Walsh, 1998). Certain individual stages may be more difficult to master, depending on one's innate characteristics and the influence of the environment.

At the family level (Carter, 1978), the vertical axis includes the family history and the patterns of relating and functioning transmitted down the generations, primarily through the mechanism of emotional triangling (Bowen, 1978). It includes all the family attitudes, taboos, expectations, labels, and loaded issues with which we grow up. These aspects of our lives are the hand we are dealt. What we do with them is the question. The horizontal flow at a family level describes the family as it moves through time, coping with the changes and transitions of the family's life cycle. This includes both the predictable developmental stresses and those unpredictable events, "the slings and arrows of outrageous fortune," that may disrupt the life-cycle process—untimely death, birth of a handicapped child, chronic illness, job loss, and so on.

At a sociocultural level, the vertical axis includes cultural and societal history, stereotypes, patterns of power, privilege and oppression, social hierarchies, and beliefs that have been passed down through the generations. A group's history, and particularly its legacy of trauma will influence families and individuals as they go through life (e.g., effects of the Holocaust on Jews and Germans; slavery on African Americans and on colonizing, slave-owning groups; homophobic crimes on homosexuals and heterosexuals). The horizontal axis relates to community connections, current events, and social policy as they impact the family and the individual at a given time, including the consequences in people's present lives of the society's "inherited" (vertical) norms of racism, sexism, classism, and homophobia, as well as ethnic and religious prejudices manifested in social, political, and economic structures that limit the options of some and support the power of others.

ANXIETY AND SYMPTOM DEVELOPMENT

As families move along, stress is often greatest at transition points from one stage to another in the developmental process as families rebalance, redefine, and realign their relationships. Hadley and his colleagues (1974) found that symptom onset correlates significantly with the normal family developmental process of addition and loss of family members (e.g., birth, marriage, divorce, remarriage, death, launching). The clinical method of

Murray Bowen (1978) tracks patterns through the family life cycle over several generations, focusing especially on nodel events and transition points to understand dysfunction at the present moment. There is the strong implication that emotional issues and developmental tasks not resolved at appropriate stages will be carried along as hindrances in future transitions and relationships (Carter & McGoldrick, 1999a). Given enough stress on the horizontal developmental axis, any family can appear extremely dysfunctional. Even a small horizontal stress on a family in which the vertical axis is full of intense stress will create great disruption in the system. The anxiety engendered on the vertical and horizontal axes where they converge, as well as the interaction of the various systems and how they work together to support or impede one another, are the key determinants of how well the family will manage its transitions through life. It becomes imperative, therefore, to assess not only the dimensions of the current life-cycle stress but also their connections to family themes and triangles coming down in the family over historical time. Although all normative change is to some degree stressful, when the horizontal (developmental) stress intersects with a vertical (transgenerational) stress, there tends to be a quantum leap in anxiety in the system (Carter, 1978). If, to give a global example, one's parents were basically pleased to be parents and handled the job without too much anxiety, the birth of the first child will produce only the normal stresses of a system expanding its boundaries. If, on the other hand, parenting was a loaded issue in the family of origin of one or both spouses, and has not been dealt with, the transition to parenthood may produce heightened anxiety for the couple. Even without any outstanding family-of-origin issues, the inclusion of a child could potentially tax a system if there is a mismatch between the child's temperament and those of the parents. Or if a child is conceived in a time of great political upheaval, forcing a family to leave its roots and culture, and migrate to another country, then the child's birth may carry with it unresolved issues.

THE CHANGING STRUCTURE OF FAMILIES

The dramatic changes in families in the United States have been described in the overview section of this book (see Walsh, Chapters 1 and 2, this volume). These changes cannot be overestimated. It is time for us as professionals to give up our attachments to the old ideals and put a more positive conceptual frame around what is: two-paycheck marriages; permanent "single-parent" households; unmarried, remarried, and gay and lesbian couples and families; single-parent adoptions; and women of all ages alone. It is past time to stop thinking of transitional crises as permanent traumas, and to drop from our vocabulary words and phrases that link us to the norms and prejudices of the past: "children of divorce," "out-of-wedlock child," "fatherless home," "working mother," and the like.

INDIVIDUAL DEVELOPMENT IN CONTEXT

Our models of individual development have been built on Freud's and Erikson's ideas of psychosocial development. Compared to Freud's narrow focus on body zones, Erikson's (1968) conceptualization of eight stages of "human" development, which actually equated human development with male development (Broverman, Vogel, Broverman, Clarkson, & Rosenkrantz, 1972), were an effort to highlight the interaction of the developing child with society. However, what Erikson's stages actually emphasize are not interdependence and the connectedness of individuals in relationships, but rather the development of individual characteristics (mostly traits of autonomy) in response to the demands of social interaction (Erikson, 1968). Thus, trust, autonomy, industry, and the formulation of an identity separate from *his* family are supposed to carry a child to young adulthood, where *he* is then presumed to know how to love, go through a middle age of caring, and develop the wisdom of aging. This discontinuity—a childhood and adolescence focused on developing one's own autonomy, supposedly in preparation for an adulthood of intimacy, caring and wisdom—is problematic as a template for "normal" human development (McGoldrick & Carter, 1999a).

Michael Kimmel, a sociologist and spokesman for the National Organization for Men Against Sexism (NOMAS) holds out to men the ideal of "democratic manhood," which "requires both private and public commitments—changing ourselves, nurturing our relationships, cherishing our families, to be sure, but also reforming the public arena to enlarge the possibilities for other people to do the same"(1996, p. 334). Kimmel welcomes feminism, gay liberation and multiculturalism as blueprints for the reconstruction of masculinity. He believes men's lives will be healed only when there is full equality for everyone.

Before feminist contributions to the developmental literature (Dinnerstein, 1976; Miller, 1976; Gilligan, 1982; McGoldrick, 1999a), most male theoreticians, such as Freud, Kohlberg, Erikson, and Piaget, tended to ignore female development or subsume it under male development, which was taken as the standard for human functioning (Notman, Klein, Jordan, & Zilbach, 1991; Broverman et al., 1972; Tavris, 1992). Separation and autonomy have been considered the primary values for male development, with values of caring and attachment, interdependence, relationship, and attention to context being primary in female development. However, we believe that all healthy development requires finding an optimal balance between connectedness and separateness, belonging and individuation, accommodation and autonomy. In general, developmental theories have failed to describe the progression of individuals in relationships toward a maturity of interdependence. Yet human identity is inextricably bound up in one's relationship with others, and the notion of complete autonomy is a fiction. Human beings cannot exist in isolation, and the most important aspects of human experience are relational.

Most developmental theorists, including feminists, have espoused psychodynamic assumptions about autonomy and separation, overfocusing on relationships with mothers as the primary factor in human development. They have assumed that masculine identity is achieved by separating from one's mother and feminine identity, by identification and attachment to her. Silverstein (1994) effectively challenged this assumption that male development requires separating from one's mother. Gilligan (1982) critiqued Piaget's conception of morality as being tied to the understanding of rights and rules, suggesting that, for females, moral development centers around the understanding of responsibility and relationships, whereas Piaget's description fits the traditional male socialization focus on autonomy (Green, 1998; McGoldrick & Carter, 1999a; Rosen, 1999). Maccoby (1990) and Miller (1976) have expanded our understandings of the power dimensions in the social context of development, suggesting a broader conception of development for both males and females.

Developing a schema that would enhance all human development by including milestones of both autonomy and emotional connectedness for both males and females from earliest childhood has drawn us, not surprisingly, to the work of those whose perspectives go beyond white male development. These include Hale-Benson (1986), who explored the multiple intelligences and other developmental features she identified in African American children; Almeida, Woods, and Messineo (1998), who have articulated a very broad-based cultural conception of human development; Comer and Poussaint (1992), who have factored racism and its effects into their blueprint for development of healthy black children; Canino and Spurlock (1994), who outline many ways that minority ethnic groups socialize their children; and the work of Borysenko (1996), whose descriptions of the stages of female development appear to have universal applicability for both males and females from all cultural groups. Borysenko's outline reflects the human need for responsible autonomy, which recent decades have granted in some measure to females, and emphasizes the importance of understanding interdependence, a concept that girls and children of color learn early, but that has been ignored in traditional Anglo-American views of male development.

NORMAL FAMILY PROCESSES IN CONTEXT

If the ideas of life-cycle norms are applied too rigidly, they lead to an anxiety that deviating from the norms is pathological. The opposite pitfall, overemphasizing the uniqueness of the "brave new world" faced by each new generation, can create a sense of historical discontinuity, devaluing the role of parenthood and the relationship between the generations. Our aim is to provide a view of the life cycle in terms of intergenerational connectedness in the family, for this is one of our greatest resources. This is not meant to oversimplify the complexity of life's transitions or to encourage stereotyping by promoting classifications of "normality" that constrict our view of human life but, rather, to expand clinicians' views of family problems and strengths.

Our classification of family life-cycle stages of American middle-class families in the beginning of the 21st century highlights our view that the central underlying processes to be negotiated are the expansion, contraction, and realignment of the relationship system to support the entry, exit, and development of family members in a functional way. Generally speaking, major life-cycle transitions require a fundamental change in the system itself rather than just incremental changes or rearrangements of the system, which go on continually throughout life. We do not see individual or family stages as "inherently" age-related (e.g., Levinson, 1978) or dependent on the structure of the traditional family (e.g., Duvall, 1977). Nor do we view healthy maturation as requiring a single sequential pathway through marriage and child rearing. We hold a pluralistic view, recognizing many valid, healthy options and relationships over the life course, in contrast to traditional views that not marrying is an "immature" choice or that women who do not have children are unfulfilled.

BETWEEN FAMILIES: YOUNG ADULTHOOD

Unlike traditional sociological depictions of the family life cycle as commencing at marriage and ending with the death of one spouse, we begin the family life cycle at the stage of "young adulthood." The primary task for this period is that young adults come to terms with their family of origin—a powerful shaper of reality, influencing who, when, how, and whether they will marry and how they will carry out all succeeding stages of the family life cycle. Adequate completion of this stage requires that the young adult separate from the family of origin without cutting off or fleeing reactively to a substitute emotional refuge. This phase is a cornerstone. It is a time to formulate personal life goals and to become a "self " before joining with another to form a new family subsystem. The more adequately young adults can differentiate themselves from the emotional program of the family of origin at this phase, the fewer vertical stressors will follow them through their new family life cycle. This is the chance for them to sort out emotionally what they will take along from the family of origin, what they will leave behind, and what they will create for themselves.

Young adults may remain in an overly dependent position, unable to leave home, or they may rebel, breaking away in a pseudoindependent cutoff from their parents and families. Whereas for women the problems at this stage more often focus on short-circuiting their definition of themselves in favor of finding and accommodating to a mate, men more often have difficulty committing themselves in relationships, forming instead an incomplete identity focused around work.

Only when the generations can shift their hierarchical relations and reconnect in a new way can the family move on developmentally. An increasing problem at this phase is the prolonged dependency that our technological society requires in order to prepare young adults for the work world, long after they would traditionally have been launched, and long after they have usually begun having intimate couple relationships. This creates a difficult situation for both parents and children, who will have difficulty establishing appropriate boundaries, because it is almost impossible to be emotionally independent when still financially dependent and in the socially ambiguous status of student.

Working with families at this phase of the life cycle is particularly rewarding because of the new options that are opened when young adults are able to move toward new life patterns. At this stage, young men can be encouraged to develop themselves emotionally and expressively, exploring their connections with family and others. For men who have had few male role models or minimal relationships with their fathers, this is a time to reconnect. Because men's socialization so often does not facilitate their learning to have intimacy even in friendship, this period can be a keystone also for being proactive about the kind of friendships they want to nurture in life. It is important to help men make connections with other men in and outside their families, without having to forsake their mothers or devalue women. Interventions directed at helping young people reevaluate the gender roles of their parents and grandparents, so that they do not replicate previous relationships of inequality or dysfunction, may be especially valuable at this crucial formative phase. For both men and women, it is important to outline all the unrecognized work that their mothers and grandmothers did to raise their families and keep a household going, in order to emphasize their courage, abilities, hard work, and strengths as role models, because mothers are too often devalued and their contributions are typically hidden from history (herstory!). In general, both men and women can be helped to draw strength from each of their parents.

THE JOINING OF FAMILIES IN MARRIAGE: THE YOUNG COUPLE

The changing role of women, the frequent marriage of partners from widely different cultural backgrounds, and the increasing physical distances between family members place a much greater burden on couples to define their relationship for themselves than was true in traditional and precedent-bound family structures (McGoldrick, 1999a). Although any two family systems always have different patterns and expectations, in our present culture, couples are less bound by family traditions and freer than ever before to develop intimate committed relationships unlike those they experienced in their families of origin. Marriage tends to be misunderstood as a joining of two individuals. It really represents the changing of two entire systems, as well as an overlapping of systems to develop a third subsystem. Women tend to turn back to their parents for more connection, whereas men may increase their separation from their families of origin, seeing the couple relationship as replacing the family of origin. In fact, a daughter is also a daughter-in-law for the rest of her life, because she typically gains responsibility for the connectedness with and care of her husband's family as well.

Achieving a successful transition to couplehood may be an extraordinarily difficult proposition in our time, when we are in the midst of a transformation of male–female relationships in the direction of partnership, educationally, occupationally, and in emotional connectedness (Eisler, 1987; see Haddock, Zimmerman, & Lyness, Chapter 12, this volume). Couples can be helped to change traditional rituals around marriage to symbolize the move toward nonsexist relationships. New rituals that allow both partners to represent their symbolic movement from their parents to their partners (rather than just the woman from her father) can potentially provide couples with the opportunity to redefine traditional family relationships in a way that may make their future marital accommodation more equitable.

The transition to marriage is an important time for helping young couples look beyond the stereotypes that have been so problematic for family development (McGoldrick, 1999a). Yet in spite of the fact that this is less of a marked transition than it used to be for many couples who are living together before marriage, many couples resist looking at the fallacies of their myths about marriage (Carter & Peters, 1997) until later, when predictable problems surface (see Olson & Gorall, Chapter 19, this volume).

The failure to renegotiate family status with the family of origin may also lead to marital failure. Nevertheless, it appears that couples are very unlikely to present with extended family problems as the stated issue. Problems reflecting the inability to shift family status are usually indicated by defective boundaries around the new subsystem. In-laws may be too intrusive, and the new couple may be afraid to set limits, or they may have difficulty forming adequate connections with the extended systems, cutting themselves off in a tight twosome. At times, the inability to formalize a marriage indicates that the partners are still too enmeshed in their own families to define a new system and accept the implications of this realignment. It is useful in such situations to help the system move to a new definition of itself rather than to get lost in the details of incremental shifts the couple may be struggling over (sex, money, time, etc.).

FAMILIES WITH YOUNG CHILDREN

With the transition to parenthood, the family becomes a threesome, which makes it a permanent system for the first time. If childless partners separate, they dissolve their family unit, but once they have children, they may end the couple bond but remain forever parents to their children, who also remain connected to both families of origin. Thus, symbolically and in reality, this transition is a key one in the family life cycle.

The shift to this stage of the family life cycle requires that adults now move up a generation and become caretakers to the younger generation. Typical problems that occur when parents cannot make this shift are struggles with each other about taking responsibility, or refusal or inability to behave as parents to their children. In some families, childhood symptoms may be more a function of the temperamental qualities and developmental needs of the child. Children who are temperamentally difficult create more discomfort for parents, make parenting more challenging, and decrease couple and family functioning.

For the modern two-paycheck family with small children, a central struggle during this stage of the life cycle is the handling of child care responsibilities and chores. The pressure of trying to find adequate child care, when affordable and satisfactory social provision is lacking, leads to several serious consequences: Two full-time jobs may fall on the woman; the family may live in conflict and chaos; child care arrangements may be less than optimal; recreation and vacations may be sharply curtailed; or the woman may give up her job to stay home, or work only part-time. The major research on the transition to parenthood indicates that it is accompanied by a general decrease in marital satisfaction, a reversion to more traditional sex roles even by dual-career couples, who previously had a more equitable relationship, and a lowering of self-esteem for women (Carter & Peters, 1997; Carter, 1999; Walsh, 1989; see also Cowan & Cowan, Chapter 16, this volume). Even when fathers do participate more actively in relating to children, mothers still tend to bear the major responsibility for seeing that children's needs are met.

In many ways, the traditional family has often not only encouraged but even required dysfunctional patterns, such as the overresponsibility of mothers for their children and the complementary underinvolvement of fathers. Society, reinforced by developmental literature and psychoanalytic models, has equated parenting with mothering, overfocusing on the mother–child relationship in the earliest years of life, to the exclusion of other relationships or later phases (McGoldrick & Carter, 1999a; McGoldrick, 1999b). There is also a great mythology involved in our assumptions about the primacy of infancy and early childhood in determining the rest of human life. The same models that stress the supreme importance of the mother–child bond also view human development as a primarily painful process in which, eventually, mothers and children are adversaries. Even the men's movement, which has been seeking to expand men's options to include more loving and nurturing behaviors, has too often focused on the idea that men need to reject their mothers and go in search of their fathers in order to find themselves and be truly liberated.

We urge a broader perspective on human development that views child development and this early stage in the life cycle in the richness of its entire context of multigenerational family relationships, as well as within its social and cultural context. For a child's complete identity and development, a shift within society must be made to value, support, and reinforce the active inclusion of fathers and to appreciate the contributions of siblings, extended family members, and other caregivers as support, resources, models, and mentors.

This is an important area for intervention when working with families at this life-cycle stage. Fathers who lack experience with small children need to learn these skills. Often, this requires time alone with children for husbands to take primary responsibility, and for mothers to let go of the responsibility. Mothers may need assistance in allowing fathers to make mistakes, giving them the opportunity to construct and discover their relationship. At this transition in the family's emerging development, grandparents must shift to a backseat from which they can allow their children to be the central parental authorities, while forming a new type of caring relationship with their grandchildren.

In working with families at this phase of life, it is important to explore boundaries and roles within the nuclear family and between the generations. How the system operates is an important variable in understanding the creation and maintenance of childhood problems. Careful history taking is imperative, examining both individual child development and the family's developmental history. Areas of assessment include problems around conception, pregnancy, and delivery; temperamental qualities of the infant; achievement of developmental milestones; and the onset and development of problems. One must carefully track the child's symptoms, inquiring about changes or stresses within the system that may relate to the problems; adjustment of all family members to the birth of the symptomatic child and to the evolution of symptoms; additional problems with other children; organization of the family; and the impact of family-of-origin issues—who the child resembles, similar problems in the extended family, and how such problems have been dealt with by others.

Inquiry about household and job responsibilities, as well as the handling of finances and the specifics of child rearing and child care can illuminate major stresses on the family and ineffective solutions. Issues of gender-role functioning weigh heavily and cannot be ignored. Men who do not develop intimate relationships with their children as they grow up will have difficulty changing the pattern later. It is also helpful to convey an awareness of what women have been doing in the family, because their role is most often taken for granted. We might ask whether both parents usually go to children's school meetings, medical appointments, and sports events; how much time each parent spends alone with each child; and how money and domestic responsibilities are divided.

FAMILIES WITH ADOLESCENTS

Although many researchers have broken down the stages of families with young children into different phases, in our view, the shifts are incremental. Adolescence, however, ushers in a new era, because it marks a new definition of the children within the family, and of the parents' roles in relation to their children. Families with adolescents must establish qualitatively different boundaries than families with younger children, a job made more difficult in our times by the lack of built-in rituals to facilitate this transition, and by the lack of community supports to provide continuity of structure as adolescents emerge beyond the structure of their families. The boundaries must now be permeable. Parents can no longer maintain complete authority. Adolescents can and do open the family to a whole array of new values as they bring friends and new ideals into the family arena. Families that become derailed at this stage may be rather closed to new values and threatened by them, frequently stuck in an earlier view of their children. This is also a time when adolescents begin to establish their own independent relationships with the extended family. Adjustments between parents and grandparents may be needed to allow and foster these new patterns.

During certain phases in development, including preschool and adolescence, children seem to adhere rigidly to sex-role stereotypes—even more so than their parents or teachers. It is important not to reinforce this stereotyping, but to instead encourage girls to develop their own opinions, values, aspirations, and interests, while discouraging them from developing competitive cliques that shun other girls. Likewise, boys need to be encouraged to communicate and express feelings, and discouraged from teasing and bullying other boys or devaluing girls.

Although conventional gender values are at an all time high during adolescence, it is also during this phase that crucial, life-shaping decisions are made. Parents may not realize how much their teenagers need them to communicate information about adult life, such as bias in the workforce, the feminization of poverty, racism, responsible sexuality, and so on, to help them make more informed choices regarding their education and relationships (Pipher, 1994). Teenage pregnancy is still viewed as the girl's responsibility. She should learn to say "no." Instead, we must teach adolescents that their sexual behavior is the responsibility of both sexes, with consequences for both.

During adolescence, daughters are particularly torn between pressures to conform to traditional societal roles as sex object and their striving for a life of their own. Our society has also encouraged distancing between mothers and sons, with pernicious messages about the negative effects of mother–son bonding. Research indicates that rebellion against parents is only one, and not the most common, way for adolescents to evolve an identity. Most teenagers of both sexes remain close to and admire their parents, and experience a minimum of conflict and rebellion (Tavris, 1992). Fathers may need help to overcome inhibitions in relating to both sons and daughters emotionally.

Commonly, the father–daughter relationship may be problematic in adolescence. Fathers often become awkward about relating to their daughters as they approach adolescence with budding sexuality. They may need encouragement to engage actively with their daughters rather than avoid them. They may interact more easily with sons and now, increasingly, also with daughters through activities such as sports, which allow companionship and pride in their offspring without pressures for intimate relating. The unavailability of fathers for their daughters may lead daughters to develop an image of the male as a romantic stranger, an unrealistic image that cannot be met when they reach adult life. The unavailability of fathers for their sons may leave sons confused about their identity and questioning their masculinity.

Clinically, when working with adolescents and their families, it is important to ask questions about the roles each one is asked to play in the family. What are the chores and responsibilities of boys and of girls? Are sons encouraged to develop social skills, or are parents focused primarily on their achievement and sports performance? Are daughters encouraged to have high academic aspirations? Are both sexes given equal responsibility and encouragement in dealing with education, athletics, aspirations for the future, extended family relationships, buying gifts, writing, calling, or caring for relatives?

We also need to help families find more positive ways of defining for their daughters the changes of the menstrual and reproductive cycle, so that they do not see themselves as "unclean" or "impure," or simply as objects for the pleasure of males. Our society still gives very different messages to daughters than to sons about their bodies, their minds, and their spirits, emphasizing for young women their physical attractiveness to men, whereas sons are still taught that their bodily changes are positive, powerful, and fulfilling aspects of their manhood, with minimum emphasis on their need for cosmetics to increase their appeal. They still too often absorb messages that they have the right to treat girls as objects for their sexual pleasure and exploitation.

A common event in the parents' relationship at this phase is the "midlife crisis" of one or both spouses, with an exploration of personal, career, and marital satisfactions and dissatisfactions. This is especially important because parents of adolescents tend to have the lowest marital satisfaction. An exclusive focus on parent–adolescent complaints by either the family or the therapist may mask an affair or a secretly pondered divorce, or it may prevent the marital problems from coming to the surface.

FAMILIES AT MIDLIFE: LAUNCHING CHILDREN AND MOVING ON

This is the newest and longest phase in the family life cycle, and for these reasons it is in many ways the most problematic of all phases. In the past, most families were occupied with raising their children for most of their active adult lives. Now, because of the low birth rate and the long life expectancy of adults, most parents launch their children almost 20 years before retirement and must then find other life activities. The difficulties of this transition can lead families to hold onto their children or can lead to parental feelings of emptiness and depression, although, especially for women, this has become increasingly a transition they welcome for the opportunity to explore new pursuits.

The most significant aspect of this phase is that it is marked by the greatest number of exits and entries of family members. It begins with the launching of grown children and proceeds with the entry of their spouses and children. It is a time when grandparents often become ill or die. This, in conjunction with the difficulties of finding meaningful new life activities, may make it a particularly stressful period. Parents must deal with the change in their own status as they make room for the next generation and prepare to move up to the position of grandparents. They must also forge a different type of relationship with their own parents, who may become dependent, giving them (particularly women) considerable caretaking responsibilities. This can also be a liberating time in that finances may be easier than during the primary years of family responsibilities, and there is the potential for moving into new and unexplored areas—travel, hobbies, new careers. For some families, this stage is seen as a time of fruition and completion, and as a second opportunity to consolidate or expand by exploring new avenues and new roles. Less commonly, it leads to disruption, a sense of emptiness, and overwhelming loss, depression, and general disintegration. The transition necessitates a restructuring of the marital relationship now that parenting responsibilities are no longer required.

Because of the changing economics of our era, there are also many families in which launching is postponed for financial reasons. Members of the younger generation cannot find ways to support themselves or they get divorced, and there is a kind of in-and-out process with the older generation.

Men and women tend to be going in opposite directions psychologically as their children move into their own lives. The divergence of interests for men and women, as well as the shift in focus of energies required at this phase, can create marital tensions, sometimes leading to divorce. The emotional limitations of work and achievement may lead men to do important soul searching at this phase. Men may be feeling the lack of intimacy in their marriages and with their children, now that they have come to realize the limitations in what their work lives can give them. They may turn to their children for closeness even as their children are moving away. Or they may turn to their wives for more intimacy. But women, who have been focused on caring for others for so many years, are likely at this stage to be enthusiastic about the opportunity they now have to focus on their own work, friendships, and other activities. Women are not nearly as sorry to see the child-rearing era end as has been assumed. Men may hope that starting over will give them a new chance to "do it better." If men do divorce, they typically miss the caretaking functions provided by their wives and remarry rather quickly, usually to a younger woman. Women who divorce at this phase are less likely to remarry. In part, this is because of the skew in availability of partners, men's preference for younger partners, and women's reluctance to "settle," particularly for a traditional relationship that would mean a return to extensive caretaking.

Therapy at this phase is often aimed at helping family members redefine their lives and relationships, along with expanding and broadening their options, many of which may be different from those of the family in which they were raised. They need to envision new pathways for their lives that their parents possibly did not experience. There is also the difficult negotiation required when children return periodically to the nest, because of the complex and difficult economics of our times and society.

THE FAMILY IN LATER LIFE

As Walsh (1999a) has pointed out, few of the visions of old age offered by our culture provide us with positive images for healthy later life adjustment within a family or social context. Pessimistic views of later life prevail. Myths persist that most elderly people have no families; or have little relationship with them and are usually set aside in institutions; or that all family interactions with older family members are minimal. On the contrary, the vast majority of adults over 65 do not live alone but with other family members. Over 80% live within an hour of at least one child (Walsh, 1999a). Another myth is that most elderly are sick, senile, and feeble, and can best be handled in nursing homes or hospitals. Only 4% of the elderly live in institutions, typically those over 85, and only after family resources are exhausted. Most individuals between ages 65 and 80 are in good health and actively engaged with life pursuits.

Among the tasks of families in later life are adjustments to retirement, which may not only create a vacuum for retiring individuals but may also put a special strain on a marriage, requiring renegotiation of household roles and postretirement plans. Financial insecurity and dependence are also special difficulties, particularly for family members who value managing for themselves. And although loss of friends and relatives is a common stress at this phase, the loss of a spouse is the most difficult adjustment. Grandparenthood can, however, offer a new lease on life.

The inability to shift status is seen when elders have difficulty accepting their lessening powers, (e.g., giving up driving when unsafe), or when the younger generation treats them as incompetent or irrelevant. Even when members of the older generation are quite frail, there is not really a reversal of roles between one generation and the next, because parents always have many more years of experience and remain models to the next generations for the phases of life ahead. Nevertheless, because older age is so devalued in our culture, family members of the middle generation often do not know how to make the appropriate shift in relational status with their parents and may feel discomfort about having to care for an incapacitated parent that was formerly a source of strength and inspiration or authority and intimidation.

Clinically, older family members rarely seek help for themselves, although they do suffer from many psychological problems, especially depression. They are more likely to consult physicians for somatic complaints that may be contextually based. Often, it is members of the next generation who seek help, and even they do not usually define their problem as relating to an elderly parent. It is often only through careful history taking that one learns of an aging grandparent just about to move in or be taken to a nursing home, only to discover that the relationship issues around the shift have been left submerged and unresolved in the family. Helping family members recognize the status changes and the need for resolving their relationships in a new balance can become critical to the family's well-being now and later.

The final phase of life might be considered "for women only," because women tend to live longer, are more stigmatized by ageism, and, unlike men, are rarely paired with younger partners, making the statistics for this life-cycle phase extremely imbalanced.

DIVORCE, SINGLE PARENTING, AND REMARRIAGE

With the divorce rate currently near 50% and the rate of redivorce at 61%, divorce is an interruption or dislocation of the traditional family life cycle that produces the kind of profound disequilibrium associated with other family life-cycle transitions, with shifts, gains, and losses in family membership (Carter & McGoldrick, 1999a). As in other life-cycle phases, there are crucial shifts in relationship status and important emotional tasks that must be dealt with by the members of divorcing families for healthy adaptation. As in other phases, emotional issues not resolved at this phase will be carried along as hindrances in future relationships.

Therefore, families in which divorce occurs must go through one or two additional phases of the family life cycle in order to restabilize and go forward developmentally at a more complex level. Many of these families go through the divorce phase and restabilize permanently as postdivorce families. Even more remarry, and these families can be said to require negotiation of an additional phase of remarriage before long-term restabilization. Divorce and postdivorce family emotional process is a roller coaster with peaks of emotional tension at all transition points, including when the couple decide to separate; when the decision is announced to family and friends; when money, custody, and visitation arrangements are discussed; when separation takes place; when the actual divorce occurs; when separated spouses have contact around money and children; when each child graduates, marries, has children, or becomes ill; and when either spouse has a new partner, marries, has other children, or dies. These emotional pressure peaks do not necessarily occur in this order—and many of them take place repeatedly over the years. Adaptation requires mourning what is lost (including hopes and dreams) and dealing with hurt, anger, blame, guilt, shame, and loss in oneself, in the spouse, in the children, and in the extended family.

Clinical work aims to minimize the tremendous tendency toward cutoff of many relationships after a divorce. It is important to help divorcing spouses continue to relate as cooperative parents and permit maximum feasible contact among children, parents, and extended family. It usually takes several years and a great deal of effort after divorce for a family to readjust to its altered structure, which may or may not include remarriage, because many families restabilize satisfactorily without a recoupling. Families in which the emotional issues of divorce are not adequately resolved can remain stuck emotionally for years, if not for generations. However, families who handle the challenges are not invariably damaged, as popular myths maintain (see Visher, Visher, & Pasley, Chapter 6, this volume).

The family emotional process at the transition to remarriage consists of struggling with fears about investment in a new marriage and a new family; dealing with hostile or upset reactions of the children, the extended families, and the ex-spouse; struggling with the ambiguity of the new family structure, roles, and relationships; handling rearousal of intense parental guilt and concerns about the welfare of children; and handling rearousal of the old attachment to ex-spouse (negative or positive). It is important for the therapist to realize that very many of the problems are structural, not personal.

A FINAL CAVEAT

Most descriptions of the typical family life cycle, including our own, fail to convey the considerable effects of culture, ethnicity, race, religion, and sexual orientation on all aspects of how, when, and in what way a family experiences various phases and transitions. Although we may ignore these variables for theoretical clarity and focus on our commonalties, a clinician working with real families in the real world cannot afford to ignore them. The definition of "family," as well as the timing of life-cycle phases and the importance of different transitions, vary depending on a family's cultural background. It is extremely important for us as clinicians to help families develop rituals (Imber-Black & Roberts, 1992; Imber-Black, 1999) that correspond to their life choices and transitions, especially those that the culture has not validated, such as in the life-cycle patterns of the gay community or the multiproblem poor. The adaptation of multiproblem poor families to a stark political, social, and economic context has produced family life-cycle patterns that vary significantly from the middle-class paradigm so often and so erroneously used to conceptualize their situation (Hines, 1999). Social class is another major definer of differences in life-cycle patterns (Kliman & Madsen, 1999), and the life cycle of gays and lesbians (Johnson & Colucci, 1999), immigrants (Hernandez & McGoldrick, 1999), those who choose single parenting (see Anderson, Chapter 5, this volume), and those who do not marry or have children (Berliner, Jacob, & Schwartzberg, 1999) offer significant variations on traditional definitions of the family life cycle that require us to expand our definitions of normality in definitions of life-cycle patterns.

REFERENCES

Ahrons, C. R. (1999). The divorce cycle: A major variation in the American family life cycle. In B. Carter & M. McGoldrick (Eds.), *The expanded family life cycle: Individual, family, and social perspectives* (3rd ed.). Boston: Allyn & Bacon.

Ahrons, C. R., & Rodgers, R. H. (1987). *Divorced families.* New York: Norton.

Almeida, R., Woods, R., & Messineo, T. (1998). Contextualizing child development theory: Race, gender, class and culture. In R. Almeida (Ed.), *Transformations of gender and race: Family developmental perspectives* (pp. 23–48). Binghamton, NY: Haworth Press.

Aries, P. (1962). *Centuries of childhood: A social history of family life.* New York: Vintage.

Berliner, K., Jacob, D., & Schwartzberg, N. (1999) The single adult and the family life cycle. In B. Carter & M. McGoldrick (Eds.), *The expanded family life cycle: Individual, family and social perspectives* (3rd ed.). Boston: Allyn & Bacon.

Borysenko, J. (1996). *A Woman's book of life.* New York: Riverhead Books.

Bowen, M. (1978). *Family therapy in clinical practice.* New York: Aronson.

Broverman, I. K., Vogel, S. R., Broverman, D. M., Clarkson, F. E., & Rosenkrantz, P. S. (1972). Sex-role stereotypes: A current appraisal. *Journal of Social Issues, 28*(2), 59–78.

Canino, I., & Spurlock, J. (1994). *Culturally diverse children and adolescents: Assessment, diagnosis and treatment.* New York: Guilford Press.

Carter, B. (1978). Transgenerational scripts and nuclear family stress: Theory and clinical implications. In R. R. Sager (Ed.), *Georgetown Family Symposium* (Vol. 3, 1975–1976, pp. 265–271). Washington, DC: Georgetown University.

Carter, B. (1999). Becoming parents: The family with young children. *The expanded family life cycle: Individual, family and social perspectives* (3rd ed.). Boston: Allyn & Bacon.

Carter, B., & McGoldrick, M. (1999a). Overview. In B. Carter & M. McGoldrick (Eds.), *The expanded family life cycle: Individual, family and social perspectives* (3rd ed.). Boston: Allyn & Bacon.

Carter, B., & McGoldrick, M. (1999b). *The expanded family life cycle: Individual, family and social perspectives* (3rd ed.). Boston: Allyn & Bacon.

Carter, B., & Peters, J. (1997). *Love, honor and negotiate: Building partnerships that last a lifetime,* New York: Pocket Books.

Comer, J., & Poussaint, A. (1992). *Raising black children.* New York: Penguin.

Crittenden, A. (2001). *The price of motherhood: Why the most important job in the world is still the least valued.* New York: Metropolitan Books/Henry Holt.

Dinnerstein. D. (1976). *The mermaid and the minotaur.* New York: Harper & Row.

Duvall, E. M. (1977). *Marriage and family development* (5th ed.). Philadelphia: Lippincott.

Eisler, R. (1987). *The chalice and the blade.* San Francisco: Harper & Row.

Elder, G. (1986). Military times and turning points in mens' lives. *Developmental Psychology, 22,* 233–245.

Elder, G. (1992). Life course. In E. Gorgatta & M. Borgatta (Eds.), *Encyclopedia of sociology* (Vol. 3, pp. 1120–1130). New York: MacMillan.

Erikson, E. (1968). *Identity: Youth and crisis.* New York: Norton.

Falicov, C. J. (1999). The Latino family life cycle. In B. Carter & M. McGoldrick (Eds.), *The expanded family life cycle: Individual, family, and social perspectives* (3rd ed., pp. 141–152). Boston: Allyn & Bacon.

Gilligan, C. (1982). *In a different voice.* Cambridge, MA: Harvard University Press.

Green, R. J. (1998). Traditional norms of masculinity. In R. Almeida (Ed.), *Transformations of gender and race: Family developmental perspectives.* Binghamton, NY: Haworth Press.

Hadley, T., Jacob, T., Milliones, J., Caplan, J., & Spitz, D. (1974). The relationship between family developmental crises and the appearance of symptoms in a family member. *Family Process, 13,* 207–214.

Hale-Benson, J. E. (1986). *Black children: Their roots, culture and learning styles.* Baltimore: Johns Hopkins University Press.

Hernandez, M., & McGoldrick, M. (1999). Migration and the family life cycle. In B. Carter & M. McGoldrick (Eds.), *The expanded family life cycle* (pp. 169–184). Boston: Allyn & Bacon.

Hess, B. B., & Waring, J. M. (1984). Changing patterns of aging and family bonds in later life. *Family Coordinator, 27*(4): 303–314.

Hines, P. (1999). The family life cycle of African American families living in poverty. In B. Carter & M. McGoldrick (Eds.), *The expanded family life cycle* (pp. 327–345). Boston: Allyn & Bacon.

Hines, P., Garcia-Preto, N., McGoldrick, M., Almeida, R., & Weltman, S. (1999). Culture and the family life cycle. In B. Carter & M. McGoldrick (Eds.), *The expanded family life cycle* (pp. 69–87). Boston: Allyn & Bacon.

Imber-Black, E. (1999). Creating meaningful rituals for new life cycle transitions. In B. Carter & M. McGoldrick (Eds.), *The expanded family life cycle* (pp. 202–214). Boston: Allyn & Bacon.

Imber-Black, E., & Roberts, J. (1992). *Rituals in family therapy*. New York: Guilford Press.

Johnson, T., & Colucci, P. (1999). Lesbians, gay men and the family life cycle. In B. Carter & M. McGoldrick (Eds.), *The expanded family life cycle* (pp. 346–361). Boston: Allyn & Bacon.

Kimmel, M. S. (1996). *Manhood in America: A cultural history*. New York: Free Press.

Kliman, J., & Madsen, W. (1999). Social class and the family life cycle. In B. Carter & M. McGoldrick (Eds.), *The expanded family life cycle* (pp. 88–105). Boston: Allyn & Bacon.

Levinson, D. (1978). *The seasons of a man's life*. New York: Knopf.

Maccoby, E. E. (1990). Gender and relationships: A developmental account. *American Psychologist, 45,* 512–520.

McGoldrick, M. (Ed.). (1998). *Revisioning family therapy: Race, culture and gender in clinical practice*. New York: Guilford Press.

McGoldrick, M. (1999a). Becoming a couple. In B. Carter & M. McGoldrick (Eds.), *The expanded family life cycle* (pp. 231–248). Boston: Allyn & Bacon.

McGoldrick, M. (1999b). Women and the family life cycle. In B. Carter & M. McGoldrick (Eds.), *The expanded family life cycle* (pp. 106–123). Boston: Allyn & Bacon.

McGoldrick, M., & Carter, B. (1999a). Self in context. The individual life cycle in systemic perspective. In B. Carter & M. McGoldrick (Eds.), *The expanded family life cycle* (pp. 27–46). Boston: Allyn & Bacon.

McGoldrick, M., & Carter, B. (1999b). Remarried families. In B. Carter & M. McGoldrick (Eds.), *The expanded family life cycle* (pp. 417–434). Boston: Allyn & Bacon.

McGoldrick, M., Gerson, R. & Schellenberger, S. (1998). *Genograms in family assessment* (2nd ed.). New York: Norton.

McGoldrick, M., Giordano, J., & Pearce, J. K. (Eds.). (1996). *Ethnicity and family therapy* (2nd ed.). New York: Guilford Press.

Miller, J. B. (1976). *Toward a new psychology of women*. Boston: Beacon Press.

Neugarten, B. (1979). Time, age and the life cycle. *American Journal of Psychiatry, 136,* 887–894.

Notman, M., Klein, R., Jordan, J., & Zilbach, J. (1991). Women's unique developmental issues across the life cycle. In A. Tasman & S. Goldfinger (Eds.), *Review of psychiatry* (Vol. 10,   ). Washington, DC: American Psychiatric Press.

Pipher, M. (1994). *Reviving Ophelia: Saving the selves of adolescent girls*. New York: Ballentine.

Rosen, E. J. (1999). Men in transition: The "new man. " In B. Carter & M. McGoldrick (Eds.), *The expanded family life cycle*. Boston: Allyn & Bacon.

Silverstein, O. (1994) *The courage to raise good men*. New York: Viking.

Sluzki, C. (1979). Migration and Family Conflict. *Family Process, 18*(4), 379–390.

Tavris, C. (1992). *The mismeasure of women.* New York: Simon & Schuster.

Taffel, R., & Blau, M. (2001). *The second family: How adolescent power is challenging the American family.* New York: St. Martin's Press.

Walsh, F. (1999). Families in later life: Opportunities and challenges. In B. Carter & M. McGoldrick (Eds.), *The expanded family life cycle.* Boston: Allyn & Bacon.

Walsh, F. (1998). *Strengthening family resilience.* New York: Guilford Press.

Walsh, F. (1999). Religion and spirituality: Wellsprings for healing and resilience. In F. Walsh (Ed.), *Spiritual resources in family therapy* (pp. 3–27). New York: Guilford Press.

Walsh, F. (1989). Reconsidering gender in the marital quid pro quo. In M. McGoldrick, C. Anderson, & F. Walsh (Eds.). *Women in families.* New York: Norton.

CHAPTER 15

FAMILY RESILIENCE
Strengths Forged
through Adversity

Froma Walsh

The concept of family resilience extends our understanding of healthy family functioning to situations of adversity. Although some families are shattered by crisis or persistent hardship, what is remarkable is that many others emerge strengthened and more resourceful, able to love fully and raise their children well. This chapter presents an overview of a family resilience framework and outlines key processes, drawing together research findings on resilience and effective family functioning. Clinical practice applications are briefly described to suggest the broad utility of this conceptual framework for intervention and prevention efforts to strengthen families facing serious life challenges.

A FAMILY RESILIENCE FRAMEWORK

Resilience—the ability to withstand and rebound from disruptive life challenges—has become an important concept in mental health theory and research over the past two decades. It involves dynamic processes fostering positive adaptation within the context of significant adversity (Luthar, Cicchetti, & Becker, 2000). These strengths and resources enable individuals and families to respond successfully to stressful crises and persistent challenges, and to recover and grow from those experiences (Cowan, Cowan, & Schultz, 1996). Some who have suffered traumatic experiences become blocked from growth or trapped in a victim position by anger or blame. In contrast, resilience involves key processes over time that foster the ability to "struggle well," heal from painful experiences, and go on to live and love fully.

A modified version of this chapter has been published: Walsh, F. (2003). Family resilience: Framework for clinical practice. *Family Process, 42*(1), 1–18.

The Relational Context of Individual Resilience

Most research to date has focused on individual resilience. In the 1980s, increasing evidence that the same adversity may result in different outcomes challenged the prevailing deterministic assumption that traumatic experiences in childhood are inevitably damaging. As Rutter (1987) noted, no combination of risk factors, regardless of severity, gave rise to disorder in more than half the children exposed. Although many lives were shattered, others overcame similar, high-risk conditions and were able to lead loving and productive lives. Studies found, for instance, that most abused children did not become abusive parents (Kaufman & Ziegler, 1987).

To account for these differences, early studies focused on personal traits for resilience, or hardiness, reflecting the dominant cultural ethos of the "rugged individual" (see Luthar & Ziegler, 1991; Walsh, 1996, for reviews of literature). Initially, resilience was viewed as innate, in the concept of "the invulnerable child," who, like a "steel doll," was thought to be impervious to stress because of character armor (Anthony & Cohler, 1987). Researchers moved toward recognition of an interaction between nature and nurture in the emergence of resilience, yet tended to hold a pessimistic, narrow view of family influence. Most studies focused on individuals who thrived despite parental mental illness or maltreatment (e.g., Wolin & Wolin, 1993) and tended to dismiss the family altogether as hopelessly dysfunctional and to seek positive extrafamilial resources to counter the negative impact. Thus, families were seen to contribute to risk, but not to resilience.

As research was extended to a wide range of adverse conditions— such as growing up in impoverished circumstances, dealing with chronic medical illness, or recovering from catastrophic life events, trauma, and loss—resilience came to be viewed in terms of an interplay of multiple risk and protective processes over time, involving individual, family, and larger sociocultural influences (Garmezy, 1991; Masten, Best, & Garmezy, 1990; Patterson, 2002; Rutter, 1987). Individual vulnerability or the impact of stressful conditions could be outweighed by mediating influences.

In a remarkable longitudinal study of resilience, Werner (1993; Werner & Smith, 1992) followed the lives of nearly 700 children raised in hardship on the Hawaiian island of Kauai. Most were born to plantation workers of diverse cultural and racial descent living in poverty. One-third were classified "at risk" because of exposure before age 2 to at least four additional risk factors, such as serious health problems and familial alcoholism, violence, divorce, or mental illness. By age 18, about two-thirds of the at-risk children had done as poorly as predicted, with early pregnancy, needs for mental health services, or trouble in school or with the law. However, one-third of those at risk had developed into competent, caring, and confident young adults, with the capacity "to work well, play well, and love well," as rated on a variety of measures. In later follow-ups through age 40, all but two of these individuals were still living successful lives. Many had outperformed Kauai children from less harsh backgrounds: more were stably married and employed, and fewer were traumatized by a hurricane that destroyed much of the island. Of note, several who had been poorly functioning in adolescence turned their lives around in adulthood, most often crediting supportive relationships and religious involvement. These findings showed that despite troubled childhood or teen years, there is potential for developing resilience at later points in life.

Notably, Werner's research and other emerging studies of individual resilience all remarked on the crucial influence of significant relationships with kin, intimate partners, and mentors, such as coaches or teachers, who supported their efforts, believed in their potential, and encouraged them to make the most of their lives. Still, the prevailing focus on parental pathology blinded many to the family resources that can be found and strengthened in family networks, from sibling bonds to couple relationships and extended family networks, even when a parent's functioning is seriously impaired. A family resilience perspective, grounded in a systemic orientation, fundamentally alters that deficit-based lens from viewing troubled families as *damaged* and beyond repair to seeing them as *challenged* by life's adversities, with potential for fostering healing and growth in its members.

Family Stress, Adaptation, and Resilience

The concept of family resilience extends beyond seeing individual family members as potential resources for individual resilience to focus on risk and resilience in the family as a functional unit (Walsh, 1996). A basic premise in this systemic view is that stressful crises and persistent challenges have an impact on the whole family, and in turn, key family processes mediate the recovery of all members and their relationships. These processes enable the family system to rally in times of crisis, buffering stress, reducing the risk of dysfunction, and supporting optimal adaptation.

Built on theory and research on family stress, coping, and adaptation (Hill, 1958; McCubbin & Patterson, 1983; Patterson, 1988, 2002), family resilience entails more than managing stressful conditions, shouldering a burden, or surviving an ordeal. It involves the potential for personal and relational transformation and growth that can be forged out of adversity (Boss, 2001). Tapping into key processes for resilience, families can emerge stronger and more resourceful in meeting future challenges. Members may discover or develop new insights and abilities. A crisis can be a wake-up call, heightening attention to what matters. It can become an opportunity for reappraisal of priorities, stimulating greater investment in meaningful relationships and life pursuits. Many families report that through weathering a crisis together, their relationships were enriched and more loving than they might otherwise have been (Stinnett & De-Frain, 1985).

Social and Developmental Contexts of Risk and Resilience

A family resilience framework combines ecological and developmental perspectives to view family functioning in relation to its broader sociocultural context and evolution over the multigenerational life cycle.

Ecological Perspective

From a *biopsychosocial systems orientation,* risk and resilience are viewed in light of multiple, recursive influences involving individuals, families, and larger social systems. Problems are seen as resulting from an interaction of individual—and family—vulnerability to the impact of stressful life experiences and social contexts. Symptoms may be primarily biologically based, as in serious illness (Rolland, 1994; see Chapter 17, this volume), or largely influenced by sociocultural variables, such as barriers of poverty and discrimination for African American and immigrant families (McCubbin, McCubbin, McCubbin, & Futrell, 1998; McCubbin, McCubbin, Thompson, & Fromer, 1998). Family distress may result from unsuccessful attempts to cope with an overwhelming situation. Symptoms may be generated by a crisis event, such as traumatic loss in the family, or the wider impact of a large-scale disaster. The family, peer group, community resources, school or work settings, and other social systems can be seen as nested contexts for nurturing and reinforcing resilience.

Each family's crisis experience will have common (typical) and unique features. Falicov's (1995) useful multidimensional framework for considering cultural diversity locates each family within a complex ecological niche, sharing borders and common ground with other families, as well as differing positions related to such variables as gender, economic status, life stage, and position vis-à-vis the dominant culture. A holistic assessment includes the varied contexts, and aims to understand the constraints and possibilities in each family's position. A family resilience framework, likewise, seeks not only to identify common elements in a crisis situation and effective family responses but also takes into account each family's unique perspectives, resources, and challenges.

Developmental Perspective

Life crises and persistent stresses can derail the functioning of a family system, with ripple effects to all family members and their relationships. In turn, family processes for dealing with challenges over time mediate coping and adaptation. Some families may do well in a short-term crisis but buckle under the strains of persistent adversity. A developmental perspective is essential in understanding and fostering family resilience.

Unfolding challenges and responses over time. Most major stressors are not simply a short-term single event, but rather, a complex set of changing conditions with a past history and a future course (Rutter, 1987). Such is the experience of divorce, from an escalation of predivorce tensions, to separation and reorganization of households and parent–child relationships; most move on to remarriage and stepfamily integration (see Greene, Anderson, Hetherington, Forgatch, & DeGarmo, Chapter 4 and Visher, Visher, & Pasley, Chapter 5, this volume). Give this complexity, no single coping response is invariably most successful; a variety of strategies may prove useful in meeting different challenges that unfold over time.

Family resilience thus involves varied adaptational processes extending over time, from a threatening event on the horizon, through disruptive transitions, and subsequent shockwaves in the immediate aftermath and beyond. For instance, how a family approaches an anticipated loss, buffers stress and manages disruption, effectively reorganizes, and reinvests in life pursuits will influence the immediate and long-term adaptation for all members and their relationships (Walsh & McGoldrick, 1991).

Pile-up of stressors. A pile-up of internal and external stressors can overwhelm the family, heightening vulnerability and risk for subsequent problems (Boss, 2001; Masten & Coatsworth, 1998; McCubbin & Patterson, 1983; Patterson, 2002). One couple's escalating conflict and the husband's heavy drinking brought them to therapy. It was essential to situate these symptoms in the context of the family's cascade of strains and losses over two years: in the midst of raising three small children, one with disabilities, the husband's brother died suddenly in a car crash. Overwhelmed by the tragedy, the paternal grandfather suffered a stroke, requiring extensive caregiving; the husband then lost his job as his company downsized, leaving the family without income or health insurance. Reeling from one cirsis to the next, these cumulative pressures on the family were overwhelming. Therapy helped them to recover from their losses, locate resources, and support each other in mastering ongoing challenges.

A family life-cycle perspective. Functioning and symptoms of distress are assessed in the context of the multigenerational family system as it moves forward across the life cycle (see McGoldrick & Carter, Chapter 14, this volume). At each developmental stage, the balance shifts between stressful events that heighten vulnerability and protective processes that enhance resilience, as well as the relative influence of family, peers, and other social forces. A family resilience framework focuses on family adaptation around nodal events including both predictable, normative transitions, such as the birth of the first child (see Cowan & Cowan, Chapter 16, this volume) and unexpected events, such as the untimely death of a young parent.

It is crucial to note symptoms that are concurrent with recent or impending events that have disrupted or threatened the family. For instance, a son's sudden drop in school grades may be precipitated by his father's recent job loss, although family members may not initially note any connection. Frequently, symptoms of a child coincide with stressful transitions, such as parental remarriage, that pose new challenges and require boundary shifts and role redefinition (Walsh, 1983). It is important to attend to the extended kin network beyond the immediate household. One woman's depression was triggered by the death of her godmother, who had been her mainstay through a difficult childhood. In assessing the impact of stressful events, it is essential to explore how family members handled the situation: their proactive stance, immediate response, and long-term "survival" strategies. Some approaches may be functional in the short term but may rigidify and become dysfunctional over time. For instance, with a sudden illness, a family must mobilize resources and pull together to meet the crisis, but later must shift gears with chronic disability and attend to other members' needs over the long haul (see Rolland, Chapter 17, this volume).

Legacies of the past. Distress is heightened when current stressors reactivate painful memories and emotions from the past, as in posttraumatic stress reactions for refugee families. The convergence of developmental and multigenerational strains increases the risk for complications (Carter and McGoldrick, 1999). Unresolved past losses often resurface with a current or threatened loss. Family members may lose perspective, conflating immediate situations with past events, and become overwhelmed or cut off from painful feelings and contacts. Family stories of past adversity influence future expectations, from an optimistic outlook to catastrophic fears. Many families function well until they reach a point in the life cycle that had been traumatic to the previous generation (Walsh, 1983).

To assess the symptoms of distress in a temporal context, as well as in family and social contexts, a family time line and a genogram (McGoldrick, Gerson, & Shellenberger, 1998) are valuable tools for clinicians and researchers to schematize relationship information, track system patterns, and guide intervention planning. Whereas clinicians typically use genograms to focus on problematic family-of-origin patterns, a resilience-based approach also searches for positive influences, such as resourceful ways a family dealt with past adversity and models of resilience in the kin network that might inspire efforts to master current challenges.

Advantages of a Family Resilience Framework

Assessment of healthy family functioning is fraught with dilemmas. Clinicians and researchers bring their own assumptive maps into every evaluation and intervention, embedded in cultural norms, professional orientations, and personal experience (see Walsh, Chapter 2, this volume).

Moreover, with the social and economic transformations of recent decades and a growing multiplicity of family arrangements, no single model of family health fits all (see Walsh, Chapter 1, this volume). In fact, family diversity has been common throughout history and across cultures, and the growing body of research in this volume reveals that well-functioning families and healthy children can be found in a variety of formal and informal kinship arrangements. What matters most in dealing with adversity are effective family *processes,* involving the quality of caring, committed relationships.

Systems-oriented family process research over the past two decades has provided some empirical grounding for assessment of healthy couple and family functioning. However, family assessment typologies tend to be static and acontextual, offering a snapshot of interaction patterns but not connecting them to a family's resources and constraints and their emerging challenges over time. In clinical practice, families most often come in periods of crisis, when distress and differences from norms are too readily assumed to be signs of family pathology.

A family resilience framework offers several advantages. First, by definition, it focuses on strengths forged under stress in the midst of crisis, or in overcoming adversity. Second, it is assumed that no single model fits all families or their situations. Functioning is assessed in context: relative to each family's values, resources, and life challenges. Third, processes for optimal functioning and the well-being of members are seen to vary over time as challenges unfold and families evolve across the life cycle. Although no single model of family health fits all, a family resilience perspective is grounded in a deep conviction in the potential for family recovery and growth out of adversity.

KEY PROCESSES IN FAMILY RESILIENCE

The family resilience framework I have developed to guide clinical practice is informed by clinical and social science research seeking to understand crucial variables contributing to individual resilience and well-functioning families (Walsh, 1996, 1998). It serves as a conceptual map to identify and target key family processes that can reduce stress and vulnerability in high-risk situations, foster healing and growth out of crisis, and empower families to overcome persistent adversity. The framework draws together findings from numerous studies, identifying and synthesizing key processes within three domains of family functioning: family belief systems, organization patterns, and communication processes. Table 15.1 presents an outline of key processes for family resilience, which are described very briefly here (see Walsh, 1998, for fuller elaboration and clinical application).

TABLE 15.1. Key Processes in Family Resilience

Belief systems

1. Make Meaning of Adversity
   - View resilience as relationally based—vs. "rugged individual."
   - Normalize, contextualize adversity and distress.
   - Sense of coherence: crisis as meaningful, comprehensible, manageable challenge.
   - Causal/explanatory attributions: How could this happen? What can be done?

2. Positive Outlook
   - Hope, optimistic bias; confidence in overcoming odds.
   - Courage and en-*courage*-ment; affirm strengths and focus on potential.
   - Active initiative and perseverence (can-do spirit).
   - Master the possible; accept what can't be changed.

3. Transcendence and Spirituality
   - Larger values, purpose.
   - Spirituality: faith, congregational support, healing rituals.
   - Inspiration: envision new possibilities; creative expression; social action.
   - Transformation: learning, change, and growth from adversity.

Organizational patterns

4. Flexibility
   - Open to change: rebound, reorganize, adapt to fit new challenges.
   - Stability through disruption: continuity, dependability, follow-through.
   - Strong authoritative leadership: nurturance, protection, guidance.
     - Varied family forms: cooperative parenting/caregiving teams.
     - Couple/Co-parent relationship: equal partners.

5. Connectedness
   - Mutual support, collaboration, and commitment.
   - Respect individual needs, differences, and boundaries.
   - Seek reconnection, reconciliation of wounded relationships.

6. Social and Economic Resources
   - Mobilize kin, social, and community networks; seek models and mentors.
   - Build financial security; balance work/family strains.

Communication/problem solving

7. Clarity
   - Clear, consistent messages (words and actions).
   - Clarify ambiguous information; truth seeking/truth speaking.

8. Open Emotional Expression
   - Share range of feelings (joy and pain; hopes and fears).
   - Mutual empathy; tolerance for differences.
   - Take responsibility for own feelings, behavior; avoid blaming.
   - Pleasurable interactions; humor.

9. Collaborative Problem solving
   - Creative brainstorming; resourcefulness.
   - Shared decision making; conflict resolution: negotiation, fairness, reciprocity.
   - Focus on goals; take concrete steps; build on success; learn from failure.
   - Proactive stance: prevent problems; avert crises; prepare for future challenges.

Family Belief Systems

Family belief systems powerfully influence how we view a crisis, our suffering, and our options (Wright, Watson, & Bell, 1996). Shared constructions of reality emerge through family and social transactions; in turn, these belief systems organize family processes and approaches to crisis situations, and they can be fundamentally altered by such experiences (Reiss, 1981). Whether a personal tragedy or a major catastrophic event, adversity generates a crisis of meaning and potential disruption of integration (Patterson & Garwick, 1994). Resilience is fostered by shared facilitative beliefs that increase options for problem resolution, healing, and growth. They help members make meaning of crisis situations, facilitate a hopeful, positive outlook, and offer transcendent or spiritual connections.

Making Meaning of Adversity

High-functioning families have a strong affiliative orientation (Beavers & Hampson, 1990; see Chapter 20, this volume). Fundamental to resilience, they approach adversity as a *shared* challenge and hold a *relational view* of strength in contrast to the American cultural ethos of the "rugged individual." "We shall overcome," the rallying song of the 1960s Civil Rights Movement, expresses this core belief: In joining together, individuals strengthen their ability to overcome adversity.

Well-functioning families have an evolutionary sense of time and becoming—a continual process of growth and change across the life cycle and the generations (Beavers & Hampson, 1990). A family life-cycle orientation helps members to see disruptive transitions also as milestones on their shared life passage. By *normalizing* and *contextualizing* distress, family members can enlarge their perspective to see their reactions and difficulties as understandable in the face of an overwhelming situation or daunting obstacles. The tendency toward blame, shame, and pathologizing is reduced if the family is able to view their complicated feelings and dilemmas as "normal," that is, common and expectable among families facing similar predicaments.

In grappling with adversity, families do best when helped to gain a *sense of coherence* (Antonovsky, 1987; Antonovsky & Sourani, 1988), by recasting a crisis as a challenge that is comprehensible, manageable, and meaningful to tackle. It involves efforts to clarify the nature and source of problems and available options. The meaning of adversity and beliefs about what can be done vary with different cultural norms; some are more fatalistic, whereas others stress personal responsibility (Walsh, 1998). Family members' subjective appraisal of a crisis situation and their resources influences their coping response and adaptation (Lazarus & Folkman, 1984). Family members attempt to make sense of how things have happened through *causal or explanatory attributions*. When a crisis event strikes like a bolt out of the blue, as did the terrorist attacks on 9/11, ambiguity about the causes and the human casualties, along with uncertainties about future security, complicate the challenges of meaning making and recovery. Efforts to clarify ambiguous losses, to learn whether and how a loved one died, and to recover the remains of a body facilitate the healing process (Boss, 1999). Communal rituals assist survivors in coming to terms with unbearable grief.

Positive Outlook

Considerable research documents the strong effects of a positive outlook in coping with stress, recovery from crisis, and overcoming barriers to success (Seligman & Csikszentmihalyi, 2000). *Hope* is to the spirit what oxygen is to the lungs: It fuels energy and efforts to rise above adversity. Hope is a future-oriented belief: No matter how bleak the present, a better future can be envisioned. In problem-saturated conditions, it is essential to rekindle hopes and dreams in order to see possibilities, tap into potential resources, and strive to surmount obstacles. Hope for a better life for their children keeps many struggling parents from being defeated by their immediate plight.

High-functioning families have been found to hold a more optimistic view of life (Beavers & Hampson, 1990). Seligman's (1990) concept of *learned optimism* has particular relevance for resilience. His earlier research on "learned helplessness" showed that with repeated experiences of futility and failure, people stop trying and become passive and pessimistic, generalizing the belief that bad things always happen to them, and that nothing they can do will matter. Seligman then reasoned that optimism could be learned, and helplessness and pessimism unlearned, through experiences of successful mastery, building confidence that one's efforts can make a difference. He cautions, however, that a positive mind-set is not sufficient for success if life conditions are relentlessly harsh, with few opportunities to rise above them. As Aponte (1994) notes, many families who feel trapped in impoverished, blighted communities lose hope, suffering a deprivation of both "bread" and "spirit." This despair robs them of meaning, purpose, and a sense of future possibility. To be sustained, a positive outlook must be reinforced by successful experiences and a nurturing community context.

Similar to an optimistic bias, epidemiologists find that "positive illusions" sustain hope in dealing with adversity, such as a life-threatening illness (Taylor, 1989; Taylor, Kemeny, Reed, Bower, & Gruenwald, 2000). Unlike denial, people are aware of a grim reality, such as a poor prognosis, and choose to believe they can overcome the odds against them. This belief fuels efforts that maximize their chances of success. As an example, when one family was told that their child had an illness with only a 10%

rate of recovery, the parents reasoned, "Someone has to be in that 10%, so why not us? Let's do all we can to get there."

Affirming family strengths and potential in the midst of difficulties helps families to counter a sense of helplessness, failure, and blame as it reinforces pride, confidence, and a "can do" spirit. Encouragement bolsters courage to take initiative and to persevere in efforts to master a harrowing ordeal. The courage and determination shown in facing hardships in the everyday life of ordinary families often go unnoticed. One young girl remarked on her mother's resilience: "I watch her in wonder. How does she do it? How does she always remember to give me lunch money and tell me she loves me? How does she work all night and run errands all day? She never, ever, gives up."

Resilience is bolstered by unwavering shared confidence through an ordeal: "We always believed we would find a way." This conviction fuels initiative and perseverance, and makes family members active participants in a relentless search for solutions. By showing confidence that they will each do their best, they support one another's efforts and build competencies. One man credited his endurance in recovery from a spinal cord injury to his wife's unfailing encouragement and their rock-solid relationship. At times when he felt like giving up on life, this restored his determination to engage in every means to regain functioning as fully as possible.

Mastering the art of the possible is a hallmark of resilience (Higgins, 1994). For families, it involves taking stock of their situation—the challenges, constraints, and resources—and then focusing energies on making the best of their options. This requires acceptance of that which is beyond their control and can't be changed, such as a catastrophic event. Instead of being immobilized, or trapped in a powerless victim position, focus is directed toward ongoing and future possibilities. Although past events can't be changed, they can be recast in a new light that fosters greater comprehension and healing. When immediate problems are overwhelming, family members can be encouraged to carve out parts that they can master. For instance, family members may not be able to influence the outcome of a terminal illness, but they can become meaningfully engaged in the dying process: to actively participate in caregiving and end-of-life preparations, ease suffering, and make the most of the time they have left. Families with an Eastern philosophical or religious orientation tend to have greater ease in accepting things beyond their control or comprehension, whereas those with a Western mastery orientation must shift from instrumental problem-solving tendencies and the need to be in control. Family members often report that by being more fully present with loved ones, this most painful time became the most precious in their relationship. In the aftermath of loss, survivors are helped to find ways to transform the living presence of a loved one into cherished memories, stories, and deeds that carry on the spirit of the deceased and their relationship.

Transcendence and Spirituality

Transcendent beliefs provide meaning and purpose beyond ourselves, our families, and immediate troubles (Beavers & Hampson, 1990). Most families find strength, comfort, and guidance in adversity through connections with their cultural and religious traditions (Walsh, 1999b; see Chapter 13, this volume). Suffering and, often, the injustice or senselessness of it are ultimately spiritual issues (Wright et al., 1996). Spiritual resources, through deep faith, rituals and ceremonies, practices such as prayer and meditation, and religious/congregational affiliation have all been found to be wellsprings for resilience (e.g., Werner & Smith, 1992). Many find spiritual nourishment outside formal religion, such as through deep personal connection with nature, music, or a higher power. Studies of successful African American families find that strong faith and congregational involvement bolster their efforts to rise above barriers of poverty and racism (see Boyd-Franklin, Chapter 10, this volume). In health crises, medical studies suggest that faith, prayer, and spiritual rituals can actually strengthen healing through the influence of emotions on the immune and cardiovascular systems (e.g., Dossey, 1993; Weil, 1994). Although faith can make a difference, we must be cautious not to attribute failures to overcome adversity to insufficient spiritual piety or positive beliefs.

The paradox of resilience is that the worst of times can also bring out our best. A crisis can yield learning, transformation, and growth in unforeseen directions. It can be a wake-up call or epiphany, awakening family members to the importance of loved ones, or jolting them into healing old wounds and reordering priorities for more meaningful relationships and life pursuits. Resilient individuals and families commonly emerge from shattering crises with a heightened moral compass and sense of purpose in their lives, gaining compassion for the plight of others (Coles, 1997). The experience of adversity and suffering can inspire creative expression through the arts or spark commitment to action on behalf of others, and even a life course dedicated to helping others or working for social justice.

Family Organizational Patterns

Contemporary families, with their diverse forms, must organize in varied ways to meet the challenges they face. In family organization, resilience is bolstered by flexible structure, connectedness (cohesion), and social and economic resources.

Flexibility: Bouncing Forward

Flexibility is a core process in resilience. Often, the ability to rebound is thought of as "bouncing back," like a spring, to a preexisting shape or norm. However, in the aftermath of most major transitions and crisis events, families can't return to "normal" life as they knew it. A more apt metaphor for resilience might be "bouncing forward," changing to meet new challenges (Walsh, 2002b). Families often need help in navigating uncharted waters and in undergoing structural reorganization. With such occurrences as parental disability or divorce, families must construct a new sense of normality as they recalibrate and reorganize patterns of interaction to fit new demands. For instance, a father's disability may require a traditional couple to alter gender-based roles as the mother becomes the sole breadwinner and he assumes household and child-rearing responsibilities.

At the same time, families need to buffer and counterbalance stressful changes through efforts to maintain continuity and restore stability (see Olson & Gorall, Chapter 19, this volume). For instance, the adaptation of immigrant families is fostered by finding ways to sustain connections with valued customs, kin, and community left behind (see Falicov, Chapter 11, this volume).

Firm yet flexible authoritative leadership is most effective for family functioning and the well-being of children. Through stressful times, it is especially important for parents and other caretakers to provide nurturance, protection, and guidance. With a disruptive transition or crisis, continuity, security, and predictability are most needed by children and other vulnerable members. For instance, children's adaptation to divorce is facilitated by strong parental leadership and dependability as new single-parent household structures, visitation schedules, rules, and routines are set in place.

Connectedness

Connectedness, or cohesion, is essential for effective family functioning (see Olson & Gorall, Chapter 19; Beavers & Hampson, Chapter 20, this volume). A crisis can shatter family cohesion if members are unable to turn to one another. Resilience is strengthened by mutual support, collaboration, and commitment to weather troubled times together. At the same time, family members need to respect each other's individual differences, separateness, and boundaries. They may have quite varied reactions to the same event, or may need more or less time to process the experience, depending on such variables as the age of a child or the meaning of a lost relationship.

The complex challenges in stepfamily integration contribute to the high risk of divorce in remarriage (see Visher, Visher, & Pasley, Chapter 6, this volume). Families do best if they can forge workable parenting coalitions across household boundaries and knit together biological and steprelations, including step- and half-siblings and extended family. When children are placed in foster care, although it may not be safe for them to live with a parent, there are many ways they can sustain vital connections with their family network through photos, keepsakes, e-mail, letters, visits with siblings and extended kin, and links to their cultural and religious heritage.

With the death of a parent, children need reassurance that other significant relationships will be sustained. In the French film *Ponette,* a small girl survives a car crash in which her mother was fatally injured. As her father takes her to stay with her aunt and cousins while he must go away for his work week, he gives her his watch to wear while he is gone. He shows her how to tell when it is seven o'clock, the time he promises to call her each day. He tells Ponette that whenever she misses him, she should listen to the tick tock of the watch and think of his beating heart and his love for her. He asks if he might take something of hers with him. She considers giving him her favorite teddy bear but decides she needs it too much, so she gives him a favorite toy instead. This symbolic exchange sustains connection to ease the first transition of many that lie ahead.

Social and Economic Resources

Kin and social networks are vital lifelines in times of trouble, offering practical and emotional support. The significance of role models and mentors for resilience of at-risk youth is well documented. The importance of strong friendships has not been sufficiently appreciated. Involvement in community groups and religious congregations also strengthens resilience. Families who are more isolated can be helped to mobilize these potential resources.

Community-based coordinated efforts, involving local agencies and residents, are essential to meet the challenges of a major disaster and widespread trauma and to prepare to avert future threats. Such multisystemic approaches facilitate both family and community resilience (Landau, 2002). In one model program, multifamily groups and parent–teacher networks were organized in lower Manhattan neighborhoods directly affected by the 9/11 terrorist attacks, proving to be a valuable resource for families to share their experiences, respond to the concerns of their children, support one another, and mobilize concerted action in recovery efforts (Saul, 2002).

The importance of financial security for resilience should not be neglected. A serious or chronic illness can drain a family's economic resources. Persistent unemployment or the loss of a breadwinner can be devastating. Many studies find that financial strain is the most common factor in single-parent families in which children fare poorly. Most importantly, the concept of family resilience should not be misused to blame families that are unable to rise above harsh conditions, by simply labeling them as not resilient. Just as individuals need supportive relationships to thrive, family resilience must be supported by social and institutional policies and practices that encourage the ability to thrive, such as flexible work schedules for parents and quality, affordable health, child-, and elder-care services.

Communication/Problem-Solving Processes

Communication processes foster resilience by bringing clarity to crisis situations, encouraging open emotional expression and fostering collaborative problem solving. It must be kept in mind that cultural norms vary considerably in the sharing of sensitive information and expression of feelings.

Clarity

Clarity and congruence in messages facilitate effective family functioning (see Epstein, Ryan, Bishop, Miller, & Keitner, Chapter 21, this volume). Often, family members have different bits and pieces of information or hearsay and then they fill in the blanks, often with their worst fears. *Clarifying and sharing crucial information* about crisis situations and future expectations, such as a medical condition, facilitates meaning making, authentic relating, and informed decision making, whereas ambiguity or secrecy can block understanding, closeness, and mastery (Boss, 1999). Shared acknowledgment of the reality and circumstances of a painful loss fosters healing, whereas denial and cover-up, especially in stigmatized circumstances such as suicide, can impede recovery and lead to estrangement (Walsh & McGoldrick, 1991).

When acknowledgment and discussion of life-threatening situations is shut down, anxiety may be expressed in a child's symptoms: In one family, a mother brought her 5-year-old son, Terell, for an evaluation, fearing he had been sexually abused because his mother repeatedly found him fondling himself. Finding no indication of sexual abuse, the therapist asked if there had been any stressful events in the family in recent months. The mother reported that several months earlier, her husband had had exploratory surgery for "stomach pains." A cancerous tumor and a large portion of his stomach were removed. At discharge from the hospital, he told his wife: "OK, they said they got it all; I just want to go back to life as normal and not talk about it." To respect her husband's wishes, the mother told the children, "Daddy's fine," and no more was said. Because the children hadn't asked any questions, she assumed they weren't worried about it. Then, she recalled that when the family had said grace before dinner recently, Terell had added: "And please God, take care of Daddy's tummy." The parents were seen together to help them open their communication about the life-threatening event and were then helped in deciding how to discuss it with their children.

Commonly, well-intentioned parents avoid painful or threatening topics, wishing to protect children or frail elders from worry, or they wait until they are certain about a precarious situation, such as a medical prognosis or a decision to divorce. However, their anxieties about something hard to talk about show through and may generate catastrophic fears. Parents can be helpful at least by giving assurance that they will keep the children and others informed as the situation develops, and that they are open at any time to discuss any questions or concerns. Parents may need guidance on age-appropriate ways to share information and can expect that, as children mature, they may revisit issues to gain greater comprehension or bring up emerging concerns. When a mother has breast cancer, conversations with her 8-year-old daughter may focus on concerns about loss; at puberty, they may need to talk about the daughter's worries that she, too, could get breast cancer.

Emotional Expression

Open communication, supported by a climate of mutual trust, empathy, and tolerance for differences, enables family members to share a wide range of feelings that can be aroused by crisis events and chronic stress. Family members may be out of sync over time; one may continue to be quite upset when others feel ready to move on. A breadwinner or single parent may suppress strong emotional reactions in order to keep functioning for the family; children may try to help out by stifling their own feelings and needs, or by trying to cheer up parents. When emotions are intense, conflict is likely to erupt. When family members feel out of control in a crisis situation, they may attempt to control each other.

Gender differences are common, with men tending more to withdraw or become angry, whereas women are more likely to become very emotional and sad. Masculine stereotypes of strength often constrain men from showing fear, vulnerability, or sadness, which are framed pejoratively as "losing control" and "falling apart." When strong emotions can't be shared with loved ones, there are increased risks of substance abuse, symptoms such as depression, self-destructive behaviors, and relational conflict or estrangement. Couples that have lost a child are at heightened risk for divorce, yet those who support each other through the painful ordeal often find their relationship strengthened through the process. For relational resilience, couples and families can be encouraged to share their feelings and comfort one another. Finding pleasure and moments of humor in the midst of pain can offer respite and lift spirits.

Collaborative Problem Solving

Collaborative problem solving and conflict management are essential for family resilience. Creative brainstorming opens new possibilities for overcoming adversity and for healing and growth to emerge out of tragedy. Shared decision making and conflict resolution involve negotiation of differences with fairness and reciprocity over time, so that partners and family members accommodate one another. In bouncing forward, resilient families set clear goals and priorities, and take concrete steps toward achieving them. They build on small successes and use failures as learning experiences. Families become more resourceful when they are able to shift from a crisis-reactive mode to a proactive stance, anticipating and preparing for future clouds on the horizon. It's most important to help families in problem-saturated situations to envision a better future, and help those whose hopes and dreams have been shattered to seize opportunities for repair and growth.

Families must find their own pathways through adversity that fit their situation, their cultural orientation, and their personal strengths and resources. In one remarkably resilient family, following the shooting death of their oldest son by a gang member in their neighborhood, the mother's deep faith led her to show compassion and forgiveness to the boy who had murdered her son. Although the father was initially too angry to share her feelings, he respected her decision, and both were able to tolerate and honor each other's positions and work together to help the surviving children with their overwhelming pain. Aided by conversations with a priest and a supportive faith congregation, the father became increasingly able to share his own sorrow with his wife. Facing the killer's mother at a hearing, he embraced her, acknowledging the painful reality that they both had lost their sons: his to a grave and hers to prison. The father channeled his anger productively by launching a community action program for gun control to stop violence and prevent such tragedies for other families.

Clinical Utility of a Family Resilience Framework

Over the past two decades, the field of family therapy has refocused attention from family deficits to family strengths (see Walsh, Chapter 2, this volume). The therapeutic relationship has become more collaborative and empowering of client potential, with recognition that successful interventions depend more on tapping into family resources than on therapist techniques (Karpel, 1986). Assessment and intervention are redirected from how problems were caused to how they can be resolved, identifying and amplifying existing and potential competencies. This positive, future-oriented stance refocuses on how families can succeed rather than how they failed.

A family resilience framework builds on these developments to strengthen families in overcoming adversity (Walsh, 1998). A basic premise guiding this approach is that stressful crises and persistent challenges impact the whole family, and, in turn, key family processes mediate the adaptation of all members and the family unit. Therapist and clients work together to find new possibilities in their problem-saturated situation and overcome impasses to change. A family resilience framework can serve as a valuable conceptual map to guide intervention efforts to identify and strengthen key processes as problems are addressed, thereby reducing risk and vulnerability. As families become more resourceful, they are better able to meet future challenges. Thus, building resilience is also a preventive measure.

Rather than rescuing so-called "survivors" from "dysfunctional families," this approach to practice engages distressed families with respect and compassion for their struggles, affirms their reparative potential, and seeks to bring out their best qualities. Efforts to foster family resilience aim both to avert or reduce dysfunction and to enhance family functioning and individual well-being (Luthar et al., 2000). Such efforts have the potential to benefit all family members as they fortify relational bonds and strengthen the family unit.

A family resilience framework can be applied in a wide range of crisis situations and persistent life challenges. Families most often come for help in crisis, but often they don't initially connect presenting problems with relevant stress events. One inner-city mother sought help for her daughter's school problems. During the assessment, it was learned that the eldest son in the family had recently been shot and killed in gang crossfire. The family cohesion had been shattered, with each member going off separately to deal with the loss: The father isolated himself and drank; a brother sought revenge in the streets; the daughter showed her upset at school; and the mother, alone in her unbearable grief, focused on her daughter's school problems. Family sessions focused on building mutual support for the family to surmount this tragedy together.

Family resilience-oriented interventions utilize principles and techniques common among strength-based approaches but attend more centrally to links between presenting symptoms and significant family stressors, identifying and fortifying key processes for resilience. Resilience does not mean bouncing back unscathed, but involves struggling well, effectively working through and learning from adversity, and attempting to integrate the experience into the fabric of family life (Higgins, 1994). We encourage family members to share their stories of adversity, often breaking down walls of silence or secrecy around painful or shameful events, to build mutual support and empathy. This approach readily engages so-called "resistant" families, who are often reluctant to come for mental health services out of beliefs (often based on prior experience) that they will be judged as disturbed or deficient and blamed for their problems. Instead, family members are viewed as intending to do their best for one another and struggling with an overwhelming set of challenges. Therapeutic/counseling efforts are directed at mastering those challenges through collaborative efforts.

We encourage efforts toward reconciliation of past relational wounds. A son, who finds it difficult to give care to his dying mother because of lingering anger at her alcohol abuse and neglect during his childhood, is helped to see her in a new light through learning more about her early life abandonment, gaining compassion for her struggles and courage alongside her limitations. Not all family members may be successful in surmounting obstacles, but all are seen to have dignity and worth.

A multisystemic assessment may lead to a variety of interventions or a combination of individual, couple, family, and multifamily group modalities, depending on the relevance of different systems levels to problem resolution. In putting an ecological view into practice, interventions may involve community agencies, workplace, school, and health care or other larger systems. Resilience-based family interventions can be adapted to a variety of formats, including periodic family consultations or more intensive family therapy. Psychoeducational multifamily groups emphasize the importance of social support and practical information, offering concrete guidelines for crisis management, problem solving, and stress reduction as families navigate through stressful periods and face future challenges (Steinglass, 1998). Therapists help families identify specific stresses and develop effective coping strategies, measuring success in small increments and maintaining family morale. Brief, cost-effective psychoeducational "modules" timed for critical phases of an illness or life challenge encourage families to accept and digest manageable portions of a long-term coping process (Rolland, 1994).

Innovative Family Resilience-Oriented Programs

Clinical training and community projects at the Chicago Center for Family Health are grounded in a family resilience orientation. Faculty members have developed several innovative programs applying a family resilience framework for training and practice with major disruptive crisis experiences, such as meeting the challenges of serious illness, disability, and loss (see Rolland, Chapter 17, this volume), and family-centered recovery from terrorist-related trauma and uncertainty. The framework is valuable in programs addressing a range of challenges: adaptation with divorce, single-parenting, and stepfamily reorganization; family stresses and resources with job loss and transition; navigation of parenting and workplace challenges; family–school partnerships for the success of at-risk youth; and challenges of stigma for gay and lesbian families (see Walsh, 2002a, for a brief overview of these programs).

One ongoing project is directed at recovery efforts from war-related trauma and loss in Bosnia and Kosovo. In 1998, resilience-based, multifamily groups were developed for Bosnian refugees in Chicago and, in the following year, for ethnic Albanians arriving from Kosovo. As a result of the Serbian genocidal campaign of "ethnic cleansing," families in both regions experienced the devastating bombing and destruction of homes and communities; they suffered and witnessed widespread atrocities, including brutal torture, rape, murder, and the disappearance of loved ones.

Our family resilience approach was sought out because refugees would not use traditional mental health services, which they experienced as pathologizing in their narrow focus on individual symptoms and use of psychiatric diagnostic categories. They found a resilience framework to be respectful, healing, and empowering. This program, called CAFES for Bosnian and TAFES for Kosovar families (Coffee/Tea and Family Education, Support), utilized a 9-week multifamily group format, tapping into the strong family-centered orientation in their culture. It offered a compassionate setting for families to share their stories of suffering and struggle while drawing out and affirming family resources, such as their courage, endurance, and faith; their strong kinship networks and deep concern for loved ones; and their determination to rise above their tragedies to forge a new life. Paraprofessional facilitators were trained to colead groups to foster a spirit of collaboration and develop resources within their community.

These projects led to the development of the Kosovar Family Professional Educational Collaborative (KFPEC), an ongoing partnership between mental health professionals in Kosovo, and a team of American family therapists.[1] This project provides resilience-based, family-focused training in Kosovo to enhance capacities to address overwhelming service needs in the war-torn region by strengthening family coping and recovery in the wake of trauma and loss. Coleaders Rolland and Weine (2000) noted that most international programs do not conceptualize or operationalize a family approach to mental health services in meaningful ways. Recognizing that the psychosocial needs of refugees, other trauma survivors, and vulnerable persons in societies in transition far exceed the individual and psychopathological focus of conventional trauma mental health approaches, their approach builds on family and cultural strengths.

One team member told of a family in which the mother had listened to the gunshots as her husband, two sons, and two grandsons were murdered in the yard of their farmhouse. She and her surviving family members talked with team members in their home about what has kept them strong.

> The surviving son in the family responded, "We are all believers. One of the strengths in our family is from God. . . . Having something to believe has helped very much."
> "What do you do to keep faith strong?" the interviewer asked.
> "I see my mother as the 'spring of strength' . . . to see someone who has lost five family members—it gives us strength just to see her. We must think about the future and what we can accomplish. This is what keeps us strong. What will happen to him (pointing to his five-year-old nephew) if I am not here? If he sees me strong, he will be strong. If I am weak, he will become weaker than me."
> "What do you hope your nephew will learn about the family as he grows up?" asked the interviewer.

"The moment when he will be independent and helping others and the family—for him, it will be like seeing his father and grandfather and uncles alive again." (in Becker, Sargent, & Rolland, 2000, p. 29)

In this family, the positive influence of belief systems was striking, in particular, the power of religious faith and the inspiration of strong models and mentors. Other families saw their resilience as strengthened by their connectedness/cohesiveness and adaptive role flexibility:

"Everyone belongs to the family and to the family's homeland, alive or dead, here or abroad. Everyone matters and everyone is counted and counted upon. . . . When cooking or planting everyone moves together fluidly, in a complementary pattern, each person picking up what the previous person left off. . . . A hidden treasure in the family is their adaptability to who fills in each of the absented roles. Although the grief about loss is immeasurable, the ability to fill in the roles . . . [is] remarkable." (in Becker et al., 2000, p. 29)

Since 2000, teams of American family therapists have conducted a series of weeklong training sessions in collaboration with Kosovar counterparts. Bringing varied orientations to family therapy, such as structural and narrative approaches, all emphasized a resilience-based perspective to address family challenges, recognizing that Kosovar professionals will adapt the framework and develop their own practice models to fit best their culture and service needs. Unlike many international projects in which foreign "experts" descend on a crisis zone to dispense knowledge, this program has emphasized ongoing collaboration, with respect for local professionals' and community members' knowledge about their own culture, values, and service needs.

Navigating New Challenges in a Changing World

A family resilience framework is especially timely in helping families with unprecedented challenges as they and the world around them are changing at an accelerated pace (see Walsh, Chapter 1, this volume). Family cultures and structures are becoming increasingly diverse and fluid. Over an extended family life cycle, adults and their children are moving in and out of increasingly complex family configurations, each transition posing new adaptational challenges. Amid social, economic, and political upheavals worldwide, families are dealing with many losses, disruptions, and uncertainties.

Many families are showing remarkable resilience in creatively reworking their family life. Yet stressful transitions and attempts to navigate uncharted territory can contribute to individual and relational distress. Nostalgia for idealized family models and for simpler and more secure times in the past makes adaptations more difficult. A resilience-oriented approach assesses individual, couple, and family distress in relation to this larger context of social change. Families may need help to grieve their actual and symbolic losses as they bounce forward in their changing world. Therapists can help families find coherence in the midst of complexity, and maintain continuities in the midst of upheaval to assist in their journey into the future.

CONCLUSION

With widespread concern about the breakdown of the family, useful conceptual models such as a family resilience framework are needed more than ever to guide efforts to strengthen couple and family relationships. Family research and practice must be rebalanced from a focus on how families fail to how families, when challenged, can succeed, if the field is to move beyond the rhetoric of promoting family strengths to support key processes in intervention and prevention efforts. Both quantitative and qualitative research contributions are useful in informing such approaches. As Werner, a leading pioneer in resilience research, recently affirmed: (1) Resilience research offers a promising knowledge base for practice; (2) the findings of resilience research have many potential applications; and (3) building bridges between clinicians, researchers, and policymakers is of utmost importance (Werner & Johnson, 1999).

This chapter has presented an overview of a research-informed family resilience framework, developed as a conceptual map to guide intervention and prevention efforts. A family resilience metaperspective involves a crucial shift in emphasis from family deficits to family challenges, with conviction in the potential for recovery and growth out of adversity. By targeting interventions to strengthen key processes for resilience, families become more resourceful in dealing with crises, weathering persistent stresses, and meeting future challenges. This conceptual framework can be usefully integrated with many strength-based practice models and applied in a range of crisis situations, with respect for family and cultural diversity. Resilience-oriented services foster family empowerment as they bring forth shared hope, develop new and renewed competencies, and strengthen family bonds.

NOTE

1. The Kosovar Family Professional Educational Collaborative was organized through the auspices of the University of Pristina; the University of Illinois Project on Genocide, Psychiatry, and Witnessing; the Chicago Center for Family Health; and the American Family Therapy Association.

REFERENCES

Anthony, E. J., & Cohler, B. J. (Eds.). (1987). *The invulnerable child*. New York: Guilford Press.

Antonovsky, A. (1987). *Unraveling the mystery of health*. San Francisco: Jossey-Bass.

Antonovsky, A., & Sourani, T. (1988). Family sense of coherence and family adaptation. *Journal of Marriage and the Family, 50,* 79–92.

Aponte, H. (1994). *Bread and spirit: Therapy with the poor*. New York: Norton.

Beavers, W. R. & Hampson, R. B. (1990). *Successful families: Assessment and intervention*. New York: Norton.

Becker, C., Sargent, J., & Rolland, J. S. (2000). Kosovar Family Professional Education Collaborative. *AFTA Newsletter, 80,* 26–30.

Boss, P. (1999). *Ambiguous loss*. Cambridge, MA: Harvard University Press.

Boss, P. (2001). *Family stress management: A contextual approach*. Newbury Park, CA: Sage.

Carter, B., & McGoldrick, M. (1999). *The expanded family life cycle: Individual, family, and social perspectives* (3rd ed.). Needham Hill: Allyn & Bacon.

Coles, R. (1997). *The moral intelligence of children*. New York: Random House.

Cowan, P., Cowan, C. P., & Schulz, M. (1996). Thinking about risk and resilience in families. In E. M. Hetherington & E. Blechman (Eds.), *Stress, coping, and resiliency in children and families* (pp. 1–38). Mahwah, NJ: Erlbaum.

Dossey, L. (1993). *Healing words: The power of prayer and the practice of medicine*. New York: Harper.

Falicov, C. (1995). Training to think culturally: A multidimensional comparative framework. *Family Process, 34,* 373–388.

Garmezy, N. (1991). Resiliency and vulnerability to adverse developmental outcomes associated with poverty. *American Behavioral Scientist, 34,* 416–430.

Hetherington, E. M., & Kelly, J. (2002). *For better or for worse: Divorce reconsidered*. New York: Norton.

Higgins, G. O. (1994). *Resilient adults: Overcoming a cruel past*. San Francisco: Jossey-Bass.

Hill, R. (1958). Generic features of families under stress. *Social Casework, 49,* 139–150.

Karpel, M. (1986). *Family resources: The hidden partner in family therapy*. New York: Guilford Press.

Kaufman, J., & Ziegler, E. (1987). Do abused children become abusive parents? *American Journal of Orthopsychiatry, 57,* 186–192.

Landau, J. (2002, June 29). *Enhancing family, community, and spiritual connectedness for accessing resilience: Overview of the Linking Human Systems (LINC) Model*. Plenary presentation, American Family Therapy Academy, 24th Annual Meeting, New York.

Lazarus, R., & Folkman, S. (1984). *Stress, appraisal, and coping*. New York: Springer.

Luthar, S. S., Cicchetti, D., & Becker, B. (2000). The construct of resilience: A critical evaluation and guidelines for future work. *Child Development, 71,* 543–562.

Luthar, S. S., & Ziegler, E. (1991). Vulnerability and competence: A review of research on resilience in childhood. *American Journal of Orthopsychiatry, 61,* 6–22.

Masten, A. S., Best, K. M., & Garmezy, N. (1990). Resilience and development: Contributions from the study of children who overcame adversity. *Developmental Psychopathology, 2,* 425–444.

Masten, A., & Coatsworth, J. 1998). The development of competence in favorable and unfavorable environments. *American Psychologist, 53*(2), 205–220.

McCubbin, H., McCubbin, M., McCubbin, A., & Futrell, J. (Eds.). (1998). *Resiliency in ethnic minority families: Vol. 2. African-American families.* Thousand Oaks, CA: Sage.

McCubbin, H., McCubbin, M., Thompson, E., & Fromer, J. (Eds.). (1998). *Resiliency in ethnic minority families: Vol. 1. Native and immigrant families.* Thousand Oaks, CA: Sage.

McCubbin, H. & Patterson, J. M. (1983). The family stress process: The Double ABCX model of adjustment and adaptation. *Marriage and Family Review, 6*(1–2), 7–37.

McGoldrick, M., Gerson, R., & Shellenberger, S. (1998). *Genograms: Assessment and intervention* (2nd. ed.) New York: Norton.

Patterson, J. (1988). Families experiencing stress: The family adjustment and adaptation response model. *Family Systems Medicine, 5*(2), 202–237.

Patterson, J. (2002). Integrating family resilience and family stress theory. *Journal of Marriage and the Family,*

Patterson, J., & Garwick, A. (1994). Levels of family meaning in family stress theory. *Family Process, 33,* 287–304.

Reiss, D. (1981). *The family's construction of reality.* Cambridge, MA: Harvard University Press.

Rolland, J. S. (1994). *Families, illness and disability: An integrative treatment model.* New York: Basic Books.

Rolland, J. S., & Weine, S. (2000). Kosovar Family Professional Educational Collaborative. *AFTA Newsletter, 79,* 34–35. Washington, DC: American Family Therapy Academy.

Rutter, M. (1987). Psychosocial resilience and protective mechanisms. *American Journal of Orthopsychiatry, 57,* 316–331.

Saul, J. (2002, June 29). *Promoting community recovery in lower Manhattan post-September 11.* Plenary presentation, American Family Therapy Academy 24th Annual Meeting, New York.

Seligman, M. E. P. (1990). *Learned optimism.* New York: Random House.

Seligman, M. E. P., & Csikszentmihalyi, M. (2000). Positive psychology. [Introduction to special issue]. *American Psychologist, 55*(1), 5–14.

Steinglass, P. (1998). Multiple family discussion groups for patients with chronic medical illness. *Family Systems Medicine, 16*(1–2), 55–70.

Stinnett, N., & DeFrain, J. (1985). *Secrets of strong families.* Boston: Little, Brown.

Taylor, S. (1989). *Positive illusion: Creative self-deception and the healthy mind.* New York: Basic Books.

Taylor, S., Kemeny, M., Reed, G. Bower, J., & Gruenwald, T. (2000). Psychological resources, positive illusions, and health. *American Psychologist, 55*(1), 99–109.

Walsh, F. (1983). The timing of symptoms and critical events in the family life cycle. In H. Liddle (Ed.), *Clinical implications of the family life cycle* (pp. 120–133). Rockville, MD: Aspen.

Walsh, F. (1996). The concept of family resilience: Crisis and challenge. *Family Process, 35,* 261–281.

Walsh, F. (1998). *Strengthening family resilience.* New York: Guilford Press.

Walsh, F. (Ed.). (1999b). *Spiritual resources in family therapy.* New York: Guilford Press.

Walsh, F. (2002a). A family resilience framework: Innovative practice applications. *Family Relations, 51*(2), 130–137.

Walsh, F. (2002b). Bouncing forward: Resilience in the aftermath of September 11. *Family Process, 40*(1), 34–36.

Walsh, F., Jacob, L., & Simon, V. (1995). Facilitating healthy divorce processes: Therapy and mediation approaches. In N. Jacobson & A. Gurman (Eds.), *Clinical handbook of couple therapy* (pp. 340–365). New York: Guilford Press.

Walsh, F., & McGoldrick, M. (Eds.). (1991). *Living beyond loss: Death in the family.* New York: Norton.

Weil, A. (1994). *Spontaneous healing.* New York: Knopf.

Werner, E. E. (1993). Risk, resilience, and recovery: Perspectives from the Kauai longitudinal study. *Development and Psychopathology, 5,* 503–515.

Werner, E. E., & Johnson, J. L. (1999). Can we apply resilience? In M. D. Glantz & J. L. Johnson (Eds.), *Resilience and development: Positive life adaptations* (pp. 259–268). New York: Kluwer Academic/Plenum.

Werner, E. E., & Smith, R. (1992). *Overcoming the odds.* Ithaca, NY: Cornell University Press.

Wolin, S., & Wolin, S. (1993). *The resilient self: How survivors of troubled families rise above adversity.* New York: Villard Books.

Wright, L., Watson, W. L., Bell, J. M. (1996). *Beliefs: The heart of healing in families.* New York: Basic Books.

CHAPTER 16

NORMATIVE FAMILY TRANSITIONS, NORMAL FAMILY PROCESSES, AND HEALTHY CHILD DEVELOPMENT

Philip A. Cowan
Carolyn Pape Cowan

In this chapter, we review both what we know and what we still need to know about family processes that shape children's development. We first examine the concept of "transition," offer a working definition, and explore the meaning of transition for a *family*. Our emphasis on "normative transitions"—those that are predictable and expectable for a substantial number of families—is not meant to imply that our interest is restricted to "normal" or nonclinical families. We attempt to show that because developmental challenges bring family coping strategies into sharp relief, the choice to study or intervene with families as they face major life transitions is an excellent strategy for identifying family processes that facilitate or impede the healthy development of children.

Next, we present a conceptual model that describes six domains of family functioning that we believe are likely to be disequilibrated during major family life transitions. We use our own family studies and those of others' to show how a dynamic combination of individual and interpersonal transactions in each domain predicts posttransition adaptation in children. We then include findings from a systematically evaluated, family-based intervention that lend weight to the claim that these family processes influence children's development and adaptation.

We focus here on the processes involved in two quite different normative family transitions—when married partners become parents, and when the first child makes the transition to elementary school—and speculate about how our theoretical formulation might be applied to other normative and non-normative transitions. We conclude by discussing the implications of our formulation for designing preventive, family-based interventions, with the ultimate goal of enhancing development in the early years of children's lives.

NORMATIVE FAMILY TRANSITIONS

The Definition of Major Life Transitions

Core Meanings

"Transition" is a frequently used word with varied meanings. Women are in transition as their roles change from stay-at-home mothers to full-time corporate executives. Adolescents becoming adults are in transition. Men and women are in transition as they become fathers and mothers. Unemployed workers seeking jobs are in transition. Families undergoing divorce are in transition. Part of the core meaning involves, first, a "passage or change from one place or state or act or set of circumstances to another" (*Oxford English Dictionary*). A second aspect is that it involves "extended periods of change and disequilibrium between periods of stability, balance, and relative quiescence" (P. A. Cowan, 1991, p. 3). A third, often implicit, assumption about a major transition is that the traveler will experience some internal conflict on leaving one shore for another. No matter how positive the prospect of the new, there is some discomfort or loss when old patterns no longer fit and adaptive patterns to meet new challenges have not yet been created (Hill, 1949).

Major transitions at any level—societies, communities, families, couples, or individuals—do not occur in a day. In our studies, we learned that transitions to parenthood may have begun years earlier, when individuals first contemplated the possibilities of parenthood for themselves, and the transitions were often not completed for some time after the child's birth (C. P. Cowan & Cowan, 2000). This is also true for the impact of negative or even catastrophic events. Despite the fact that transitions are usually described as finite, sudden changes, they involve a set of linked processes that unfold over time.

Different Kinds of Transitions

The metaphor of transition as a voyage between stable states was originally used to describe the early years of development (Erikson, 1950; Freud, 1938; Piaget, 1968) and included the notion that the passage from one stage to another *requires* a transitional period in which there is change, disequilibrium, and some psychological stress or confusion. A number of theorists then found this term useful to describe turning points in a life trajectory as a person takes on new life tasks (e.g., Neugarten, 1965; Vaillant & Koury, 1993). Yet unlike childhood transitions, those in adulthood, such as leaving school, entering the work force, selecting a mate, or having a child, are expectable, have some degree of choice, and do not necessarily occur in sequence, especially given the departures from traditional family patterns over recent decades.

Studies tend to focus on either normative or non-normative transitions. Normative transitions are expectable and predictable based on biological, psychological, or social norms. Non-normative transitions are statistically more unusual and often unexpected, but this distinction is not always so clear in practice. Moreover, what is normative in one subculture (e.g., adolescents becoming autonomous from parents) may not be normative in another. Here, we focus primarily on transitions that are normative in contemporary American society and leave open the question of applicability of our conclusions for other cultures. We also focus primarily on the psychosocial aspects of transition.

The Distinction between Change and Transition

We have proposed that major life transitions for individuals involve qualitative reorganizations of the self and the inner world, social roles, and close relationships (P. A. Cowan, 1991).

The Self and the Inner World. A developmental transition in childhood or adulthood involves a restructuring of one's psychological sense of self. Children entering kindergarten see themselves as becoming a "big kid" (P. A. Cowan, Cowan, Ablow, Johnson, & Measelle, in press). Adolescents develop a new identity structure that extends back into the past and forward into the future (Erikson, 1950). Entering parenthood (C. P. Cowan & Cowan, 2000) and old age (Vailliant & Koury, 1993) involves shifts in the definition of who we are and will become. Shifts in one's assumptive world occur (Parkes, 1971). Transitions essentially shift the lenses through which we process information about the world (e.g., Piaget, 1967). Losing a job or becoming a grandparent can change one's assumptions about the nature of the world as cruel or nurturant. Transitions involve the need to cope with new challenges and losses. In addition to the specific knowledge and skills required to meet particular challenges, all transitions involve a shift in the balance of internal regulation of affect.

Roles. Life transitions involve a qualitative shift in roles and the definition of appropriate behaviors for persons occupying given positions. The entrance to elementary school signals a shift in the kind of behavior expected of children. New parenthood involves a marked redefinition of how both partners apportion the energy they devote to juggling involvement in family and work domains.

Roles change in different ways—by addition (e.g., becoming a parent), subtraction (e.g., widowhood), and revision (e.g., job reclassification). In all cases, consistent with a systemic view of individuals and their social environments, changes in an individual's major role require reorganization of other roles in the individual's life and in the network of roles in central relationships. An example of internal reorganization can be seen in our study of couples becoming parents (C. P. Cowan & Cowan, 2000). We asked each partner as an expectant parent, and then after the birth, to fill out an instrument called The Pie by dividing a circle into the salient aspects of self and identity. We found that both men and women experienced a significant increase in the Parent aspect of self from pregnancy to 6 and 18 months postpartum, with women's Parent piece of the pie increasing twice as much as men's (C.P. Cowan et al., 1985). As the parental aspect of men's and women's identity grew larger, the Partner/Lover piece grew significantly smaller. (For men, this decline was correlated with their drop in marital satisfaction.)

The Quality of Close Relationships. A shift in one's inner world and identity, and a reorganization of major life roles are almost inevitably accompanied by disequilibrium in one's central relationships inside and outside the family. As children enter elementary school, they become members of a much larger social system, with new peers, teachers, and rules to master.

Transitional change, then, involves substantial, qualitative, psychological, and social change in one's sense of self, in one's roles, and in the quality of one's relationships. Because transitions are unfolding processes and not discrete events, an individual may pass a major life milestone without making a major life transition. The biological and social fact of becoming a parent does not *necessarily* imply a psychological transition to parenthood, unless the new mother or father makes an actual shift in both inner and outer aspects of life. Similarly, transition from midlife to old age is not marked simply by chronological aging but by shifts in worldview, social roles, and relationships.

The Meaning of Transition for a Family

When an individual, or a couple, grapples with major life change, there are repercussions throughout the family system (e.g., Walsh, 1998). For example, in our study of couples becoming parents, the addition of a new identity as parent and the reduction in identity as "partner" was paralleled by changes in the nature and quality of the division of family work for both spouses and shifts in the quality of their relationship.

Similar intrapsychic and interactional reorganizations of roles may occur with any major life transition. From the perspective of family life, adding, subtracting, or refashioning one's identity and the system of family roles has an impact on the frequency, intensity, quality, and content of family transactions. As the family shifts from dyad to triad when partners become parents, new fathers and mothers often experience an unwelcome drop in the temperature of their relationship (C. P. Cowan & Cowan, 2000). Although it may seem obvious that life transitions can affect the quality of family relationships, explanations of why *positive* changes can have a negative impact have not gone much beyond recognition that the stress of major change can have a debilitating effect on interactions (McCubbin & Patterson, 1983) and the flow of negative emotion (Gottman, 2001; Gottman, Katz, & Hooven, 1997; see Driver et al., Chapter 18, this volume).

Using Transitions and Interventions as a Lens for Viewing Family Processes

The study of transitions provides three important opportunities for family researchers and clinicians. First, because transitions involve the dynamic unfolding of processes from before to after a complex event, they function as "natural experiments" that help us to build conceptual causal models of family adaptation. For example, researchers set up a study in an area of the country rife with economic difficulties and a fairly high risk of job loss. They find that compared to families whose parents maintained their job, families in which parents lost their job showed increased parent–teen conflict (see Flanagan, 1990). We can begin to make some inferences about one factor in deteriorating relationships between parents and their teenage children.

Such inferences must be made cautiously. Most studies of life transitions do not involve a systematic clinical trial with randomized assignment to transition or no-transition conditions. In this case, it is possible that chronic family conflict precipitates the job loss. Nevertheless, observation and comparison of changes in two groups, one experiencing job loss and the other not (the natural experiment), allow us to make stronger inferences about cause and effect than single-time or even longitudinal studies that are not keyed to analyses of transition and change.

Second, because transitions disrupt the status quo, the usual individual and family resistances to change may be lower, and openness to trying new ways of coping may be higher. Thus, life transitions signal opportune moments to consider preventive or therapeutic interventions that could be helpful in moving families closer to adaptive positions on their life trajectories (Caplan, 1964). Third, as we show later, just as intervention studies provide potential benefits for family processes, they also allow researchers to test hypotheses about the impact of family processes on children's adaptation (P. A. Cowan & Cowan, 2001); that is, planned interventions (randomized clinical trial experiments) add weight to the natural experiments triggered by life transitions and help us understand some of the mechanisms explaining how family processes affect children's development.

A SYSTEMS MODEL OF FAMILY PROCESSES DURING MAJOR LIFE TRANSITIONS

In our two longitudinal research and preventive intervention studies of (1) couples making the transition to parenthood (C. P. Cowan & Cowan, 2000) and (2) families with a first child making the transition to elementary school (P. A. Cowan, Cowan, Ablow, et al., in press), we have been testing a six-domain model of family functioning. Based on a variety of descriptions of family systems (McGoldrick & Carter, 1988; Walsh, 1993), the model is consistent with other family researchers' attempts to show that understanding adaptation in one domain (e.g., the couple relationship or the child's development) requires an ecological (Bronfenbrenner, 1979) or contextual analysis of multiple aspects of family life (e.g., Belsky, 1984, Cox, Owen, Lewis, & Henderson, 1989; Heinicke, 1991).

The six interacting domains of family life in our model are (1) the well-being or distress of individual family members; (2) the quality of relationship between parents and *their* parents; (3) the quality of relationships between each parent and child(ren); (4) the quality of relationships between siblings; (5) the balance of life stress and social supports available to the parents, children, and family; and the central focus in our own studies, (6) the quality of relationship *between* the parents.

Figure 16.1 presents a schematic representation of the connections among five of the six family domains. We have omitted sibling relationships because of our initial focus on the first child, but we do not mean to discount the important influence of sibling relationships in children's development (e.g., Dunn & Plomin, 1990). The model represented in Figure 16.1 contains central features of family systems approaches to analysis of development and psychopathology (Wagner & Reiss, 1995). The structure or organization of family relationships affects the quality of the relationship between any two family members and vice versa. The double-headed arrows signify that causality is circular rather than linear; parents affect children, and children affect parents; marital relationships affect parenting, and parenting affects marital relationships; grandparents from both "sides" of the family affect parents and children, and vice versa. Like cybernetic systems, family systems are self-regulating in that a perturbation of the system sets forces in motion that attempt to reach a new and more adaptive equilibrium.

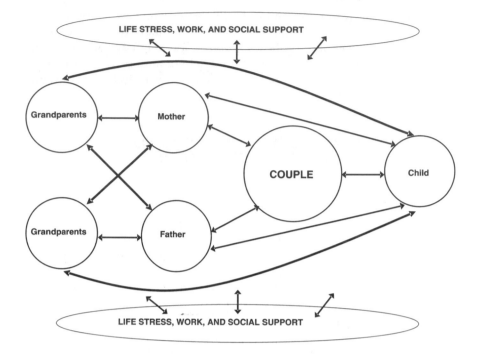

FIGURE 16.1. Domains of family life associated with children's development.

One important feature of the systemic model is that family relationships have both direct and indirect effects. A cold, unforgiving relationship between grandparent and parent can affect the grandchild directly in terms of what the child observes and indirectly in its impact on the parents as individuals, as a couple, and the way they treat the child. We use this model to look at two major family transitions—when couples are becoming parents, and when children enter the elementary school system—to show how variation in multiple domains contributes to our understanding of the dynamic connections among marital adaptation, parent–child relationship quality, and children's development.

NORMAL FAMILY PROCESSES IN COUPLES BECOMING PARENTS

Over 40 years ago, sociologist LeMasters (1957) made the startling claim that having a first child produced a moderate or severe crisis in the marriages of 83% of the couples he interviewed, a view that generated wide controversy (C. P. Cowan et al., 1985). Early debates were based on retrospective studies, but by the 1980s, a rash of prospective longitudinal studies followed couples through the transition to parenthood (see also Belsky & Pensky, 1988). Here, we provide a selective update of this literature from our previous reviews (C. P. Cowan & Cowan, 1995). In all, we found close to 40 systematic longitudinal studies of the transition to parenthood, with most focusing on the period from late pregnancy through the first postpartum year, and a few extending further. Studies were conducted in the United States and abroad; those in the United States include both European American and African American samples. Most studied couples in their mid- to late 20s, with teen parents rarely included. Single parents and poor families have rarely been followed through this major transition. Demographically, the families in most studies might be considered "low risk." However, this term is misleading when the realities of the participants' lives are examined closely.

What Happens to Men, Women, and Marriage around the Birth of a First Child?

We consider all of the family domains represented in Figure 16.1.

Shifts in the Sense of Self

Using a model of development derived from Erikson (1980), many writers have suggested that the disequilibration involved in the transition to parenthood can precipitate an intrapsychic crisis leading either to adaptation or dysfunction (Grossman, Eichler, & Winickoff, 1980). On the positive side, becoming a parent can lead to an increased sense of maturity and a more mature approach to life—more differentiated and integrated, with more perspective on the connections between oneself and the world, increased vitality and commitment, and a greater ability to control one's own impulses in the service of caring for others (e.g., P. A. Cowan, 1988). For others, becoming new parents can reawaken inner conflicts from early family relationships (Anthony & Benedek, 1970) and increase risk for depression and other maladjustment (Cutrona, 1982).

Most of the assertions about the impact *on the individual* of having a child, either positive or negative, remain untested in systematic research. Very few longitudinal studies have compared couples having a baby with others on measures of self-concept or individual functioning, and none has directly tested hypotheses about parenthood as a facilitator of adult development. A comprehensive summary of research on the transition to parenthood and individual functioning (Antonucci & Mikus, 1988) suggested many possibilities for positive change in new parents, but only a few studies actually provided data concerning increases in self-confidence and self-worth.

As noted earlier, our own longitudinal study found a significant increase in the proportion of subjects' identity as parents, with a much greater increase for new mothers than new fathers. In some, the increased salience of identity as a parent was welcome and a source of joy. In others, the intense preoccupation with figuring out the best way to parent a newborn was a source of some anxiety, strain, and depression. In contrast with older parents (ages 31–40), who showed stable self-esteem over the transition to parenthood, younger men's and women's (ages 21–30) self-esteem showed a significant decline (C. P. Cowan & Cowan, 2000), trends that require replication before generalizations can be made about the impact of the transition on the individual parents.

Despite extensive writing about the reawakening of inner conflicts (Anthony & Benedek, 1970), the only well-established finding about negative effects of the transition on individual adaptation is an increased risk of clinical depression in postpartum women, approximately 10% of women in one study (Campbell, Cohn, Flanagan, & Popper, 1992). Other longitudinal research finds an increase in depressive symptoms from pregnancy into the first year of parenthood for both partners (Cox, Paley, Payne, & Burchinal, 1999; Pancer, Pratt, Hunsberger, & Gallant, 2000).

Clearly, for many new parents, this transition represents a marked restructuring of the self and a shifting sense of well-being. Nevertheless, an emphasis on change obscures the fact that people are likely to be consistent over time; expectant parents with low self-esteem before the birth were most likely to be low in self-esteem as new parents at 6- and 18-months postpartum (C. P. Cowan et al., 1985).

More research is needed to understand the differences between parents who become depressed in the postpartum months and those who do not. The consequences for infants' development are obvious (Seifer & Dickstein, 2000). There is also a need for more research on the growth-producing potential for men and women having children. The consequences for children and the family as a whole are equally obvious. With more empirical evidence, we assume that it will still be consistent with Erikson's formulation: The transition to parenthood presents opportunities for individual development and risks for difficulties and distress.

Shifts in Relationships with Families of Origin

Bringing a first child into the family requires a shift in family roles and relationships (see McGoldrick & Carter, Chapter 14, this volume). As the baby's due date approaches, and especially after the birth, there tends to be more contact between the new parents and their families of origin (C. P. Cowan & Cowan, 2000). The increased calls and visits are not always positive, especially if the relationships were strained or ambivalent before the pregnancy (Hansen & Jacob, 1992). We found several common sources of stress between the generations in the early postpartum period, especially for couples who lived far from their families of origin. Many new parents in our couples groups were troubled by questions of (1) how and when to arrange visits, and (2) how to respond to grandparents' criticism about their handling of the baby or (3) whether or when mothers planned to return to work. Many new parents expected that relationships between the generations would improve with the birth of a child. Although the hoped-for improvement happened in a few cases (e.g., one new father reestablished phone contact with his parents after not talking to them for 10 years), on the whole, these relationships continued pretty much as they had before the babies were born; that is, there are notable shifts in the intensity of the connection, but the underlying positive or negative valence of the relationship tends to remain unchanged.

Shifts in Relation to the Child

Forming a new family unit by adding a child to the couple system leads to a structural change in the family (from dyad to triad and a new generation) that adds new roles (mother, father) and new relationships (parent–child, grandparent–grandchild) to the system. Family processes may be affected not only by the parents' reaction but also by the child's biological and psychological characteristics (see Towers, Spotts, & Reiss, Chapter 22, this volume). An infant's quiet or wiry temperament makes a difference to parental equilibrium and is related to both individual and marital adaptation in the early postpartum months (Klinnert, Gavin, Wamboldt, & Mrazek, 1992). Later in this chapter, we show how the family relationship context—parents' individual adaptation, their relationships with their own parents, and their relationships as couples—is linked with the quality of the relationships that parents establish with their child.

Changes in Stress and Social Support

In our study, men and women described no significant increase in overall stressful life events *outside* the nuclear family between pregnancy and 6- and 18-months postpartum (C. P. Cowan & Cowan, 2000). However other researchers (Levy-Shiff, Dimitrovsky, Shulman, & Har-Even, 1998) found an increase in parental stress from pregnancy to 1-month postpartum, a decline in stress by 6-months postpartum, followed by another decline 6 months later.

One central issue for couples to resolve is their level of involvement in work outside the home during their child's first months of life. On The Pie, psychological involvement in work and actual hours of work increased for fathers and declined for mothers (C. P. Cowan & Cowan, 2000). Most husbands described their work involvement as stemming directly from their desire to be good providers, but wives often viewed their husbands' work as an avoidance of involvement in the family. In the context of contemporary U.S. culture, where working outside the home is now normative for mothers of young children, mothers who went back to work during the first 18 postpartum months (about 50%) reported feeling torn by wanting to care for their infants and toddlers, and mothers who stayed home by choice felt conflicting desires to care for their children, to ease the family's new financial burdens, and to pursue their careers (Hochschild & Machung, 1990). (See Fraenkel, Chapter 3, this volume.)

Changes in the Couple

We have noted that the increased psychological space allocated to men's and women's identity as new parents seemed to come at the expense of the aspect of the self they labeled "partner" or "lover." Data from The Pie were buttressed by each parent's reports of placing their relationship on the back burner to cope with the realities and ambiguities of life with a newborn, whose requests for nurturance required extensive decoding, and whose sleep and waking patterns were often unpredictable. Parental fatigue and anxiety, the need to juggle family and work life, and simply the presence of a new resident in the household certainly reduced the time, opportunity, and actual investment in marital intimacy.

A number of investigators have found that the role arrangements that constitute a couple's division of family labor become more traditional when partners become parents. Despite a growing ideology of egalitarianism in marriage over the past 40 years, men do less family work after the birth of a baby than they did before, and fewer of the daily tasks of caring for the children than they predicted they would (Belsky, Lang, & Huston, 1986; C. P. Cowan & P. A. Cowan, 1988; Crohan, 1996). This shift in roles appears to spill over into communication between husbands and wives as marital conflict increases and the "Who does what?" of daily life becomes the number one issue of conflict between them (C. P. Cowan et al., 1985).

Not surprisingly, then, for average couples making the transition to first-time parenthood, marital satisfaction declines from pregnancy into the early child-rearing years—for women in the first year of parenthood, and for men in the second. Let us be clear: New parents' satisfaction with marriage does not plummet from the heights of happiness to the depths of despair. The average decline is quite modest but very consistent across studies. It is also important to note that marital satisfaction rises for 18–30% of couples after having a baby, which is a significant proportion (C. P. Cowan & Cowan, 1995). Nevertheless, except for three studies that report no significant change, in more than 30 longitudinal studies conducted between the late 1970s and the turn of the 21st century in different regions of the United States, Israel (Levy-Shiff et al., 1998), England (Parr, 1997), and Germany (Engfer, Heinig, & Gavranidou, 1998; Gloger-Tippelt & Huerkamp, 1998; Schneewind, 1983), a majority of couples show significant declines in marital satisfaction after having a first baby.

The data from quantitative studies of nonclinical families are remarkably consistent with descriptions based on observations of couples in therapy. For example, in Walsh's (1989) account of how gendered role prescriptions for men and women influence the "marital quid pro quo" (rules for the relationship), she suggests that the transition to parenthood presents a special challenge for couples with egalitarian ideologies, who commonly find themselves sliding back into traditional patterns of stereotyped expectations for masculine (dominant, privileged, breadwinner role) and feminine (accommodating, self-sacrificing, nurturant) behavior. Workplace inflexibility and gendered inequities in job status and salary complicate efforts to share parenting and household demands equitably.

Two methodological points about research on the transition to parenthood are worth noting. First, it is rare for studies to include a comparison group of couples that have not had a baby, to control for the possibility that marital decline is attributable to the erosion of intimacy over time. Our own results (C. P. Cowan et al., 1985) and those of Shapiro, Gottman, and Carrere (2000) reveal that, compared with childless couples, new parents showed a sharper drop in marital satisfaction over the 2-year period surrounding the transition to parenthood. Two studies that began with young newlyweds (Lindahl, Clements, & Markman, 1998; McHale & Huston, 1985) found similar declines in marital satisfaction in both groups but did not follow couples beyond the early postpartum months; we would expect to see some later divergence between parent and nonparent couples.

Relatively little is known about the transition to parenthood in samples defined as high risk by virtue of youth, low income, and/or single parenthood (C. P. Cowan & Cowan, 1995). A number of studies have been conducted with high risk mothers; many are single-time cross sectional studies (Brooks-Gunn & Chase-Lansdale, 1995) and a few have longitudinal designs (Olds et al., 1998), but all begin after childbirth, and none compare new mothers with childless women in the same general life circumstances. Therefore, we have almost no information about how much of the stress attributed to low-income single mothers is attributable to the normative challenges involved in making the transition to parenthood, and how much additional stress can be explained by the economic and social conditions associated with poverty (see Anderson, Chapter 5, this volume). Furthermore, it is important to investigate not only what happens to the mothers themselves as they become parents, but also what happens to their intimate relationships. Studies have ignored the fact that a majority of contemporary single mothers giving birth are in romantic relationships with the child's father, making it possible to study the impact of the transition on the couple (Harknett, Hardman, Garfinkel, & McLanahan, 2001).

In summary, findings from many studies demonstrate clearly that becoming a parent is a major life transition, with significant changes in men's and women's self-view, roles, and relationships. Despite the pleasures associated with this transition, many recent studies document changes in new parents' relationships, especially in their couple relationships, in the direction of conflict, dissatisfaction, and disappointment. The myriad stresses and changes described here appear to be obvious sources of difficulty for couples in this transtion.

In addition, two prebaby risk factors for marital decline emerged in our study and others. First, the ways couples collaborated on the planning of the pregnancy was predictive of what happened subsequently to their relationship. Approximately 50% of the couples deliberately planned the timing of their first pregnancy, and 20% accepted the news of a pregnancy as "fate." All of these couples did reasonably well in terms of their satisfaction as a couple in the first 3 years of parenthood. Another 20% of the couples described moderate ambivalence about the prospect of becoming parents in their sixth or seventh month of pregnancy; they showed a sharp decline in marital satisfaction in the early years of parenthood. Another 10% of the couples, interviewed in their third trimester of pregnancy, were still divided, with one partner wanting a child and the other not feeling ready. Out of those nine couples, two, in which the man wanted the baby and the woman was the reluctant partner, reported high marital conflict 3 years later. In all seven couples in which the woman wanted the baby but the man did not feel ready to become a father, the partners had divorced by the time the child entered kindergarten. Cox and her colleagues (1999) report data that support the same conclusion: Disagreement on whether or when to have a child signals risk for the parents' couple relationship during the early child-rearing years.

Second, how the marriage fares is closely connected with individual well-being, especially for new mothers. Depressive symptoms are more likely when prebaby expectations of partner support fail to materialize after the baby arrives (C. P. Cowan & Cowan, 2000; Cox et al., 1999). This would also contribute to overload for the mother, another factor in depression, and may explain why depression and marital dissatisfaction tend to be correlated in the early child-rearing years (Cox et al., 1999). A bright spot in this gloomy picture is that social support from grandparents and others provides a buffer to the family system by reducing life stress for new parents, who feel they have available, positive support (Fischer, 1988; Levy-Shiff et al., 1998).

Of course, what happens after the birth also contributes to the direction of change in marital satisfaction, and here the regulation of emotion in marital interaction appears to play a central role. In a study of 43 couples in transition to parenthood, Shapiro et al. (2000) found that husbands' expression of fondness toward their wives predicted stable or increasing marital satisfaction, whereas husbands' negativity toward their wives and disappointment in their couple relationship predicted declines in wives' marital satisfaction (see Driver et al., Chapter 18, this volume).

In our own study, to our surprise, we found little direct correlation between change in any single domain of family life and declines in marital satisfaction. Rather, the more women and men diverged in the experience of their individual and mutual lives, the more their marital conflict increased and the more their satisfaction with the overall relationship declined (C. P. Cowan et al., 1985). In addition to the fact that new fathers and mothers were less likely to share family tasks than they expected, partners described growing differences in other areas as well—discrepancies in the size of the Parent piece of The Pie, satisfaction with their division of family work, parenting ideology, descriptions of their families of origin, and the balance between life stress and social support. We found that the more discrepancy there was between partners' descriptions of these aspects of their lives from pregnancy to 6 months postpartum, the more conflict they reported in their marriage. These two factors taken together predicted 30% of the variance in declines in marital satisfaction for men and 37% of women's decline. In other words, in this culture at this time, the transition to parenthood appears to propel men and women down separate tracks, and the farther apart they become, the greater their disenchantment with their marital relationship. It seems particularly poignant that in the face of these normative changes, there are no services to support families with young children, unless they are experiencing serious enough marital distress or psychopathology to seek help.

The Divorce Perspective

Another important marker of marital adaptation is the tendency for marriages to remain intact or to dissolve. Our own data correspond with national surveys, which suggest that about 20% of all divorces occur within 5 years after the birth of a first child (Bumpass & Rindfuss, 1979). *This means that almost half of all couples with children who divorce will have done so before their first child enters kindergarten.* Before rushing to conclude that the strains inherent in the transition to parenthood are responsible for early marital dissolution, the statistics on marital stability–divorce reveal that couples without children tend to divorce at an even higher rate than those in early parenthood, with the rates evening up only during the second decade of marriage. In our sample, compared with the 20% divorce rate in new parents, 50% of those who did not have a baby were separated or divorced 5 years after the study began. This suggests that despite increased marital stresses that accompany the transition to parenthood, the presence of a child appears to help keep couples together in the early family-making years.

The Developmental Continuity Perspective

Moreover, most transition to parenthood studies, including our own, find that the best predictor of marital quality after having a baby is the quality of the couple's relationship before the baby arrived (C. P. Cowan & Cowan, 1995). Babies do not bring couples together that were previously experiencing high conflict, nor do they drive couples whose relationships were highly compatible and satisfying apart. This point deserves more attention in discussions of the transition to parenthood. A central feature of life transitions is that even in a context of small but important before and after changes, the central core of individual and relationship functioning remains in place.

FAMILY PROCESSES AND CHILDREN'S DEVELOPMENT

We applied the systems model developed for our study of the transition to parenthood to our study designed to understand how family processes affect children's development in early elementary school. Our focus on the impact *of* family relationships *on* children requires some explanation. First, a basic assumption of family systems theorists, inherent in the definition of the field, is that parents influence children, and children influence parents. However, it is not always easy to identify the contributions that parents and family processes make to the development of the child. Second, we need to address Harris's (1998) recent challenges to traditional socialization theory in her argument that parents have little long-term impact on their children's personality and behavior outside the family setting.

Transition to Parenthood Research and the Direction of Effects

Despite the focus of early family systems theorists on bidirectional influences within the family, until recently, child development researchers tended to use a socialization paradigm; parents' behavior was interpreted as the major force shaping both development and adaptation of the child (Parke & Buriel, 1998). Harris (1989) challenged this view by suggesting that a vast majority of socialization researchers make causal inferences about parental influence based on concurrent correlations between parenting behavior and children's adaptation. We agree with the criticisms about correlation and causation but reject her conclusions about parental influence (P. A. Cowan & Cowan, 2002). Even longitudinal studies do not solve the problem of making inferences about parental influence on children. The fact that a parent's behavior at Time 1 predicts a child's behavior at Time 2 does not allow us to conclude that the parent's behavior is causally related to the "child outcome"; the parent may have been reacting to the child's behavior before the study began. A systemic paradigm shifts from linear causal assumptions to consider multiple, recursive influences over time.

Capitalizing on the notion of transitions as natural experiments, transition to parenthood studies provide some help in disentangling child and parent effects. First, as noted earlier, parents' individual functioning (self-esteem, depression) and marital satisfaction before the baby are highly correlated with the same measures after the baby arrives. Unlike family studies conducted only after babies are born, this design allows us to say that men and women bring a great deal of their prebaby selves into their role as parents.

Moreover, parents' characteristics during pregnancy are predictors of both their postbirth interaction with the child and the child's development. For example, Fonagy, Steele, and Steele (1991) showed that when mothers were coded as having secure working models of attachment on the Adult Attachment Interview (Main, Kaplan, & Cassidy, 1985) during pregnancy, their 1-year-old infants were more likely to be classified as securely attached in the standard Strange Situation laboratory procedure. One set of studies suggests that when expectant mothers are depressed, their subsequent interaction with their infants is less optimal, which is followed by increased risk of later problem behavior in children (Carter, Garrity-Rokous, Chazan-Cohen, Little, & Briggs-Gowan, 2001; Field, 1995; Hipwell & Kumar, 1996). A meta-analysis of observational studies in the early postpartum months (Lovejoy, Graczyk, O'Hare, & Neuman, 2000) indicates that women with other clinical diagnoses show a similar pattern. More generally, the results of these studies and a review by Heinicke (1995), lead us to conclude that mothers' prebirth adjustment predicts both the quality of their interactions with their infants and the infants' and toddlers' competence and adaptation.

The finding that marital quality is fairly consistent over time also has implications for understanding parents' contribution to children's development. Cox and her colleagues (1989) found that even when measures of psychological adjustment were statistically controlled, mothers and fathers were more positive with their 3-month-old infants if they had been in a close, confiding marriage during pregnancy. In two other studies, prebaby marital quality predicted the infants' security of attachment to their mother (Gloger-Tippelt & Huerkamp, 1998; Howes & Markman, 1989). In structural equation models of our own longitudinal data, we found that trajectories of declining marital satisfaction from pregnancy through 1½ and 3½ years postpartum were linked with low warmth and structure in our observations of mothers' and fathers' interactions with their children when they were 3½. The structural models predicted 54% of the variance in children's later academic achievement test scores, 20% of the variance in their shy withdrawn behavior, and 28% of the variance in their aggressive behavior, as perceived by their kindergarten teachers (P. A. Cowan, Cowan, Schulz, & Heming, 1994).

None of these studies prove that parents' individual and marital characteristics are *the source* of difficulties in parent–child relationships or children's maladaptation, because they cannot rule out the possibility that the connections might be attributable to genetic factors. Nevertheless, because there is substantial continuity in parents' characteristics as individuals and as couples during the transition to parenthood period, it is not possible to claim, as Harris (1998) and others do, that postbirth family processes are primarily shaped by child temperament factors, such as infant irritability. Again, this point may be obvious to family theorists, but there are very few studies that can provide empirical support.

Moreover, substantial predictability of pre- to postbirth characteristics means that it is possible to identify families and children at risk for relationship difficulties and behavior problems before the child's birth. This increases the possibility of providing targeted preventive interventions to help parents make the transition more successfully and to facilitate the healthy development of their children in the long term.

Family Factors in Children's Transition to School

In the years that follow couples' transition to parenthood, individuals and families may undergo many transitions, such as having a second child, moving, changing jobs, parents' divorcing, and children entering day care. Even so, in Western cultures, the next *universal* normative transition after the birth of a first child occurs when the child begins formal education. We focus here on children's transition to elementary school, and on the family processes that facilitate or impede their development and adaptation. We rely centrally on our own work (P. A. Cowan, Cowan, Ablow, et al., in press), because very few studies have followed families longitudinally from the preschool through the early school period, with systematic observation-based information about family processes before and after children make the transition to school. After we describe the design of the study and why we think the first child's entrance to kindergarten constitutes a major life transition for a family (albeit, with some important differences from the transition to parenthood), we report some of the correlations between family functioning and children's adaptation based on our family model. We then return to the issue of direction of effects by briefly summarizing the intervention aspect of our study.

Study Design

The Schoolchildren and their Families Project draws on a population quite similar to that of our earlier study of couples in transition to parenthood. More than 200 couples with children in preschools and day care centers in many communities in the San Francisco Bay area initially filled out a questionnaire and agreed to be interviewed. They were randomly offered a chance to participate in one of three conditions: (1) a 16-session couples group meeting weekly, led by male–female teams of trained mental health professionals who emphasized marital issues; (2) a similar 16-week couples group in which the leaders emphasized parent–child issues; and (3) a chance to consult the mental health professionals once each year over the next 3 years. The third condition constituted our "low dose" control sample. One hundred couples agreed to take part in the longitudinal study—about half of them in one of the two kinds of couples groups. We describe the groups briefly below (see P. A. Cowan, Cowan, & Heming, in press). Couples who agreed to participate were no different than those who dropped out on measures of depression, parenting stress, marital satisfaction, and concerns about their child entering school. Furthermore, there were no differences among participants in each of the experimental conditions on these preintervention measures.

As in our earlier study, about 16% of this second sample of parents were members of ethnic minorities (Hispanic, African American, Asian American), and 84% were European American. When their first child was 4 years old, the average age of the fathers was 37.9 years, and the mothers, 36.2 years. The couples lived in 27 cities and towns in the Bay area. Their median yearly total family income ($78,000) indicated a relatively affluent sample, with two qualifications: (1) Because the primary sources of recruitment were day care centers and preschools, the study attracted mostly two-job families (71% of mothers were employed at least half-time); (2) despite the sample's generally high total family income, 22% of the families were below the median family income of $58,000 for U.S. *dual-worker* families in 1990–1993. These were "nonclinical" families in the sense that the couples initially entering the study were responding to a request for participants in a study of family factors in children's adaptation to school. Only after they had filled out an initial questionnaire were they randomly assigned to couples group and consultation conditions.

Although this was not an epidemiological sample of families, the children were not significantly different from their classmates. An adaptive behavior checklist was filled out by teachers on every child in class, without knowing which child was a study participant. Those in this study were rated as slightly more academically competent than classmates in kindergarten and first grade, but at any time period, there were no significant differences between them on scales reflecting social competence, externalizing–aggressive, externalizing–hyperactive, internalizing–anxious/depressed, and internalizing–somatic symptoms.

Is the Entrance to Kindergarten a Major Life Transition for a Child?

On the first day of elementary school, it is clear that the children's sense of self and their roles and relationships are changing. They are entering a new institution with new rules and demands. Even with extensive preschool experience, they are now required to take the role of student in a larger social environment with few close friends and adults who know and understand them.

We found that a majority of the children were faring quite well, able to meet the challenges posed by kindergarten and first grade, and responding to the new, complex school environment by developing new intellectual and interpersonal skills. Nevertheless, despite their generally positive sense of competence, the children appeared to have two vulnerabilities during the transition to elementary school. First, girls' perceptions of their academic competence became more negative in the period from the last preschool year to their completion of first grade.

Reports from children, parents, and teachers of children's adaptation to kindergarten and first grade all showed substantial cross-time correlations of children's adaptation from preschool through the following two years (P. A. Cowan & Heming, in press). The data are consistent with Alexander and Entwisle's trajectory hypothesis (1988): Despite significant changes, children tend to stay in the same rank order on measures of adaptation relative to their age cohort (see also Baumrind, 1991; Bennet et al., 1999; Carlson et al., 1999). Like the adults in our transition to parenthood study, preschool children at the bottom of the adaptation continuum tend to remain in that place as they enter school.

Is This a Major Transition for Parents?

Our studies of couples with children entering school and couples becoming parents used different samples but *identical measures* of self-concept, self-esteem, work hours, social support, life stress, marital satisfaction, and family role arrangements. In contrast with men and women becoming parents, fathers and mothers of preschoolers entering elementary school did not change much in their perceptions of the salience of Parent, Partner, and Lover aspects of themselves on The Pie. Unlike new parents, there were no changes in self-esteem. As children entered kindergarten, we found significant decreases for fathers and mothers in both anxiety and depression scores on standard questionnaires. Unlike new parents, who moved toward a more traditional division of family labor and increasing dissatisfaction with their family work arrangements, parents of children entering kindergarten showed relative stability of role arrangements and *increasing satisfaction* with their division of labor (Alexandrova, 1999). Men and women becoming first-time parents described declining social support in contrast to the parents of school-age children in the current study, who reported stable social support in a context of declining life stress.

We do not conclude that the first child's transition to school has no negative effects on parents and family relationships. We had ample opportunity to hear about parents' (1) preoccupation with the choice of schools, (2) disagreements between spouses about who obtained school information and what decisions they would make, (3) worries about whether the child would "get along" with peers and teachers, (4) reawakened emotional issues about whether they could help their child in ways their own parents had not, and (5) questions about whether the child's entrance to school provided some opportunity, especially for women, to consider new work arrangements. This was also a period in which two-thirds of the families had already had second children, and several were about to have a third. Sibling relationships, too, felt the pressure of the family focus on the oldest child and the fact that the first child was now going off to the big school. In short, parents talked about concerns in each of the domains of family life represented in our six-domain model, but with one important exception: Their questionnaire responses did not show the same systematic negative changes on the same measures as new parents in the earlier study.

How do we understand the fact that despite the rather positive picture presented by parents' responses to our measures of individual adaptation and life stress, marital satisfaction showed a small but statistically significant decline during this period? We measured marital satisfaction with the widely used Marital Adjustment Test (Locke & Wallace, 1959), which has an average score of 100; a score of 120 is very high. In our earlier study of expectant parents, men and women started with an average score of 121 in late pregnancy, declining to 116 at 6 months postpartum and 110 a year later, when the children were 18 months old. In the present study, the parents of 4-year-olds began with an average score of 110 and declined to 109 in the kindergarten year (not a significant change), and to 105 when their child completed first grade. In statistical analyses similar to those in the earlier study, we found that the decline was not related to a widening gap between husbands' and wives' roles or perceptions of themselves and their life as a family. Why was marital satisfaction still declining?

Part of the answer seemed to be different for wives and husbands. Although parents' average dissatisfaction with family role arrangements remained stable, those women who became increasingly dissatisfied with the "Who does what?" of family life were more likely to be dissatisfied with the overall marital relationship. Their dissatisfaction was represented by descriptions of their husbands as taking less responsibility than anticipated for care of the child during the transition to school. Interestingly, husbands who *increased* their share of family and child-related tasks over the transition years were significantly *less* satisfied with their couple relationship by the time their child was in first grade. Our preliminary interpretation of these findings is that the child's transition to school begins to lessen some domestic pressure for women, but in the renegotiation of responsibilities for family work, the couple relationships may experience increased tension.

There is a cultural context to this internal and relationship conflict. Some of the contemporary stresses associated with the transition to parenthood in the United States stem from the pressures of traditional and nontraditional role expectations for men and women that exist side by side, and the conflicting demands of work and family life that create dilemmas for both partners that are not easy to resolve.

We had expected the impact of the child's transition to school on parents would be more similar to the transition to parenthood than we found it to be. Perhaps we might have paid more attention to several salient differences between the two transitions. First, though the child comes under the control of a school system that is more separate from the parents than the preschool had been, there is no major structural change in the family's life that is analogous to the shift from a couple dyad to a two-generational triad, with partners thrust into new roles as parents, responsible for the well-being of an infant. The structural stability of the family over early childhood may buffer the system from the potentially disequilibrating, more temporary reverberations of a child entering the culture of elementary school. Second, the challenges to parents caused by the care of a newborn, exacerbated by sleep disruptions, are of a different order of magnitude than those presented by the dilemma of trying to decide about public, private, or parochial education, or how to deal with a child's learning or social difficulties in the classroom.

Researchers studying family transitions rarely consider more than one transition. It would be valuable to begin the task of conceptualizing the dimensions of each of these transitions in order to identify their salient characteristics. These dimensions may interact with the family resources to influence how mothers, fathers, and children fare as they experience changes in themselves, their roles, and their relationships.

Family Processes Predicting Children's Adaptation to School

Most studies of family processes and children's adaptation to school measure adaptation in both settings at the same time. If we want to evaluate the impact of the family on the child, a first step is to assess family functioning before the child enters elementary school and then assess the child in kindergarten and first grade. As noted, this strategy does not provide a foolproof way of identifying family influences, but it will do as a first step. We consider next what happens when we add information from an intervention with the parents to our account of family–school adaptation.

We focused on three indices of the child's adaptation to school: (1) academic achievement, as measured by the Peabody Individual Achievement Test (Markwardt, 1989), and (2) externalizing (aggressive and hyperactive) and (3) internalizing (depressed and shy/withdrawn) behavior problems, as measured by the Child Adaptive Behavior Inventory (P. A. Cowan, Cowan, & Heming, 1995), a checklist filled out by teachers on every child in their class.

Most studies of the family context of child development begin with parenting behavior, which we assessed in a laboratory/playroom by observing mother–child and father–child interactions over a 40-minute period while they worked and played together. Our ratings of parenting style included items such as warmth, responsiveness, limit-setting, engagement, and respect for the child's autonomy. In combination, the items assess a construct that Baumrind (1989) termed "authoritative parenting." She found that parents who are both warm/responsive and limit-setting, rather than warm without setting limits (permissive), or cold, angry, and controlling (authoritarian), tend to have children who are more academically and socially competent. In our study, variations in authoritative parenting accounted for 10–15% of the variance in the children's adaptation (Hsu, in press; Mattanah, in press; Measelle, in press). In other words, when mothers or fathers responded to their preschoolers in warm, supportive ways, granting them appropriate levels of autonomy while at the same time providing help and guidance when the children needed it, the children had higher academic achievement scores, and lower levels of acting out, aggressive, or shy/withdrawn and depressed behavior in kindergarten and first grade.

The parents' marital relationship quality was assessed in three ways. First, the couple engaged in two 10-minute problem-solving discussions, using similar protocols to the marital studies of Gottman and Levenson (1986). Second, for 30 minutes, mothers, fathers, and children together engaged in tasks that were difficult for the child and several games that were meant to be fun for the family. During that time, we coded the parents' style of interacting *with each other*. Third, we asked the children in the Berkeley Puppet Interview (Ablow & Measelle, 1993) to describe whether their parents fought a lot, and whether they felt their parents' fights were about them. Adding information about the quality of the marital interaction as perceived by observers, and by the children before they entered kindergarten allowed us to account for another 10–15% of the variance in the children's adaptation to school (Ablow, in press; P. A. Cowan, Bradburn, & Cowan, in press). When parents were coded by project staff as being high in displeasure with each other, coldness, anger, disagreement, and competition, and when their children described them as fighting a lot, the children tended to score especially high in externalizing aggressive behavior in kindergarten and first grade, higher in internalizing behavior, and somewhat lower in academic achievement than children of parents with lower scores on negative interaction and fighting as a couple.

Yet another family context was provided by the parents' experiences in their families of origin, measured by systematically coding parents' memories of their early relationships with their parents on the Adult Attachment Interview (George, Kaplan, & Main, 1985). With this information, we could predict an additional 15% of the variance in the children's academic achievement and externalizing or internalizing behaviors in kindergarten and first grade (P. A. Cowan, Bradburn, et al., in press).

Finally, by including information from two additional domains of family life, we found that parents' symptoms on the Brief Symptom Inventory (Derogatis & Melisaratos, 1983) contributed especially to predictions of their children's internalizing–depression as teachers viewed it, whereas parents' perceptions of stressors in their life outside the family added a small but significant amount of predictive power to links between preschool family functioning and children's adaptation to the first 2 years of school (P. A. Cowan & Cowan, in press; Schulz, in press).

All of these longitudinal results focused on children entering kindergarten are consistent with both cross-sectional and longitudinal studies of children at other ages. Children who show positive developmental progress and positive signs of competence and well-being tend to come from families in which parents (1) show signs of mental health; (2) have positive past or present relationships with their families of origin, or at least view them in perspective; (3) have cooperative relationships as a couple, whether they are married or divorced; (4) have parenting styles that are authoritative; and (5) have low levels of life stress and high levels of social support as a family (Cummings, DeArth-Pendley, Du Rocher Schudlich, & Smith, 2001; Hetherington, 1999; Parke & Buriel, 1998).

Although our study has minimal data concerning sibling relationships (Measelle, in press), what we did find supports the multidomain model presented in Figure 16.1. When we combine information about how parents and children are faring as individuals and the quality of their relationships in the preschool period, we can explain from 32% to 65% of the variance in the children's academic competence and quality of their relationships with peers and teachers in the first 2 years of school, depending on the specific outcome and when it was measured. Missing from this account, given space limitations, is our finding that gender plays a central role in family processes and children's adaptation. We really cannot talk simply about "parents" and "children" but must specify whether we mean mothers, fathers, sons, or daughters (P. A. Cowan, Cowan, & Kerig, 1993). The story of marital relationships in these heterosexual couples is not simply one of two adults trying to make a relationship; it is colored by gender differences and disparities (Walsh, 1989).

The longitudinal data with predictors obtained from the preschool period allow us to conclude that the findings are not simply attributable to child effects (when children do well or poorly at school, there are consequences for the quality of family life). However, as we noted earlier, neither do they permit us to conclude that family processes play a causal role in children's adaptation to school. To examine that hypothesis we turn to the intervention aspect of our study design.

From Correlation to Causation: The Role of Intervention in Testing Hypotheses

In a randomized clinical trial design, we assigned couples to a group intervention or a low-dose consultation during the year before their child entered kindergarten (P. A. Cowan, Cowan, & Heming, in press). Because they entered the study not knowing about the intervention, they were not couples seeking help with problems. The couples groups, led by trained mental health professionals, were 2 hours long and met weekly for 16 weeks. Discussions in the groups, which were partially structured and partially open-ended, covered salient topics in each of the family domains in Figure 16.1 (e.g., feelings about themselves as individuals, issues with parents and in-laws, developmentally appropriate discipline of children, conflicts between siblings, stress at work, conflict between the parents). In half the groups, the leaders emphasized marital relationships in the unstructured part of the evening. For example, they might ask how a disagreement about discipline was affecting the partners' relationship as a couple. In the other half of the groups, the leaders emphasized parent–child relationships during the open-ended part of the evening. Here, they might discuss how each parent was dealing with the child's evasion of limits and work on that issue. The different emphases of the group were initially developed to explore whether a direct focus on parenting was necessary to influence children's development, or whether an improvement in the marriage would spill over in positive ways to affect parent–child relationships and, ultimately, children's adaptation to school.

Although the couples themselves offered advice, and the leaders sometimes had specific suggestions about a handling a marital or parenting issue, the structure of the groups was not didactic. The intent was to provide a safe, containing environment in which men and women could (1) listen to their partners and other parents facing similar problems and dilemmas at the same stage of family life, and (2) discuss differences and impasses under the guidance of mental health professionals who would help them to express ideas and feelings but prevent high levels of conflict from escalating in ways that tend to erode marital relationships over time (Gottman, 1994). Couples in both intervention conditions were compared with those randomly assigned to the control condition (offered the chance to meet yearly over the next 3 years with the mental health professionals who initially interviewed them).

When group couples were compared with the consultation controls, we found significant positive effects of the two kinds of interventions. Parents in the maritally focused groups were observed to fight less in front of their children in the year after the groups ended. Parents in the parenting-focused groups were observed to be warmer and more structuring (i.e., more authoritative) with their children. Children whose parents had been in either kind of couples group were at an advantage in kindergarten and first grade compared to children of controls; they had higher academic achievement, less aggression, and fewer symptoms of depression. We found that targeted aspects of the intervention (marital and parent–child relationships) were at least in part responsible for the more favorable child outcomes. Finally, *changes* in the quality of observed marital and parent–child relationships were directly associated with how well the children were faring in their first 2 years of school.

Other parent-based interventions also have been found to affect parent–child relationships and children's development (Dadds, Schwartz, &

Sanders, 1987; Webster-Stratton, 1994; Wolchik et al., 1993). In addition to demonstrating the possibilities of help for families and children, these studies illustrate how intervention designs can be used as tests of theory. First, the results provide strong support for the hypothesis that the quality of family relationships affects children's development. In response to Judith Harris's (1998) controversial assertion that parents have little impact, these results clearly indicate that parents can affect their children's adaptation (P. A. Cowan & Cowan, 2002).

Second, some of the results in our intervention study helped to clarify links between marital and parenting relationships as espoused in family systems theories. Early systemic models assumed that changes in any domain of family life affect every other domain (the double-headed arrows of Figure 16.1). However, not all members of a system have equal influence on other individuals, relationships, and the system as a whole, and change in some aspects of a relationship may be more influential than others (McGoldrick, Anderson, & Walsh, 1989). Here, we noted that when the men and women in the parenting-focused intervention improved in their parenting skills, their marital interaction did not change systematically. However, when couples in the maritally focused group reduced their conflict in front of the children, their parenting effectiveness also improved. Thus, beyond the information that marital and parent–child relationship quality is correlated, intervention designs can tell us something about how family systems operate. From the results so far, we conclude that the relationship between the parents may exert more influence on parent–child relationships than vice versa. Future research could well examine whether this marital-to-parenting influence holds at different stages of the family life cycle, for different normative and non-normative transitions.

IMPLICATIONS FOR THEORY AND PRACTICE

What Do the Findings Tell Us about Normal Family Processes? What Do We Still Need to Know?

The Major Messages

One of the major messages in this account of our own research and other family studies of major life transitions is virtually identical to core tenets endorsed by family systems clinicians all along. Various domains of family life are interconnected; to explain adaptation or dysfunction in children, we need information about relationships across the generations, and about the relationship of the parents, who have been metaphorically described as the "architects" of the family, not simply information about parenting quality. The marital relationship may also be thought of as a thermostat that regulates or dysregulates perturbations in the system to amplify or reduce their effects. In our view, it is a sign of progress when the studies of family researchers and family clinicians begin to converge in their focus, assumptions, and conclusions.

Another major message is certainly consistent with the views of family clinicians. Transitions are useful times to study families, and they signal the opportunity for preventive intervention to strengthen normal family processes in ways that facilitate children's development.

Searching for Mechanisms of Transmission

Having "explained" a substantial portion of the variation in children's adaptation to school by considering various indicators of family functioning, we must acknowledge that there is still more to explain. It seems obvious that when parents' relationships with their own parents are difficult, when the marriage is full of unresolved conflict, when the parents are permissive or authoritarian with their preschoolers, the children will have a more difficult time meeting the academic and social challenges of adapting to the demands and challenges of elementary school. Yet these generalizations do not specify the mechanisms by which this cascade of negativity comes to have an impact on the child, or, to turn the story around, how positive family relationships facilitate children's learning to read or developing relationships with teachers and other children.

Certainly, modeling and social learning play a role, with each generation likely to repeat what they have learned when parents have children, and when children become students. From a meaning-making perspective, we speculate that the "working models" of relationships developed in families of origin (Bretherton, Ridgeway, & Cassidy, 1990) help to shape both expectations and behavior in new friendships and intimate relationships. Based on Byng-Hall's writings (1999), we believe that positive family relationships can provide children with a "secure base" that they can return to in times of stress but depart from, with energy free to invest in learning about academic subjects and social relationships. And, as we noted earlier, we suspect that one of the key ingredients that determine whether negativity or positivity in one relationship spills over into another has to do with the extent to which those relationships help children learn how to regulate emotions (Gottman et al., 1997). We do not mean here that family members need to learn to keep the emotional lid on, but rather, fitting their own cultural norms, to allow a reciprocal give and take of information and emotional connection. The identification of these and other mechanisms of transmission is essential not only to flesh out our theories concerning family processes and children's adaptation but also to provide a more concrete basis for preventive and therapeutic intervention for families.

The Normality of Nonclinical Families

We return to the issue of "normal" families, raised by Walsh in each of the editions of *Normal Family Processes*. At this point in the history of family theory and research, it is not surprising to find that early family life is normally stressful and even debilitating for some new parents and their children. In the study examining the transition to school, parents did not experience increases in psychological symptoms over the 3-year study, but about 20–30% of them were over the clinical cutoff on a standard measure of depression, and a similar percentage showed low levels of marital satisfaction. Furthermore, 10% of their children had entered the mental health system for assessment or treatment by the time they had completed kindergarten.

Our research findings have led to concerns about the difficulties encountered by ordinary couples with young children getting lost in the attention paid to "families at risk"—those with the least financial, social, and psychological resources. First, too many normal, relatively advantaged families are showing strains similar to those of people already in the mental health system. Yet it is clear that resources are not being made available to them, because they are assumed to be "doing fine" or to have the resources to find and finance help if they recognize the need for assistance. Second, despite the general acceptance of biopsychosocial views of the etiology of major disorders, many researchers and clinicians who focus on problems of poverty, alcoholism, and emotional disorders, such as depression, antisocial behavior, and schizophrenia, have tended to assume that difficulties encountered in these families stem from the psychopathology of the family members. Family systems theorists may have long since regarded these views as outmoded, but a quick look at the operation of managed care provides ubiquitous examples of drug treatment for depression that is unaccompanied by any psychological or family-based intervention (Weissman, 2001).

As we have seen in the studies of nonclinical families presented here, some of the difficulties may be attributable to the expectable strain associated with moving through normative life transitions. For example, some of the stresses associated with being a single mother, with an income below the poverty line, are associated with a recent transition to parenthood (C. P. Cowan & Cowan, 1995). We do not mean to minimize the seriousness of these higher risk transitions but rather to emphasize that they have some commonalities with normative change across the lifespan. This information is essential for planning effective interventions.

Speculative Extension of This Analysis to Other Normative and Non-Normative Transitions

We have seen that although major life transitions all have some impact on views of self, on family roles, and on relationships, the two early family transitions focused on here have quite different effects on family life. We would expect that the impact of normative life transitions at other periods in the life cycle might be different yet again. Because family studies rarely provide prospective information with systematic assessments of family relationships at different points in time, we do not really know what happens to the whole family system when children become teenagers or leave home, when mothers return to work after their children are in school, or when men and women retire. And because prospective studies are even more difficult to do when the focus is on non-normative transitions (e.g., job loss, onset of physical or mental illness in a family member, death of a parent or child), there is even less solid evidence of how self, roles, and relationships change over time. An exemplary research program by Hetherington (1999) has enriched our understanding of the myriad changes and influences in divorce adaptation (see Greene, Anderson, Hetherington, Forgatch, & DeGarmo, Chapter 4, this volume).

Still, the model of family transitions we have presented could serve as a checklist for researchers and clinicians. For example, if we are concerned about the potential impact on a child of a mother's descent into depression (Field, 1995), we need to look beyond her self-image and parenting style to examine changes in the relationships with her partner, her parents and extended family members, and other potential sources of stress and support outside the family. Similarly, studies of the impact of job loss must focus not only on the prior, current, and future reactions of the individual out of work, but also on the reverberations within the worker's marriage (Howe, Caplan, Foster, Lockshin, & McGrath, 1995) and in other relationships in the family system. It may be that transitions differ systematically from each other by virtue of the subsystems affected and the pattern of reverberating effects. Findings from both research and clinical investigations using a systemic framework might have a better chance of identifying specific aspects of the family to target for preventive interventions if the hoped-for outcome is the prevention of children's distress or the enhancement of their adaptation.

Thinking about Family-Based Preventive Interventions

Based on Erikson's formulation of individual development, Hill (1949) and McCubbin and Patterson (1983) developed the ABCX model of transition and crisis as applied to families. Although "crisis" has negative connotations, this approach preserves Erikson's (1950) assumption that there is both danger and opportunity in a crisis. Consistent also with the principles of preventive psychiatry (Caplan, 1964), this view implies that transitions are turning points that may lead toward growth or toward dysfunction.

Although psychoanalytic and Piagetian perspectives on development are radically different in many respects, they concur with family systems theories on the notion that disequilibrating transitions are necessary for developmental change. Development involves progressive differentiation and integration of the internal system and of interpersonal transactions. As long as the current level of functioning is adequate, there is no need to develop more complex systems. New stimuli are understood by fitting them into existing schemas (assimilation), and change in the system (accommodation) is not required. When the person or family attempts to use available strategies of understanding and coping, and these fail to meet the new challenge, disequilibrium ensues; only then is development possible. Because therapists also hope to facilitate change in the system, helping individuals and families get past impasses, they may be more effective if the client(s) are facing a period of life change. This is one argument for the notion that major life transitions are optimal times for offering intervention programs.

The research reviewed here makes it clear that although major life transitions can produce positive change in people and their families, they often signal not opportunity but risk, which in some cases is followed by actual distress. We cannot expect that the natural experiments of nature will automatically provide challenges in the optimal form to stimulate new and more adaptive reorganization. Preventive and therapeutic interventions may be required to help some families manage apparently positive or seemingly benign life transitions given the distress we find in parents and children in apparently favorable life circumstances.

The import of this analysis is that the mental health field describes risks as if they were a property of an individual or a family. The picture we are attempting to paint here is of normative life transitions that are accompanied by stressful conditions, which for a substantial proportion of adults and children lead to increased distress and dissatisfaction for men and women and some of their children—just as they do in so-called high-risk families. The links between the quality of key family relationships and children's academic, social, and emotional development, along with the intervention results, suggest that therapeutic interventions can be targeted to reduce risk and promote resilience, in order to reduce the probability of dysfunction and increase the probability that transitions will stimulate positive developmental change for all family members.

It would be advantageous to make these interventions available to all who undergo stressful life transitions. Unfortunately, the time is not ideal for government support of large-scale intervention programs. The findings of almost every investigator mentioned in this chapter make clear that we already know how to identify individuals and families who are most likely to be in difficulty after a major life transition. Despite the fact that transitions trigger shifts in views of one's sense of self, family, roles, and close relationships, without intervention, individuals, couples, and families tend to stay in the same relative position on measures of adaptation after a transition that they held before the transition began (Caspi & Roberts,

1999). For those at the well-functioning end of the continuum, this is reassuring news. For families at the low end of the adaptation continuum, there is cause for concern.

Of course, the rule of consistency is far from absolute. Some individuals and families not faring well at one time do manage to improve the quality of their relationships or their mental health over time (Block & Haan, 1971; P. A. Cowan, Cowan, Ablow, et al., in press). Both for theory development and intervention planning, we need more research to discover which processes naturally buffer children from the negative effects of troubling family transactions (e.g., marital conflict, authoritarian parenting), and which processes increase children's vulnerability to distress, even when risks seem relatively low.

In summary, we are not arguing that all families need help with all family transitions. We are suggesting that if we want to optimize families' ability to provide the kinds of environments and processes that foster children's well-being and development, preventive and therapeutic interventions can help us to seize the opportunity during normative and non-normative transitions, when new challenges and confusion can be expected to strain family relationships and threaten family equilibrium. If these interventions help parents make positive shifts in their relationships with their children *and* with their partners, it seems clear that their children will reap the benefits academically, socially, and emotionally.

REFERENCES

Ablow, J. (in press). When parents conflict or disengage: Understanding links between marital distress and children's adaptation to school. In P. A. Cowan, C. P. Cowan, J. Ablow, V. K. Johnson & J. Measelle (Eds.), *The family context of parenting in children's adaptation to elementary school.* Mahwah, NJ: Erlbaum.

Ablow, J., & Measelle, J. (1993). *The Berkeley Puppet Interview: Administration and scoring system manuals.* Unpublished manuscript, University of California, Berkeley.

Alexander, K. L., & Entwisle, D. R. (1988). Achievement in the first 2 years of school: Patterns and processes. *Monographs of the Society for Research in Child Development, 53*(2, Serial No. 218), 157.

Alexandrova, E. O. (1999). *Who does what, why, and how it affects marital relationships during the child's transition to school.* Unpublished master's thesis, University of California, Berkeley.

Anthony, E. J., & Benedek, T. (1970). *Parenthood: Its psychology and psychopathology.* Boston: Little, Brown.

Antonucci, T. C., & Mikus, K. (1988). The power of parenthood: Personality and attitudinal changes during the transition to parenthood. In G. Y. Michaels & W. A. Goldberg (Eds.), *The transition to parenthood: Current theory and research* (pp. 62–84). New York: Cambridge University Press.

Baumrind, D. (1989). Rearing competent children. In W. Damon (Ed.), *Child development today and tomorrow* (pp. 349–378). San Francisco: Jossey-Bass.

Baumrind, D. (1991). Effective parenting during the early adolescent transition. In P. A. Cowan & E. M. Hetherington (Eds.), *Advances in family research* (Vol. 2, pp. 111–163). Hillsdale, NJ: Erlbaum.

Belsky, J. (1984). The determinants of parenting: A process model. *Child Development, 55*(1), 83–96.

Belsky, J., Lang, M., & Huston, T. L. (1986). Sex typing and division of labor as determinants of marital change across the transition to parenthood. *Journal of Personality and Social Psychology, 50*(3), 517–522.

Belsky, J., & Pensky, E. (1988). Marital change across the transition to parenthood. *Marriage and Family Review, 12*(3–4), 133–156.

Bennet, K. J., Lipman, E. L., Brown, S., Racine, Y., Boyle, M. H., & Offord, D. R. (1999). Predicting conduct problems: Can high-risk children be identified in kindergarten and grade 1? *Journal of Consulting and Clinical Psychology, 67,* 470–480.

Block, J., & Haan, N. (1971). *Lives through time.* Berkeley, CA: Bancroft Books.

Bretherton, I., Ridgeway, D., & Cassidy, J. (1990). Assessing internal working models of the attachment relationship: An attachment story completion task for 3-year-olds. In M. T. Greenberg, D. Cicchetti, & E. M. Cummings (Eds.), *Attachment in the preschool years: Theory, research, and intervention* (pp. 273–308). Chicago: University of Chicago Press.

Bronfenbrenner, U. (1979). *The ecology of human development: Experiments by nature and design.* Cambridge, MA: Harvard University Press.

Brooks-Gunn, J., & Chase-Lansdale, P. L. (1995). Adolescent parenthood. In M. H. Bornstein (Ed.), *Handbook of parenting: Vol. 3. Status and social conditions of parenting* (pp. 113–149). Hillsdale, NJ: Erlbaum.

Bumpass, L., & Rindfuss, R. R. (1979). Children's experience of marital disruption. *American Journal of Sociology, 85,* 49–65.

Byng-Hall, J. (1999). Family couple therapy: Toward greater security. In J. Cassidy & P. R. Shaver (Eds.), *Handbook of attachment: Theory, research, and clinical applications* (pp. 625–645). New York: Guilford Press.

Campbell, S. B., Cohn, J. F., Flanagan, C., & Popper, S. (1992). Course and correlates of postpartum depression during the transition to parenthood. *Development and Psychopathology, 4*(1), 29–47.

Caplan, G. (1964). *Principles of preventive psychiatry.* New York: Basic Books.

Carlson, E. A., Sroufe, L. A., Collins, W. A., Jimerson, S., Weinfield, N., Henninghausen, K., Egeland, B., Hyson, D. M., Anderson, F., & Meyer, S. E. (1999). Early environmental support and elementary school adjustment as predictors of school adjustment in middleadolescence. *Journal of Adolescent Research, 14*(1), 72–94.

Carter, A. S., Garrity-Rokous, F. E., Chazan-Cohen, R., Little, C., & Briggs-Gowan, M. J. (2001). Maternal depression and comorbidity: Predicting early parenting, attachment security, and toddler social-emotional problems and competencies. *Journal of the American Academy of Child and Adolescent Psychiatry, 40*(1), 18–26.

Caspi, A., & Roberts, B. W. (1999). Personality continuity and change across the life course. In L. A. Pervin & O. P. John (Eds.), *Handbook of personality: Theory and research* (2nd ed., pp. 300–326). New York: Guilford Press.

Cowan, C. P., & Cowan, P. A. (1988). Who does what when partners become parents: Implications for men, women, and marriage. *Marriage and Family Review, 12*(3–4), 105–131.

Cowan, C. P., & Cowan, P. A. (1995). Interventions to ease the transition to parenthood: Why they are needed and what they can do. *Family Relations: Journal of Applied Family and Child Studies, 44*(4), 412–423.

Cowan, C. P., & Cowan, P. A. (2000). *When partners become parents: The big life change for couples.* Mahwah, NJ: Erlbaum.

Cowan, P. A., Cowan, C. P., Heming, G., Garrett, E. T., Coysh, W. S., Curtis-Boles, H., & Boles, A. (1985). Transitions to parenthood: His, hers, and theirs [Special issue]. *Journal of Family Issues, 6,* 451–481.

Cowan, P. A. (1988). Becoming a father: A time of change, an opportunity for development. In P. Bronstein & C. P. Cowan (Eds.), *Fatherhood today: Men's changing role in the family* (pp. 13–35). New York: Wiley.

Cowan, P. A. (1991). Individual and family life transitions: A proposal for a new definition. In P. A. Cowan & E. M. Hetherington (Eds.), *Family transitions* (pp. 3–30). Hillsdale, NJ: Erlbaum.

Cowan, P. A., Bradburn, I. S., & Cowan, C. P. (in press). Parents' working models of attachment: The intergenerational context of problem behavior in kindergarten. In P. A. Cowan, C. P. Cowan, J. Ablow, V. K. Johnson, & J. Measelle (Eds.), *The family context of parenting in children's adaptation to elementary school.* Mahwah, NJ: Erlbaum.

Cowan, P. A., & Cowan, C. P. (1988). Changes in marriage during the transition to parenthood: Must we blame the baby? In G. Y. Michaels & W. A. Goldberg (Eds.), *The transition to parenthood: Current theory and research* (pp. 114–154). New York: Cambridge University Press.

Cowan, P. A., & Cowan, C. P. (2001). What an intervention design reveals about how parents affect their children's academic achievement and behavior problems. In M. Bristol-Power (Ed.), *Parenting and the child's world: Influences on intellectual, academic, and social-emotional development* (pp. 75–98). Mahwah, NJ: Erlbaum.

Cowan, P. A., & Cowan, C. P. (2002). What an intervention design reveals about how parents affect their children's academic achievement and behavior problems. In J. G. Borkowski, S. Ramey, & M. Bristol-Power (Eds.), *Parenting and the child's world: Influences on intellectual, academic, and social-emotional development* Mahwah, NJ: : Erlbaum.

Cowan, P. A., & Cowan, C. P. (in press). "Mega-models" of parenting in context. In P. A. Cowan, C. P. Cowan, J. Ablow, V. K. Johnson, & J. Measelle (Eds.), *The family context of parenting in children's adaptation to elementary school.* Mahwah, NJ: Erlbaum.

Cowan, P. A., Cowan, C. P., Ablow, J., Johnson, V., & Measelle, J. (Eds.). (in press). *The family context of parenting in children's adaptation to school.* Mahwah, NJ: Erlbaum.

Cowan, P. A., Cowan, C. P., & Heming, G. (1995). *Manual for the Child Adaptive Behavior Inventory (CABI).* Unpublished manuscript, University of California, Berkeley.

Cowan, P. A., Cowan, C. P., & Heming, G. (in press). Two variations of a preventive intervention for couples: Effects on parents and children during the transition to elementary school. In P. A. Cowan, C. P. Cowan, J. Ablow, V. K. Johnson, & J. Measelle (Eds.), *The family context of parenting in children's adaptation to elementary school.* Mahwah, NJ: Erlbaum.

Cowan, P. A., Cowan, C. P., & Kerig, P. K. (1993). Mothers, fathers, sons, and daughters: Gender differences in family formation and parenting style. In P. A. Cowan, D. Field, D. A. Hansen, A. Skolmick, & G. E. Swanson (Eds.), *Family, self, and society: Toward a new agenda for family research* (pp. 165–195). Hillsdale, NJ: Erlbaum.

Cowan, P. A., Cowan, C. P., Schulz, M. S., & Heming, G. (1994). Prebirth to preschool family factors in children's adaptation to kindergarten. In R. D. Parke & S. G. Kellam (Eds.), *Exploring family relationships with other social contexts: Family research consortium: Advances in family research* (Vol. 4, pp. 75–114). Hillsdale, NJ: Erlbaum.

Cowan, P. A., & Heming, G. (in press). Change, stability, and predictability in family members during children's transition to school. P. A. Cowan, C. E. Cowan, J. Ablow, V. K. Johnson, & J. Measelle (Eds.), *The family context of parenting in children's adaptation to elementary school.* Mahwah, NJ: Erlbaum.

Cox, M. J., Owen, M. T., Lewis, J. M., & Henderson, V. K. (1989). Marriage, adult adjustment, and early parenting. *Child Development, 60*(5), 1015–1024.

Cox, M. J., Paley, B., Payne, C. C., & Burchinal, M. (1999). The transition to parenthood: Marital conflict and withdrawal and parent–infant interactions. In M. J. Cox & J. Brooks-Gunn (Eds.), *Conflict and cohesion in families: Causes and consequences* (pp. 87–104). Mahwah, NJ: Erlbaum.

Crohan, S. E. (1996). Marital quality and conflict across the transition to parenthood in African American and white couples. *Journal of Marriage and the Family, 58*(4), 933–944.

Cummings, E. M., DeArth-Pendley, G., Du Rocher Schudlich, T., & Smith, D. A. (2001). Parental depression and family functioning: Toward a process-oriented model of children's adjustment. In S. R. H. Beach (Ed.), *Marital and Family Processes in depression: A scientific foundation for clinical practice* (pp. 89–110). Washington, DC: American Psychological Association.

Cutrona, C. E. (1982). Nonpsychotic postpartum depression: A review of recent research. *Clinical Psychology Review, 2*(4), 487–503.

Dadds, M. R., Schwartz, S., & Sanders, M. R. (1987). Marital discord and treatment outcome in behavioral treatment of child conduct disorders. *Journal of Consulting and Clinical Psychology, 55*(3), 396–403.

Derogatis, L. R., & Melisaratos, N. (1983). The Brief Symptom Inventory: An introductory report. *Psychological Medicine, 13*(3), 595–605.

Dunn, J., & Plomin, R. (1990). *Separate lives: Why siblings are so different.* New York: Basic Books.

Engfer, A., Heinig, L., & Gavranidou, M. (1998). Veranderungen in Ehe and Partnerschaft nach der Geburt von Kindern: Ergebnissse einer Langsschnittstudie [Changes in marriage and partnership after children's birth: Results of a longitudinal study]. *Verhaltensmodifikation und Verhaltensmedizin, 9,* 297–311.

Erikson, E. H. (1950). *Childhood and society.* New York: Norton.

Erikson, E. H. (1980). *Identity and the life cycle.* New York: Norton.

Field, T. M. (1995). Psychologically depressed parents. In M. H. Bornstein (Ed.), *Handbook of parenting: Vol. 4. Applied and practical parenting* (pp. 85–99). Hillsdale, NJ: Erlbaum.

Fischer, L. R. (1988). The influence of kin on the transition to parenthood. *Marriage and Family Review, 12*(3–4), 201–219.

Flanagan, C. A. (1990). Families and schools in hard times. *New Directions for Child Development, 46,* 7–26.

Fonagy, P., Steele, H., & Steele, M. (1991). Maternal representations of attachment during pregnancy predict the organization of infant–mother attachment at one year of age. *Child Development, 62*(5), 891–905.

Freud, S. (1938). *The basic writings of Sigmund Freud* (A. A. Brill, Trans.). New York: Modern Library.

George, C., Kaplan, N., & Main, M. (1985). *The Adult Attachment Interview.* Unpublished manuscript, University of California, Berkeley.

Gloger-Tippelt, G. S., & Huerkamp, M. (1998). Relationship change at the transition to parenthood and security of infant–mother attachment. *International Journal of Behavioral Development, 22*(3), 633–655.

Gottman, J. (2001). Meta-emotion, children's emotional intelligence, and buffering children from marital conflict. In C. D. Ryff & B. H. Singer (Eds.), *Emotion, social relationships, and health* (pp. 23–40). New York: Oxford University Press.

Gottman, J. M. (1994). *What predicts divorce?: The relationship between marital processes and marital outcomes.* Hillsdale, NJ: Erlbaum.

Gottman, J. M., Katz, L. F., & Hooven, C. (1997). *Meta-emotion: How families communicate emotionally.* Hillsdale, NJ: Erlbaum.

Gottman, J. M., & Levenson, R. W. (1986). Assessing the role of emotion in marriage. *Behavioral Assessment, 8*(1), 31–48.

Grossman, F. K., Eichler, L. S., & Winickoff, S. A. (1980). *Pregnancy, birth, and parenthood* (1st ed.). San Francisco: Jossey-Bass.

Hansen, L. B., & Jacob, E. (1992). Intergenerational support during the transition to parenthood: Issues for new parents and grandparents. *Families in Society, 73*(8), 471–479.

Harknett, K., Hardman, L., Garfinkel, I., & McLanahan, S. S. (2001). The Fragile Families Study: Social policies and labor markets in seven cities. *Children and Youth Services Review, 23*(6–7), 537–555.

Harris, J. (1998). *The nurture assumption: Why children turn out the way they do.* New York: Free Press.

Heinicke, C. M. (1991). Early family intervention: Focusing on the mother's adaptation–competence and quality of partnership. In D. G. Unger & D. R. Powell (Eds.), *Families as nurturing systems: Support across the life span* (pp. 127–142). Binghamton, NY: Haworth Press.

Heinicke, C. M. (1995). Determinants of the transition to parenting. In M. H. Bornstein (Ed.), *Handbook of parenting: Vol. 3. Status and social conditions of parenting* (pp. 277–303). Hillsdale, NJ: Erlbaum.

Hetherington, E. M. (1999). *Coping with divorce, single parenting, and remarriage: A risk and resiliency perspective.* Matwah, NJ: Erlbaum.

Hill, R. (1949). *Families under stress: Adjustment to the crises of war separation and return.* New York: Harper.

Hipwell, A. E., & Kumar, R. (1996). Maternal psychopathology and prediction of outcome based on mother–infant interaction ratings (BMIS). *British Journal of Psychiatry, 169*(5), 655–661.

Hochschild, A. R., & Machung, A. (1990). *The second shift.* New York: Avon Books.

Howe, G. W., Caplan, R. D., Foster, D., Lockshin, M., & McGrath, C. (1995). When couples cope with job loss: A strategy for developing and testing preventive interventions. In L. R. Murphy, J. J. Hurrell, Jr. & et al. (Eds.), *Job stress interventions* (pp. 139–157). Washington, DC: American Psychological Association.

Howes, P., & Markman, H. J. (1989). Marital quality and child functioning: A longitudinal investigation. *Child Development, 60*(5), 1044–1051.

Hsu, J. (in press). Effects of gendered parenting on girls' and boys' expression of problem behaviors. In P. A. Cowan, C. P. Cowan, J. Ablow, V. K. Johnson & J. Measelle (Eds.), *The family context of parenting in children's adaptation to elementary school.* Mahwah, NJ: Erlbaum.

Klinnert, M. D., Gavin, L. A., Wamboldt, F. S., & Mrazek, D. A. (1992). Marriages with children at medical risk: The transition to parenthood. *Journal of the American Academy of Child and Adolescent Psychiatry, 31*(2), 334–342.

LeMasters, E. E. (1957). Parenthood as crisis. *Marriage and Family Living, 19,* 352–355.

Levy-Shiff, R., Dimitrovsky, L., Shulman, S., & Har-Even, D. (1998). Cognitive appraisals, coping strategies, and support resources as correlates of parenting and infant development. *Developmental Psychology, 34*(6), 1417–1427.

Lindahl, K., Clements, M., & Markman, H. (1998). The development of marriage: A 9-year perspective. In T. N. Bradbury (Ed.), *The developmental course of marital dysfunction* (pp. 205–236). New York: Cambridge University Press.

Locke, H. J., & Wallace, K. M. (1959). Short Marital-Adjustment and Prediction Tests: Their reliability and validity. *Marriage and Family Living, 21,* 251–255.

Lovejoy, M. C., Graczyk, P. A., O'Hare, E., & Neuman, G. (2000). Maternal depression and parenting behavior: A meta-analytic review. *Clinical Psychology Review, 20*(5), 561–592.

Main, M., Kaplan, N., & Cassidy, J. (1985). Security in infancy, childhood, and adulthood: A move to the level of representation: Growing points of attachment theory and research. *Monographs of the Society for Research in Child Development, 50,* 66–106.

Markwardt, F. C. (1989). *Peabody Individual Achievement Test—Revised.* Circle Pines, MN: American Guidance Service.

Mattanah, J. (in press). The importance of authoritative parenting and the encouragement of autonomy during children's transition to elementary school. In J. Measelle (Ed.), *The family context of parenting in children's adaptation to elementary school.* Mahwah, NJ: Erlbaum.

McCubbin, H. I., & Patterson, J. M. (1983). The family stress process: The double ABCX model of adjustment and adaptation. *Marriage and Family Review, 6*(1–2), 7–37.

McCubbin, H. I., Thompson, E. A., Thompson, A. I., & Futrell, J. A. (Eds.). (1999). *The dynamics of resilient families.* Thousand Oaks, CA: Sage.

McGoldrick, M., Anderson, C. M., & Walsh, F. (Eds.). (1989). *Women in families: A framework for family therapy.* New York: Norton.

McGoldrick, M., & Carter, E. A. (1988). *The changing life cycle: A framework for family therapy* (2nd ed.). Boston: Allyn & Bacon.

McHale, S. M., & Huston, T. L. (1985). The effect of the transition to parenthood on the marital relationship. *Journal of Family Issues, 6,* 409–435.

Measelle, J. (in press). The role of young children's self-perceptions in links between early family relationships and social adjustment to kindergarten. In P. A. Cowan, C. P. Cowan, J. Ablow, V. K. Johnson, & J. Measelle (Eds.), *The family context of parenting in children's adaptation to elementary school.* Mahwah, NJ: Erlbaum.

Neugarten, B. L. (1965). Personality and patterns of aging. *Anthropology and Medicine, 13*(4), 249–256.

Olds, D., Henderson, C. R., Jr., Cole, R., Eckenrode, J., Kitzman, H., Luckey, D., Pettit, L., Sidora, K., Morris, P., & Powers, S. (1998). Long-term effects of nurse home visitation on children's criminal and antisocial behavior: 15-year follow-up of a randomized controlled trial. *Journal of the American Medical Association, 280*(14), 1238–1244.

Pancer, S. M., Pratt, M., Hunsberger, B., & Gallant, M. (2000). Thinking ahead: Complexity of expectations and the transition to parenthood. *Journal of Personality, 68*(2), 253–280.

Parke, R. D., & Buriel, R. (1998). Socialization in the family: Ethnic and ecological perspectives. In N. Eisenberg (Ed.), *Social, emotional, and personality development* (5th ed., Vol. 3, pp. 463–552) New York: John Wiley & Sons, Inc.

Parkes, C. M. (1971). Psycho-social transitions: A field for study. *Social Science and Medicine, 5*(2), 101–115.

Parr, M. (1997). Adjustment to family life. In C. Henderson (Ed.), *Essential midwifery* (pp. 131–140). London: Times/Mirror.

Piaget, J. (1968). *Six psychological studies* (A. Tenzer, Trans.) New York: Random House.

Schneewind, K. A. (1983). Konsequenzen der Erstelternschaft. *Psychologie in Erziehung und Unterricht, 30*(3), 161–172.

Schulz, M. (in press). Parents' work experiences and children's adjustment to kindergarten. In P. A. Cowan, C. P. Cowan, J. Ablow, V. K. Johnson, & J. Measelle (Eds.), *The family context of parenting in children's adaptation to elementary school.* Mahwah, NJ: Erlbaum.

Seifer, R., & Dickstein, S. (2000). Parental mental illness and infant development. In C. H. Zeanah, Jr. (Ed.), *Handbook of infant mental health* (2nd ed., pp. 145–160). New York: Guilford Press.

Shapiro, A. F., Gottman, J. M., & Carrere, S. (2000). The baby and the marriage: Identifying factors that buffer against decline in marital satisfaction after the first baby arrives. *Journal of Family Psychology, 14*(1), 59–70.

Vaillant, G. E., & Koury, S. H. (1993). Late midlife development. In G. H. Pollock & S. I. Greenspan (Eds.), *The course of life: Vol. 6. Late adulthood* (rev. and exp. ed., pp. 1–22). Madison, CT: International Universities Press.

Wagner, B. M., & Reiss, D. (1995). Family systems and developmental psychopathology: Courtship, marriage, or divorce? In D. Cicchetti & D. J. Cohen (Eds.), *Developmental psychopathology* (Vol. 1, pp. 696–730). New York: Wiley.

Walsh, F. (1989). Reconsidering gender in the marital quid pro quo. In M. McGoldrick, C. M. Anderson, & F. Walsh (Eds.), *Women in families: A framework for family therapy* (pp. 267–285). New York: Norton.

Walsh, F. (1998). *Strengthening family resilience.* New York: Guilford Press.

Walsh, F. (Ed.). (1993). *Normal Family Processes* (2nd ed.). New York: Guilford Press.

Webster-Stratton, C. (1994). Advancing videotape parent training: A comparison study. *Journal of Consulting and Clinical Psychology, 62*(3), 583–593.

Weissman, M. M. (Ed.). (2001). *Treatment of depression: Bridging the 21st century.* Washington, DC: American Psychiatric Press.

Wolchik, S. A., West, S. G., Westover, D., Sandler, I. N., Martin, A., Lustig, J., Tein, J., & Fisher, (1993). The children of divorce parenting intervention: Outcome evaluation of an empirically based program. *American Journal of Community Psychology, 21*, 293–330.

CHAPTER 17

MASTERING FAMILY CHALLENGES IN SERIOUS ILLNESS AND DISABILITY

John S. Rolland

A NORMATIVE SYSTEMIC HEALTH PARADIGM

Illness, disability, and death are universal experiences in families. The real question is not "if" we will face these issues, but when in our lives, what kinds of conditions, how serious they will be, and for how long. With major advances in medical technology, people with formerly fatal conditions are living much longer. Cancer, heart disease, diabetes, and now AIDS are just a few examples. Many children with chronic conditions that were previously fatal or necessitated institutional life are now reaching adulthood, and, with the help of new policies, they are assimilating into mainstream adult life. This means that ever-growing numbers of families are both living with chronic disorders over an increasingly long time span and coping with a greater number of chronic conditions, often simultaneously.

The extension of later life has heightened the strain on sons and daughters who must contend with divided loyalties and a complex juggling act between caregiving for aging parents, child rearing, and providing financially for the family. They must achieve these ends in a society in which families are geographically dispersed and health care is exorbitant and inadequate.

Given these changes, how can we best describe the normative challenges of serious illness and optimal family coping and adaptation? We are advancing past stereotypical definitions of "the family" and the view of normal family life as "problem-free" to recognize that all families are challenged by adversity. In the same way, when serious illness strikes, we need to move beyond an outdated, rigid, and often romanticized version of coping.

This chapter provides a normative, preventive model for psychoeducation, assessment, and intervention with families facing chronic and life-threatening conditions (Rolland, 1984, 1987a, 1987b, 1990, 1994, 1998, 1999, 2002). This model offers a systemic view of healthy family adaptation to serious illness as a developmental process over time in relation to the complexities and diversity of contemporary family life, modern medicine, and existing flawed models of health care delivery and access to care. First, before I describe the model, some basic constructs are useful.

As a first step to constructing a normative model, we need to redefine the unit of care in terms of the family or caregiving system as distinct from the ill individual (McDaniel, Hepworth, & Doherty, 1992). Defined in systems terms, an effective biopsychosocial model needs to encompass all persons affected psychosocially. This is a departure form the medical model's narrow focus on the patient receiving care. By using a broad definition of family as the cornerstone of the caregiving system, we can describe a model of successful coping and adaptation based on family system strengths.

Second, we need to describe the complex mutual interactions among illness, ill family member, and family within a normative framework. There is a vast literature describing the impact of chronic disorders on individuals and families. However, the impact of individual and family dynamics on disease has historically been defined in terms of psychosomatic processes and almost invariably in pathological terms. The definition of a condition as "psychosomatic" is a shameful label associated with a number of pejorative cultural meanings that imply character or family weakness.

An alternative framework would describe psychosomatic processes in more holistic, interactive, and normative terms. All illnesses can be viewed as having a psychosomatic interplay, in which the relative influence of biological and psychosocial factors vary over a range of disorders and phases of an illness. From this perspective, a psychosomatic interplay provides an opportunity for psychosocial factors, not just biomedical interventions, to be important influences in healing. When professionals take this approach, they help to undercut pathologizing family and cultural beliefs, and help families approach a psychosomatic interaction as an opportunity to make a difference. This increases their sense of control and overall quality of life.

Family research in the arena of chronic illness, like studies of the individual, has tended to emphasize pathological family dynamics associated with poor disease course or treatment compliance (Campbell & Patterson, 1995). This leads to paradigms that emphasize illness-based family systems and psychosomatic families. By defining pathological systems at one end of a continuum, we do not clarify what constitutes healthy family coping and adaptation to illness.

At the other end of the continuum, especially in the popular literature, there has been a focus on the exceptional patient (Siegel, 1986; Simonton, Mathews-Simonton, & Sparks, 1980). Numerous personal accounts highlight the superstar patient or family. Although these provide a
refreshing relief from descriptions of pathological patients and families,
they often err toward superhuman epic descriptions that leave the average
family without a reference point. The average family is vulnerable to double jeopardy. Its members can feel pathological either by noting any similarities with severely dysfunctional families or by not measuring up to the
exceptional one. This leaves families with a view of healthy adaptation that
is rarely achieved and perpetuates self-judgments about performance that
are infused with blame, shame, and guilt. The inspirations of the exceptional and the warning signs of dysfunction need to be grounded by descriptions of typical experiences. Only recently have investigators shifted
attention toward the efficacy of social support and a range of family dynamics that enhance coping and adaptation. This has led to a beginning
literature examining the impact of individual and family strengths on the
quality of life for all family members and on disease course and outcome
(Weihs, Fisher, & Baird, 2001).

Finally, definitions of what constitutes normal families are integral to
defining healthy caregiving systems. Outdated, rigid, gender-based models
of the family invariably define a narrow range of acceptable roles and strategies for coping with illness and disability. Traditional models of patient and
caregiver roles shackle families in the face of the protracted strains of illness
and threatened loss. A rich and broad multigenerational and multicultural
definition of family that evolves over the life cycle (Carter & McGoldrick,
1998) is essential to constructing a normative model.

By viewing the family as the unit of care, in which a broad range of
family forms and dynamics are normative, we can develop a model that
uses as its central reference point the idea of goodness of fit over time.
From this perspective, for example, high versus low family cohesion is not
viewed as inherently healthy or unhealthy. Rather, the organizing principle becomes relative: What degree of family cohesion will work optimally
with this illness now, and how might that change in future phases of the
condition?

In situations of chronic disorders, a basic task for families is to create
a meaning for the illness situation that preserves their sense of competency and mastery. At the extremes, competing ideologies can leave families
with a choice between a biological explanation or one of personal responsibility (bad things happen to bad people). Families desperately need reassurance that they are handling the illness normally (bad things do happen
to good people). These needs often occur in the context of a vague or
nonexistant psychosocial map. Many families, particularly those with untimely disorders, find themselves in unfamiliar territory and without
guides. This highlights the need for a preventive, psychoeducational ap-

proach that helps families anticipate normative illness-related developmental tasks over time in a fashion that maximizes a sense of control and mastery.

To create a normative context for their illness experience, families need the following foundation. First, they need a psychosocial understanding of the condition in systems terms. This means learning the expected pattern of practical and affective demands of a disorder over the life course of the condition. This includes a time frame for disease-related developmental tasks associated with different phases of the unfolding disorder. Second, families need to understand themselves as a systemic functional unit. Third, they need an appreciation of individual and family life-cycle patterns and changes to facilitate their incorporation of changing developmental demands for the family unit and individual members in relation to the demands of a chronic disorder. Finally, families need to understand the cultural, ethnic, spiritual, and gender-based beliefs that guide the type of caregiving system they construct. This includes guiding principles that delineate roles, rules of communication, definitions of success or mastery, and fit with beliefs of the health care providers. Family understanding in these areas facilitates a more holistic integration of the disorder and the family as a functional family-health/illness system evolving over time.

FAMILY SYSTEMS HEALTH MODEL

A normative, preventive model has been developed for psychoeducation, assessment, and intervention with families facing chronic and life-threatening disorders (Rolland 1984, 1987a, 1987b, 1990, 1994, 1998). This model is based on the concept of a systemic interaction between an illness and family that evolves over time. The goodness of "fit" between the psychosocial demands of the disorder and the family style of functioning and resources is a prime determinant of successful versus dysfunctional coping and adaptation. The model distinguishes three dimensions: (1) psychosocial "types" of disorders, (2) major phases in their natural history, and (3) key family system variables (Figure 17.1). A scheme of the systemic interaction between illness and family might look like the diagram in Figure 17.2. Family variables given particular emphasis include (1) the family and individual life cycles, particularly in relation to the time phases of a disorder; (2) multigenerational legacies related to illness and loss; and (3) belief systems.

Psychosocial Types of Illness

The standard disease classification used in medical settings is based on purely biological criteria that are clustered in ways to establish a medical diagnosis and treatment plan, rather than on the psychosocial demands

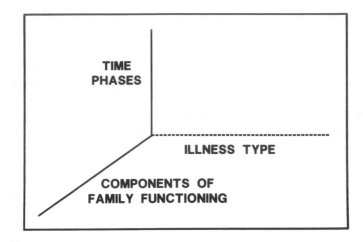

FIGURE 17.1. Three-dimensional model representing the relationship between illness type, time phases, and family functioning. (From Rolland, 1987a, with permission.)

on patients and their families. I have proposed a different classification scheme that provides a better link between the biological and psychosocial worlds, and thereby clarifies the relationship between chronic illness and the family (Rolland, 1984, 1994). The goal of this typology is to define meaningful and useful categories with similar psychosocial demands for a wide array of chronic illnesses affecting individuals across the lifespan.

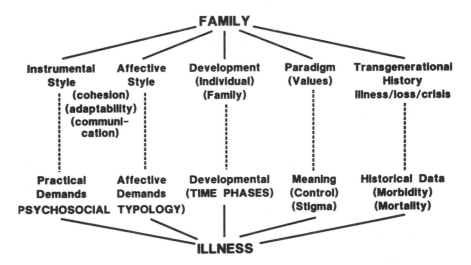

FIGURE 17.2. Interface of chronic illness and the family. (From Rolland, 1987a, with permission.)

Onset

Illnesses can be divided into those that have either an acute onset, such as strokes, or gradual onset, such as Alzheimer's disease. For acute-onset illnesses, affective and practical changes are compressed into a short time, requiring of the family more rapid mobilization of crisis management skills. Families able to tolerate highly charged emotional situations, exchange roles flexibly, problem-solve efficiently, and utilize outside resources will have an advantage in managing acute-onset conditions.

Course

The course of chronic diseases can take three general forms: progressive, constant, or relapsing/episodic. With a *progressive* disease such as Alzheimer's disease, the family is faced with a perpetually symptomatic family member whose disability worsens in a stepwise or gradual way. The family must live with the prospect of continual role change and adaptation to continued losses as the disease progresses. Increasing strain on family caregiving is caused by exhaustion, with few periods of relief from demands of the illness, and by new caregiving tasks over time.

With a *constant*-course illness, the occurrence of an initial event is followed by a stable biological course. A single heart attack and spinal cord injury are examples. Typically, after an initial period of recovery, the illness is characterized by some clear-cut deficit or limitation. The family is faced with a semipermanent change that is stable and predictable over a considerable time span. The potential for family exhaustion exists without the strain of new role demands over time.

Relapsing- or *episodic*-course illnesses, such as disk problems and asthma, are distinguished by the alternation of stable low-symptom periods with periods of flare-up or exacerbation. Families are strained by both the frequency of transitions between crisis and noncrisis, and the ongoing uncertainty of *when* a recurrence will occur. This requires family flexibility to alternate between two forms of family organization. The wide psychological discrepancy between low-symptom periods versus flare-up is a particularly taxing feature unique to relapsing diseases.

Outcome

The extent to which a chronic illness leads to death or shortens one's lifespan has profound psychosocial impact. The most crucial factor is the *initial expectation* of whether a disease is likely to cause death. On one end of the continuum are illnesses that do not typically affect the lifespan, such as disk disease or arthritis. At the other extreme are clearly progressive and fatal illnesses such as metastatic cancer. An intermediate, more unpredictable category includes both illnesses that shorten the lifespan, such as heart disease, and those with the possibility of sudden death, such as hemophilia. A major difference between these kinds of outcome is the degree to which the family experiences anticipatory loss and its pervasive effects on family life (Rolland, 1990).

Incapacitation

Disability can involve impairment of cognition (e.g., Alzheimer's disease), sensation (e.g., blindness), movement (e.g., stroke with paralysis), stamina (e.g., heart disease), disfigurement (e.g., mastectomy), and conditions associated with social stigma (e.g., AIDS) (Olkin, 1999). The extent, kind, and timing of disability imply sharp differences in the degree of family stress. For instance, the combined cognitive and motor deficits caused by a stroke necessitate greater family role reallocation than for a spinal cord injury in which cognitive abilities are unaffected. For some illnesses, such as stroke, disability is often worst at the beginning. For progressive diseases, such as Alzheimer's disease, disability looms as an increasing problem in later phases of the illness, allowing a family more time to prepare for anticipated changes and an opportunity for the ill member to participate in disease-related family planning while still cognitively able (Boss, 1999).

By combining the kinds of onset, course, outcome, and incapacitation into a grid format, we generate a typology that clusters illnesses according to similarities and differences in patterns that pose differing psychosocial demands (Table 17.1).

The *predictability* of an illness, and the degree of uncertainty about the specific way or rate at which it unfolds, overlays all other variables. For illnesses with highly unpredictable courses, such as multiple sclerosis, family coping and adaptation, especially future planning, are hindered by anticipatory anxiety and ambiguity about what family members will actually encounter. Families able to put long-term uncertainty into perspective are best prepared to avoid the risks of exhaustion and dysfunction.

Time Phases of Illness

Too often, discussions of "coping with cancer," "managing disability," or "dealing with life-threatening illness" approach illness as a static state and fail to appreciate the dynamic unfolding of illness processes over time. The concept of time phases provides a way for clinicians and families to think longitudinally and to understand chronic illness as an ongoing process with normative landmarks, transitions, and changing demands. Each phase of an illness poses its own psychosocial demands and developmental tasks that require significantly different strengths, attitudes, or changes from a family. The core psychosocial themes in the natural history of chronic disease can be described as three major phases: crisis, chronic, and terminal (Figure 17.3).

TABLE 17.1. Categorization of Chronic Disorders by Psychosocial Type

		Incapacitating		Nonincapacitating	
		Acute	Gradual	Acute	Gradual
FATAL	Progressive		Lung cancer CNS metastases Bone marrow failure Amyotrophic lateral sclerosis	Acute leukemia Pancreatic cancer Metastatic breast cancer Malignant melanoma Lung cancer Liver cancer, etc.	Cystic fibrosis[a]
	Relapsing			Cancers in remission	
POSSIBLY SHORTENED LIFE SPAN or FATAL	Progressive		Emphysema Alzheimer's disease Multi-infarct dementia AIDS Multiple sclerosis (late) Chronic alcoholism Huntington's chorea Scleroderma		Juvenile diabetes[a] Malignant hypertension Insulin-dependent adult-onset diabetes
	Relapsing	Angina	Early multiple sclerosis Episodic alcoholism	Sickle cell disease[a] Hemophilia[a]	Systemic lupus erythematosus[a]
	Constant	Stroke Moderate/severe myocardial infarction	PKU and other inborn errors of metabolism	Mild myocardial infarction Cardiac arrhythmia	Hemodialysis-treated renal failure Hodgkin's disease

(continued)

Table 17.1. *Continued*

	Incapacitating		Nonincapacitating	
	Acute	Gradual	Acute	Gradual
Progressive		Parkinson's disease Rheumatoid arthritis Osteoarthritis		Non-insulin-dependent adult-onset diabetes
Relapsing	Lumbosacral disk disease		Kidney stones Gout Migraine Seasonal allergy Asthma Epilepsy	Peptic ulcer Ulcerative colitis Chronic bronchitis Other inflammatory bowel diseases Psoriasis
Constant	Congenital malformations Spinal cord injury Acute blindness Acute deafness Survived severe trauma and burns Posthypoxic syndrome	Nonprogressive mental retardation Cerebral palsy	Benign arrhythmia Congenital heart disease	Malabsorption syndromes Hyper/hypothyroidism Pernicious anemia Controlled hypertension Controlled glaucoma

N O N F A T A L

Note. Excerpted from Rolland (1984), with permission.
[a]Early.

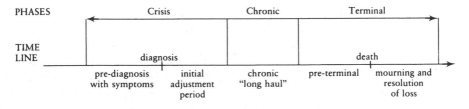

FIGURE 17.3. Timeline and phases of illness. (From Rolland, 1984, with permission.)

The *crisis* phase includes any symptomatic period before diagnosis and the initial readjustment period after a diagnosis and initial treatment planning. This phase holds a number of key tasks for the ill member and family. Moos (1984) describes certain universal, practical, illness-related tasks, including (1) learning to cope with any symptoms or disability; (2) adapting to health care settings and any treatment procedures; and (3) establishing and maintaining workable relationships with the health care team. Also, there are critical tasks of a more general, existential nature. Family members needs to (1) create a meaning for the illness that maximizes a sense of mastery and competency; (2) grieve for the loss of "life" before illness; (3) gradually accept the illness as permanent while maintaining a sense of continuity between their past and future; (4) pull together to cope with the immediate crisis; and (5) in the face of uncertainty, develop flexibility toward future goals.

During this initial crisis period, health professionals have enormous influence over a family's sense of competence and the methods devised to accomplish these developmental tasks. Initial meetings and advice given at the time of diagnosis can be thought of as a "framing event." Because families are so vulnerable at this point, clinicians need to be extremely sensitive in their interactions with family members. They need to be aware of messages conveyed by their behavior with the family. Who is included or excluded (e.g., patient) from a discussion can be interpreted by the family as a message of how a family should plan their communication for the duration of the illness. This "framing event" has a powerful influence on families deciding what is normal. For instance, a clinician may meet with family members separately from the patient to give them information about the illness diagnosis and prognosis. At this vulnerable moment, family members may assume they are being instructed implicitly to exclude the patient from any discussion of the illness. Clinicians also need to be careful not to undercut a family's attempt to sustain a sense of competence by implicitly blaming the patient or the family for an illness (e.g., delay in seeking an appointment, negligence by parents, poor health habits) or by distancing themselves from the family.

The *chronic* phase, whether long or short, is the time span between the initial diagnosis/readjustment and the third phase, when issues of death and terminal illness predominate. This era can be marked by constancy, progression, or episodic change. It has been referred to as "the long haul," or "the day-to-day living with chronic illness" phase. Often the patient and family have come to grips psychologically and organizationally with permanent changes and have devised an ongoing coping strategy. The ability of the family to maintain the semblance of a normal life with a chronic illness and heightened uncertainty is a key task of this period. If the illness is fatal, this is a time of "living in limbo." For certain highly debilitating but not clearly fatal illnesses, such as a massive stroke or dementia, the family can feel saddled with an exhausting problem "without end." Paradoxically, a family may feel its hope to resume a "normal" life can only be realized after the death of its ill member. The maintenance of maximum autonomy for all family members in the face of protracted adversity helps offset these trapped, helpless feelings.

For long-term disorders, customary patterns of intimacy for couples become skewed by discrepancies between the ill member and the well spouse/caregiver. As one young husband lamented about his wife's cancer, "It was hard enough two years ago to absorb that, even if Ann was cured, her radiation treatment would make pregnancy impossible. Now, I find it unbearable that her continued slow, losing battle with cancer makes it impossible to go for our dreams like other couples our age." Normative ambivalence and escape fantasies often remain underground and contribute to "survivor guilt." Psychoeducational family interventions that normalize such emotions related to threatened loss can help prevent destructive cycles of blame, shame, and guilt.

In the *terminal* phase of an illness, the inevitability of death becomes apparent and dominates family life. Now the family must cope with issues of separation, death, mourning, and resumption of "normal" family life beyond the loss (Walsh & McGoldrick, 1991). Families that adapt best to this phase are able to shift their view of mastery from controlling the illness to a successful process of "letting go." Optimal coping involves emotional openness as well as dealing with the myriad practical tasks at hand. This includes seeing this phase as an opportunity to share precious time together to acknowledge the impending loss, to deal with unfinished business, to say good-byes and to begin the process of family reorganization. If they have not decided beforehand, the patient and key family members need to decide about such things as a living will; the extent of medical heroics desired; preferences about dying at home, in the hospital, or at hospice; and wishes about a funeral or memorial service and burial.

Critical *transition periods* link the three time phases. Transitions in the illness life cycle are times when families reevaluate the appropriateness of their previous life structure in the face of new illness-related developmental demands. Unfinished business from the previous phase can complicate or block movement through the transitions. Families can become permanently frozen in an adaptive structure that has outlived its utility (Penn, 1983). For example, the usefulness of pulling together in the crisis phase can become maladaptive and stifling for all family members in the chronic phase.

The interaction of the time phases and typology of illness provides a framework for a normative psychosocial developmental model for chronic disease that resembles models for human development. The time phases (crisis, chronic, and terminal) can be considered broad developmental periods in the natural history of chronic disease. Each period has certain basic tasks independent of the type of illness. Each "type" of illness has specific supplementary tasks.

Clinical Implications

This model provides a framework for assessment and clinical intervention by facilitating an understanding of chronic illness and disability in psychosocial terms. Attention to features of onset, course, outcome, and incapacitation provides markers that focus clinical assessment and intervention with a family. For instance, acute-onset illnesses demand high levels of adaptability, problem solving, role reallocation, and balanced cohesion. In such circumstances, helping families to maximize flexibility enables them to adapt more successfully.

An illness time line delineates psychosocial developmental phases of an illness, each phase with its own unique developmental tasks. It is important for families to address normative phase–related tasks in sequence to optimize successful adaptation over the long haul of a chronic disorder. Attention to time allows the clinician to assess family strengths and vulnerabilities in relation to the present and future phases of the illness.

The model clarifies treatment planning. Goal setting is guided by awareness of the components of family functioning most relevant to the particular type or phase of an illness. Sharing this information with the family and deciding on specific goals provides a better sense of control and realistic hope to the family. This process empowers families in their journey of living with a chronic disorder. Also, this knowledge educates family members about warning signs that should alert them to call at appropriate times for brief, goal-oriented treatment.

The framework is useful for timing family psychosocial checkups to coincide with key transition points in the illness life cycle. Preventively oriented family psychoeducational or support groups for patients and their families (Gonzalez, Steinglass, & Reiss, 1989; Steinglass, 1998) can be designed to deal with different types of conditions (e.g., progressive, life-threatening, relapsing). Also, brief psychoeducational "modules," timed for critical phases of particular "types" of diseases, enable families to digest manageable portions of a long-term coping process. Modules can be tailored to particular phases of the illness and to family coping skills necessary to confront disease-related demands. This provides a cost-effective preventive service that also can identify high-risk families.

FAMILY ASSESSMENT

As chronic illnesses become incorporated into the family system and all its processes, family coping is influenced by illness-oriented family dynamics that concern the dimension of time and belief systems.

Multigenerational Legacies of Illness, Loss, and Crisis

A family's current behavior, and therefore its response to illness, cannot be adequately comprehended apart from its history (Boszormenyi-Nagy & Spark, 1973; Bowen, 1978; Byng-Hall, 1995; Carter & McGoldrick, 1998; Framo, 1992; Walsh & McGoldrick, 1991). Clinicians can use historical questioning and construct a genogram and time line (McGoldrick, Gerson, & Schellenberger, 1999) to track key events and transitions to gain an understanding of a family's organizational shifts and coping strategies as a system in response to past stressors, and more specifically, to past illnesses. Such inquiry helps explain and predict the family's current style of coping, adaptation, and creation of meaning. A multigenerational assessment helps to clarify areas of strength and vulnerability. It also identifies high-risk families burdened by past unresolved issues and dysfunctional patterns that cannot absorb the challenges presented by a serious condition.

A chronic illness–oriented genogram focuses on the organization of a family in terms of past stressors and tracks the evolution of family adaptation over time. It focuses on how a family organized itself as an evolving system specifically around previous illnesses and unexpected crises. A central goal is to bring to light areas of consensus and "learned differences" (Penn, 1983) that are sources of cohesion and conflict. Patterns of coping, replications, discontinuities, shifts in relationships (i.e., alliances, triangles, cutoff), and sense of competence are noted. These patterns are transmitted across generations as family pride, myths, taboos, catastrophic expectations, and belief systems (Walsh & McGoldrick, 1991). Also, it is useful to inquire about other forms of loss (e.g., divorce, migration), crisis (e.g., lengthy unemployment, rape, a natural disaster), and protracted adversity (e.g., poverty, racism, war, political oppression). These experiences can provide transferable sources of resilience and effective coping skills in the face of a serious health problem (Walsh, 1998).

Illness Type and Time Phase Issues

Whereas a family may have certain standard ways of coping with any illness, there may be critical differences in their style and success in adaptation to different "types" of diseases. It is important to track prior family illnesses for areas of perceived competence, failures, or inexperience. Inquiry about different types of illness (e.g., life threatening vs. non-life threatening) may find, for instance, that a family dealt successfully with non-life-threatening illnesses but reeled under the weight of metastatic cancer. Such a family might be well equipped to deal with less severe conditions, but it might be particularly vulnerable if another life-threatening illness were to occur.

Tracking a family's coping capabilities in the crisis, chronic, and terminal phases of previous chronic illnesses highlights legacies of strength as well as complication in adaptation related to different points in the "illness life cycle." One man grew up with a partially disabled father with heart disease and witnessed his parents successful renegotiation of traditional gender-defined roles when his mother went to work, while his father assumed household responsibilities. This man, now with heart disease himself, has a positive legacy about gender roles from his family of origin that facilitated a flexible response to his own illness. Another family with a member with chronic kidney failure functioned very well in handling the practicalities of home dialysis. However, in the terminal phase, their limitations with emotional expression left a legacy of unresolved grief. Tracking prior illness experiences in terms of time phases helps clinicians see both the strengths and vulnerabilities in a family, which counteracts the assignment of dysfunctional labels that emphasize the difficult periods. Clinicians need to ask specifically about positive family-of-origin experiences with illness and loss that can be used as models to adapt to the current situation.

For any significant illness in either adult partner's family of origin, a clinician should try to get a picture of how those families organized to handle the range of disease-related affective and practical tasks. What role did each play in handling these tasks, and did they emerge with a strong sense of competence or failure? Such information can help to anticipate areas of conflict, consensus, and similar patterns of adaptation. Hidden strengths, not just unresolved issues, can remain dormant in a marriage and suddenly reemerge when triggered by a chronic illness in the current family unit.

Although many families facing chronic disease have healthy multigenerational family patterns of adaptation, any family may falter in the face of multiple, superimposed disease and nondisease stressors that impact in a relatively short time. With progressive, incapacitating diseases or the concurrence of illnesses in several family members, a pragmatic approach that focuses on expanded or creative use of supports and resources outside the family is most productive.

Interface of the Illness, Individual, and Family Life Cycles

A life-cycle lens provides a powerful way to construct a normative framework for serious illness. To place the unfolding of chronic disease into a developmental context, it is crucial to understand the intertwining of three evolutionary threads: the illness, individual, and family life cycles.

Life cycle and *life structure* are central concepts for both family and individual development. "Life cycle" means there is a basic sequence and unfolding of the life course within which individual, family, or illness uniqueness occurs. "Life structure" refers to the core elements (e.g., work, child rearing, caregiving) of an individual's or family's life at any phase of the life cycle. Illness, individual, and family development have in common the notion of phases (each with its own developmental tasks) and are marked by the alternation of life structure–building/maintaining (stable) and life structure–changing (transitional) periods linking developmental phases (Levinson, 1986). The primary goal of a building/maintaining period is to form a life structure and enrich life within it based on the key choices an individual/family made during the preceding transition period. Transition periods are potentially the most vulnerable, because previous individual, family, and illness life structures are reappraised in the face of new developmental tasks that may require major, discontinuous change rather than minor alterations (Hoffman, 1989; see Cowan & Cowan, Chapter 16, this volume).

The concepts of centrifugal and centripetal family styles are useful in integrating illness, individual, and family development (Beavers & Hampson, 1990). Combrinck-Graham (1985) describes a family life spiral model, envisioning a three-generational family system oscillating over time between centripetal and centrifugal phases. Centripetal periods of the family life cycle, such as when raising young children, are marked by family developmental tasks that require intense bonding or an inside-the-family focus. Centrifugal periods, such as rearing adolescents and launching, are characterized by looser boundaries around the family, often emphasizing individual members' activities and interests outside the family. In life-cycle terms, centripetal and centrifugal periods suggest the fit between family developmental tasks and the relative need for family members to direct their energies inside the family to work together to accomplish those tasks.

Several key life-cycle concepts provide a foundation for understanding the experience of chronic disorders. The life cycle contains alternating transition and life structure–building/maintaining periods. And particular periods can be characterized as either centripetal or centrifugal in nature, as diagrammed in Figure 17.4.

The notion of centripetal and centrifugal modes is useful in linking the illness life cycle to those of the individual and family. In general, serious disorders exert an inward cohesive pull on the family system. Analogous to the addition of a new family member, illness onset sets in motion an inside-the-family focused process of socialization to illness. Symptoms, loss of function, the demands of shifting or acquiring new illness-related roles, and the fear of loss through death all require a family to focus inward.

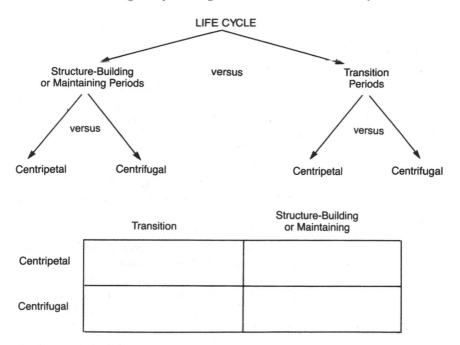

FIGURE 17.4. Periods in the family and individual life cycles. (From Rolland, 1987a, with permission.)

The need for family cohesion varies enormously with different illness types and phases. The tendency for a disease to pull a family inward increases with the level of disability or risk of progression and death. Progressive diseases over time inherently require a greater centripetal focus than constant-course illnesses. The ongoing addition of new demands as an illness progresses keeps a family's energy focused inward, often impeding or halting the natural life-cycle evolution of other members. After an initial period of adaptation, a constant-course disease (without severe disability) permits a family to get back on track developmentally. Relapsing illnesses alternate between periods of drawing a family inward and of release from immediate demands of disease. But, the on-call nature of many such illnesses keeps part of the family focus in a centripetal mode despite asymptomatic periods, hindering the natural flow between phases of the family life cycle.

If illness onset coincides with a centrifugal period in the family's development, it can derail the family from its natural momentum. Illness or disability in a young adult may require a heightened dependency and return to the family of origin for disease-related caregiving. The autonomy and individuation of parents and child are diminished, and separate interests and priorities are relinquished or put on hold. Family dynamics, as well as disease severity, will influence whether the family's reversion to a centripetal life structure is a temporary detour or a permanent reversal.

When the inward pull of disease onset coincides with a centripetal period in the family life cycle (e.g., early child rearing), it can prolong this period. The research of Minuchin, Rosman, and Baker (1978) with "psychosomatic" families has documented the risk of vulnerable families dealing with childhood disorders becoming permanently enmeshed and developmentally stuck. On the other hand, in situations of chronic disorders, there is a risk of labeling enmeshment when the normative lengthening of developmental phases for child and family is disregarded. Often, families coping with a chronically ill child are tentative about giving more autonomy, not because of inherent family dysfunction, but, rather, because of chronic anticipation of further loss coupled with a lack of preventive psychoeducation from professionals.

With major health conditions, definitions concerning normative family structure need to be reconsidered. Enmeshment with blurred generational boundaries is touted as the hallmark of family dysfunction. Yet the very real demands on older children and adolescents to assume adult functions, in the interest of family survival, need to be distinguished from rigid pathological descriptions of "parentified" children. For instance, when a parent develops a serious disorder during a child-rearing phase of development, a family's ability to stay on course is most severely taxed. The impact is twofold: A new family burden is added as a parent is "lost," analogous to becoming a single-parent family with an added child. To meet simultaneous child-rearing and caregiving needs, an older child or grandparent may need to assume parental responsibilities. These forms of family adaptation are appropriate if structural realignments are flexible, shared and sensitive to competing age-related developmental needs.

The onset of a serious disorder forces a family into a transition in which one of the family's main tasks is to accommodate the anticipation of further loss and possibly untimely death. When illness onset coincides with a transition in the individual or family life cycle, issues related to previous, current, and anticipated loss will tend to be magnified. Transition periods are often characterized by upheaval, rethinking of prior commitments, and openness to change. As a result, those times hold a greater risk for the illness to become unnecessarily embedded or inappropriately ignored in planning for the next developmental phase. During a transition period, the very process of loosening prior commitments often brings to the forefront family rules regarding loyalty through sacrifice and caregiving. These "vulnerable" nodal points provide opportunities for clinicians to help family members clarify and resolve divided and competing loyalty demands.

Illness onset that coincides with a life structure–building/maintaining period in individual or family development presents a different challenge. These periods are characterized by living out choices made during the preceding transition period. Relative to transition periods, family members try to protect their own and the family unit's current life structure. Milder conditions may require some revision of individual/family life structure, but not a radical restructuring that would necessitate a return to a transitional period. A severe chronic illness will force families into a more complete transition at a time when individual/family inertia is to preserve the momentum of a stable period. To navigate this kind of crisis successfully, family adaptability requires the ability to transform the entire life structure to a prolonged transitional state.

From a systems viewpoint, at the time of diagnosis, it is important to know the phase of the family life cycle and the stage of individual development of all family members, not just the ill member. Chronic disease in one family member can profoundly affect developmental goals of another member. For instance, an infant disability can be a serious roadblock to parents' preconceived ideas about competent child rearing, or a life-threatening illness in a young married adult can interfere with the well spouse's readiness to become a parent. Also, family members frequently do not adapt equally to chronic illness. Each member's ability to adapt, and the rate at which he or she does so, is related to his or her own developmental stage and role in the family (Ireys & Burr, 1984). When family members are in tune with each other's developmental processes, while promoting flexibility and alternative means to satisfy developmental needs, successful long-term adaptation is maximized.

The timing of chronic illness in the life cycle can be normative (e.g., expectable in relation to chronological and social time) or non normative (e.g., "off-time"). Coping with chronic illness is considered a normally anticipated task in late adulthood, whereas its occurrence earlier is "out of phase" and developmentally more disruptive (Neugarten, 1976). For instance, chronic diseases that occur in the child-rearing period can be most challenging because of their potential impact on family financial and child-rearing responsibilities. The actual impact will depend on the "type" of illness and preillness family roles. Families governed by flexible gender-influenced rules about who is the financial provider and caregiver of children will tend to adjust better.

The notion of "out of phase" illnesses can be conceptualized in a more refined way that highlights patterns of strain related to time. First, because diseases have a centripetal influence on most families, they can be more disruptive to families in a centrifugal phase of development. Second, if the particular illness is progressive, relapsing, increasingly incapacitating, and/or life-threatening, then the unfolding phases of the disease will be punctuated by numerous transitions. Under these conditions, a family will need to alter its structure more frequently to accommodate shifting and increasing demands of the disease. This level of demand and uncertainty keeps the illness in the forefront of a family's consciousness, constantly impinging on its attempts to get back "in phase" developmentally.

Finally, the transition from the crisis to the chronic phase is the key juncture at which the intensity of the family's socialization to living with chronic disease can often be relaxed. In this sense, it offers a "window of opportunity" for the family to recover its developmental course.

With chronic disorders, an overarching family goal is to deal with the developmental demands of the illness without family members sacrificing their own or the family's development as a system over time. It is important to determine whose life plans were cancelled, postponed, or altered, and when plans put on hold and future developmental issues will be addressed. In this way, clinicians can anticipate life-cycle nodal points related to "autonomy within" versus "subjugation to" the condition. Family members can be helped to strike a healthier balance, with life plans that resolve feelings of guilt, overresponsibility, and hopelessness, and find family and external resources to enhance freedom both to pursue personal goals and to provide needed care for the ill member.

HEALTH/ILLNESS BELIEF SYSTEM

When illness strikes, a primary developmental challenge for a family is to create a meaning for the illness experience that promotes a sense of mastery and competency. Because serious illness is often experienced as a betrayal of our fundamental trust in our bodies and belief in our invulnerability (Kleinman, 1988), creating an empowering narrative can be a formidable task. Family health beliefs help us grapple with the existential dilemmas of our fear of death, our tendency to want to sustain our denial of death, and our attempts to reassert control when suffering and loss occur. They serve as a cognitive map guiding decisions and action; they provide a way to approach new and ambiguous situations for coherence in family life, facilitating continuity between past, present, and future (Antonovsky & Sourani, 1988; Reiss, 1981). Our inquiry into and curiosity about family beliefs is perhaps the most powerful foundation stone of collaboration between families and health professionals (Wright, Watson, & Bell, 1996). Beliefs are the fiber that weaves a resilient, collaborative relationship.

In the initial crisis phase, it is essential for clinicians to inquire about key family beliefs that shape the family's narrative and coping strategies. This includes tracking (1) beliefs about normality; (2) mind–body relationship, control, and mastery; (3) meanings attached by a family, ethnic group, religion, or the wider culture to symptoms (e.g., chronic pain), types of illnesses (e.g., life-threatening), or specific diseases (e.g., AIDS); (4) assumptions about what caused an illness and what will influence it's course and outcome; (5) multigenerational factors that have shaped a family's health beliefs; and (6) anticipated nodal points in the illness, individual, and family life cycles when health beliefs will be strained or need to shift. A clinician should also assess the fit of health beliefs within the family and its various subsystems (e.g., spouse, parental, extended family), as well as between the family and health care system, and the wider culture.

Beliefs about Normality

Family beliefs about what is normal or abnormal, and the importance members place on conformity and excellence in relation to the average family, have far-reaching implications for adaptation to chronic disorders. Families whose values allow having a "problem" without self-denigration have a distinct advantage, enabling them to seek outside help, yet maintain a positive identity in the face of chronic conditions. Families who define help-seeking as weak and shameful undercut this kind of resilience. Essentially, with chronic disorders in which problems are to be expected and the use of professionals and outside resources are necessary, a belief that pathologizes this normative process adds insult to injury.

Two useful questions to elicit these beliefs are, "How do you think other *average* families would deal with a similar situation to yours?" and "How would a *healthy* family ideally cope with your situation?" Families with strong beliefs in high achievement and perfectionism are prone to apply accustomed standards of control that are impossible to achieve in a situation of illness. Particularly with untimely conditions that occur early in the life cycle, there are additional pressures to keep up with normative, socially expectable developmental milestones of age peers or other young couples. The fact that life-cycle goals may take longer or need revision requires a flexible belief about what is normal and healthy. To effectively sustain hope, particularly in situations of long-term adversity, families need to embrace a flexible definition of normality.

The Family's Sense of Mastery Facing Illness

It is critical to determine how a family defines mastery or control in general, and in situations of illness. Mastery is similar to the concept of health locus of control (Lefcourt, 1982), which can be defined as the belief about influence over the course/outcome of an illness. It is useful to distinguish whether a family's beliefs are based on the premise of internal control, external control by chance, or external control by powerful others.

An internal locus of control orientation means that individuals or families believe they can affect the outcome of a situation. In illness, such families believe they are directly responsible for their health and have the power to recover from illness (Wallston & Wallston, 1978). An external orientation entails a belief that outcomes are not contingent on the individual's or family's behavior. Families that view illness in terms of chance believe that when illness occurs, it is a matter of luck and that fate determines recovery. Those who see health control as being in the hands of powerful others view health professionals, God, or sometimes "powerful" family members as exerting control over their bodies and illness course.

A family may adhere to a different set of beliefs about control when dealing with biological as opposed to typical day-to-day issues. Therefore, it is important to assess both a family's basic value system and beliefs about control for illnesses in general, chronic and life-threatening illness, and finally, the specific disease facing the family. For instance, regardless of the actual severity or prognosis in a particular case, cancer may be equated with "death" or "no control" because of medical statistics, cultural myth, or prior family history. On the other hand, families may have enabling stories about a member or friend, who in spite of cancer and a shortened life-span, lived a "full" life centered on effectively prioritizing the quality of relationships and goals. Clinicians can highlight these positive narratives as a means to help families counteract cultural beliefs that focus exclusively on control of biology as defining success.

A family's beliefs about mastery strongly affect the nature of its relationship to an illness and to the health care system. Beliefs about control can affect treatment compliance and a family's preferences about participation in their family member's treatment and healing process. Families that view disease course/outcome as a matter of chance tend to establish marginal relationships with health professionals, largely because their belief system minimizes the importance of their own or the professional's impact on a disease process. Also, poor minority families may receive inadequate care or lack insurance or access, leading to a fatalistic attitude and lack of engagement with health care providers, who may not be trusted to help. Just as any psychotherapeutic relationship depends on a shared belief system about what is therapeutic, a workable accommodation among the patient, family, and health care team in terms of these fundamental values is essential. Families that feel misunderstood by health care professionals are often reacting to a lack of joining at this basic value level. Too often, their healthy need to participate was ignored or preempted by a professional needing unilateral control.

The goodness of fit between family beliefs about mastery can vary depending on the time phase of the condition. For some disorders, the crisis phase involves protracted care outside the family's direct control. This may be stressful for a family that prefers to tackle its own problems without outside control and "interference." The patient's return home may increase the workload but allow members to reassert more fully their competence and leadership. In contrast, a family guided more by a preference for external control by experts can expect greater difficulty when their family member returns home. Recognition of such normative differences in belief about control can guide an effective psychosocial treatment plan tailored to each family's needs and affirming rather than disrespecting its core values.

In the terminal phase, a family may feel least in control of the biological course of the disease and the decision making regarding the overall care of the dying member. Families with a strong belief about being involved in a family member's health care may need to assert themselves more vigorously with health providers. Effective decision making about the extent of heroic medical efforts or whether a patient will die at home or at an institution or hospice requires a family–provider relationship that respects the family's basic beliefs.

With illness and disability, we must be cautious about judging the relative usefulness of positive illusions (Taylor, 1989) or minimization versus direct confrontation with and acceptance of painful realities. Often, both are needed. The healthy use of minimization or selective focus on the positive and timely uses of humor should be distinguished from the concept of denial, regarded as pathological. The skilled clinician must thread the needle supporting both the usefulness of exaggerated hope and the need for treatment to control the illness or a new complication. There is greater incentive for a family to confront denial of an illness or its severity both when there is hope that preventive action or medical treatment can affect the outcome, and when an illness is entering a terminal phase. Yet to cope with an arduous, uncertain course, families often need simultaneously to acknowledge the condition itself and to minimize treatment risks or the likelihood of a poor outcome.

Family Beliefs about the Cause of an Illness

When a significant health problem arises, all of us wonder, "Why me (or us)?" and "Why now?" We invariably construct an explanation or story that helps organize our experience. With the limits of current medical knowledge, tremendous uncertainties persist about the relative importance of myriad factors, leaving individuals and families to make idiosyncratic attributions about what caused an illness. A family's beliefs about the cause of an illness need to be assessed separately from its beliefs about what can affect the outcome. It is important to ask each family member for his or her explanation. Responses will generally reflect a combination of medical information and family mythology. Beliefs about cause might include punishment for prior misdeeds (e.g., an affair), blame of a particular family member ("Your drinking made me sick!"), a sense of injustice ("Why am I being punished? I have been a good person."), genetics (e.g., cancer runs on one side of the family), negligence of the patient (e.g., careless driving) or of parents (e.g., sudden infant death syndrome), or simply bad luck.

Optimal family narratives respect the limits of scientific knowledge, affirm basic competency, and promote the flexible use of multiple biological and psychosocial healing strategies. In contrast, causal attributions that invoke blame, shame, or guilt are particularly important to uncover. Such beliefs make it extremely difficult for a family to cope and adapt in a functional way. With a life-threatening illness, a blamed family member is implicitly, if not explicitly, held accountable if the patient dies. Decisions about treatment then become confounded and filled with tension. A mother who feels blamed by her husband for their son's leukemia may be less able to stop a low-probability experimental treatment than the angry, blaming husband. A husband who believes his drinking caused his wife's coronary and subsequent death may increase self-destructive drinking in his profound guilt.

Belief System Adaptability

Because illnesses vary enormously in their responsiveness to psychosocial factors, *both families and providers need to make distinctions* between beliefs about their overall participation in a long-term disease process, and beliefs about their ability to control the biological unfolding of an illness and the flexibility with which they can apply these beliefs. Families' experience of competence or mastery depends on their grasp of these distinctions. Optimal family and provider narratives respect the limits of scientific knowledge, affirm basic competency, and promote the flexible use of multiple biological and psychosocial healing strategies.

A family's belief in its participation in the total illness process can be thought of as independent of whether a disease is stable, improving, or in a terminal phase. Sometimes, mastery and the attempt to control biological process coincide, as when a family tailors its behavior to help maintain the health of a member with cancer in remission. This might include changes in family roles, communication, diet, exercise, and balance between work and recreation. Optimally, when an ill family member loses remission, as the family enters the terminal phase of the illness, participation as an expression of mastery is transformed to a successful process of letting go that eases suffering and allows palliative care to be provided.

Families with flexible belief systems are more likely to experience death with a sense of equanimity rather than profound failure. The death of a patient whose long, debilitating illness has heavily burdened others can bring relief as well as sadness to family members. Because relief over death goes against societal conventions, it can trigger massive guilt reactions that may be expressed through symptoms such as depression and family conflict. Clinicians need to help family members accept ambivalent feeling they may have about the death as natural.

Thus, flexibility both within the family and the health professional system is a key variable in optimal family functioning. Rather than linking mastery in a rigid way with biological outcome (survival or recovery) as the sole determinant of success, families can define control in a more "holistic" sense, with involvement and participation in the overall process as the main criteria defining success. This is analogous to the distinction between curing "the disease" and "healing the system." Healing the system may influence the course and outcome, but a positive disease outcome is not necessary for a family to feel successful. This flexible view of mastery permits the quality of relations within the family, or between the family and health care professional, to become more central to criteria of success. The health care provider's competence becomes valued from both a technical and caregiving perspective not solely linked to the biological course (Reiss & Kaplan De-Nour, 1989).

Ethnic, Religious, and Cultural Beliefs

Ethnicity, race, and religion strongly influence family beliefs concerning health and illness (McGoldrick, Giordano, & Pearce, 1996; Walsh, 1999; Zborowski, 1969). Significant ethnic differences regarding health beliefs typically emerge at the time of a major health crisis. Health professionals need to be mindful of the belief systems of various ethnic, racial, and religious groups in their community, particularly as these translate into different behavioral patterns. Cultural norms vary in such areas as the definition of the appropriate "sick role" for the patient; the kind and degree of open communication about the disease; who should be included in the illness caregiving system (e.g., extended family, friends, professionals); who is the primary caretaker (almost always wife/mother/daughter/daughter-in-law); and the kind of rituals viewed as normative at different stages of an illness (e.g., hospital bedside vigils, healing, and funeral rituals). This is especially true for minority groups (e.g., African American, Asian, Hispanic) that experience discrimination or marginalization from prevailing white Anglo culture. Illness provides an opportunity to encourage role flexibility and shift from defining one female member as the caregiver to a collaborative caregiving team that includes male and female siblings/adult children.

Clinicians need to be mindful of these cultural differences among themselves, the patient, and the family as a necessary step to forging a workable alliance that can endure a long-term illness (Seaburn, Gunn, Mauksch, Gawinski, & Lorenz, 1996). Disregarding these issues can lead families to wall themselves off from health care providers and available community resources—a major cause of noncompliance and treatment failure. Sometimes professionals may need the flexibility to suspend their need to prevail, especially in relation to family/cultural beliefs that proscribe certain standard forms of medical care (e.g., blood products for Jehovah's Witness). This requires an acceptance that the patient, not the physician, retains final responsibility for decisions about his or her body.

Fit among Clinicians, Health Systems, and Families

It is a common, but unfortunate, error to regard "the family" as a monolithic unit that feels, thinks, believes, and behaves as an undifferentiated whole. Clinicians should inquire both about the level of agreement and tolerance for differences among family members' beliefs, and between the family and the health care system. Is the family rule "We must agree on all/some values," or are diversity and different viewpoints acceptable? How much do family members feel the need to stay in sync with prevailing cultural or societal beliefs, or family tradition?

Family beliefs that balance the need for consensus with diversity and innovation are optimal and maximize permissible options. If consensus is the rule, then individual differentiation implies disloyalty and deviance. If the guiding principle is "We can hold different viewpoints," then diversity is allowed. This is adaptive because it facilitates bringing to the family novel and creative forms of problem solving that may be needed in a situation of protracted adversity, such as serious illness. Families also need open communication and effective conflict resolution when members differ on major health care/treatment decisions.

To assess the fit between the family and health care team, the same questions concerning beliefs asked of families are relevant to the medical team members:

1. What are their attitudes about their own and the family's ability to influence the course/outcome of the disease?
2. How do the health care team members see the balance between their own versus the family's participation in the treatment process?
3. If basic differences in beliefs about control exist, how can these differences be reconciled?

Because of the tendency of most health facilities to disempower individuals and thereby foster dependence, utmost sensitivity to family values is needed to create a therapeutic system. Many breakdowns in relationships between "noncompliant" or marginal patients and their providers can be traced to natural disagreements at this basic level that were not addressed.

Normative differences among family members' health beliefs may emerge into destructive conflicts during a health crisis, as in the following case: When Stavros H., a first-generation Greek American, became ill with heart disease, his mother kept a 24-hour bedside vigil in his hospital room, so she could tend to her son at any hour. His wife, Dana, from a Scandinavian family, greatly resented the "intrusive behavior" of her mother-in-law, who in turn criticized Dana's emotional "coldness" and relative lack of concern. Stavros felt caught between his warring mother and wife, and complained of increased symptoms.

In such situations, clinicians need to sort out normative cultural differences from pathological enmeshment. In this case, all concerned behaved according to their own cultural norms. In Greek culture, it is normal to maintain close ties to one's family of origin after marriage and expected that a mother would tend to her son in a health crisis. A son would be disloyal not to allow his mother that role. This sharply differs from the northern European traditions of the wife. Each side pathologizes the other, creating a conflictual triangle, with the patient caught in the middle. In such situations, the clinician who affirms normative multicultural differences promotes a transformation of process from blaming or pathologizing to one of accommodating different, equally legitimate cultures.

It is common for differences in beliefs or attitude to erupt at any major life-cycle or illness transition. For instance, in situations of severe disability or terminal illness, one member may want the patient to return home, whereas another prefers long-term hospitalization or transfer to an extended care facility. Because the chief task of patient caretaking is usually assigned to the wife/mother, she is the one most apt to bear the chief burdens in this regard. A family able to anticipate the collision of gender-based beliefs about caregiving with the potential overwhelming demands of home-based care for a dying family member and flexibly modify its rules would avert the risk of family caretaker overload, resentment, and deteriorating family relationships.

The murky boundary between the chronic and terminal phase highlights the potential for professionals' beliefs to collide with those of the family. Physicians can feel bound to a technological imperative that requires them to exhaust all possibilities at their disposal, regardless of the odds of success. Families may not know how to interpret continued lifesaving efforts, assuming real hope where virtually none exists. Health care professionals and institutions can collude in a pervasive societal wish to deny death as a natural process truly beyond technological control (Becker, 1973). Endless treatment can represent the medical team members' inability to separate a general value placed on controlling diseases from their beliefs about participation (separate from cure) in a patient's total care.

CONCLUSIONS

Facing the risks and burdens of a serious illness, the "healthiest" families are able to harness that experience to improve the quality of life. Families can achieve a healthy balance between accepting limits and promoting autonomy. For illnesses with long-range risks, families can maintain mastery in the face of uncertainty by enhancing the following capacities: acknowledge the possibility of loss, sustain hope, and build flexibility into family life-cycle planning that conserves and adjusts major goals, and helps circumvent the forces of uncertainty. The systemic model described here, which integrates the psychosocial demands of disorders over time with individual and family life cycles and belief systems, provides a foundation for such a normative perspective.

A serious illness or brush with death provides an opportunity to confront catastrophic fears about loss. This can lead family members to develop a better appreciation and perspective on life that results in clearer priorities and closer relationships. Seizing opportunities can replace procrastination for the "right moment" or passive waiting for the dreaded moment. Serious illness, by emphasizing life's fragility and preciousness, provides families with an opportunity to heal unresolved issues and develop more immediate, caring relationships. For illnesses in a more advanced stage, clinicians should help families emphasize quality of life by defining goals that are attainable more immediately and that enrich their everyday lives.

Writings (Imber-Black, Roberts, & Whiting, 1988; Imber-Black, 1991) in the family therapy field have underscored the lack of rituals for many families dealing with chronic and life-threatening disorders. Heightened uncertainty and loss increase awareness that each family gathering and ritual may be the last together. Clinicians can help families dealing with serious illness by promoting the timely creation and use of rituals of celebration and inclusion. A family reunion can invigorate a family and serve to coalesce its healing energies to support the ill member and key caretakers. With a serious illness, traditional celebrations offer an opportunity to affirm, strengthen, and repair all family relationships.

As the genetic revolution unfolds, families and clinicians are facing unprecedentedly complex clinical and ethical challenges (Miller, McDaniel, Rolland, & Feetham, in press). Families will increasingly be able to choose genetically informed knowledge of their future health risks or fate. Some key questions include the following: Which individuals and families will benefit by genetic risk screening and knowledge of their health risks or fate? How can we best help family members reach decisions about whether to pursue predictive testing? Who are the relevant family members to include in these decisions? Spouses or partners? Extended family? Our societal fixation on "the perfect healthy body" could meld seamlessly with technology and eugenics, forcing families living with disability, illness, or genetic risk to hide their suffering further, in order to demonstrate the value of their lives and avoid increased stigmatization (Rolland, 1997, 1999b).

Finally, clinicians need to consider their own experiences and feelings about illness and loss (McDaniel, Doherty, & Hepworth, 1997). Awareness and ease with our own multigenerational and family history with illness and loss, our health beliefs, and our current life-cycle passage will enhance our ability to work effectively with families facing serious illness.

REFERENCES

Antonovsky, A., & Sourani, T. (1988). Family sense of coherence and family adaptation. *Journal of Marriage and the Family, 50,* 79–92.

Beavers, W. R., & Hampson, R. (1990). *Successful families: Assessment and intervention.* New York: Norton.

Becker, E. (1973). *The denial of death.* New York: Free Press.

Boss. P. (1999). *Ambiguous loss: Learning to live with unresolved grief.* Cambridge, MA: Harvard University Press.

Boszormenyi-Nagy, I., & Spark, G. (1973). *Invisible loyalties.* New York: Harper & Row.

Bowen, M. (1978). *Family therapy in clinical practice.* New York: Aronson.

Byng-Hall, J. (1995). *Rewriting family scripts.* New York: Guilford Press.

Campbell, T. L., & Patterson, J. M. (1995). The effectiveness of family interventions in the treatment of physical illness. *Journal of Marital and Family Therapy, 21*(4), 545–583.

Carter, E. A., & McGoldrick, M. (Eds.). (1998). *The evolving family life cycle: Individual, family, and social perspectives* (3rd ed.). Boston: Allyn & Bacon.

Combrinck-Graham, L. (1985). A developmental model for family systems. *Family Process, 24*(2), 139–150.

Framo, J. (1992). *Family-of-origin therapy: An intergenerational approach.* New York: Brunner/Mazel.

Gonzales, S., Steinglass, P., & Reiss, D. (1989). Putting the illness in its place: Discussion groups for families with chronic medical illness. *Family Process, 28,* 69–87.

Hoffman, L. (1988). The life cycle and discontinuous change. In E. Carter & M. McGoldrick (Eds.), *The changing family life cycle: A framework for family therapy* (2nd ed.). Boston: Allyn & Bacon.

Imber-Black, E. (1991). Rituals and the healing process. In F. Walsh & M. McGoldrick (Eds.), *Living beyond loss: Death in the family.* New York: Norton.

Imber-Black, E., Roberts, J., & Whiting, R. (Eds.). (1988). *Rituals in families and family therapy.* New York: Norton.

Ireys, H. T., & Burr, C. K. (1984). Apart and a part: Family issues for young adults with chronic illness and disability. In M. G. Eisenberg, L. C. Sutkin, & M. A. Jansen (Eds.), *Chronic illness and disability through the life span: Effects on self and family.* New York. Springer.

Kleinman, A. M. (1988). *The illness narratives: Suffering, healing and the human condition.* New York. Basic Books.

Lefcourt, H. M. (1982). *Locus of control* (2nd ed.). Hillsdale, NJ: Erlbaum.

Levinson, D. J. (1986). A conception of adult development. *American Psychologist, 41,* 3–13.

McDaniel, S. H., Hepworth, J., & Doherty, W. J. (1992). *Medical family therapy.* New York: Basic Books.

McDaniel, S., Hepworth, J., & Doherty, W. (Eds.). (1997). *The shared experience of illness: Stories of patients, families, and their therapists.* New York: Basic Books.

McGoldrick, M., Gerson, R., & Schellenberger, S. (1999). *Genograms in family assessment* (2nd ed.). New York: Norton.

McGoldrick, M., Giordano, J. & Pearce, J. K. (Eds.). (1996). *Ethnicity and family therapy* (2nd ed.). New York: Guilford Press.

Miller, S., McDaniel, S., Rolland, J., & Feetham, S. (Eds.). (in press). *Individuals, families, and the new genetics.* New York: Norton.

Minuchin, S., Rosman, B. L., & Baker, L. (1978). *Psychosomatic families.* Cambridge, MA: Harvard University Press.

Moos, R. H. (Ed.). (1984). *Coping with physical illness: Vol. 2. New perspectives.* New York: Plenum Press.

Neugarten, B. (1976). Adaptation and the life cycle. *Counseling Psychologist, 6*(1), 16–20.

Olkin, R. (1999). *What psychotherapists should know about disability.* New York: Guilford Press.

Penn, P. (1983). Coalitions and binding interactions in families with chronic illness. *Family Systems Medicine, 1*(2), 16–25.

Reiss, D., & Kaplan De-Nour, A. (1981). *The family's construction of reality.* Cambridge, MA: Harvard University Press.

Reiss D. (1989). The family and medical team in chronic illness: A transactional and developmental perspective. In C. N. Ramsey, Jr. (Ed.), *Family systems in family medicine.* New York: Guilford Press.

Rolland, J. S. (1984). Toward a psychosocial typology of chronic and life-threatening illness. *Family Systems Medicine, 2*(3), 245–263.

Rolland, J. S. (1987a). Chronic illness and the life cycle: A conceptual framework. *Family Process, 26*(2), 203–221.

Rolland, J. S. (1987b). Family illness paradigms: Evolution and significance. *Family Systems Medicine, 5*(4), 467–486.

Rolland, J. S. (1990). Anticipatory loss: A family systems developmental framework. *Family Process, 29*(3), 229–244.

Rolland, J. S. (1994). *Families, illness, and disability: An integrative treatment model.* New York: Basic Books.

Rolland, J. S. (1997). The meaning of disability and suffering: Socio-political and ethical concerns. *Family Process, 36*(4), 437–440.

Rolland, J. S. (1998). Families and collaboration: Evolution over time. *Families, Systems and Health* (formerly *Family Systems Medicine*), *16*(1), 7–25.

Rolland, J. S. (1999a). Families and parental illness: A conceptual framework. *Journal of Family Therapy, 21*(3), 242–267.

Rolland, J. S. (1999b) Families and genetic fate: A millennial challenge. *Families, Systems, and Health, 16*(1), 123–133.

Rolland, J. S. (2002). Managing chronic illness. In M. Mengel, W. Holleman, & S. Fields (Eds.), *Fundamentals of clinical practice: A textbook on the patient, doctor and society* (2nd ed.). New York: Plenum Press.

Seaburn, D., Gunn, W., Mauksch, L., Gawinski, A., & Lorenz, A. (Eds.). (1996). *Models of collaboration: A guide for mental health professionals working with physicians and health care providers.* New York: Basic Books.

Siegel, B. S. (1986). *Love, medicine and miracles.* New York: Harper & Row.

Simonton, C. O., Mathews-Simonton, S., & Sparks, T. F. (1980). Psychological intervention in the treatment of cancer. *Psychosomatics, 21*(3), 226–233.

Steinglass, P. (1998). Multiple family discussion groups for patients with chronic medical illness. *Families, Systems, and Health, 16*(1–2), 55–71.

Taylor, S. (1989). *Positive illusions: Creative self-deception and the healthy mind.* New York: Basic Books.

Wallston, K. A., & Wallston, B. S. (1978). Development of the Multidimensional Health Locus of Control (MHLC) Scales. *Health Education Monographs, 6*(2), 160–170.

Walsh, F. (1998). *Strengthening family resilience.* New York: Guilford Press.

Walsh, F. (Ed.). (1999). *Spiritual resources in family therapy.* New York: Guilford Press.

Walsh, F., & McGoldrick, M. (Eds.). (1991). *Living beyond loss: Death in the family.* New York: Norton.

Weihs, K. Fisher, L., & Baird, M. (2001). *Families, health, and behavior.* Commissioned report: Institute of Medicine, National Academy of Sciences. Washington, DC: National Academy Press.

Wright, L. M., Watson, W. L., & Bell, J. M. (1996). *Beliefs: The heart of healing in families and illness.* New York: Basic Books.

Zborowski, M. (1969). *People in pain.* San Francisco: Jossey-Bass.

PART V

Healthy Couple and Family Processes: Mapping the Complexity

CHAPTER 18

INTERACTIONAL PATTERNS IN MARITAL SUCCESS OR FAILURE

Gottman Laboratory Studies

Janice Driver
Amber Tabares
Alyson Shapiro
Eun Young Nahm
John M. Gottman

Our research team at the Gottman Laboratory has devoted over three decades to identifying the patterns that distinguish masters of marriage—happy, stable couples—from unhappy couples headed for divorce. Although a great deal of marital research has been based on survey methods such as questionnaires and self-reports, our research also includes detailed, in-depth observations. Traditionally, our research has focused on marital conflict, which we believe is an important and necessary part of both happy and unhappy marriages. We have found that the success or failure of a marriage depends not on whether there is conflict, but rather how conflict is handled when it does occur. This research has enabled us to expose existing myths about marriage.

Through the years, we have expanded our observational style to include nonconflict studies of couples during daily interactions and couple interviews. By looking at partners in these three distinct settings, we have identified marked differences between happy and unhappy relationships. We have also learned what factors contribute to the friendship at the foundation of happy marriages. We summarize the major results of these findings in this chapter.

DEMOGRAPHICS

This summary is based on six different longitudinal studies with a total of 667 married couples. As required by the National Institute of Mental Health, each of these studies matched the major racial and ethnics groups of the area in which the research was conducted. Approximately 30% of the total sample across all six studies was from nonwhite ethnic groups. Although our sample includes ethnic minorities, we do not make racial distinctions in our summary. This kind of future research would require oversampling a particular ethnic group to observe differing patterns in couple interactions.

Throughout this summary, we refer to couples as happily married, unhappily married, or divorced. The classification of happy or unhappy was based on marital satisfaction questionnaires given to each of the partners at various time points throughout the study. For a couple to be classified as happy, both partners had to be satisfied with the marriage. To be considered unhappy or distressed, one or both partners had to be dissatisfied with the marriage. If one partner was happy in the marriage and the other was unhappy, we considered the couple to be unhappy or distressed. In all of our studies, we have followed the couples longitudinally to determine whether they remained married. The divorce category includes all couples who went on to divorce.

FOUR HORSEMEN

One consistent characteristic of distressed couples who are headed for divorce is the expression of specific negative behaviors we call the Four Horsemen of the Apocalypse (Gottman, 1994). Although negativity is part of any marital conflict, these are specific predictors of impending doom to a relationship. The Four Horsemen are criticism, contempt, defensiveness, and stonewalling.

The first of the Four Horsemen, criticism, is very common in distressed relationships. All couples have complaints of some kind during an argument, but criticism goes much further and is more damaging to the relationship than a simple complaint. Criticism is more global and includes character attacks such as "You didn't take the trash out last night. Why can't you ever remember to do it? You're so lazy!" A complaint, on the other hand, remains specific to a situation, such as "I'm annoyed that you didn't take the trash out last night." The added personality attack of criticism escalates negativity and causes damage to the relationship over time.

In addition to character attacks, criticism includes global complaints, which can be identified by words such as "You always . . ." and "You never . . . ," or it can include a laundry list of complaints that imply "always" or "never." For example, "I noticed you didn't get a chance to clean the bathroom like you said you would. It was the same thing last week, when you said you'd organize the shelves and get up early to help make lunch for the kids." Again, the focus of the speaker is on a character defect rather than a specific behavior.

Contempt, the next of the Four Horsemen, is the most corrosive. It is more destructive than criticism, because it conveys disgust and disrespect between spouses. A contemptuous comment might include sarcasm, mockery, insults, eye rolls, scowls, and hostile humor to belittle the partner. The attitude conveyed by contempt is one of disdain or superiority. One spouse may show condescension by taking a higher moral ground: "Did you really think showing up for just one soccer game all season would really be enough? That's an involved parent for you." Contempt is a type of scorn that often hinders any conciliatory attempts by the other spouse and may severely escalate negativity on both sides.

The third of the Four Horsemen is defensiveness. Although defensiveness seems a natural way to protect oneself against a perceived attack, our research shows that it usually becomes a counterattack, which further escalates negativity. Defensiveness is ineffective, because it becomes a way for one spouse to blame the other for his or her own behavior. One person might start with contempt: "Well that was pretty immature to go barhopping with your friends." To which a defensive spouse would respond, "You did the same thing last week." Defensiveness frequently takes on a childish tone, with the partners trying to shield themselves from both attack and personal responsibility.

Stonewalling is the fourth of the Four Horsemen. After many arguments with high levels of contempt, criticism, and defensiveness, it is easy for one spouse to feel overwhelmed by the conflict. At this point, the overwhelmed spouse begins stonewalling by conveying to the speaker that he or she does not want to interact, and appearing not to listen at all. There is no eye contact, no back-channeling, and no verbal response. The speaker is actively ignored. Stonewalling appears after the emergence of what Christensen and Heavey (1990) call the demand–withdraw pattern. This pattern shows clear gender differences, with the wife commonly demanding and the husband withdrawing, each reacting to the other as the couple becomes increasingly polarized. Stonewalling follows this same pattern, with husbands stonewalling more often than wives. Surprisingly, although the stonewaller appears to be hostile, his primary thoughts during this interaction are usually self-protective: "When is she going to quit talking?" "I can't stand arguing about this anymore." "If I'm quiet, she'll leave me alone." This kind of self-protection requires a great deal of energy and makes it impossible to listen, even if the comments are constructive and helpful.

When all of the four horsemen are present during a conflict discussion, we are able to predict divorce with 94% accuracy, even with newlywed couples (Carrère, Buehlman, Coan, Gottman, & Ruckstuhl, 2000; Buehlman, Gottman, & Katz, 1992). These truly are danger signals for any relationship. When used habitually during conflict, they erode the marriage and create hostility. Although some happily married couples occasionally use defensiveness, criticism, or even stonewalling, they rarely use contempt. We believe that the disrespect characteristic of contempt is the most harmful to the relationship overall. A high frequency of all the Four Horsemen, however, creates lasting damage and, most likely, the eventual ruin of the marriage.

EMOTIONAL DISENGAGEMENT

Whereas the interactional patterns we call the Four Horsemen are detrimental to a marriage, it is also damaging for a couple to display emotional disengagement (Gottman, 1994). Emotionally disengaged couples do not display extreme levels of negativity and are unlikely to include the Four Horsemen, but they also show a complete lack of positive affect. Characteristically, they demonstrate little of the interest, affection, humor, and concern characteristic of happy couples. Emotional disengagement is an interesting phenomenon because the couples appear fine on the surface but are actually highly distressed. Emotionally disengaged couples are attempting to enclave the problem, so that it does not poison the entire relationship. However, the cost of this avoidance is the erosion of intimacy and the absence of shared positive affect in their interaction. They begin editing out parts of their personality and become hidden from their partners. This further erodes their intimate connection. Couples who appear emotionally disengaged may exhibit higher levels of physiological arousal during conflicts as a result of suppressing negative affect. Gross and Levenson (1997) reported that the suppression of negative affects increases physiological arousal. In this way, emotionally disengaged couples may also expend tremendous physical effort to act as if everything is okay.

Both emotional disengagement and the Four Horsemen predict divorce, but there is a marked difference in the timing of divorce for each of these negative styles. Gottman and Levenson (2000) found that couples who frequently use contempt, criticism, defensiveness, and stonewalling tend to divorce earlier in the marriage, most within 7 years. Emotionally disengaged couples, however, tend to divorce after 7–14 years. It seems that these relationships slowly atrophy as the partners become more and more distant.

FLOODING

When a conflict is tainted by the Four Horsemen pattern or by emotional disengagement, it is common for one or both partners to become emotionally and physically overwhelmed (Gottman, 1994; Gottman & Levenson, 1983). In our physiological research, we find that at this point of "flooding," their palms begin to sweat, their heart rate increases to over 90 beats per minute, and their breathing becomes shallow or irregular. With these physiological symptoms, the partner is unable to think clearly or participate in constructive conversation. The primary focus of the flooded spouse is reduced to self-preservation, with thoughts such as "I can't stand this anymore" or "Why is she attacking me?" At this point, it is impossible to take in new information. Even positive interactions, such as an apology or a humorous moment, are subdued as the partner tries to protect himself from a perceived attack. Although flooding is more common for men than women, it can happen to either partner during an argument.

Flooding, an emergency state during a conflict, must be treated with respect and concern. The best antidote to flooding is to take a break from the conflict for at least 20 minutes. Taking a break, however, does not mean going to separate rooms and preparing for another attack. The person who feels flooded needs to engage in a soothing activity, such as going for a walk, reading, or listening to music. It is essential during this time to concentrate on thoughts other than the argument. To ruminate on the conflict or brood over being an innocent victim will only maintain a flooded state.

As important as it is to take time out when flooded, it is equally important to return to or reschedule the conflict discussion as soon as possible. If the couple does not return to the argument, a break to relieve flooding becomes a way to stonewall. Thus, the respite, which is intended to improve the marriage, can become a way to damage it.

NEGATIVE RECIPROCITY

Criticism, contempt, defensiveness, and stonewalling are specific types of negative conflict that signal danger, but not all negativity is damaging to the relationship. One pattern of marital conflict we have studied is that of negative reciprocity (Gottman, Coan, Carrère, & Swanson, 1998; Gottman, Markman, & Notarius, 1977), in which one spouse responds to the other's negativity with more negativity. There has long been a myth that this pattern is harmful to relationships; but we have found that there are two types of negative reciprocity, only one of which predicts divorce (Gottman et al., 1998).

The more harmful of the two is the pattern of negative escalation, in which negativity is responded to with increased negativity. There is an escalation of the conflict when each partner uses a more hurtful or severe response. In watching these interactions, it is as if each partner is trying to get back at the other by trying to "win." This type of negative escalation is often found in conjunction with the Four Horsemen. A lower level of negative affect, such as anger or sadness, from one spouse will be reciprocated with contempt, criticism, or defensiveness. This specific pattern of combative escalation, along with the Four Horsemen, predicts divorce (Gottman et al., 1998).

The second type of negative reciprocity is characteristic of all marriages, including happy ones. This pattern of negative reciprocation matches negativity for negativity. One partner will respond to anger with anger, and to sadness with sadness. This does not include, however, those couples that respond to contempt with contempt. We consider this to be escalation of the negativity. When couples are able to match low-level negativity the argument will be negative but not harmful. It is important to understand from this finding that negative emotions are a natural part of conflict and are not all perilous to marriage.

CONFLICT STYLES OF HAPPY COUPLES

As with the myth that all negative reciprocity is destructive, an opposite myth exists regarding happy couples. This is the belief that all happily married couples talk about their problems in a way that validates each other's views. Not all satisfied couples argue in this way, however. We have found three different conflict styles (or couple types) that seem to work well for happy couples: validators, volatiles, and avoiders (Gottman, 1993, 1994).

Validators "talk out" their problems. These partners are very adept at validating their spouse's emotions and opinions. They are very good friends and, when questioned about their relationship, tend to emphasize "we" over "me" or "I." Validators are also noncoercive and tend to have few disagreements. But when disagreements do arise, there is a strong sense of mutual respect between these spouses. Rarely if ever, would validators raise their voices during conflict. They are very skilled at compromise and use these skills to resolve their differences.

A different approach to dealing with conflict is seen in couples with a volatile style, who have a more explosive approach to handling conflict. Their arguments tend to be higher energy and more heated than disagreements between validators. In volatile couples, both partners are highly involved in the argument, viewing each other as equals. Volatiles give significance to their own individuality and feel marriage should strengthen and accentuate their distinctiveness. During arguments, volatiles express both negative and positive emotions with vigor, though their arguments rarely contain the Four Horsemen. Volatiles tend to be passionate, however, and their displays of warmth and affection counterbalance the negativity. In fact, all stable couple types, including volatiles, exhibit five times more positive interactions than negative ones. For every negative behavior, there are five positive behaviors (Gottman & Levenson, 1992). The key to the success of volatile couples is the overall warm and loving environment they maintain in their marriage despite their negative and explosive moments.

On the opposite end of the conflict scale is the third style, the avoiders. Avoiders minimize their problems and thus avoid conflict. They emphasize any positive aspects of the marriage, while downplaying or completely ignoring any complaints. When ignoring differences is not possible, they often agree to disagree. The marital style of conflict avoiders has been the most difficult for the psychological community to accept, because there is a pervasive myth that "avoiding conflict will ruin your marriage." We have found that some couples prefer to avoid disagreements, but they describe themselves as satisfied with their marriages and share a deep love for each other.

All three conflict styles can be equally effective. Whereas some couples avoid all arguments, others jump into the conflict with shouting, and still others discuss disagreements and find compromise. No one style is better or worse for a marriage, but it is important to understand that it has to work for both spouses. When people of differing styles get married, it can be a difficult situation. For example, if one spouse tends to avoid conflict, he or she is not likely to be happy with someone who argues loudly and vigorously. Thus, an avoider can be happily married to another avoider but would be unhappily married to a volatile. This does not mean that partners are hopeless and destined for divorce if they have differing styles, but the relationship will require tremendous effort and patience on the part of both spouses

It would be interesting for future research to focus on the cultural differences related to these conflict styles. Each culture may have strong preferences in dealing with interpersonal conflict, but there may also be great variability within each system.

Regardless of the style of handling conflict, it is important to remember that each couple must offset disagreements with positive interactions. As we mentioned earlier, all couples, regardless of style, must counter each negative behavior with five positive behaviors. Maintaining this level of positive interaction is crucial to sustain a happy and stable relationship.

SOLVABLE VERSUS UNSOLVABLE PROBLEMS

Yet another myth about happily married couples is the belief that they are able to resolve all their disagreements. We have found, however, that both happy and unhappy marriages have unsolvable as well as solvable problems. In fact, we have found that all conflict can be reduced to these two categories. Solvable problems have a solution, whereas unsolvable problems are ongoing issues that may never be resolved. Unsolvable or perpetual problems often arise from fundamental personality, cultural, or reli-

gious differences, or essential needs of each spouse. One partner may love
to hike and camp, while the other enjoys city attractions.

Both successful and unsuccessful marriages have disagreements, but
happily married couples seem to understand the distinction between the
two types of problems and handle them differently. Satisfied couples deal
with perpetual problems much the way aging adults deal with persistent
back pain. It may irritate them, but they learn to accept it. The aim in discussing a perpetual problem is to create an atmosphere of acceptance of
the partner's viewpoint rather than creating a condition of "gridlock." So
the goal is not to solve the problem, but for the couple to find a way to
gain some degree of peace around it.

Robert and Anna Maria have opposing views on how to spend their
weekends.

> ANNA MARIA: It's just that we have different ideas about what it
>   means to relax. I like to sleep late and take it slow,
>   while you jump out of bed and straight into your run-
>   ning shoes.
> ROBERT: No! I usually put on my socks first. (*They both laugh.*)
> ANNA MARIA: I do like it when you bring me back some coffee.
> ROBERT: That's good. That's my secret to jump-start our day.

Anna Maria may never enjoy getting up early, and Robert may never
sleep in, but they are able to live with each other's style. Successful couples
try to understand what is at the foundation of the differences that are causing conflicts and use this understanding to communicate amusement and
affection while learning to cope with their perpetual issue. The positive affect in these discussions is in direct contrast to gridlocked discussions of
perpetual problems.

Greg and Kimberly also discuss how they spend their weekends, but
they become gridlocked around the problem.

> GREG: We didn't get a chance to relax all weekend. You're con-
>   stantly going from one thing to the next.
> KIMBERLY: What do you mean? We went on that bike ride on Satur-
>   day. That was relaxing.
> GREG: Relaxing? That was exhausting! You dragged me half way
>   around the city.
> KIMBERLY: Well, I wouldn't have to drag you if you were in better
>   shape.

Partners who are gridlocked are firmly planted in their respective positions. As a result their discussions include very little positive affect and
one or more of the Four Horsemen. Over time, these couples feel rejected, overwhelmed, and hopeless about ever reaching any sort of a compro-

mise. Gridlocked couples seem to focus on the unsolvable problem rather than on the underlying meaning that contributes to the opposing views.

ACCEPTING INFLUENCE

One way that masterful couples deal with gridlocked conflict is by accepting "influence" from each other. This is a term we use to describe each partner's willingness to yield during an argument, in order to "win" in the relationship. The best analogy for accepting influence is city driving. You are driving home in traffic when someone stops and illegally parks in your lane. You can't move unless one of two things happens: Either the other driver moves his car or you change lanes and drive home. It would be a waste of time and energy to park behind the offender, shout threats of traffic violations, and summon a police officer, when simply changing lanes will achieve your greater purpose. Accepting influence is similar to this idea of changing lanes and driving home. By learning to find a point of yielding, even a minor point, the spouse wins the desired purpose of a close and satisfying relationship.

Yielding to win, however, should not be mistakenly translated into a complete surrender of oneself to the other's whims. Instead, accepting influence is the ability to find a point of agreement in the other's position. It is important to note that both partners need to accommodate the other, or the relationship becomes skewed. Often, this agreement is only achieved when each partner tries to understand the meaning of the other's perspective in the conflict.

Vincent and Alicia, for example, often argued about how to spend their vacation. Vincent wanted to visit his family in Virginia, and Alicia preferred that they go somewhere alone as a couple. This problem had been a continuing area of disagreement in their 10-year relationship. Each had decided that his or her position was correct, so the couple considered taking separate vacations. Vincent would go to visit his family, while Alicia would go somewhere with her best friend. To look at this problem from the standpoint of accepting influence, both Vincent and Alicia needed to understand why the other was entrenched (or parked) in their position.

Vincent only saw his family once a year and found it easy to relax and enjoy himself in their company. Alicia's family lived nearby, so he saw them often (at least once a week) and felt he deserved to see his family more regularly. Alicia, on the other hand, didn't get along with Vincent's mother and found it difficult to spend an entire week with her. She also had a very stressful job and wanted go somewhere more relaxing. Each partner had good reasons for remaining in their fixed position. This inflexibility, however, made it impossible to move toward an agreeable solution.

In contrast, if they were able to accept influence from each other, they could move from positions that were rigid and unyielding to ones of compromise and collaboration. Vincent would be able to see that Alicia needed a break from her demanding schedule. Alicia would be able to understand Vincent's desire to spend time with his family. If they could acknowledge some part of the other's viewpoint, they could see the problem differently. The issue would no longer be where to go, but how to achieve both goals.

Although accepting influence is difficult at times, it has tremendous power for the marital relationship. When partners learn to yield on certain points of a conflict, they realize that they can cooperate and work together as a couple. The problem itself becomes an issue that they can conquer together as a team. This creates cohesiveness in other areas of their life as well, and they learn to move through time together.

This ability for both partners to accept influence is a skill that discriminates between happily married, unhappily married, and divorced couples in our research. In fact, we found that abusive husbands *never* accepted influence from their wives (Coan, Gottman, Babcock, & Jacobson, 1997). Although these abusive husbands are the extreme, their inability to accept influence highlights its importance for healthy relationships. Gottman, et al. (1998) reported that in nonviolent marriages, once again it was the *husband's* rejection of influence from his wife that predicted divorce and not the wife's rejection of influence from her husband. Wives were accepting influence at high rates in all the marriages. This finding speaks to general issues of women's power and powerlessness in heterosexual relationships (Walsh, 1989).

REPAIR ATTEMPTS

In addition to accepting influence, happy couples also manage conflict and miscommunication with what we call "repair attempts," which we have defined as interactions that decrease negative escalation. Because disagreements are a natural part of any relationship, even happy relationships, the ability to repair is crucial. This is especially true when couples are engaged in conflict. The actual issue, whether finances, in-laws, or housework, is less important than the way the couple engages in the dispute. Miscommunication during these conflicts often leads to negative escalation and erosion of the relationship; so it is important to repair the miscommunication during the conflict.

For the last 2 years, we have studied repair attempts in an effort to understand their role in preventing and reducing increased negativity. Examples of repair attempts include apologies, humor, affection, and changing the subject. These interactions are not necessarily related to the content of the argument but may simply provide a brief reprieve from it. For instance, one husband suddenly stopped in the middle of a heated debate and said, "After this, I need to stop by my sister's house to drop off the radio we borrowed." The wife went along with his repair by saying, "Okay. We can drop it off before we pick up the kids." This seemingly unimportant change of subject gave the husband a brief diversion from the intensity of the conflict. Once they talked about the radio, he seemed more relaxed and was able to return to the argument. Happy couples tend to give their partner the opportunity to maneuver in the discussion. They allow the conflict to ebb and flow, with occasional unrelated topics interspersed in the conflict.

Unhappy couples frequently respond to these types of repairs by interpreting the interaction in a negative way. Rather than allowing the change of subject, an unhappy spouse may respond, "You're not listening to me!" or "Who cares about the stupid radio?" As a result, unhappy couples may remain adamantly fixed on the discussion topic and not allow breaks in the argument. This rigid adherence to the conflict seems to escalate further negativity. Allowing a change of topic, however, must not be misconstrued as avoiding the topic. Happy couples return to the argument and do not allow the reprieve to derail their discussion, even if the topic is uncomfortable or tense.

In addition to accepting the repairs, we have seen that couples who use repairs early in the conflict prevent it from becoming too negative. Happily married couples tend to use repairs throughout their discussion, whereas distressed couples wait until the argument is heated and divisive. When the argument is at a point of severe negativity, repair attempts are often less effective and may even backfire. One couple was in the middle of a heated and hostile debate about finances, when the husband tried to lighten the moment with a joke about a stain on his T-shirt. Rather than reducing the negative tone of the conflict, this attempt at humor enraged the wife, who responded with increased anger and contempt. Repairs do not always have this backlash effect during high negativity, but it is common for unhappy spouses to ignore or reject them when the conflict is too intense. We are currently exploring this area further to see if certain repairs are better able to relieve these highly charged moments. At this point, however, we've found that using repairs early and often is more effective than waiting until the conflict is more severe.

When there is a balance of repair attempts between the spouses, the conflict also tends to maintain a lower level of negativity. If, however, one partner is making repair after repair, while the other plunges on with the conflict, the argument will continue to escalate. This pattern of uneven repair attempts seems characteristic of distressed couples.

Another important component of repair attempts is each partner's ability to respond in a positive way when a repair is made. If one partner recognizes a repair and allows his or her spouse to lighten the moment or gain a reprieve, the overall conflict is more positive. For example, one couple in our lab was involved in an intense disagreement about the husband's disappointment with their oldest son. During a brief pause in the argument, the husband commented, "I do admire the fact that you're able to stay calm no matter what he says." The wife smiled and simply said, "Thanks." After this moment of affection (compliment), both the husband and wife returned to the conflict discussion. As this example shows, repairs do not avoid the conflict or demean the partner, but they interject some positive moments into difficult discussions. Repair attempts are tools that can be used effectively to reduce negativity and provide a break from the argument. The conflict will continue in a more positive manner when repairs are used often and accepted well.

TURNING TOWARD

We believe that one of the most important leaps we made in our way of thinking occurred when we started studying marriages in the day-to-day moments outside of conflict. By observing couples' interactions in our apartment laboratory at the University of Washington, and by interviewing couples about the history of their relationship, we have discovered several key factors we attribute to successful marriages.

In couple therapy, there is often an emphasis on the major events in the couple's lives, such as conflict discussions. However, the minor, every-day moments for a couple may determine how the partners interact when major events unfold. As a foundation for approaching major events, daily interactions are a crucial component for marital success. Imagine, for example, that a husband gives his wife a dozen roses for Valentine's Day. These roses have a completely different meaning, depending on daily interactions: whether the husband has been aloof, crabby and absent or attentive, positive and helpful. In the first instance, the roses would be an inadequate attempt to make up for his neglect; in the second, they would be a loving and romantic gesture. The giving of roses comes with current and ongoing contexts.

To understand these daily interactions, we designed one of our studies to accommodate couples in an apartment laboratory setting. We asked the couples to live in a studio-type apartment and videotaped them for 12 of the 24 hours they stayed there. We allowed them to bring anything from home that would help them feel comfortable, such as groceries, CDs, videos, and work. One couple even brought their cat. The only instruction we gave to each couple was to ask them to live as they would at home.

To capture their everyday interactions, we created an observational coding system that categorizes ways in which couples initiate and respond to each other on a moment-to-moment basis. We defined an invitation to interact as a "bid." For each bid, we noted the needs and demands involved, from information exchange to sharing emotional support. The responses to these bids ranged from mere eye movement to playfulness and were categorized as "turning toward," "turning away," and "turning against."

From these data, we found that each time one partner initiates an interaction (or "bids" for attention), the other spouse is given a choice that will improve or erode the marriage. Ignoring the interaction or responding in a negative way fosters distance and separation, whereas even a minor response helps promote emotional connection and friendship. Suppose, for example, that Stephanie and Carl are sitting in the living room reading. Stephanie looks up and comments that there's a sparrow outside their window. At that moment, Carl faces a series of choices for his response. He can ignore the comment and continue reading (turning away); he can comment that he thinks bird watching is a waste of time (turning against); he can momentarily set aside his book to look at the bird (low-level turning toward); or he can look at the bird and comment on its activity (enthusiastic turning toward). If Carl responds by ignoring Stephanie or making a negative comment, it discourages her from making further attempts to interact. Such responses lead to reduced bidding and connection. On the other hand, if Carl responds by looking at the bird and making a comment, he is welcoming her interaction, which will lead to increased interactions and increased marital connection.

We have found that happily married couples rarely ignore their partners. Nearly 85% of their bids were met with some kind of positive response. What is interesting about these responses is that they were not always overly attentive or enthusiastic. One partner may simply look up and smile. Acknowledging the bid in some way seemed to play an important role in maintaining a healthy relationship. This does not mean, however, that satisfied couples always made low level responses. Their responses ranged from low-level to playful. With this variety, spouses expressed their willingness and interest to interact.

Having an eagerness to interact, we believe, creates more interaction and increased friendship. In fact, our happily married couples made up to 77 bids in 10 minutes. Contrast this to some distressed couples that made 10–20 bids in 10 minutes. A positive response to a bid appears to lead to increased bidding and strengthened friendship.

Playful bidding was another characteristic of happy couples. We defined "playfulness" as good-natured teasing with some physical sparring. For example, a husband might throw a crumpled napkin at his wife in a mock snowball fight. Such playful interactions were nonexistent for distressed couples. What was important, however, was that couples who used playfulness and enthusiasm in their daily interactions had better access to humor and affection during their conflict discussions (Driver & Gottman, 2001). In a longitudinal study of middle-aged and senior couples in first marriages, humor and affection during conflict was a characteristic of happily married, stable, older couples (Carstensen, Gottman, & Levenson, 1995). Thus, if daily interactions contribute to more positive affect during conflict, the overall quality of the relationship is affected by these minor moments.

REWRITING THE PAST

Another nonconflict situation we have studied is the way that couples describe their relationship. We have found that a couple's description of the past predicts the future of the marriage (Buehlman et al., 1992; Carrère et al., 2000; Shapiro, Gottman, & Carrère, 2000). Over and over again, we have seen that partners who are deeply entrenched in a negative view of their spouse and their marriage often revise the past, such that they only remember and talk about the negative things that have happened in their relationship. Happy couples, in contrast, highlight their good memories. This revision of their marital history has allowed us to predict stability in marriage versus divorce with 88–94% accuracy (Carrere et al., 2000; Buhelman et al., 1992). These historical descriptions have also allowed us to identify buffers that appear to protect couples from decline in marital satisfaction during the stressful adjustment to parenting (Shapiro et al., 2000).

To engage the couple in a description of their marital history, we use the Oral History Interview (OHI), developed in our laboratory by Buehlman and Gottman (1996). This interview asks couples about the beginnings of their relationship, their philosophy of marriage, how their relationship has changed over time, and what marriage was like in their family of origin. By interviewing the couples in this way, we are able to capture the dynamics of their marital journey and their identity as a couple. Although they may tell us about their past in great detail, our focus is not on content, but rather on how the couples describe their relationship (Buehlman & Gottman, 1996).

Most couples enter marriage with high hopes and great expectations. When a marriage is not going well, however, history gets rewritten for the worst. In a distressed marriage, the wife is more likely to recall that her husband was 30 minutes late to the ceremony. He, in a similar way, may focus on all the time she spent talking to his best man and may even speculate that she was actually flirting with him.

Along with remembering the worst, unhappy couples find the past difficult to remember. It's as though the memory is unimportant or painful and they've let it fade away. Their lack of appropriate detail, along with their negative perspective, gives us tremendous insight into their marital distress.

In happy marriages, couples tend to look back on their early days with fondness. Even if the wedding wasn't perfect, they emphasize the highlights rather than the low points, and even joke about the low points and imperfections. This is also true for the way they remember and describe each other. They reminisce about how positive they felt early on, how excited they were when they first met, and how much admiration they had for each other. When they talk about the tough times, they emphasize the strength they drew from each other rather than the specific struggles.

Through categorizing couples' descriptions during the OHI, we have been able to separate the masters of marriage from the disasters. Unhappy spouses headed toward divorce were negative to each other, thought of their lives as chaotic, and expressed disappointment in the marriage. Happy couples used fondness during their interview, used expressions of "we-ness," were expansive in their descriptions, showing their awareness of each other's worlds, and tended to glorify any hardships. We would like to describe each of these categories in more detail.

UNHAPPY COUPLES

Negativity toward Spouse

Distressed spouses tended to express negativity and criticism toward each other, even when remembering such pleasant events as their wedding or honeymoon. A husband describing the honeymoon might only remember tension and unpleasant experiences: "It seems like all we did was fight; she nagged me all the time. . . . Oh, and the mosquitoes were terrible. I could barely step foot outside." Unhappy spouses may also be vague and unclear about what attracted them to their spouse. The husband and wife may wrack their brains to think of a single quality they admired about their spouse before they were married, and sometimes what they remember is not very flattering. One wife's first impression of her husband was "Well, I guess I thought he was cute enough but, boy was he a bad dresser!"

Chaotic Perceptions

Many couples face struggles such as financial loss or stress at work. When these events occur, however, unhappy couples tend to view their lives as out of control or chaotic. They see themselves as pummeled by outside events: "It's just one thing after another. It seems like one of us is always needed somewhere. If it's not our families, it's the kids or one of our jobs. There's pressure from every angle and there's no way to stop it. We can't do anything about our situation." There is a helpless quality to these chaotic perceptions; couples feel unable to overcome stress and hardship. Often these couples are dealing with major-stresses, such as sick parents, but the critical thing that defines their relationships is hopelessness. They believe that there is no solution.

Disappointment/Disillusionment

One final pattern of unhappy couples is their disappointment and disillusionment with their relationship. Each partner has given up on their marriage and expresses depression about the relationship: "We used to be such good friends and now we don't agree about anything. This is not what I expected." A tone of sadness and resignation often accompanies these statements. Unhappy couples also seem unable to articulate what makes a successful marriage. It's as if their personal disappointment alters their general view of marriage, making it difficult to define a happy relationship. During the relationship interviews, negativity and chaos were predictive of divorce, but this tendency toward disappointment was the strongest divorce predictor (Buehlman et al., 1992; Carrère et al., 2000).

HAPPY COUPLES

Fondness and Admiration

Happy couples that were still "in love" also showed unique characteristics in the way they described their marital past. Fondness and admiration are two of the most crucial elements in a rewarding and lasting romance. Partners conveyed a fundamental sense that their spouse was worthy of admiration, respect, and love. In a marriage with much fondness and admiration, a wife may recall her first impressions of her husband as being "perfect, like a dream." In a marriage with less fondness, the wife might describe him being "a nice, stable guy." Although even happily married couples have times of frustration with their partners' flaws, they still remember that the person they married is worthy of honor and respect. When this sense is completely missing from a marriage, we believe the relationship cannot be revived.

Awareness or Love Maps

Along with fondness and admiration, happy spouses usually show an awareness of each other and their relationship. This is clear in the way expansive couples describe the details of their past. They are expressive and descriptive during the interview, and will often finish each other's sentences.

For example, Richard and Judy describe their first date:

JUDY: He took me to a fun restaurant with a Polynesian theme. There were palm trees and hammocks inside. I was wearing my favorite dress.
RICHARD: The dress was red and black—she looked great.
JUDY: He was dressed up too, which at the time was rare to see. . . .
RICHARD: I use to be in construction, so I usually wore jeans and a t-shirt.

This dimension shows not only each spouse's expressiveness, but how both respond to and expand on their partner's comments. In contrast, distressed spouses respond to questions with just a few short sentences, seem withdrawn, and don't add to the description. An unhappy spouse would describe the same first date by saying, "We went out to dinner."

Happy spouses are also intimately familiar with their partner's world. They remember the major events in each other's history and keep updating these facts/feelings as their partner's world changes. We call this a richly detailed "love map." When she orders him a salad, she knows to ask for his favorite dressing. We believe that this type of awareness works together with fondness and admiration to create a satisfying relationship. Suppose, for example, that the wife is having a difficult time with her boss at work. If the husband is aware of his wife's distress, he may respond by expressing warmth and emotional support. Thus, the level of awareness is directly related to his ability to express comfort.

Glorifying the Struggle

In contrast to couples who are unhappy in their marriage, happy couples approach hardships as trials to be overcome together and believe that these struggles make their relationship stronger (Walsh, 1998; see Walsh, Chapter 15, this volume). They emphasize how they conquered their difficulties together as a couple: "It was really hard at first when he was laid off, but we managed to support each other and things started to work out." Sometimes the hardships are even about the relationship or adjusting to marriage: "Marriage is the hardest job you'll ever have, but it's worth it." Happy couples emphasize both the difficulty of their experiences and pride in how they managed through it all. Their struggles bring them closer together as they endure challenging outside events and work to prevail.

We-ness

When happy couples describe their marital past, each partner tends to use the words "we" and "us" as opposed to "he or she" or "I." This simple pattern reflects the degree to which couples perceive themselves as a team rather than as individuals: "We oversaw the remodeling of our house. It was difficult at times, but we were able to work it out." If this same couple were low in we-ness, each partner would talk about the remodeling in individual terms: "The remodeling was difficult, but I was able to work with the contractor." Couples who use "we" more often also tend to emphasize the same beliefs, values, and goals.

Although happy couples tend to use the terms "we" and "us," this does not describe their level of differentiation. For example, happy partners may phone each other daily and spend most of their free time together. Other equally happy partners may rarely call during the day, have separate friends, and enjoy different interests. Regardless of their level of independence, happy couples will continue to talk about their relationship in terms of teamwork and collaboration. These couples maintain their desired level of unity or separateness, while referring to themselves as "we" and "us." It is their perception of we-ness that is important.

TRANSITION TO PARENTHOOD

After the arrival of a new baby, there is often a dramatic decline in marital satisfaction for women. In fact, 67% of the wives in our study showed this trend (Shapiro et al., 2000). Not all of these couples experienced a decline in martial satisfaction, however. So we again turned to the OHI to better understand why some couples are vulnerable, while others are resilient during transition to parenthood (see also Cowan & Cowan, Chapter 16, this volume). By looking at the way couples talked about their marital past, we were able to predict this decline in marital satisfaction. It is particularly interesting that this prediction was based on OHIs with couples when they were newlyweds and not on prebirth interviews.

Our classifications of couples in the OHIs can be seen as reflecting the health of the couples' marital friendship. We have found that this friendship can be seen in the early months of marriage and becomes an important buffer when the couple encounters stresses such as the transition to parenthood.

VULNERABLE COUPLES

Based on the newlywed interviews, we have been able to identify two warning signs of couples who are vulnerable to marital decline with the arrival of the first baby: First, the husbands tended to express negativity toward their wives; and second, the partners were likely to view their lives as chaotic. Although these were newlywed and not prebirth interviews, these patterns provided valuable information about couples at risk for marital decline.

When husbands were critical and negative toward their wives in the newlywed interview, the marital satisfaction of both partners plummeted with the arrival of the first baby. Early in their marriage, these husbands tended to express negativity toward their wives and disappointment in the marriage. Here, again, we see the corrosiveness of criticism and negativity eating away at the quality of the marriage. We found that wives were particularly sensitive and vulnerable to their husbands' negativity and marital disappointment when they became parents. Thus, a habit of negativity seems to effect greater damage after the baby is born.

As mentioned earlier, unhappy partners tend to view their lives as chaotic and out of control. This feeling was exacerbated with the disorder that often accompanies life with a new infant. The feelings of chaos expressed by distressed newlywed couples make them particularly vulnerable in coping with the additional duties necessary for parenting. They were more likely to see parenting challenges as problems beyond their control that throw their lives and their relationship into disarray. Difficulties such as getting up in the middle of the night seemed insurmountable and overwhelming.

RESILIENT COUPLES

Stable couples, in contrast, used awareness, with fondness and admiration, to buffer the marriage through this stressful period. A husband with a high level of awareness or a detailed love map of his wife's world would know when she was feeling overwhelmed by the challenges she was facing as a new mother. He would then respond to her stress by expressing his fondness and admiration for her and increasing his level of participation in child care and household tasks. A wife who was highly aware of her husband's world would also sympathize with her husband's frustrations and increasingly support him as well. Regardless of the level of participation prior to becoming parents, the *increased* activity of both spouses predicted stable relationships.

THE INFLUENCE OF NEW FATHERS

It is interesting to note that the most important sign of continuing relationship satisfaction after the first baby is born is the husband's descriptions during the newlywed OHI. Wives are most vulnerable to a decline in marital satisfaction over the transition to parenthood, probably because the wife traditionally bears the bulk of the child-rearing responsibilities. They are expected to know naturally how to be good mothers. It is, however, the husband's fondness, awareness, and lack of negativity and disappointment during the newlywed interview that buffers his wife's decline in martial satisfaction when the first baby arrives.

Overall, the OHI provides a dynamic index to the marital relationship. The quality of the couple's friendship makes stressful periods, such as the transition to parenthood, either more difficult or smoother. Disappointment in the marriage, negativity towards one's spouse, and the feeling of chaos in a couple's lives may reflect vulnerabilities in the relationship that become particularly problematic during stressful periods. On the other hand, qualities such as fondness, admiration, and awareness seem to act as buffers in protecting the relationship during stressful changes.

CONCLUSIONS

Through careful, observational research, we have identified patterns that determine both happy and unhappy marriages. The relationships that end in divorce tend to gravitate toward the Four Horsemen of the Apocalypse and negative reciprocity during conflict discussions. This leads to the dysfunctional coping mechanisms of flooding and eventual emotional disengagement as partners struggle to protect themselves. Likewise, in their daily interactions, they reject bid attempts and become more and more distant. When stressors such as parenthood come along, these relationships are vulnerable and the couples become distressed in response to the added pressure.

In contrast, masters of marriage use repair attempts and accepting influence to moderate their negativity. The use of these skills keeps their arguments from escalating out of control and allows them to stay engaged in the conflict. This, in turn, allows them to find possible solutions to their disagreements. If their conflicts are over issues without resolution, they use humor and acceptance to arrive at some peace with the issue. In their daily lives, they encourage interaction and stay emotionally connected. As they encounter life stressors, they are more aware of each other's struggles and use this awareness to support and encourage one another. Later, when the stress has subsided, these couples emphasize their teamwork in conquering the problem.

We believe that finding these clear differences between unhappy and happy couples is the first step toward effecting lasting change for distressed couples. The next step in our marital research involves developing useful interventions aimed at improving couples' marital friendship by increasing positive affect in their daily lives. Our goal is to combine clinical practice with research to create effective, empirically based interventions that are tailored to each couple's needs and values.

REFERENCES

Buehlman K. T., & Gottman, J. M. (1996). The Oral History Coding System. In J. Gottman (Ed.), *What predicts divorce: The measures* (pp. OH11–OH118). Hillsdale, NJ: Erlbaum.

Buehlman, K. T., Gottman, J. M., & Katz, L. F. (1992). How a couple views their past predicts their future: Predicting divorce from an oral history interview. *Journal of Family Psychology, 5,* 295–318.

Carrère, S., Buehlman, K. T., Coan, J., Gottman, J. M., & Ruckstuhl, L. (2000). Predicting marital stability and divorce in newlywed couples. *Journal of Family Psychology, 14*(1), 42–58.

Carstensen, L. L., Gottman, J. M., & Levenson, R. W. (1995). Emotional behavior in long-term marriage. *Psychology and Aging, 10*(1), 140–149.

Christensen, A., & Heavey, C. C. (1990). Gender and social structure in the demand/withdrawal pattern of marital conflict. *Journal of Personality and Social Psychology, 59,* 73–81.

Coan, J., Gottman, J. M., Babcock, J., & Jacobson, N. (1997). Battering and the male rejection of influence from women. *Aggressive Behavior, 23*(5), 375–388.

Driver, J. L., & Gottman, J. M. (2001). *Daily marital interactions during dinnertime in an apartment laboratory and positive affect during marital conflict among newlywed couples.* Manuscript submitted for publication.

Gottman, J. M. (1993). The roles of conflict engagement, escalation, and avoidance in marital interaction: A longitudinal view of five types of couples. *Journal of Consulting and Clinical Psychology, 61*(1), 6–15.

Gottman, J. M., (1994). *What predicts divorce? The relationship between marital processes and marital outcomes.* Hillsdale, NJ: Erlbaum.

Gottman, J. M., Coan, J., Carrere, S., & Swanson, C. (1998). Predicting marital happiness and stability from newlywed interactions. *Journal of Marriage and the Family, 60,* 5–22.

Gottman, J. M., & Levenson, R. W. (1983). Marital interaction: Physiological linkage and affective exchange. *Journal of Personality and Social Psychology, 45*(3), 587–597.

Gottman, J. M., & Levenson, R. W. (1992). Marital processes predictive of later dissolution: Behavior, physiology, and health. *Journal of Personality and Social Psychology, 63*(2), 221–233.

Gottman, J. M., & Levenson, R. W. (2000). The timing of divorce: Predicting when a couple will divorce over a 14-year period. *Journal of Marriage and the Family, 62*(3), 737–745.

Gottman, J. M., Markman, H., & Notarius, C. (1977). The topography of marital conflict: A sequential analysis of verbal and nonverbal behavior. *Journal of Marriage and the Family, 39*(3), 461–477.

Gross, J. J., & Levenson, R. W. (1997). Hiding feelings: The acute effects of inhibiting negative and positive emotion. *Journal of Abnormal Psychology, 106*(1), 95–103.

Shapiro, A. F., Gottman, J., M., Carrère, S. (2000). The Baby and the marriage: Identifying factors that buffer against decline in marital satisfaction after the first baby arrives. *Journal of Family Psychology, 14*(1), 59–70.

Walsh, F. (1989). Reconsidering gender in the marital quid pro quo. In M. McGoldrick (Eds.), C. M. Anderson, & F. Walsh (Eds.), *Women in families: A framework for family therapy* (pp. 267–285). New York: Norton.

Walsh, F. (1998). *Strengthening family resilience.* New York: Guilford Press.

CHAPTER 19

CIRCUMPLEX MODEL OF MARITAL AND FAMILY SYSTEMS

David H. Olson
Dean M. Gorall

This chapter presents an update of the 25-year journey of development and refinement of both the Circumplex Model of Marital and Family Systems and the related assessment scales of the Family Adaptability and Cohesion Evaluation Scales (FACES) and the Clinical Rating Scale (CRS). Over 700 studies have been published on the Circumplex Model using the self-report family assessment called FACES (Kouneski, 2001), making it one of the most researched family model. The model has also been used with diverse couple and family systems in terms of ethnicity/race, marital status (cohabitating, married), family structure (single parent, stepfamilies), sexual orientation (gay and lesbian couples), stage of family life cycle (newlywed to retired couples), and social class and educational levels. This chapter reviews the past research and theory development, and the clinical applications that use the Circumplex Model.

The Circumplex Model, its historical roots, basic concepts, and dimensions, are grounded in systems theory. An updated graphic representation of the Circumplex Model is called the Couple and Family Map. Changes that families go through developmentally and in reaction to stressors are illustrated with the model. Research regarding the validity of the model and the clinical usefulness of both the self-report (FACES) and observational assessment (CRS) are described. The model is also incorporated into the PREPARE/ENRICH Program to prepare couples for marriage and to treat troubled marriages.

Significant updates include a revision of the graphic representation called the Couple and Family Map, with additional levels that provide a more useful assessment of couple and family systems. FACES IV is a significant revision to the self-report assessment designed to tap Circumplex Model dimensions. This revised version of the FACES is designed to address concerns that past versions of the FACES instrument. FACES IV was designed to tap the high and low extremes of the dimensions of cohesion and flexibility, as well as the moderate regions that had been tapped by previous versions of FACES. The instrument did tap key dimensions of family functioning. An updated assessment package, the Family Inventories Package, includes FACES IV and other family dynamics that have been found to be central to family functioning (family stress, strengths, communication, and satisfaction). It is hoped that this step in the journey of the development of the model and instruments will continue to generate continued research, theory development, and clinical application, as it has over the history of the Circumplex Model.

DEVELOPMENT OF THE MODEL OVER TIME

The Circumplex Model of Marital and Family Systems was initially developed in an attempt to bridge the gap that typically exists between research, theory and practice (Olson, Russell, & Sprenkle, 1989). The Circumplex Model is particularly useful as a "relational diagnosis," because it is focused on the relational system and integrates three dimensions that have repeatedly been considered highly relevant in a variety of family theory models and family therapy approaches (see Table 19.1). Family cohesion, flexibility, and communication, the three dimensions in the Circumplex Model, emerged from a conceptual clustering of over 50 concepts developed to describe marital and family dynamics. The model is specifically designed for family research, clinical assessment, treatment planning, and outcome effectiveness of marital and family therapy (Olson, 2000).

A variety of other therapists and theorists have focused independently on variables related to the cohesion, flexibility, and communication dimensions. Table 19.1 summarizes the historical research of 10 family theorists who have worked on describing marital and family systems. Most of these models have been developed in the last 20 years by individuals who utilize a family systems perspective. One source of evidence regarding the value and importance of these three dimensions is the fact that these theorists have independently concluded that these dimensions are critical for understanding and treating marital and family systems.

TABLE 19.1 Theoretical Models Using Cohesion, Flexibility, and Communication

	Cohesion	Flexibility	Communication
Beavers & Hampson (1990)	Stylistic dimension	Adaptability	Affect
Benjamin (1977)	Affiliation	Interdependence	
Epstein & Bishop (1993)	Affective involvement	Behavior control, problem solving	Communication, affective responsiveness
Gottman (1994)	Validation	Contrasting	
Kantor and Lehr (1975)	Affect	Power	—
Leary (1975)	Affection, hostility	Dominance, submission	—
Leff & Vaughn (1985)	Distance	Problem solving	
Parsons & Bales (1955)	Expressive role	Instrumental role	—
Reiss (1981)	Coordination	Closure	—
Walsh (1998)	Connectedness	Flexibility	Communication belief systems

COUPLE AND FAMILY COHESION (TOGETHERNESS)

Family cohesion is defined *as the emotional bonding that couple and family members have toward one another.* Within the Circumplex Model, some of the specific concepts or variables used to diagnose and measure the family cohesion dimensions are emotional bonding, boundaries, coalitions, time, space, friends, decision making, interests, and recreation (see Clinical Rating Scale in Appendices 19.1–19.3 for how each concept is operationally defined). *Cohesion focuses on how systems balance separateness versus togetherness.*

There are five levels of cohesion ranging from *disengaged/disconnected* (extremely low) to *somewhat connected* (low to moderate), to *connected* (moderate), to *very connected* (moderate to high), to *enmeshed/overly connected* (extremely high). The terms "disengaged" and "enmeshed," used for consistency with previous versions of the model, are used primarily throughout this chapter; the terms "disconnected" and "overly connected" are introduced to be used with clients/patients in order to simplify terminology and reduce pathological terms (see Figure 19.1).

This five-level approach for each dimension is a change from previous versions of the model that had only four levels. There are now three balanced levels and two unbalanced levels. It is hypothesized that the three central or *balanced* levels of cohesion (somewhat connected, connected,

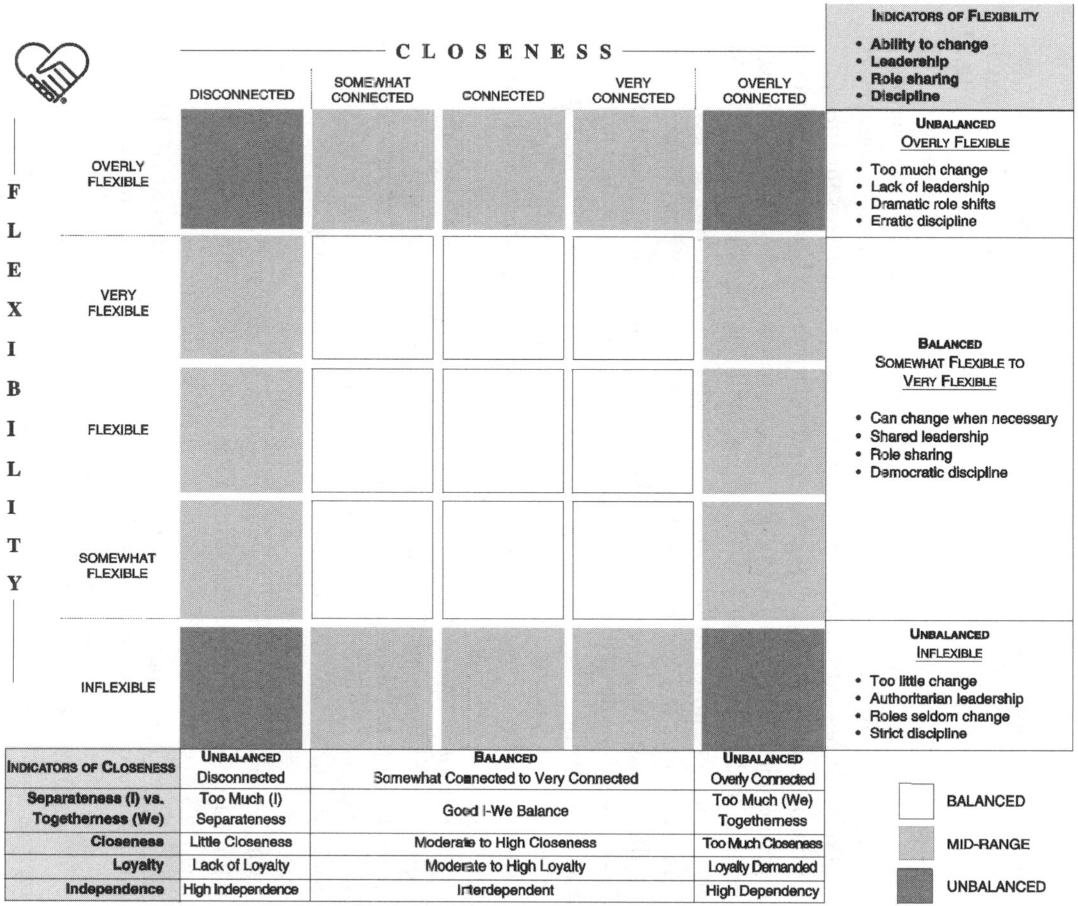

FIGURE 19.1. Couple and family map.

INDICATORS OF FLEXIBILITY
- Ability to change
- Leadership
- Role sharing
- Discipline

UNBALANCED
OVERLY FLEXIBLE
- Too much change
- Lack of leadership
- Dramatic role shifts
- Erratic discipline

BALANCED
SOMEWHAT FLEXIBLE TO VERY FLEXIBLE
- Can change when necessary
- Shared leadership
- Role sharing
- Democratic discipline

UNBALANCED
INFLEXIBLE
- Too little change
- Authoritarian leadership
- Roles seldom change
- Strict discipline

Legend: BALANCED / MID-RANGE / UNBALANCED

CLOSENESS (columns): DISCONNECTED · SOMEWHAT CONNECTED · CONNECTED · VERY CONNECTED · OVERLY CONNECTED

FLEXIBILITY (rows): OVERLY FLEXIBLE · VERY FLEXIBLE · FLEXIBLE · SOMEWHAT FLEXIBLE · INFLEXIBLE

INDICATORS OF CLOSENESS	UNBALANCED Disconnected	BALANCED Somewhat Connected to Very Connected	UNBALANCED Overly Connected
Separateness (I) vs. Togetherness (We)	Too Much (I) Separateness	Good I-We Balance	Too Much (We) Togetherness
Closeness	Little Closeness	Moderate to High Closeness	Too Much Closeness
Loyalty	Lack of Loyalty	Moderate to High Loyalty	Loyalty Demanded
Independence	High Independence	Interdependent	High Dependency

and very connected) make for optimal family functioning. The extremes or *unbalanced* levels (disengaged or enmeshed) are generally seen as problematic for relationships over the long term.

In the model's *balanced* area of cohesion, families are able to strike equilibrium, moderating both separateness and togetherness. Individuals are able to be both independent from and connected to their families. Couples and families that present for therapy services often fall into one of the extremes or *unbalanced* areas of too much separateness and togetherness. When cohesion levels are very high (enmeshed systems), there is too much consensus/emotional closeness within the family and too little independence. At the other extreme (disengaged systems), family members "do their own thing," with limited attachment or commitment to their family.

Balanced couple and family systems (somewhat connected, connected, and very connected types) tend to be more functional across the life cycle. More specifically, a somewhat connected relationship has some emotional separateness but is not as extreme as the disengaged system. Although time apart is more important, there is some time together, some joint decision making and marital support. Activities and interests are generally separate, but a few are shared. A connected relationship is characterized by the greatest degree of balance between connectedness and separateness. A very connected relationship has emotional closeness and loyalty to the relationship. There is an emphasis on togetherness; time together is more important than time alone. There are not only separate friends but also friends shared by the couple. Shared interests are common with some separate activities (see Appendix 19.1, Family Cohesion).

Unbalanced levels of cohesion are at the extremes of being either extremely low (disengaged) or extremely high (enmeshed). A *disengaged relationship* often has extreme emotional separateness. There is little involvement among family members and a great deal of personal separateness and independence. Individuals often do their own thing; separate time, space, and interests predominate; and members are unable to turn to one another for support and problem solving. In an *enmeshed relationship,* there is an extreme amount of emotional closeness, and loyalty is demanded. Individuals are very dependent on and reactive to one another. There is a lack of personal separateness, and little private space is permitted. The energy of the individuals is focused almost exclusively inside the family, and there are few outside individual friends or interests.

In summary, extremely high levels of cohesion (enmeshed) and extremely low levels of cohesion (disengaged) tend to be problematic for individuals and relationship development in the long run. On the other hand, relationships having moderate scores are able to balance being separate and together in a more functional way. Although there is no absolute best level for any relationship, many will have problems if they function at either extreme levels for too long. Also, it is expected that couple and family systems will change levels of cohesion over time.

COUPLE AND FAMILY FLEXIBILITY

Family flexibility is the *amount of change in its leadership, role relationships, and relationship rules.* The specific concepts include leadership (control, discipline), negotiation styles, role relationships, and relationship rules (see Clinical Rating Scale in Appendices 19.1–19.3 for how each concept is defined). *Flexibility concerns how systems balance stability with change.*

The five levels of flexibility range from *rigid/inflexible* (extremely low) to *somewhat flexible* (low to moderate), to *flexible* (moderate), to *very flexible* (moderate to high), to *chaotic/overly flexible* (extremely high). The terms "rigid" and "chaotic" used throughout this chapter are consistent with previous versions of the model. The terms "inflexible" and "overly flexible" were introduced to be used with clients/patients in order to simplify terminology (see Figure 19.1). As with cohesion, it is hypothesized that central or balanced levels of flexibility (somewhat flexible, flexible, and very flexible) are more conducive to good couple and family functioning, with the extremes (rigid and chaotic) being the most problematic for families as they move through their life cycle.

Basically, flexibility focuses on the change in a family's leadership, roles, and rules. Early application of systems theory to families emphasized the rigidity of the family and its tendency to maintain the status quo. Subsequently, the importance of potential for change and flexibility of systems was realized (Olson & Olson, 2000). Couples and families need both stability and change. The ability to change, when appropriate, is one of the characteristics that distinguishes functional couples and families from dysfunctional ones.

Couple and family systems balanced on flexibility are able to manage both stability and change. A *somewhat flexible relationship* tends to have democratic leadership characteristics, with some negotiations including the children. Roles are stable, with some role sharing, and rules are firmly enforced, with few changes. There are few rule changes, with rules firmly enforced. A *flexible relationship* has an equalitarian leadership with a democratic approach to decision making. Negotiations are open and actively include the children. Roles are shared and there is fluid change, when necessary. Rules can be changed and are age-appropriate. A *very flexible relationship* has a tendency toward frequent change in leadership and roles. Rules are very flexible and adjusted readily when there is a need for change (see Appendix 19.2, Family Flexibility).

Unbalanced couples and families tend to be either at the extreme of too much stability (rigid) or of too much change (chaotic). In a *rigid relationship,* one individual is in charge and is highly controlling. There tend to be limited negotiations with most decisions imposed by the leader. Roles are strictly defined, and rules do not change. A *chaotic relationship* has erratic or limited leadership. Decisions are impulsive and not well thought out. Roles are unclear and often shift from individual to individual.

In summary, extremely high (chaotic) and extremely low levels of flexibility (rigid) tend to be problematic for individuals and relationship development in the long run. Relationships having moderate scores (structured and flexible) are able to balance change and stability in a more functional way. Although there is no absolute best level for any relationship, many relationships tend to have problems if they always function at either extreme of the model (rigid or chaotic) for an extended period of time.

COUPLE AND FAMILY COMMUNICATION

Communication, the third dimension in the Circumplex Model, is considered a facilitating dimension. Communication is considered critical for facilitating couples and families to alter their levels of cohesion and flexibility. Using positive communication skills enables couples and families to alter their levels of cohesion and flexibility to meet developmental or situational demands. Because it is a facilitating dimension, communication is not graphically included in the model along with cohesion and flexibility (see Clinical Rating Scale in Appendix 19.3 for assessment of communication).

Couple and family communication is measured by focusing on the family as a group with regard to its listening skills, speaking skills, self-disclosure, clarity, continuity tracking, and respect and regard. Listening skills include empathy and attentive listening. Speaking skills include speaking for oneself and not speaking for others. Self-disclosure relates to sharing feelings about oneself and the relationship. Tracking refers to staying on topic, and respect and regard refer to the affective aspects of communication. Several studies investigating communication and problem-solving skills in couples and families have found that systems balanced on cohesion and flexibility tend to have very good communication, whereas systems unbalanced on these dimensions tend to have poor communication.

CIRCUMPLEX MODEL: A COUPLE AND FAMILY MAP

Another way to consider the model is as a descriptive Couple Map and Family Map of 25 types of couple and family relationships (Figure 19.1). This graphic representation of the model is an expansion of an earlier 16-type graphic representation. The expansion was implemented by increasing the number of balanced or healthy levels for each of the dimensions of cohesion and flexibility, thus increasing the number of balanced family types from four to nine.

The type of marriage is illustrated in the Couple Map (see Figure 19.1). Couples need to balance their levels of separateness–togetherness on cohesion and their levels of stability–change on flexibility. When partners differ in their preferences regarding the balance on these dimensions, these levels can be altered by a couple to achieve a level that is acceptable to each individual. In other words, the levels are dynamic, in that they can and do change over time.

The Family Map is useful not only for describing how the family is but also for addressing past and future multigenerational dynamics and issues. Knowing one's family is important, because people often use their own family of origin as a reference for the type of marriage and family they either want or do not want. Individuals often either attempt to recreate the type of family system they had as a child or react to this family of origin by attempting to do the opposite. If partners come from two quite different family systems or prefer different types of family dynamics, it is more difficult to create a compatible relationship style that works for them. Thus, the fit between individuals and their respective families of origin is a critical variable in determining how functional and satisfying a relationship system is likely to be.

An important distinction in the Circumplex Model is between *balanced* and *unbalanced* types of couple and family relationships. There are nine *balanced* types that exhibit somewhat connected, connected, or very connected levels on cohesion and somewhat flexible, flexible, or very flexible levels on flexibility. Figure 19.1 illustrates the nine balanced and the four extreme or unbalanced relationship types. Unbalanced relationship types are characterized by either extremely high or extremely low cohesion levels, combined with either extremely high or extremely low levels of flexibility: *chaotically disengaged, chaotically enmeshed, rigidly disengaged,* and *rigidly enmeshed.* The nine midrange family types consist of families that are balanced on one dimension and extremely high or low on the other dimension.

HYPOTHESES DERIVED FROM
THE CIRCUMPLEX MODEL

One value of a theoretical model is that hypotheses can be deduced from that model and tested in order to evaluate and further develop the model. The following hypotheses are derived from the Circumplex Model:

1. *Balanced type couples and families will generally function more adequately across the family life cycle than unbalanced types.* An important issue in the Circumplex Model relates to the concept of balance. Individuals and family systems need to balance their "separateness versus togetherness" on cohesion and their level of "stability versus change" on flexibility. Even though a *balanced* family system is placed at the three central levels of the model, these families do not always operate in a "moderate" manner. Being *bal-*

anced means that a family system can experience the extremes on the dimension when appropriate, but they do not typically function at these extremes for long periods of time.

Couples and families in the balanced area of the cohesion dimension allow their members to experience being both independent from and connected to their family. On flexibility, balance means maintaining some level of stability in a system with openness to some chance when it is necessary. Being extreme on these two dimensions might be appropriate for certain stages of the life cycle or when a family is under stress, but it can be problematic when families are stuck at the extremes.

1a. *If a couple's/family's expectations or subcultural group norms support more extreme patterns, families can function well as long as all family members desire the family to function in that manner.* Ethnicity has a large influence on the functioning of families and needs to be seriously considered in assessing family dynamics. What might appear to be an "enmeshed" ethnic family to a Caucasian outsider may be a normative style of functioning for an ethnic group. Unbalanced types of family systems are not necessarily dysfunctional, especially if the family in question belongs to a ethnic group (e.g., Hmong) or religious groups (e.g., Amish, Mormon) in which the norms support these more extreme behavior patterns.

2. *Positive communication skills will enable balanced types of couples/families to change their levels of cohesion and flexibility.* In general, positive communication skills are seen as helping family systems facilitate and maintain a balance on the two dimensions. Conversely, poor communication impedes movement in *unbalanced* systems and increases the likelihood these systems will remain extreme.

3. *Couples/families will modify their levels of cohesion and/or flexibility to deal effectively with situational stress and developmental changes across the family life cycle.* This hypothesis deals with the capacity of the couple/family system to change (second-order change) in order to deal with stress or to accommodate changes in members' development and expectations. The Circumplex Model is dynamic in that it assumes that couples and families will change levels of cohesion and flexibility, and thus family system type, and it is hypothesized that change is beneficial to the maintenance and improvement of couple and family functioning.

When one member's needs or preferences change, the system must somehow respond. For example, wives increasingly seek to develop more autonomy from their husbands (cohesion dimension), and also want more power and equality in their relationships (flexibility dimension). If their husbands are unwilling to understand and change in accordance with these expectations, these marriages will suffer from increasing levels of stress and dissatisfaction. Another common example of changing expectations occurs when a child reaches adolescence and wants more freedom, independence, and power in the family system. These pressures to change the family system by one member can facilitate change in the family despite family resistance.

DYNAMIC BALANCE ON THE CIRCUMPLEX AND SKIING: AN ANALOGY

An analogy can be made between *balanced* versus *unbalanced* family systems and professional versus novice skiers, a comparison first made in an article by Walsh and Olson (1989). Professional skiers function more like a *balanced* system, whereas novice skiers function more like an *unbalanced* system. In terms of cohesion, couples and families need to balance *separateness versus togetherness*. These two areas can be compared to the legs of a skier. Professional skiers keep their legs together and smoothly shift between their legs and the edges of the skis, creating a balance on separateness and togetherness. Similarly, *balanced* couples and families are also able to shift between being apart and being connected in a fluid manner. Conversely, novice skiers tend to keep their legs too far apart (too much separateness) or too close together (enmeshed), thereby creating an unbalanced system. Unbalanced couples and families also tend to be stuck at either extreme of separateness or togetherness and are unable to find a balance.

In terms of flexibility, couples and families need to balance *stability and change*. These two areas can be equated to the movements of the body of the skier. In watching professional skiers come down a ski slope, one sees fluidity in their movement left and right; they move their legs up and down to absorb the moguls while keeping the upper part of their body upright. In other words, there is both stability in the body and the ability to change. Likewise, in balanced couples and families, there is the ability not only to maintain stability but also to change, when necessary. Conversely, novice skiers tend to keep their body rather rigid; then, when they hit a mogul, they become even more rigid (unbalanced), which often results in a chaotic fall. Unbalanced couples and families also seem to be either too focused on stability (leading to rigidity) or too open to change (leading to chaos).

In regard to communication, there is also a clear analogy between skiing and couple/family systems. Professional skiers are very much "in touch" with all aspects of the hill, including the moguls and type of snow conditions, and they use this feedback to make good decisions. Likewise, *balanced* couples and families are open to communication and feedback from other sources, so that they can better adjust their levels of cohesion and flexibility. Conversely, novice skiers are often unaware of the conditions of the hill or how to use that information. Lacking the feedback and information they need, they fail to improve their skiing. *Unbalanced* couples and families also ignore or are unable to accept feedback from others that could help them improve their ability to change their level of cohesion and flexibility.

Stress clearly highlights the differences between professional and novice skiers, and balanced versus unbalanced couples/families. Professional skiers, like *balanced* systems, are able to become more cohesive and flexible under stress. On the other hand, like *unbalanced* systems, novice skiers become stuck at the extremes of cohesion and flexibility, which only adds to their lack of success in managing the stress or crises. So, as with skiing, couples and families need to become more cohesive and flexible in order to cope successfully with life's moguls.

CHANGES IN COUPLE AND FAMILY SYSTEMS OVER TIME

The Circumplex Model allows one to integrate systems theory and family developmental theory. Building on the family development approach, it is hypothesized that the stage of the family life cycle and composition of the family will have considerable impact on the type of family system. It is hypothesized that at any stage of the family life cycle, there will be diversity in the types of family systems as described in the Circumplex Model. Nevertheless, it is predicted that at different stages of the family life cycle, many of the families will cluster together—in some types more frequently than others.

The Circumplex Model is dynamic in that it assumes that changes can and do occur in family types over time. Families can move in any direction that the situation, stage of the family life cycle, or socialization of family members may require. The model can be used to illustrate developmental change of couples as they progress from dating to marriage; to pregnancy, childbirth and child rearing; to raising and launching adolescents, and moving into life as a couple again.

Figure 19.2 illustrates the changes one young couple experienced in a period of only 5 years, from dating to having their first child, and up to the time the child was 4 years old. During the dating period (1), the couple had a *very flexible/very connected* relationship. They felt close (very connected) and had a very flexible style in terms of leadership and decision making. If dating moves them toward marriage, they often become increasingly close and try out different ways of operating as a couple in term of flexibility.

During the first year of marriage (2), the newlywed couple can best be described as *flexible/overly connected*. They are generally flexible, because they are still getting more organized in terms of their roles and leadership. Being in love and enjoying maximum time together, they are still in the "honeymoon" phase and emotionally enmeshed.

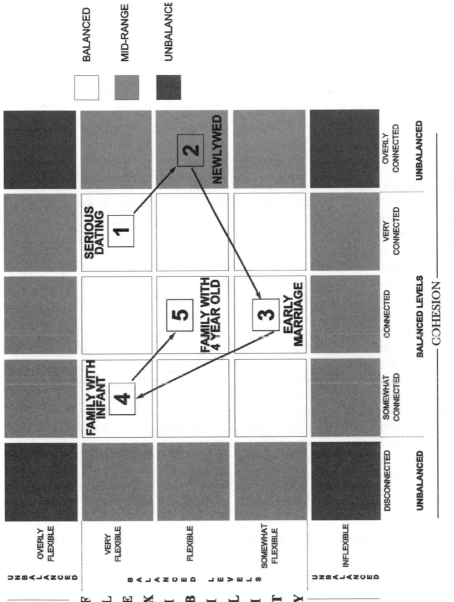

FIGURE 19.2. Dating and early marriage: Couple and family map.

525

By the end of their second year of marriage (3), the so-called "honeymoon" effect has worn off, and the couple becomes *somewhat flexible/connected*. The excitement with each other is not as great as it has been, and their togetherness has become more balanced, with each getting more into his or her individual life. They also develop more routines in their roles and life style and are now *somewhat flexible*.

During the third year of the marriage, the couple has a baby (4). The infant dramatically changes the couple relationship and they become a *very flexible/somewhat connected* family. Change is high at this time, and the couple is forced to adapt to the new challenges of parenting. Their life is in relative turmoil because they are up each night to feed and attend to the baby. The infant's unpredictable behavior often creates chaos and it is very difficult for the couple to keep on a fixed routine; hence, they become a *very flexible* family. The baby's presence initially increases the sense of bonding between the husband and wife, who feel united in their goal of rearing their child. But the infant takes a great deal of the mother's time and energy, and the couple finds it difficult to spend time to stay connected as a couple. Although the mother and infant are very close, the couple becomes *somewhat connected*.

By the time the child is 4 years old, life has stabilized for this family (5). They are now functioning as a *flexible/connected* family and experiencing very few changes. Formerly a dual career couple, they have shifted toward more traditional gender roles, with the mother staying at home, but she has now returned to work part-time. Although he spends a little time with the infant, the husband is more focused on his job and seeking a promotion. Both their closeness and flexibility have dropped one level and life is now more manageable for them both.

In summary, this example illustrates how a couple's relationship can change from dating across the early stages of marriage. The changes can occur gradually over months or more rapidly, after the birth of a child. These changes often occur without specific planning. However, couples can negotiate the type of relationship they want and be more proactive in creating the type of relationship they both prefer. These changes in a couple/family system are a snapshot version of the changes that occur in couple/family levels of cohesion and flexibility over their family life cycle.

FAMILY SYSTEM CHANGES AND FAMILY STRESS FROM THE "ATTACK ON AMERICA"

One hypothesis of the Circumplex Model relates to how family systems adapt to major stressors. *Balanced types of families will more effectively manage stress than unbalanced types, because they are able to change their system (second-order change) in order to cope with the stressor.*

An example of how a family system reacts to stress can be drawn from the tragic attack on America on September 11, 2001. Let us consider the hypothetical Greenberg family before and after the bombing of the Twin Towers of the World Trade Center (see Figure 19.3). The father, Henry, worked on the 92nd floor and it was initially unclear whether he was able to escape. Married for 26 years, he had three children ages 22, 20, and 17.

Before the bombing attack (point A), the family was *flexible/somewhat connected,* which is appropriate for their stage of the life cycle. Hours after the bombing attack (point B), the family system became *overly flexible/overly connected* (chaotically enmeshed), because the family did not know if the father had escaped from his office. The family, along with close relatives and friends, gathered at their home and huddled together in a mutually supportive way. A very high level of closeness and bonding was created, and uncertainty regarding the father's survival created a great deal of chaos in their family (Boss, 1999). This is an example of how levels of cohesion or flexibility that would otherwise be hypothesized as problematic for family functioning can indeed be highly functional.

During the next day or two after the bombing, family members stayed together and were emotionally enmeshed, but they developed a highly structured style of operating, creating a *somewhat flexible/overly connected* system (point C). They got very organized as a group in an attempt to find out what happened to Henry. This added structure was an attempt to bring some order to the chaos. They decided that their home would be the headquarters, and everyone needed to be in touch by phone. They divided up into teams so they could better find out what happened to Henry. Some family members went to the bombing site, others went to check out the hospitals, and still others stayed at home. They checked in at home every few hours.

On the third day, a miracle occured, from their point of view. They found that Henry was in a downtown hospital but severely injured in one leg and arm, and he had some memory loss. He could not remember his phone number but did know his name, which enabled the hospital to post his name on the second day.

Two weeks later, he was home, and the family then shifted again, becoming a *somewhat flexible/very connected* system (point D). They were still rather organized in order to care for him and to start to get back to their normal routines. Some of the closeness decreased from extreme levels. Yet the family was closer and more organized than before the attack, which is a useful style while the family recovers from the stress that they all experience.

This example illustrates one family's ability to adapt to a crisis. The family changed system levels several times over the few weeks following the attack, and these changes were beneficial in helping them to deal more effectively with this major trauma. The ability of the family to change in a fluid manner rather than stay stuck in a particular level is very functional, since it enables them to adapt more adequately to the major events.

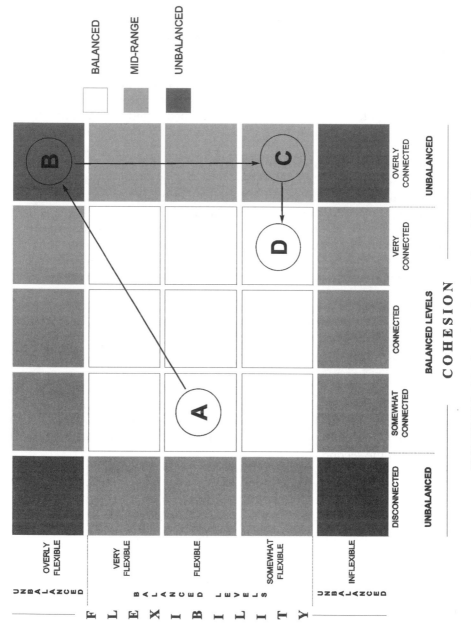

FIGURE 19.3. Attack on America: Couple and family map.

The following general principles of stress-related change were developed after studying the impact of stress on several hundred couples and families with the Couple and Family Map (Olson, 2000). First, under stress, couples and families often become more extreme on both flexibility (a move toward a more chaotic system) and on cohesion (a move toward a more enmeshed system). Second, communication almost always increases during a stressful event. Third, once the stress has abated, couples and families usually return to a similar—but rarely to the same—type of system they had in place before the stress. Fourth, couples and families often require a minimum of 6 months to a year to adjust to a major stress. Fifth, *balanced* couple and family systems tend to become *unbalanced* during the stress and then return to another *balanced* system type.

In summary, it is expected that family systems will change in response to a crisis. As hypothesized in the Circumplex Model, *balanced* families have the resources and skills to shift their system in an appropriate way to cope more effectively with a crisis. In contrast, *unbalanced* families lack the resources needed to change their family and, therefore, have more difficulty adapting to a crisis. Balanced families, therefore, possess greater ability to achieve second-order change, because they are able to alter their family system to adapt to family crises.

STUDIES VALIDATING THE CIRCUMPLEX MODEL

Balanced versus Unbalanced Families

A central hypothesis derived from the model is that balanced couples and families function more adequately than unbalanced couples and families. More than 250 studies (Kouneski, 2001; Olson, 2000) have supported this major hypothesis. These studies have generally compared families with a variety of emotional problems and symptoms to nonclinical families. Most of these studies have used the self-report scale, FACES, in which higher scores on cohesion and flexibility represent balanced couples and families. This means that there is a linear relationship between healthy functioning and scores on FACES (Olson, 2000). Earlier versions of FACES did not tap the enmeshment) chaos, but FACES IV achieves this goal.

Strong support for the major hypothesis that balanced families function more adequately are from about 10 studies using the CRS, the observational assessment designed to assess Circumplex Model dimensions (Kouneski, 2001). In contrast to FACES, the CRS does tap the full continuum of the cohesion and flexibility dimensions and reveals a curvilinear relationship with family functioning (Thomas & Olson, 1993; Thomas & Ozechowski, 2000).

Balanced Couples/Families and Communication

Another hypothesis is that balanced couples and families have more positive communication skills than unbalanced families. Communication can be measured at both the marital and family levels.

In a national survey of 21,501 married couples who took the ENRICH couple inventory, it was found that the most happy marriages were balanced on cohesion and flexibility and had very good communication (Olson & Olson, 2000). In a review of over 20 studies of families, Kouneski (2001) found that most of the studies provided strong support for the hypothesis that balanced families have more positive communication than unbalanced families.

ASSESSMENT: MULTIMETHOD, MULTIPERSON, MULTITRAIT, AND MULTISYSTEM

Multimethod assessment utilizes self-report scales, which provide an "insider's perspective" on the family relationship, and the therapists' or observers' ratings, which provide an "outsider's perspective" on that same system. That these two approaches often provide different perspectives provides an important rationale for why both approaches should be used in work with families (Olson, 2000).

In order to assess the three major dimensions of the Circumplex Model and other related family concepts, (Olson, Gorall, and Tiesel (2002) developed a variety of self-report instruments, which are described later in this chapter. The self-report instrument package, called the Family Inventories Package (FIP), provides the insider's perspective, whereas the CRS completed by the researcher or therapist provides the outsider's perspective. Both perspectives are useful, but they often yield apparently conflicting data. Used together, however, they help capture the complexity of marital and family systems.

Multiperson assessment is also important, because family members often do not agree in describing their family system. This is understandable, because an adolescence, marriage, and family occupy unique locations in the family system, which gives each person a unique experience and perspective on that system. Assessment using multiple family members, therefore, provides a more complete picture of how various family members view the system and the level of agreement or disagreement between them.

Multitrait assessment is based on the three central dimensions of the Circumplex Model: cohesion, flexibility, and communication. Although other traits can be incorporated into couple and family assessment, these three dimensions provide the foundation and central core of these relationship systems.

Multisystem assessment ideally focuses on the individual, the couple system, the parent–child system, and the total family—including extended family relationships. *One important question to ask family members is whom they each consider to be members of their family.* It is surprising to us how often family members disagree regarding who are the current members in their family system. This question becomes even more important when we consider the increasing complexity of families today, with so much divorce and increasing numbers of stepfamilies. These changes raise important questions about boundary issues and who is psychologically and/or physically present in a given family system (Boss, 1999). This is especially important given the increasing diversity of family forms, particularly with respect to the changes accompanying divorce and remarriage.

UPDATED FAMILY INVENTORIES PACKAGE (FIP)

The new FIP is the latest in a series of self-report assessments based on the Circumplex Model (Olson et al., 2002). This procedure is multidimensional in that it assesses the three Circumplex Model dimensions of cohesion, flexibility and communication. In addition, there are scales measuring family satisfaction, stress, and strengths.

FACES I, II, and III

The FACES self-report instrument has gone through multiple revisions over the past 20 years, with alterations that attempt to improve the reliability and validity of the instrument. Critiques of the instrument and of the Circumplex Model have encouraged these revisions, which continue to the present day. FACES IV was created because the earlier versions of the instrument (FACES I, II, and III) had *linear relationships* with family functioning rather than the curvilinear relationship, as hypothesized by the Circumplex Model. The earlier versions of FACES did not adequately capture the high extremes of cohesion (enmeshment) or flexibility (chaos). FACES IV was developed in an attempt to address this limitation.

FACES IV

The FACES IV instrument (Olson et al., 2002) was developed to tap the *full range* of the cohesion and flexibility dimensions. Work was done to develop items to tap the high and low extremes (unbalanced) of the dimensions (Tiesel, 1994). These items were then added to the moderately worded items of the previous versions of FACES in an attempt to develop scales to tap the full theoretical range of the dimensions (Gorall, 2002). Reliabilities for FACES IV and validation scales are shown in Table 19.2.

TABLE 19.2. Alpha Reliability of FACES IV Scales and Validity Scales

Scale	Cronbach Alpha
Unbalanced Scales	
Disengaged Scale	.87
Enmeshment Scale	.77
Rigid Scale	.83
Chaos Scale	.85
Balanced Scales	
Closeness Scale	.89
Change Scale	.80
Dimensional Scales	
Cohesion Scale	.90
Flexibility Scale	.83
Validity Scales	
Family Satisfaction	.93
Self Report Family Inventory (SFI)	.93
Family Assessment Device (FAD)	.91

The FACES IV scales have been found to be reliable and valid for research use and clinical use. The FACES IV scales have also been shown to discriminate between healthy and problematic-functioning families, showing clinical validity (Gorall, 2002; see Table 19.3). These findings are based on an ethnically representative sample of the metropolitan area in which the research was conducted.

Family Communication

Communication is assessed by the Family Communication Scale, which is a revised version of the Parent–Adolescent Communication Scale (Barnes & Olson, 1989). Family communication focuses on the free-flowing exchange of information, both factual and emotional. It deals with the lack of constraint and degree of understanding and satisfaction experienced in family communication interactions. The Family Communication Scale has been used in a wide variety of studies examining family communication in conjunction with other family dynamics (Friedman, Terras, & Kreisher, 1995; Henry, Sager, & Plunkett, 1996; Tulloch, Blizzard, & Pinkus, 1997; White, 1996).

Family Satisfaction

Satisfaction with the current family system is assessed by the Family Satisfaction Scale (Olson & Wilson, 1989), specifically designed to assess satisfaction with family functioning, which is a sparsely studied area compared to the voluminous studies on marital satisfaction. The items in the scale are specifically designed to tap individuals' satisfaction with levels of cohe-

TABLE 19.3. Discriminant Analysis of Problem and Nonproblem Families

Scale	Top vs. Bottom 50% On SFI & FAD	Top vs. Bottom 40% On SFI & FAD	Top vs. Bottom 50% on Family Satisfaction	Problem Plus Therapy[a]
N for Each Group	Top = 199 Bottom = 192 Missing = 76	Top = 142 Bottom = 149 Missing = 178	Top = 231 Bottom = 228 Missing = 10	No Problems = 163 Problems & Therapy = 134
Unbalanced				
Disengaged Subscale	86	89	76	67
Chaos Subscale	80	85	60	65
Enmeshed Subscale	64	65	53	50
Rigid Subscale	54	55	75	54
Balanced				
Closeness Subscale	89	94	80	68
Change Subscale	74	80	72	64
Dimension Scales				
Cohesion Scale	89	94	79	67
Flexibility Scale	79	85	78	63
Validation Scales				
SFI	—	—	82	72
FAD	—	—	82	69
Family Satisfaction	88	93	—	68

[a]Subject identified physical, sexual, emotional, or chemical abuse as a problem in their family as well as identifying the receipt or need for therapy services for the problem group, and identified none of these as problems or the receipt or need for therapy for the no-problems group.
—Not reported because the groups for discriminant analysis are based on the same scale(s).

sion and flexibility in their family. It has been used widely in family research in studies both in conjunction with the FACES instrument and as a stand-alone assessment of family satisfaction (Cashwell & Vance, 1996; Kusada, 1995; Pillay & Wassenaar, 1997).

Family Strengths

The Family Strengths Scale (Olson, Larsen, & McCubbin, 1989) is included to focus specifically on those family characteristics and dynamics that enable families to show resilience and deal successfully with family problems. It specifically taps the subdimensions of Pride and Accord. The Pride subscale incorporates pride, loyalty, trust, and respect, whereas the Accord subscale is designed to assess a family's sense of competency. The scale has been used in a variety of studies focused on issues of strengths within families (Brage & Meredith, 1994; Kashani, Canfield, Soltys, & Reid, 1995; Meske, Sanders, Meredith, & Abbott, 1994).

Family Stress

As described previously, families often react to stressful situations by altering their level of cohesion and/or flexibility. In order to assess the current levels of stressors with which a family is dealing, and thus assess the impact on their levels of cohesion and flexibility, an assessment of family stress is included in the FIP. The Family Stress Scale is designed to tap the levels of stress currently being experienced by family members within their family system. It is adapted from the Coping and Stress Profile (CSP) (Olson, 1997).

CLINICAL RATING SCALE

The CRS was initially developed in 1980 to operationalize the three dimensions of the Circumplex Model. The observational scale describes specific indicators for each level of the three dimensions. The current CRS was modified several times by Olson (1990). It was designed to be used by therapists and researchers for rating couple and family systems based on clinical interviews or observations of their interaction.

The CRS has been validated in an extensive study by Thomas and Olson (1993). A recent study revealed a curvilinear relationship between the dimensions of cohesion and flexibility in relation to family functioning (Thomas & Ozechowski, 2000). Recent research has also shown that the scale produces the same factor structure when raters using the scale are researchers or therapists (Lee, Jager, Whiting, & Kwantes, 2000).

This scale is a useful training device both for helping individuals learn more about the Circumplex Model and for family assessment and treatment planning. Lee et al. (2000) found that the CRS is a useful tool in training family therapists to examine family dynamics and develop treatment plans. (A list of the key concepts in the CRS is included in Appendices 19.1–19.3.)

GOALS OF FAMILY THERAPY USING THE CIRCUMPLEX MODEL

Family therapists' central goal of reducing presenting problems and symptoms of family members is achieved by interventions focused on changing dysfunctional patterns in the couple and/or family system. The basic assumption is that the current family system dynamics are helping to maintain symptomatic behaviors. Such patterns of interaction need to be changed before the symptoms or presenting problems can be alleviated.

Table 19.4 summarizes the specific goals of family therapy based on the Circumplex Model. The first goal is ultimately to reduce any problems and symptoms. Because most dysfunctional families coming for therapy represent midrange or *unbalanced* family types, change often involves trying to shift the system one level on cohesion and one level on adaptability toward the *balanced* levels. It is, therefore, typically assumed that the family will function more adequately if the marital and/or family system is moved toward the *balanced* types.

Because the model is dynamic, intervention on either cohesion or flexibility often has a ripple effect, influencing the system on the other dimension. In terms of cohesion, problems in families often occur because of family members' difficulty in balancing separateness (autonomy) and togetherness (intimacy). In couples coming for therapy, often there is a difference in the amount of separateness and togetherness the two partners experience or desire. For example, in disengaged couples, one or both individuals have emphasized looking out for themselves; thus, they have not maintained their emotional bond of intimacy.

In troubled families, the dynamics of cohesion are often more complicated. One family might have an enmeshed mother–adolescent coalition with a disengaged father. In this case, the marital dyad would not be emotionally close. Increasing their marital/parental collaboration is an effective strategy for breaking up the strong parent child coalition.

In terms of flexibility, couples and families with problems often have difficulty balancing stability and change. These relationships are either too rigid or too chaotic. With rigid systems, the behavioral repertoire is often very narrow. When confronted with increasing stress, family members tend to become more rigid and inflexible. These families can often benefit from learning and using more democratic decision-making and better problem-solving skills. On the other hand, chaotic relationships often need in-

---

TABLE 19.4 . Goals of Marital and Family Therapy Based on Circumplex Model

Goals regarding symptoms
- Reduce presenting problems and symptoms.

Goals regarding system (couple and/or family)
- Change system one level on cohesion and one level on flexibility toward balanced types.
- On cohesion, balancing togetherness and separateness.
- On flexibility, balancing stability and change.
- Improve communication skills.

Metagoal regarding system (preventative)
- Increase ability to negotiate system change over time.

creased structure and can also benefit from improved problem-solving skills.

Increasing the positive communication skills of couples and families can also facilitate systems change. Individuals in troubled families often need to learn how to be more assertive in expressing their wants and desires. They usually gain from learning how to express their feelings in a constructive manner, and how to listen and give empathetic feedback to each other.

However, improving the communication skills in a family is a necessary but not sufficient condition for change on the dimensions of cohesion and adaptability. Communication skills can help increase awareness of current needs and preferences. Systems change on cohesion and adaptability is more difficult and complex. Good communication skills enable families to express more clearly their relationship preferences. One desirable goal of couple and family therapy is ultimately not only to deal with their current issues but also to help families develop the necessary skills to negotiate system change over time. It is an assumption of the model that couples and families need to alter their system as their individual needs and preferences change. Being able to articulate and negotiate these changes on cohesion and adaptability will also enable couples or families to cope more adequately with stress and other problematic issues they encounter over time. This important preventive goal moves beyond dealing with the current presenting symptoms. Unfortunately, this metagoal is often not achieved in therapy, because most families, and even some therapists, are too focused on reducing the presenting problems.

TREATMENT PLANNING USING THE CIRCUMPLEX MODEL

The Circumplex Model is a valuable resource in assessment-based treatment planning with severely dysfunctional families. A major task for outcome research is to determine which elements of intervention are most appropriate and effective with specific presenting problems and elements of family functioning. The Circumplex Model and accompanying self-report scale (FACES IV) and CRS offer an empirically based family assessment tool that can be used for treatment planning and outcome evaluation.

The model provides a conceptual framework for assessing family system functioning on two fundamental dimensions of family organization: cohesion and flexibility. This descriptive typology of transactional patterns can be used to determine a family's current level and style of functioning on each dimension and to guide treatment planning to strengthen particular components of functioning toward clearly specified and realistic objectives. Thus, family therapy is not limited to reduction or interruption of extreme dysfunctional patterns, but is directed systematically toward promotion of more functional patterns (Walsh & Olson, 1989).

For families assessed at either extreme on the dimensions, intervention strategies can be targeted to fit their particular pattern of organization and to guide change in a stepwise progression toward a more *balanced* system. A common therapeutic error with very dysfunctional families is to assume that patterns are unchangeable or that change toward the opposite pattern is necessary and desirable. In most significantly troubled families, a reachable therapeutic goal would be to move the family one level, from enmeshed to very connected. It would also be unrealistic to attempt to change family patterns more than two levels, such as moving a disengaged family to become very connected.

Chronically dysfunctional families often assume such extreme all-or-none positions regarding change. They are likely to alternate between feelings of hopelessness that any change can occur and unrealistic expectations for goals that are unlikely to be met. They commonly fluctuate between extremes of enmeshed/disengaged and of rigidity/chaos. An enmeshed family may resist a clinician's efforts to promote physical separation, such as leaving home at launching, when they hold catastrophic expectations that any separation will result in a total cutoff.

Opposite extremes may also be found in different family subsystems. In many enmeshed families, some siblings may disengage completely from the family in order to avoid fusion, assuming positions of pseudoautonomy that dissolve in contact with the family. Clinicians must be cautious not to collude with presuppositions of the all-or-none position. Fears of runaway change or loss of patterns considered to be essential to individual or family survival are common sources of "resistance" to change and therapy dropouts. Clinicians need to be alert to prevent extreme family oscillation, which can occur much like a "short-circuiting" process. A therapist must actively structure and monitor family interaction to block or interrupt the all-or-none tendency in these families to flip to the opposite extreme. It is essential to set modest, concrete objectives to be reached through small increments of change, in order to reduce anxiety to a manageable level, to prevent extreme fluctuations, and to help the family modulate and moderate changes than can be maintained over time.

PREPARE/ENRICH PROGRAM: COUNSELING PREMARITAL AND MARRIED COUPLES

The PREPARE/ENRICH Program was developed to help couples prepare for marriage (PREPARE Program) and for marriage enrichment and marital therapy (ENRICH Program). The PREPARE/ENRICH Program is currently used by over 50,000 counselors with couples, and over 1,000,000 couples have taken the program nationally. It was originally developed in 1979 and has been modified and expanded four times since then by David Olson and colleagues (Olson, Fournier, & Druckman, 1986; Olson & Olson, 1999). The Program is available in seven other languages (Chinese, French, German, Korean, Japanese, Spanish, and Swedish) and in 12 other countries (Australia, Canada, England, Germany, Hong Kong, Korea, Japan, New Zealand, Singapore, South Africa, Sweden, and Taiwan). Computer scoring is done via the Internet. To learn more about the program, go to the website: www.lifeinnovations.com.

In the first step, the couple takes one of five PREPARE/ENRICH Couple Inventories (PREPARE, PREPARE—Cohabiting Couple, PREPARE—Marriage with Children, ENRICH for married couples, and MATE for couples over 50). The counselor receives the inventory computer score and receives a 15-page computer report on the couple and a 25-page workbook for the couple called *Building a Strong Marriage*. Feedback from the computer report is integrated into counseling with the couple.

The counselor uses the feedback from the computer report to work with the couple. A semistructured feedback process was developed; it has six goals and matching couple exercises (see Table 19.5). The six couple exercises are designed to identify couple strengths, to teach couples assertiveness and active listening skills, and to learn how to effectively resolve conflict, deal with family-of-origin issues and financial planning, and achieve goals.

The Couple and Family Map is used to look at the couple dynamics and how they relate to the family of origin of each partner. Each person describes the couple relationship and his or her own family of origin. The findings are plotted onto the Map. The similarities and differences in families of origin are discussed. The spouses also discuss what they would like (proactively) to bring from their families into their couple/family, and what they do not want to bring (repeat). Couples enjoy this discussion and learn a great deal about their families and how they often repeat what they did in their family of origin.

TABLE 19.5. Six Goals and Couple Exercises with PREPARE/ENRICH Program

- Explore relationship strength and growth areas.
- Strengthen couple communication skills, including assertiveness and active listening.
- Resolve couple conflict using the Ten-Step Procedure.
- Explore family-of-origin issues using Couple and Family Map (Circumplex Model).
- Develop a workable budget and financial plan.
- Develop personal, couple, and family goals.

Predictive Validity of Couple Scales

The five PREPARE/ENRICH scales tap 20 individual and couple content areas that have been found to be critical to the healthy or problematic functioning of couple relationships. The 20 areas each contain a 10-item scale and are organized into the following categories: Personality—4 scales (e.g., self confidence); Intrapersonal—5 scales (e.g., marriage expectation, spiritual beliefs); Interpersonal—5 scales (e.g., communication and conflict resolution); External—2 scales (e.g., financial); Couple and Family System—4 scales (e.g., closeness and flexibility). PREPARE, for premarital couples, has been found to predict couple satisfaction and which couples will divorce with 80–85% accuracy in 3-year longitudinal studies (Fowers & Olson, 1986; Larsen & Olson, 1989). ENRICH, designed for married couples, is able to discriminate happy, nonclinical couples from clinical couples with 90% accuracy (Fowers & Olson, 1989).

Couple Types

Using data from 5,030 premarital couples that took PREPARE, Fowers and Olson (1993) identified the four types of premarital couples: vitalized, harmonious, traditional, and conflicted (see Figure 19.4). Five types of married couples were identified using a sample of 6,267 married couples (Olson & Fowers, 1993) who took ENRICH. The same four premarital types were found in married couples, along with one additional type: devitalized.

- *Vitalized couples* were the happiest couple type, because they had many strengths (high Positive Couple Agreement [PCA] scores) and few growth areas (low PCA scores).
- *Harmonious couples* had many strengths, but fewer than the vitalized couples. They had high PCA scores in many areas, but often had low scores in the Children and Parenting area.
- *Traditional couples* had more strengths in traditional areas such as Children and Parenting, Family and Friends, Traditional Roles, and Spiritual Beliefs. However, they had lower scores on internal dynamics, where they indicated problems with Personality Issues, Communication, and Conflict Resolution.
- *Conflicted couples* had numerous growth areas and few relationship strengths. They are called conflicted because they had low scores on Communication, Conflict Resolution, and many other areas. Conflicted premarital couples are at high risk for divorce. Married couples of this type commonly seek therapy (Fowers, Montel, & Olson, 1996).
- *Devitalized couples* (only from ENRICH) had growth areas in almost all aspects of their relationship. They were typically very unhappy, had few strengths as a couple. They are a common type of couple that seeks marital therapy.

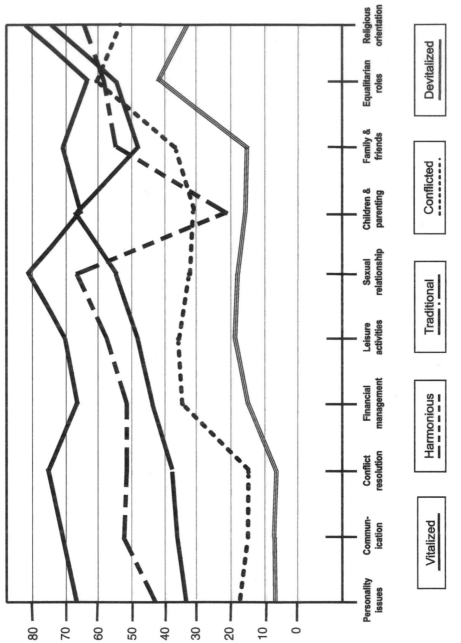

FIGURE 19.4. Five types of married couples based on ENRICH.

Validity of Couple Types

In order to validate the four premarital types, 328 premarital couples were followed for 3 years after marriage to assess their marital success (Fowers et al., 1996). These couples were classified into the four premarital types. The outcome measure 3 years after marriage was whether they were happily married or separated/divorced.

The most significant validation of the typology was the finding related to the marital outcomes of the premarital couples. As hypothesized, the Vitalized couples had the highest percentage of happily married couples (60%) and the lowest percentage of separated and divorced couples (17%). Conversely, Conflicted couples had the most separated/divorced couples (49%) and the lowest number of happily married couples (17%). Traditional couples had the lowest percentage of separated/divorced couples (6%) but the highest percentage of unhappily married couples (50%).

There were also 89 couples who cancelled their wedding plans after taking PREPARE and receiving feedback. As predicted, the highest percentage of those who cancelled their wedding plans were Conflicted couple types (40%), followed by the Traditional couple type (26%), the Harmonious couple type (22%) and the Vitalized couple type (12%).

A study comparing the Couple and Family Map with the couple typology based on ENRICH by Ed Kouneski (2002) demonstrated a linear relationship between couple cohesion and couple flexibility in the five types. More specifically, Vitalized/Harmonious couples had the highest level of couple cohesion and flexibility, whereas Conflicted/Devitalized couples had the lowest levels.

SUMMARY

In summary, the Circumplex Model is both a theoretical model with testable hypotheses and a descriptive model for understanding couple and family functioning. The Model has been used increasingly in clinical work and research with diverse samples of couples and families in terms of ethnicity/race, family structure, sexual orientation, and social class. The Couple and Family Map is also designed for clinical assessment, treatment planning, and evaluation of therapeutic outcome. An assessment package includes both the self-report scales in the FIP and the observer (therapist/researcher) rating, the CRS. The ultimate goal of the Circumplex Model is to bridge research, theory, and clinical practice.

REFERENCES

Barnes, H., & Olson, D. H. (1989). Parent–adolescent communication scale. In D. H. Olson, H. I. McCubbin, H. Barnes, A. Larsen, M. Muxen, & M. Wilson

(Eds.), *Family inventories.* St. Paul, MN: Family Social Science, University of Minnesota.

Beavers, W. B., & Hampson, R. B. (1990). *Successful families: Assessment and intervention.* New York: Norton.

Benjamin, L. S. (1977). Structural analysis of a family in therapy. *Journal of Counseling Clinical Psychology, 45,* 391–406.

Boss, P. (1999). *Ambiguous loss: Learning to live with unresolved grief.* Cambridge, MA: Harvard University Press.

Brage, D., & Meredith, W. (1994). A causal model of adolescent depression. *Journal of Psychology , 128,* 455–468.

Cashwell, C. S., & Vance, N. A. (1996). Familial influences on adolescent delinquent behavior. *Family Journal: Counseling and Therapy for Couples and Families, 4,* 217–225.

Epstein, N. B., & Bishop, D. S. (1993). The McMaster Assessment Device (FAD). In F. Walsh (Ed.), *Normal family processes.* New York: Guilford Press.

Fowers, B. J., Montel, K. H., & Olson, D. H. (1996). Predicting marital success for premarital couple types based on PREPARE. *Journal of Marital and Family Therapy, 22*(1), 103–119.

Fowers, B. J., & Olson, D. H. (1993). Five types of marriage: Empiricial typology based on ENRICH. *Family Journal, 1*(3), 196–207.

Fowers, B. J., & Olson, D. H. (1986). Predicting marital success with PREPARE: A predictive validity study. *Journal of Marital and Family Therapy, 12,* 403–413.

Fowers, B. J., & Olson, D. H. (1989). ENRICH marital inventory: A discriminant validity and cross-validation assessment. *Journal of Marital and Family Therapy, 15*(1), 65–79.

Friedmand, A. S., Terras, A., & Kreisher, C. (1995). Family and client characteristics as predictors of outpatient treatment outcome for adolescent drug abusers. *Journal of Substance Abuse, 7,* 345–356.

Gorall, D. (2002). *FACES IV and Circumplex Model.* Unpublished doctoral dissertation, Family Social Science, University of Minnesota, St. Paul.

Gottman, J. M. (1994). *Why marriages succeed or fail.* New York: Simon & Schuster.

Henry, C. S., Sager, D. W., & Plunkett, S. W. (1996). Adolescent's perceptions of family system characteristics, parent-adolescent dyadic behaviors, adolescent qualities, and adolescent empathy. *Family Relations, 45,* 283–292.

Kantor, D., & Lehr, W. (1975). *Inside the family.* San Francisco: Jossey-Bass.

Kashani, J. H., Canfield, L. A., Soltys, S. M., & Reid, J. C. (1995). Psychiatric inpatient children's family perceptions and anger expression. *Journal of Emotional and Behavioral Disorders, 3,* 13–18, 39.

Kouneski, E. (2001). Circumplex Model and FACES: Review of literature. Available online at http://www.lifeinnovations.com/familyinventoriesdatabase.html.

Kouneski, E. (2002). *Five types of marriage based on ENRICH: Linking intrapersonal and interpersonal factors.* Unpublished doctoral dissertation, Family Social Science, University of Minnesota, St. Paul.

Kusada, H. (1995). A study of figures of family relationships. *Japanese Journal of Counseling Science, 28,* 21–27. [in Japanese]

Larsen, A. S., & Olson, D. H. (1989). Predicting marital satisfaction using PREPARE: A replication study. *Journal of Marital and Family Therapy, 15*(3), 311–322.

Leary, T. (1975). *Interpersonal diagnosis of personality.* New York: Ronald Press.

Lee, R. E., Jager, K. B., Whiting, J. B., & Kwantes, C. T. (2000). Clinical assessment using the Clinical Rating Scale: Thomas and Olson revisited. *Journal of Marital and Family Therapy, 26,* 535–537.

Leff, J., & Vaughn, C. (1985). *Expressed emotion in families.* New York: Guilford Press.

Meske, C., Sanders, G. F., Meredith, W. H., & Abbott, D. A. (1994). Perceptions of rituals and traditions among elderly persons. *Activities, Adaptation and Aging, 18,* 13–26.

Olson, D. H. (1990). *Clinical rating scale for Circumplex Model.* St. Paul: Family Social Science, University of Minnesota.

Olson, D. H. (1997). Family stress and coping: A multi-system perspective. In S. Dreman (Ed.), *The family on the threshold of the 21st century* (pp. 258–282). Mahwah, NJ: Erlbaum.

Olson, D. H. (2000). Circumplex Model of marital and family systems. *Journal of Family Therapy, 22*(2), 144–167.

Olson, D. H., & Fowers, B. J. (1993). Five types of marriage: Empirical typology based on ENRICH. *Family Journal: Counseling and Therapy for Couples and Families, 1*(3), 196–207.

Olson, D. H., Fournier, D., & Druckman, J. (1986). *PREPARE/ENRICH Inventories.* Minneapolis: Life Innovations.

Olson, D. H., Gorall, D., & Tiesel, J. (2002). *Family inventories package.* Minneapolis: Life Innovations.

Olson, D. H., Larsen, A., & McCubbin, H. I. (1989). Family strengths. In D. H. Olson, H. I. McCubbin, H. Barnes, A. Larsen, M. Muxen, & M. Wilson (Eds.), *Family Inventories.* St. Paul: Family Social Science, University of Minnesota.

Olson, D. H., & Olson, A. K. (1999). PREPARE/ENRICH Program: Version 2000. In R. Berger & M. T. Hannah (Eds.), *Preventive approaches in couple therapy* (pp. 196–216). Philadelphia: Brunner/Mazel.

Olson, D. H., & Olson, A. K. (2000). *Empowering couples: Building on your strengths.* Minneapolis: Life Innovations.

Olson, D. H., Russell, C. S., & Sprenkle, D. H. (1989). *Circumplex Model: Systemic assessment and treatment of families.* New York: Haworth Press.

Olson, D. H., & Wilson, M. (1989). Family satisfaction. In D. H. Olson & H. I. McCubbin (Eds.), *Family inventories.* St. Paul: Family Social Science, University of Minnesota.

Parsons, T., & Bales, R. F. (1955). *Family socialization and interaction process.* Glencoe, IL: Free Press.

Pillay, A. L., & Wassenaar, D. R. (1997). Recent stressors and family satisfaction in suicidal adolescents in South Africa. *Journal of Adolescence, 20,* 155–162.

Reiss, D. (1981). *The family's construction of reality.* Cambridge, MA: Harvard University Press.

Thomas, V., & Olson, D. H. (1993). Problem families and the Circumplex Model: Observational assessment using the Clinical Rating Scale. *Journal of Marital & Family Therapy, 19,* 159–175.

Thomas, V., & Ozechowski, T. J. (2000). A test of the Circumplex Model of marital and family systems using the Clinical Rating Scale. *Journal of Marital and Family Therapy, 26,* 523–534.

Tiesel, J. (1994). *FACES IV: Reliability and validity.* Unpublished doctoral dissertation, Family Social Science, University of Minnesota, St. Paul.

Tulloch, A. L., Blizzard, L., & Pinkus, Z. (1997). Adolescent–parent communication in self-harm. *Journal of Adolescent Health, 21,* 267–275.

Walsh, F. (1998). Strengthening family resilience. New York: Guilford Press.

Walsh, F., & Olson, D. H. (1993). Utility of the Circumplex Model with severely dysfunctional family systems. In D. H. Olson, C. S. Russell, & D. H. Sprenkle (Eds.), *Circumplex Model: Systemic assessment and treatment of families* (2nd ed., pp. 104–137). New York: Haworth Press.

White, F. A. (1996). Parent–adolescent communication and adolescent decision-making. *Journal of Family Studies, 2,* 41–56.

APPENDIX 19.1. Couple and Family Cohesion

Couple/Family Score	DISCONNECTED (disengaged)		SOMEWHAT CONNECTED		CONNECTED		VERY CONNECTED		OVERLY CONNECTED (ENMESHED)	
	1	2	3	4	5	6	7	8	9	10
EMOTIONAL BONDING	Extreme emotional separateness. Lack of family loyalty.		Emotional separateness. Limited closeness. Occasional family loyalty.		Emotional closeness. Some separateness. Good loyalty to family.		High emotional closeness. Some separateness. High loyalty to family.		Extreme emotional closeness. Little separateness. Loyalty demanded.	
FAMILY INVOLVEMENT	Very low involvement or interaction.		Involvement acceptable. Personal distance preferred.		Good family involvement. Some personal distance		Involvement emphasized. Personal distance allowed.		Very high involvement. Fusion, overdependency.	
MARITAL RELATIONSHIP	Infrequent affective responsiveness. High emotional separateness. Limited closeness.		Some affective responsiveness. Emotional separateness. Some closeness.		Good affective responsiveness. Emotional closeness. Some separateness		Affective interactions encouraged and preferred. High emotional closeness. Low separateness.		High responsiveness and control. Extreme closeness, fusion. Limited separateness.	
PARENT–CHILD RELATIONSHIP	Low parent–child closeness. Rigid generational boundaries.		Some parent–child closeness. Somewhat clear generational boundaries.		Good parent–child closeness. Generally clear generational boundaries.		High parent–child closeness. Clear generational boundaries.		Excessive parent–child closeness. Lack of generational boundaries.	

(continued)

APPENDIX 19.1. *Continued*

Couple/Family Score	DISCONNECTED (disengaged)		SOMEWHAT CONNECTED		CONNECTED		VERY CONNECTED		OVERLY CONNECTED (ENMESHED)	
	1	2	3	4	5	6	7	8	9	10
INTERNAL BOUNDARIES	**Separateness dominates.**		**More separateness than togetherness.**		**Balance of togetherness and separateness.**		**More togetherness than separateness.**		**Togetherness dominates.**	
TIME (Physical & Emotional)	Time apart maximized. Rarely time together.		Time alone important. Some time together.		Good balance of time together and apart.		Time together important. Time alone permitted.		Time together maximized. Little time alone permitted.	
SPACE (Physical & Emotional)	Separate space needed and preferred.		Separate space preferred. Sharing of family space.		Good sharing of space. Private space respected.		Sharing family space. Private space respected.		Little private space permitted.	
DECISION MAKING	Individual decision making emphasized.		Individual decision making but joint possible.		Mainly joint but also individual decisions.		Joint decisions preferred.		Decisions by parents, imposed on children.	
EXTERNAL BOUNDARIES	**Mainly focused outside the family.**		**More focused outside than inside family.**		**Balanced focus inside and outside of family.**		**More focused inside than outside family.**		**Mainly focused inside the family.**	
FRIENDS	Individual friends seen alone.		Individual friends seldom shared with family.		Individual friends shared sometimes with family.		Individual friendships often shared with family.		Family friends preferred. Limited individual friends.	
INTERESTS	Disparate interests.		Separate interests.		Some joint interests.		Many joint interests.		Joint interests mandated.	
ACTIVITIES	Mainly separate activities.		More separate than shared activities.		Balance of shared and individual activities.		More shared than individual activities.		Separate activities seen as disloyal.	
COHESION	**Very Low Unbalanced**		**Low to Moderate Balanced**		**Moderate Balanced**		**Moderate to High Balanced**		**Very High Unbalanced**	

APPENDIX 19.2. Couple and Family Flexibility

Couple/Family Score	INFLEXIBLE (RIGID)		SOMEWHAT FLEXIBLE		FLEXIBLE		VERY FLEXIBLE		OVERLY FLEXIBLE (CHAOTIC)	
	1	2	3	4	5	6	7	8	9	10
LEADERSHIP	Authoritarian leadership.		Primarily authoritarian, but some egalitarian leadership.		Generally egalitarian leadership.		Egalitarian leadership with fluid changes.		Limited and/or erratic leadership.	
DISCIPLINE (for families only)	Autocratic "law and order." Strict, rigid consequences. Not lenient.		Somewhat democratic Predictable consequences. Seldom lenient.		Often democratic. Often negotiated consequences. Somewhat lenient.		Usually democratic. Usually negotiated consequences. Generally lenient.		Laissez-faire and ineffective. Inconsistent consequences. Very lenient.	
NEGOTIATION	Limited negotiations. Decisions imposed by parents.		Structured negotiations. Decisions made by parents.		Flexible negotiations. Generally agreed-upon decisions.		Flexible negotiations. Agreed-upon decisions.		Endless negotiations. Impulsive decisions.	
ROLES	Limited repertoire. Strictly defined roles. Unchanging routines.		Roles stable, but may be shared. Few changes of roles. Routines seldom change.		Role sharing. Some changes of roles. Routines sometimes change.		Role sharing and making. Fluid changes of roles. Routines often change.		Lack of role clarity. Role shifts and role reversals. Few routines.	
RULES	Unchanging rules. Rules strictly enforced.		Few rule changes. Rules firmly enforced.		Some rule changes. Rules generally enforced.		Often rule changes. Rules flexibly enforced.		Frequent rule changes. Rules inconsistently enforced.	
FLEXIBILITY	Very Low Unbalanced		Low to Moderate Balanced		Moderate Balanced		Moderate to High Balanced		Very High Unbalanced	

APPENDIX 19.3. Couple and Family Communication

| | Low ←——— | | Facilitating ——— | | ———→ High | |
Couple/Family Score	1	2	3	4	5	6
LISTENER'S SKILLS Empathy Attentive listening	Seldom evident Seldom evident		Sometimes evident Sometimes evident		Often evident Often evident	
SPEAKER'S SKILLS Speaking for self Speaking for others* *Note reverse scoring	Seldom evident ***Often evident (reversed)**		Sometimes evident **Sometimes evident**		Often evident **Seldom evident**	
SELF-DISCLOSURE		Infrequent discussion of self, feelings, and relationships	Some discussion of self, feelings, and relationships		Open discussion of self, feelings, and relationships.	
CLARITY		Inconsistent and/or unclear verbal messages. Frequent incongruences between verbal and nonverbal messages.	Some degree of clarity, but not consistent across time or across all members. Some incongruent messages.		Verbal messages very clear. Generally congruent messages.	
CONTINUITY/TRACKING	Little continuity of content.	Irrelevant/distracting nonverbals and asides frequently occur. Frequent/inappropriate topic changes.	Some continuity, but not consistent across time or across all members. Some irrelevant/distracting nonverbals and asides. Topic changes not consistently appropriate.		Members consistently tracking. Few irrelevant/distracting nonverbals and asides. Facilitative nonverbals. Appropriate topic changes.	
RESPECT AND REGARD		Lack of respect for feelings or message of other(s). Possibly overtly disrespectful or belitting attitude.	Somewhat respectful of others, but not consistent across time or across all members. Some incongruent messages.		Consistently appears respectful of other's feelings and messages. Few incongruent messages.	

MEASURING FAMILY COMPETENCE

The Beavers Systems Model

W. Robert Beavers
Robert B. Hampson

O ur studies of family processes have evolved over more than 40 years of clinical and research work with a wide range of individuals and families. Given the many aspects of "normal" family processes, our interest has been primarily in here-and-now functioning abilities. Through observing, interviewing, and assessing families across a broad spectrum—various socioeconomic groups, ethnic groups, and styles of functioning, we have developed a variety of measures and core constructs of interactional family functioning that clearly differentiate healthy from less healthy families. This is an assessment made at a particular moment in a family's life in a cross-sectional rather than longitudinal view. These assessments, then, are simply the functioning of families, which includes their biology, their experiences and skills, and their current stressors. We have found that such observations can be most helpful both in determining intervention possibilities and in providing some concepts of optimal functioning.

This research does not attempt to sort out contributions from biology and experience. Indeed, one of our systems views is that a difficult child can produce an angry parent, and an angry parent can produce a difficult child. Determining causality is not our goal, but rather, developing practical information regarding a family's functioning from either 10 minutes of family observation or from a short pencil-and-paper report of individual perceptions of family strengths.

Systems thinking properly recognizes data from neurotransmitters, genetics, individual functioning, family functioning, and broader social phenomena. The meticulous studies of Reiss (see Chapter 22, this volume) have begun to tease out the significance of genetic versus environmental variables in the functioning of adolescents. That task can be contrasted with our efforts to identify family strengths and processes. The results of many variables of each individual's reality converge in a display of immediate family response to a simple stimulus. "Discuss what you would like to see changed in your family" is the stimulus we use to observe family activity in research, clinical, and emergency room settings. This is a question that seems appropriate even to families in acute turmoil. A series of statements based on our observational research has evolved into our Self-Report Family Inventory (SFI), which is a series of statements that an individual family member fills out regarding his or her perceptions of that family. The SFI has been evaluated with good results for reliability and validity over many years.

It is emphasized to our trainees that the observational or self-report is only one source of vital information about families: the first from an outsider's (i.e., researcher/clinician's) perspective; the second from an insider's (i.e., family member's) perceptions. Indeed, it is my firm belief that because family interactions are varied and subtle, no clear and coherent statement can be "true." As Korzybski said, "a map is not the territory" (1933, p. 17). Yet without a map, one can be hopelessly lost in unfamiliar surroundings; our intention has been and remains to offer a clear enough map to help clinicians stay focused on the task at hand, defined by the clients, and not to become lost in a cacophony of techniques, subjective opinions, countertransference possibilities and fads that pop up from time to time. Our evaluations are appropriate for whoever refer to themselves as "family." We have studied (and treated) nuclear, divorced, single-parent, remarried, and quite unconventional families with diverse configurations and have found the methodology appropriate.

Since 1960, we have worked with various groups of researchers to determine cornerstone criteria of family competence as observed at this moment in time. The first published study (Beavers, Blumberg, Timken, & Weiner, 1965) investigated communication patterns in family members of psychiatrically hospitalized adolescents. The Timberlawn study of healthy families (Lewis, Beavers, Gossett, & Phillips, 1976) was the first published report of a detailed examination of well-functioning families that used an interactional, systemic viewpoint. From these and our continuing studies of nonlabeled and clinical families (Beavers, 1982, 1985; Beavers & Voeller, 1983; Beavers, Hampson, & Hulgus, 1985; Hampson & Beavers, 1988, 1996a, 1996b; Hampson, Beavers, & Hulgus, 1988, 1989; Beavers & Hampson, 1990, 2000; Hampson, Hulgus, & Beavers, 1991; Hampson, Hyman, & Beavers, 1994; Hampson, Prince, & Beavers, 1999), some cornerstone criteria for the study of family competence emerge. These concepts, central to the Beavers systems model, are as follows:

1. Family *functioning*—observable, live, interactional functioning— takes precedence over symptoms or typology. Attempting to label clinical typologies, such as "schizophrenic," "addictive," or "codependent," yields little clinically useful information about the functional strengths and vulnerabilities of families and their members.

2. Family *competence,* ranging from effective, healthy family functioning through midrange to severely dysfunctional patterns is viewed along a progressive continuum rather than in segmented categories. This concept promotes the view that observable and measurable growth and adaptation in families is possible.

3. Several families at similar competence levels may show different functional and behavioral *styles* of relating and interacting. The most competent families are able to shift their functional style as developmental changes occur, whereas the most dysfunctional families show a marked rigidity in functional style.

4. Family *assessment* involves perceptions of family events from at least two sources: the observer/therapist ("outsider") and each family member ("insider") (Hampson et al., 1989).

5. Competence in small tasks (such as discussing an issue or resolving a conflict) is related to competence in the larger areas of living, raising children, and managing a family (Beavers, 1977; Lewis, Beavers, Gossett, & Phillips, 1976).

The major constructs and instruments of the Beavers systems model have emerged from this framework. In this chapter, we present the constructs of competence and style, which define levels of family functioning. Next, we present clinically useful groupings of families based on the assessment model. Finally, we present related studies to emphasize the model's validity and clinical utility.

FAMILY COMPETENCE AND STYLE

The Beavers Model emphasizes family competence, that is, how well a family as an interactional unit performs the necessary and nurturing tasks of organizing and managing itself. The major theme of this dimension is the structure of the family unit: The ability of the adults to negotiate and share leadership, and of the family to establish strong, clear generational boundaries is indicative of competence. Conversely, weak adult coalitions, which may include a parent–child coalition and ineffective leadership are indicators of lower levels of system competence. It is important that family members know who is parent and who is child, and operate accordingly.

Highly related to competence is the development of confidence and self-esteem in individual family members, which carries with it increasing trust, clear and direct communication, and the ability to resolve or accept differences. Competent families are more readily able to resolve conflict and communicate openly and directly. These fortunate families are also quite spontaneous, show a wide range of feelings, and are generally optimistic, whereas less functional families show more limited ranges of feelings and more pessimism.

In assessing family competence, it is important to recognize that some families may perform certain tasks better than they do others, but we have not seen one family show extremely competent interaction in one area and dysfunctional levels at all others (Beavers & Hampson, 1990). Hence, a rating of family competence that includes several variables is a useful common denominator of the components of family competence.

When assessed observationally, family competence is measured using the Beavers Interactional Competence Scale. This scale has changed over the years and was reevaluated and renormed several times. Currently, our interrater reliabilities for trained raters are consistently high for both the subscales and for the global score. In terms of validity, scores on the competence scale successfully discriminate clinical from nonclinical families (Beavers et al., 1990) and even between diagnostic subsamples of clinical families (Beavers & Hampson, 1990). We have found no significant differences among nonlabeled Anglo, African American, and Mexican American families on global competence (Hampson, Beavers, & Hulgus, 1990), which suggests that the measures are relatively culturally fair.

As the model evolved, we emphasized the assessment of family style. Style here refers to the degree of centripetal (CP) or centrifugal (CF) qualities in the family. CP family members seek satisfaction more often from within the family, and children are slower to leave home. A specific example would be the family that chooses to home-school their children, believing the home experience superior to that provided by outside institutions and school socialization. CF family members look for satisfaction in the outside world, and the children often leave home earlier than the developmental norm. "It's 10 P.M.—do you know where your children are?" CP families know; CF families often do not. Erikson (1963) used this stylistic dimension in his description of Native American tribes, as did Stierlin (1972) in describing binding versus expelling patterns of families whose adolescents were separating.

CP family members, looking for satisfaction within the family, are somewhat less trustful of the world beyond the family boundaries. CF family members, in contrast, seek gratification from outside the family unit more than from within it. Mixed feelings in family members are handled quite differently in that CP families try to repress, suppress, or deny negative or hostile feelings and play up the positive, caring ones (hence, the "glue" in the CP style that holds children closer and later). In contrast, CF family members are wary of affectionate messages and are more comfortable with negative or angry feelings (hence, the force for outward movement). Extremely CP families tend to bind children and make emancipation difficult, whereas extremely CF families tend to expel children before individuation is complete. These prematurely expelled children often, however, do return home after they have found the outside world more threatening and demanding than they have been able to tolerate. It's not surprising, then, that our studies find more internalizing (anxious, depressive) disorders in extreme CP families and more externalizing (conduct, aggressive) disorders in extreme CF families (Beavers & Hampson, 1990; Hampson & Pierce, 1993).

The Beavers Interactional Style Scales are used observationally to measure the family style (Beavers & Hampson, 1990); this is a revision and update of the previously published Centripetal/Centrifugal Family Style Scale (Kelsey-Smith & Beavers, 1981). Seven observational ratings and a global style rating (ranged 1 to 5, with 1 being highly CP and 5 being highly CF) are completed following the rater's completion of the Competence scale. The rating points represent behavioral correlates of CP or CF styles (Beavers, 1977) and are based on the present observation of the family's response to dependency needs of offspring, overt adult conflict, physical spacing and proximity (when given the choice, CP families tend to sit closer together than CF families), concern about social presentation to outsiders, professed family closeness, degree of expression of angry/hostile feelings, and the balance/skew of positive and negative feelings.

Our studies indicate acceptable to high interrater reliabilities for trained raters. Studies of clinical families also show significant differences between CP and CF families in the distribution of DSM-III-R diagnoses, with significantly more anxiety and unipolar depression in individual patients with CP families, and more conduct and externalizing disorders in individuals with CF families (Hampson & Pierce, 1993). Family style differs slightly among ethnic groupings, with Mexican American families rated as slightly more CP than Anglo or African American families (Hampson et al., 1990). However, style is more clearly related to socioeconomic status of the family than to ethnicity; lower socioeconomic levels are associated with more CF style ratings (Hampson et al., 1990).

In addition to the observational instruments, we have developed the Self-Report Family Inventory (SFI; Beavers & Hampson, 1990), which is able to access individual family members' perceptions of family competence, style, and several related qualities. The 36-item questionnaire (Appendix 20.1) is fairly simple to complete, so that children age 11 have little difficulty completing the items independently. The SFI provides a Competence score for each member and a Cohesion score, which is used as an estimate of Family Style. This factor addresses closeness, togetherness, and tendencies to enjoy time and activities together; as such, it is an approximation of some of the major family themes related to style. In addition, clinically useful scales of Conflict, Leadership, and Emotional Expressiveness can be derived from the questionnaire.

When included with the observational information, the SFI allows a comparison of "insider" and "outsider" perspectives on the family. It also serves as a brief and useful screening device to identify potential family dysfunction. The correlations between observational and self-report Competence scores are very high at the more dysfunctional end of the continuum. The determination of healthy family functioning by self-report has been more elusive, because individual family members at the higher end of functioning may disagree significantly in terms of their views of family health. We continue to study within-family agreement levels and patterns of self-report scores in healthy versus dysfunctional families (Hampson et al., 1994).

BEAVERS SYSTEMS MODEL

Regardless of whether the assessment procedure utilizes observational instruments, self-report scales, or both, the dimensions of competence and style provide a useful map for identifying levels of family health/dysfunction. The observational subscales include overt power, parental coalitions, closeness, mythology, goal-directed negotiation, clarity of expression, responsibility, permeability, range of feelings, mood and tone, unresolvable conflict, and empathy. The style subscales include dependency need, overt/covert conflicts, physical spacing, concerns/lack of concerns of appearance to the outside, profession of closeness, degree of assertiveness/aggressiveness, and ease of expression of positive–negative feelings. Figure 20.1 illustrates this systems model.

The horizontal axis represents the continuum of Family Competence, ranging from optimal functioning (ratings of 1 or 2, on the right) to severely dysfunctional (ratings of 9 or 10, on the left). This continuum of Family Competence shows regression from the capacity for equal powered successful transactions through marked dominance–submission patterns to extreme rigidity (chaotic, with little coherent interaction).

The vertical axis represents Family Style, ranging from highly CP (rating of 1, lower end) to highly CF (rating of 5, upper end). This representation is intended to suggest more extreme styles to be found in the more dysfunctional families, and blended and flexible style in more competent families. Therefore, the figure is in the shape of an arrow, representing the clinical and empirical findings that healthy families show a flexible and blended family style, such that they can adapt stylistic behavior as developmental, individual, and family needs change over time. At the most dysfunctional end of the competence dimension are the most extreme and inflexible family styles. Here, extreme rigidity and limited coping skills preclude variation in style. The V-shaped "notch" on the left repre-

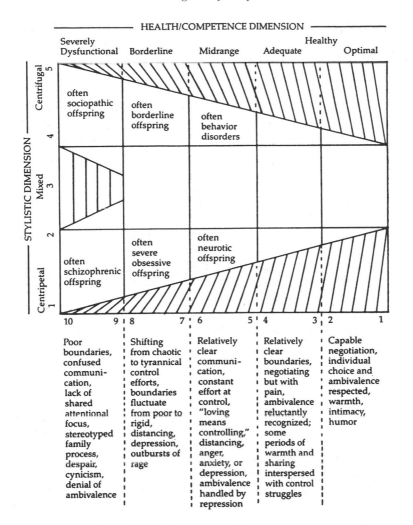

─────────── HEALTH/COMPETENCE DIMENSION ───────────

Severely   Healthy
Dysfunctional Borderline   Midrange   Adequate   Optimal

STYLISTIC DIMENSION

Centrifugal 5

often
sociopathic   often
offspring   borderline
                offspring   often
                                behavior
4   disorders

Mixed 3

2

                often   often
                severe   neurotic
often   obsessive   offspring
schizophrenic   offspring
offspring

Centripetal 1

| 10 | 9 | 8 | 7 | 6 | 5 | 4 | 3 | 2 | 1 |

Poor	Shifting	Relatively	Relatively	Capable
boundaries,	from chaotic	clear	clear	negotiation,
confused	to tyrannical	communi-	boundaries,	individual
communi-	control	cation,	negotiating	choice and
cation,	efforts,	constant	but with	ambivalence
lack of	boundaries	effort at	pain,	respected,
shared	fluctuate	control,	ambivalence	warmth,
attentional	from poor to	"loving	reluctantly	intimacy,
focus,	rigid,	means	recognized;	humor
stereotyped	distancing,	controlling,"	some	
family	depression,	distancing,	periods of	
process,	outbursts of	anger,	warmth and	
despair,	rage	anxiety, or	sharing	
cynicism,		depression,	interspersed	
denial of		ambivalence	with control	
ambivalence		handled by	struggles	
		repression		

FIGURE 20.1. Beavers model of family functioning.

sents the finding that severely disturbed families show more extreme and inflexible styles, with no moderation or blending of stylistic behavior. All our empirical studies support this observation: System rigidity is system sickness (von Bertalanffy, 1969).

This model and its assessment tools offer a snapshot of current family functioning, and the assessment offers useful guidance to the therapist especially in terms of information on strengths and weaknesses, and guidelines on most effective joining and structuring strategies (Hampson & Beavers, 1996b). The scales used in observational evaluation may be obtained from the authors.

CLINICALLY USEFUL GROUPINGS OF FAMILIES

Optimal Families

Systems Orientation

Families that score highest on our observational and self-report measures have members with what we describe as a *systems orientation,* which includes at least five basic assumptions:

1. An individual needs a group, a human system, for identity, support, and satisfaction.
2. Causes and effects are circular; either can become the other.
3. Any human behavior is the result of many variables rather than one "cause"; therefore, simplistic solutions are questioned.
4. Human beings are limited and finite. No one is absolutely helpless or absolutely powerful in a relationship.
5. Conflict is inevitable, just as is ambivalence (mixed feelings), in individuals. These are not evidence of dysfunction. The ability to *resolve* conflict or mixed feelings is necessary for health and competence in individuals and families.

First, optimal family members know that people do not do well alone; human needs are satisfied in relationships. As children develop and mature, they leave their families, not for isolated independence but for other human systems. Whether they enter college or marriage, the military or a fast track career, the need for community continues, and interpersonal skills are required to adapt to these various networks. Some infants are more "cuddly," others are more active, are "movers and shakers." Less adaptive families often perceive both of these as abnormal—the cuddly infant might be considered passive, and the active one can be experienced as avoiding or rejecting a loving parent. More competent families, able to incorporate children with various styles and define them as normal, are therefore capable of accepting wide variations in basic personalities. We have seen many such families, for example, incorporate a child with Down's syndrome and lovingly accept and integrate this child into family life (Beavers, Hampson, Hulgus, & Beavers, 1986).

The second hallmark of a systems view, the recognition that causes and effects are circular, is equally significant. Optimal family members know, for example, that hostility in one person promotes attack or withdrawal in the other, which in turn promotes hostility. Efforts at tyrannical control increase the possibility of angry defiance, just as uncooperative defiance invites tyrannical control. Thus, stimuli become responses and responses stimuli, in a process with shape and form but no clearly defined villains or victims.

Less fortunate or less knowledgeable families can become enmeshed in a triangular victim–persecutor–rescuer pattern. All members accept this view of their plight, but no participant will agree as to who is victim, who is persecutor, and who is rescuer. Linear thinking and a lack of appreciation of subjective views of reality produce never-ending, never-resolved conflictual relationships.

The third concept, that human behavior results from many variables, is possessed by optimal families but painfully absent in dysfunctional families. For instance, when a child of three spills milk at the table, possible explanations include the following:

1. The incident happens accidentally, and no motive should be attached to the behavior.
2. The incident has interpersonal meaning; for example, the child has "a score" to settle with the mother or wishes to provoke her.
3. The child is attempting to express hostile, destructive drives unrelated to the mother.
4. The child is tired or anxious and therefore apt to make mistakes.
5. The problem is mechanical; the glass is too large for the child's small hands.

A characteristic of dysfunctional families is that they believe one or another of these explanations almost exclusively. In contrast, optimal family members consider all these possibilities and make every effort to find the explanation most likely to resolve a particular problem.

Fourth, a systems orientation includes an awareness that humans are finite, that they have limited power, and that self-esteem comes from achieving relative competence rather than from absolute control. Optimal family members know that success in human endeavors depends on variables beyond anyone's control; yet they believe that if they possess goals and purpose, they can make a difference in their own and in others' lives. People are terribly vulnerable if they try to control others absolutely. Negotiation is essential for success in human enterprise, and individual choice must be taken into account. These family members accept that people have the capacity to envision perfection yet are destined to flounder, make mistakes, get scared, and need reassurance. This encourages a sense of humor and an appreciation of paradox. We seek a measure of control over our children, so that they can become adult decision makers; we reach for closeness and support, so that we can define ourselves as separate. We are never free from having mixed feelings about important people and things. We want our children to leave home, but we fear the loneliness their leaving engenders. We resolve mixed feelings by determining action *on balance*—the greater good or lesser evil. No compulsively linear thinkers need apply for entrance into optimal functioning families!

Finally, conflict and ambivalence, or mixed feelings, are inevitable;

they do not indicate either health or illness, competence or incompetence. It is necessary, however, for the conflict and ambivalence to be resolved for families and individuals to function well, and these two concepts are related. It is most difficult for family members to resolve conflict if the individuals have significant unresolved mixed feelings. Discussions are apt to degenerate into arguments that go nowhere, just as individuals who can't make up their minds about important things cannot progress and grow. For example, many adolescents argue for more freedom, yet behave in such a way that encourages limit setting. Parents must have clearly resolved mixed feelings about their roles and their expectations to help the adolescent get words and behavior in harmony.

Clear Boundaries

A useful parallel to the external boundary of an optimal family system is that of a living cell, which possesses enough strength and integrity to allow a highly involved interaction within its borders, yet is permeable to the outside world, to allow a satisfying interchange. Optimal family members are actively involved in the world beyond the family, relate to it with optimism and hope, and from their encounters outside bring varied interests and excitement back into the family. Openness to other viewpoints, lifestyles, and perceptions contribute to the congruent mythology seen in the optimal families studied. Their perceptions of their own family strengths and weaknesses are usually close to observations of outside raters. In addition, optimal families have clear boundaries among members. It is easy to distinguish a mother's feelings from a father's and one child's view of a situation from another child's view. Negotiation consists of accepting differences and working toward shared goals. In such a differentiated family unit, individual choice is expected, family members speak up, and even the youngest children are respected as significant, unique individuals who make valuable contributions.

In addition, there are definite generational boundaries. Though overt power is shared freely, there is no question as to who is parent and who is child. No parents feel obligated to disclaim their adult power, and no children feel called upon to assume a premature responsibility. Parents understand their function of helping children grow up and do not lean on these children for emotional support that is appropriately received from other adults.

Contextual Clarity

In any social context—family, friendship, and patient–therapist—there is a useful rule of thumb in defining the degree of craziness or sanity: How clear is the context? When an optimal family interacts, it is generally clear

to whom comments are addressed and the nature of the relationship between the speaker and the audience. There is a shared theme, and members can continue discussions over a period of time with effective results.
Social roles, though flexible, are clear.

An example of clarifying context is the necessity for parents to resolve
their own competitiveness and rivalries. In dysfunctional families, a child
may be constantly used in parental battles; even a warm "hi, Dad" or "Boy,
that was a good dinner, Mom" can fuel a parental battle. It is necessary for
parents to work out their own conflicts and refuse to triangulate children.
Parents in optimal families assist children in accepting role limitations and
understanding the context of being children by presenting clarity in generation boundaries.

Relatively Equal Power and the Process of Intimacy

A human being, when frightened, seeks some kind of power. Two choices
are available:

1. The power of a loving relationship with others—the experiencing
   of closeness without coercion.
2. The power of control—controls over one's inner self and/or control over others.

In an optimal family, there is a clear hierarchy of power, with leadership in
the hands of the adults who form a coalition with shared power. Children
are less overtly powerful than their parents, but their contributions influence decisions, and their share of overt power increases as they grow toward adulthood. Frustrating, self-defeating power struggles seldom occur,
and family tasks are undertaken with good-humored effectiveness. These
fortunate individuals have learned to deal with fear by relating rather than
by controlling.

Parents in two-parent families have relatively equal overt power and
need complementary interaction in order to avoid competitive conflict.
Perhaps we need to describe more clearly this awkward phrase "equal
overt power." It is reasonable to believe that every family member has as
much power as another. For example, an ill child may control the whole
family, not through overt power but through helplessness. In dysfunctional interaction, power is frequently of the helpless kind or, conversely, an
attempt to be absolutely controlling (omnipotent). The helpless role is
covert power, and this is why we use the admittedly awkward term "equal
overt power."

Generations ago, in two-parent families, the complementary was
defined by tradition as "We are partners in this family endeavor—you
make the living, I will make a home." In these more complex times, fa-

thers and mothers are both very apt to work, and the home activities become a matter of necessary negotiation. Departing from traditional guidelines, each couple necessarily develops its own system of complementarity. Here is the job to be done. How do we work out an equitable arrangement of tasks that we both feel allows for personal dignity and negotiated choice?

Optimal functioning couples are up to this challenge. They do not depend on outworn rules nor rebel from them. (We have seen as many disturbed couples, with men who insist that the wife work whether she wants to or not, as women who adamantly refuse to be domestic.)

The conflictual aspects of systemetrical solutions ("You take the baby when she cries this night, and I will take the baby the next night; you vacuum this week, and I will vacuum the next") was brought home to me by an airline pilot and his spouse, who made the bargain "We will be equal" (i.e., symmetrical). There was endless bickering and unresolved conflict as they both confused sameness with equity in cooperatively accomplishing necessary tasks.

From both clinical work and families research, it is clear that couples in the 21st century must negotiate rules and tasks; both must feel they are valued and not coerced by tradition, social pressures, or their partner. The negotiation goes on as children come into the mix, and chores are increasingly shared as youngsters become more capable. Single-parent families do not have the double edge of necessary negotiation with partners but still must negotiate with offspring to accomplish necessary tasks. Optimal functioning families carry off this task well and offer much information for clinicians in helping less successful families.

These optimal functioning families show the least amount of sexual stereotyping. Though mothers are usually somewhat more involved in child care than fathers in intact families, the fathers are quite involved in ensuring the children's welfare. For children, instead of gender dictating character (females becoming grown-up emotional children, males stoic and oblivious of feelings), birth order is more significant (Beavers, 1977). Oldest children generally have more controlled emotional expression, better discipline, and are more achievement-oriented. Second children show more affective openness, spontaneity, and less concern with achievement or personal discipline. Younger children are often slower in social development and may show more emotion.

Operating with equal overt power fosters intimacy. It is only when power differences are thrown aside that people can experience the sharing of their innermost selves achieved by the dropping of pretense in the presence of trust and the absence of fear. This experience is at once liberating and empowering. It provides a true "launching pad" for family members, enabling parents to go into the community with energy and confidence, and allowing children to approach their developmental tasks of leaving home with exceptional drive and performance.

Autonomy

Optimal family members take responsibility for their own thoughts, feelings, and behavior. They are open to communication from others and respect the unique and different subjective views of reality found in any human group. They express feelings and thoughts clearly, show a relative absence of blame and personal attack, and there is no scapegoating of family members. Because optimal family systems accept uncertainty, ambivalence, and disagreement, members risk little in being known and open. These families recognize people as mistake makers. Parents can issue pronouncements that later prove to be erroneous with little defensiveness. Children can fail without being attacked or defined as inadequate. Tolerance of uncertainty, ambivalence, and imperfection allows family members to be honest, creating a climate in which mutual trust flourishes. Lying is unnecessary if people are not punished for telling the truth as they have experienced it.

Joy and Comfort in Relating

Transactions among optimal functioning family members are notable not only for their warm, optimistic tone of feeling but also for their intensity. Empathy for each other's feelings, interest in what each other has to say, and expectation of being understood encourage members to respond to each other with concern and action. Their orientation is affiliative; each person expects satisfaction and reward from relationships, and this reinforces involvement with and investment in each other. Assessment of this affiliative attitude in a family is based on a complex synthesis of behavior, voice tone, verbal context, and communicative patterns.

As a corollary to an affiliative expectation, optimal functioning family members see human nature as essentially benign. Human needs for sexual expression, intimacy, and assertiveness are recognized with an absence of apprehension. People are understood to be struggling to do as well as possible under their particular circumstances, rather than to be fundamentally hostile or destructive. There is variability in the extent to which people outside the family are seen as benign, but all optimal functioning families include at least their own members in this assumption. The belief that the other is basically benign and of good will is essential to the success of any effort at achieving closeness. Indeed, this is where we begin in working with couples and families. Without this leap of faith, no useful work will occur.

Skilled Negotiation

In shared tasks, optimal functioning family members excel in their capacity to accept directions, organize themselves, develop input from each other, negotiate differences, and reach closure coherently and effectively. Parents act as coordinators, bringing out others' ideas and voicing their own. They usually alternate this role several times in a short planning session. All the variables important in family systems come into play, including clarity of context, relatively equal power, affiliative expectations, and encouragement of choice. Family performance in specified small-scale tasks correlates with overall competence in parenting. This negotiating skill is present is all groups of optimal functioning families that we have studied—middle-class white, disadvantaged white, African American, Hispanic, single-parent, and unconventional family groups (Hampson et al., 1990).

Significant Transcendent Values and Beliefs

Capable families accept change. Children grow up, themselves becoming parents. Parents grow old and die. To accept the inevitable risks and losses of loving and being close, families and individuals appear to require a system of values and beliefs that transcends the limits of their experience and knowledge. With such transcendent beliefs and values, families and their members can view their particular reality, which may be painful, uncertain, and frightening, from a perspective that makes some sense of events and allows for hope. Without such beliefs and perspective, families and individuals are vulnerable to hopelessness and despair.

The ability to accept change and loss is closely tied to the acceptance of the idea of one's own mortality. Only by using the human capacity for symbolism, defining oneself as part of a meaningful whole, can one's own death and that of loved ones be faced openly and courageously. Just as no individual person can survive and prosper without relating to an organizational unit—usually a family—no family can survive and prosper without a larger system. A transcendent value system, whether conventional or unique, allows individuals and families to define themselves and their activities as meaningful and significant (see Walsh & Pryce, Chapter 13, this volume).

Implicit in the behavior and relationships of all families are certain attitudes about human nature and the nature of truth. For optimal functioning families, these attitudes encompass a positive view of humanity as essentially good, or at least as neutral, and of human behavior as a response to experiences and an effort to deal with problems. The behavior and relationships of these family members also imply an understanding of truth as relative rather than as absolute; or, expressed another way, they permit family members to approach reality as subjective and different for each person. With these two underlying assumptions about people and reality, healthy families are able to relate with trust, without erecting ponderous interpersonal defenses.

Limits to This Rosy Picture of Optimal Families

It is important to put the foregoing description of optimal families in perspective. Yes, these skills are present, and these attitudes are found, but the overall description suggests a near perfection that is wondrously absent! Healthy families, like other healthy organisms, have defects and weaknesses resulting from the very processes that produce this health. Along with the capabilities are also fears of the unusual, or a need to control through affluence, or concerted efforts to blot out what is nonnormative or disturbing. Such flaws are a part of the health and the vibrancy of any competent family. These real limitations represent vulnerability; no family can be confident that its skills can encompass all possible environmental stresses.

Indeed, in our original group of volunteer families, some of the most effective families fell upon hard times. The father in one of those families became unemployed. He began to drink more, and his wife was forced to take a job. On remeasure of the SFI, the family was at the low midrange. Another optimal family, 3 years after observation, placed the youngest child, at age 17, in a psychiatric hospital for depression. The boy may have been biologically vulnerable, lost in a high school jungle, or perhaps the parents were resisting the loss of active parenting, but this stressed adolescent put great strain on the family. In another optimal family, all went well for several years, but then the marriage broke up after the children left home. Some couples do much better when there are lively youngsters at home.

The optimal families studied were fortunate in not having very much illness or early death in the family. The foregoing qualities of optimal families, then, are to be cherished but may not be sustained throughout a family lifecycle. In fact, as we have given lectures on family health in recent years, *luck* has risen in significance, because families can be blindsided by loss of job, illness, or unexpected deaths, which can precipitate a marked drop in functioning. Indeed, pediatrician E. James Anthony (1969) found family regression similar to that shown in Figure 20.1, from optimal to midrange to severely dysfunctional, in describing the impact of a child with leukemia on the family. Today's optimal families may decline in function depending on biological contributions of its members and contextual, environmental circumstances. Families have limits, and stresses may occur that are beyond the adaptive capabilities of the family.

Adequate Families

Adequate families have also been found to be relatively effective, competent systems. Their boundaries are clear, and a gratifying presence of both intimacy and individual responsibility is encouraged. They contrast optimal families, however, in a greater emphasis on control efforts; conflicts are more often resolved through intimidation rather than negotiation.

The parental coalition in intact families is less effective; the emotional needs of each adult are shortchanged, although the parents characteristically cooperate in parenting efforts. These families also exhibit more evidence of stress and emotional pain than do optimal functioning ones. Family interaction produces less joy, less intimacy and trust, and is less spontaneous than in optimal functioning families. Role stereotyping, particularly in sex roles, is more evident and approaches that seen in midrange families. These families do, however, develop children that test as competent as those from optimal functioning families, apparently because of family members' strong belief in the importance of family life. Thus, tenacity and genuine caring prove effective despite more modest parenting and negotiating skills. They certainly can be called "normal."

Midrange Families

Midrange families constitute the most numerous of family groups; hence, they also can be called "normal" in the sense of average. Both parents and children are more susceptible to psychiatric illness. They evidence obvious pain and difficulty in functioning over the lifecycle. Characteristically, an emphasis on control efforts reduces possibilities for intimacy.

Boundary problems are most evident in the abiding efforts of family members to control one another's thoughts and feelings: "You shouldn't think that way," "You will disgrace the family by talking that way," and "Loving means controlling" represent midrange family mottos, whether expressed openly or not, derived from a pervasive belief that people are basically evil, and that caring is shown by controlling oneself and others. Thus, there will be a "war" in the nursery, with loving parenting understood as controlling the inborn antisocial impulses of the young.

There are frequently subtle or broad evidences of unresolved generation boundaries. Coalitions between parent and child that are stronger than parental bonds are often accepted as natural. These both produce and result from parental conflict and make it more difficult for children to fulfill the immensely important task of leaving home.

In this group of families, one sees the most slavish repetition of cultural stereotyping. Stoic, insensitive males and emotional, overtly dependent females abound. Healthier families are freer to make up their own minds about their roles in this society; very disturbed families are alienated from the culture and, hence, are less influenced by it. It is the broad group of midrange families that continues to validate and pass on cultural stereotypes.

Midrange family members acknowledge mixed feelings in themselves and others but tend to condemn these feelings. Fears of the outside world are defined as cowardice. Needs for independence are often characterized as willfulness and disrespect for elders. In addition, these families have a hard time dealing with infants who, though normal, do not fit within the parents' expected range. Sometimes there is more passivity or more aggressiveness that falls outside the parenting range of these families, and difference can be interpreted as abnormal.

Negotiating becomes far more difficult due to the greater problems with boundaries, accepting ambivalence, and the need for autonomy. More decisions are unilateral, and more solutions are based on power plays and intimidation.

Midrange family members have a self-definition that is coherent but quite vulnerable because of its limited nature. Repression is a common way of handling the condemned half of mixed feelings, and the return of that which is repressed remains a continuing threat to emotional health. Children in these families grow up with many developmental tasks only partially completed. Leaving home is difficult in any style of midrange families, and the children may fall prey to the development of neuroses or behavior disturbances.

Midrange Centripetal Families

These families manifest great concern for rules and authority; they expect overt, authoritarianism to be successful in controlling the base impulses of family member. Because expressions of hostility and overt anger are disapproved and expressions of "love" and "caring" approved, raised and vented feelings of frustration and conflict are infrequent. Therefore, conflict resolution, clarity of expression, and competent negotiation are compromised. Only modest spontaneity shines through the web of concern for rules, order, and authority. Sex stereotyping is very strong in these families: Dependent, emotional women and strong, silent, authority-based men are predominant. Hence, the marital relationship is a male-led unit, often with depressed wives carrying out the vast majority of household and child-rearing duties.

These families promote internalization and repression to deal with distress and upset. When psychiatric illness occurs, it is usually manifested in anxiety disorders, mild depression, and somatizing disorders. Concern for properness and authority make them "good" patients who pay their bills, work hard, and keep their problems well hidden from the community.

Midrange Centrifugal Families

Like midrange CP families, midrange CF families attempt to control by authority and intimidation; however, they find over time that such control is ineffective and come to expect that their control efforts will not be successful. Hence, the belief evolves that outsiders will discover their inadequacies. These family members deal with this inevitable lack of control with frontal assaults and blame, usually spread across all members from time to time. Anger and derogatory blame are far more frequent manifestations of emotion than warmth or sharing. Adults spend little time in the home, and unresolved power and control struggles are commonplace. Children observe that one survives through maneuvering and blaming others; they move out into the streets earlier than the norm and often have difficulty with authority figures. When they manifest psychiatric difficulties, these usually take the form of acting-out behaviors such as vandalism, sexual precocity, substance abuse, and conduct disorders. They rarely voluntarily present for treatment, because they have a reliance on action and a distrust of words and relationships.

Midrange Mixed Families

This group of families displays competing and alternating CP and CF behavior, which reduces the rigidity of the more extreme style but concomitantly increases inconsistency and uncertainty of position in the family. The attempts at control are consistent, but the effects vary at different times or with different children, depending on internal scapegoating patterns. Couples in this group experience role tension and struggles; they can present well socially but engage in blaming and hostile attacks on other occasions or in private. They distance through work or independent social activities. It is common for one child to manifest internalizing symptoms while another is openly defiant and hostile.

Borderline Families

These families are more concerned about control issues than are midrange families. CP borderline families pursue control more effectively than do the CF group, but both family groupings are preoccupied with control to near exclusion of concerns for joy, satisfaction, or intimacy. Individual family members find little emotional support from the family. Developmental tasks are difficult to accomplish in these surroundings; resolution of ambivalence about important issues is accomplished infrequently, and both separation and individuation are compromised.

These families alternate between earnest efforts at control and a peculiar "zaniness," in which the focus of conversation or interaction is lost and incoherence results. Boundary problems are quite apparent, both of the "You should" variety (efforts to control another's thinking and feeling) and the "You *really* think (or feel)" (invasions of another's experience of self). These invasions are, however, much less frequent than those seen in severely dysfunctional families. The mood of the family varies from overt depression to overt rage, with little evidence of joy.

Borderline Centripetal Families

These families represent a difficult challenge for family therapists. They are well-enough organized to attempt control of the outside world, including therapists, as well as to pursue controlling efforts within the family.

Ambivalence is only reluctantly recognized or admitted, which leads to the frequent demonstration of incoherence in interactions (what we have termed "zaniness"). In watching this group of families, it is usual to see effective domination and control disintegrate into confusion and disorganization characteristic of severely dysfunctional families, and this disarray in turn chaotically reverts to controlled interaction.

Offspring are typically compulsive, whether defined as symptomatic or not. Symptom complexes include severe obsessive–compulsive states, depression, and anorexia. The modal patient with anorexia has dynamics quite isomorphic with the family dynamics—seeming to have given up hope or expectation of enjoyment to efforts for total control, which is always out of reach and often self-destructive; that is, one can never control others except by thwarting them. Children who succeed in controlling parents defeat themselves and any efforts to grow up and leave home.

Borderline Centrifugal Families

These families are much more open than borderline CP families in the expression of anger, with ample leave taking and frequent direct assaults. The parental coalition is loosely connected, and stormy battles occur with high regularity. These systems produce a sense of "no-man's land," where children are left with little or no nurturance or support. Each individual is on his or her own to try to derive whatever satisfaction can be gained by manipulation or reckless attention seeking. Ambivalence is dramatically evident but unacknowledged. Desired nurturance is never obtained, and the resulting impetus toward depression is masked by anger and rebelliousness. Children learn to manipulate within this unstable oscillating system. Many receive a label of "borderline personality disorder" as they carry these behaviors into the outside world.

Severely Dysfunctional Families

These families are the most limited in negotiating conflicts and in adapting to developmental demands and situational crises. Family members have the most trouble resolving ambivalence and defining goals. The main lack, and the greatest need, is coherence in interaction. Such families have a poorly defined power structure; unclear, ineffective, and unsatisfying communication; extreme problems in interpersonal boundaries; few negotiation skills; and a pervasively depressed or cynical tone. The family power structure is difficult to define, and communication is chronically ineffective. Family members characteristically lack a shared focus of attention, and any parental coalition is in shambles.

Family members in severely dysfunctional families deny the passage of time and its implications for growth and development, aging and death. Behavior and feelings are quite often unresponsive to the changing abilities of family members, who have great difficulty in looking forward to the future and making effective plans. Ambivalence is typically expressed in a sequential fashion; that is, family members tend to express first one side and then another of the strong mixed feelings that they have toward one another. There is little "glue" in these ambivalent communications, and the listener is left to interpret and make some sense out of quite opposite communications (Beavers, Blumberg, Timken, & Weiner, 1965).

The lack of individuality or differentiation of self in these families leads to profound difficulties in members' ability to decide on and move toward goals, as well as in their capacity to resolve conflicts and deal with pressing problems. The system wallows like a rudderless ship. The mood and tone of feeling are the most painful found in any of the family classifications. Expressions of warmth and affirmation are rare. Severely disturbed families feel chronically disappointed, frustrated, angry, resentful, and guilty. In these families and individuals, a basic developmental task, that of evolving trust, remains unfinished.

The child growing up in such families develops a quite incomplete sense of self or identity, because choice is so important in the development of the self. Sharing powerful feelings with family members and reaching out to friends and loved ones are necessary to mourn the inevitable losses that accompany growth and development, aging and death. With the lack of a shared focus of attention, the boundary defects, and the communicational obscurity and isolation, no one in such families deals well with loss. Finally, dysfunctional patterns become cyclical, because such unmourned loss blocks the next generation's efforts to develop competent families.

Severely Dysfunctional Centripetal Families

This group of severely disturbed families has a tough, nearly impermeable outer boundary. The family is usually seen as strange or odd by neighbors, and family loyalty requires remaining in the family and either physically or emotionally never leaving home. Family members are expected to think and feel alike, with no comprehension of uniquely subjective human responses to the world. There are severe boundary problems. Children receive few clear messages and many confusing ones. Parents speak for children ("You don't really mean that; you really love your sister. You don't hate her"). Family members are unable to experience or express a sense of individual identity.

The coalition between family adults always functions poorly. Relationships are maintained through polite role playing, although the adults' inability to relate to each other closely is obvious on direct observation. Generational boundaries are unclear; there are continually confusing contexts, and the result is communicational obscurity. Due to the lack of a shared focus of attention and the pervasive communicational obscurity, dealing with loss by sharing is quite impossible.

Children in these families are characteristically quite inhibited and overcontrolled; for them, one result of the conflict between developmental pressures toward separation and family rules of remaining loyal and static is an extremely low level of functioning, as is found in schizophrenia in families that have a genetic predisposition to such illness.

Severely Dysfunctional Centrifugal Families

These families are characterized by an extremely diffuse boundary with the outside world. Family organization is unstable. Parents move in and out, children run away, and the very definition of who constitutes the family is often ambiguous. Family interaction is marked by competition, teasing, manipulation, and open conflicts that are never resolved. Interpersonal skills are so limited that children and even parents may leave home but, usually unsuccessful in personal and occupational endeavors, return to the family as needful and hostile as before.

Parental discipline is attempted through intimidation but usually fails because of the shifting, ineffective power structure and the lack of positive relationships. Family members are unreceptive to each other's efforts to communicate, and there is a marked lack of empathy. The quarrelsome, angry family interaction and the hostile, antisocial behavior of individual members can be seen as a defense against the pain and sadness of emotional deprivation. These family members find hostility easy to express, but tenderness, loneliness, and emotional pain are difficult or impossible to admit. Physical abuse is common in these families. Inept parenting and relating lead to great frustration, and family members' control of impulses is often inadequate.

These families may produce sociopathic offspring (antisocial personalities). Children can find no way to be loved by obeying the rules, because the rules shift, and no behavior patterns are rewarded consistently by closeness or caring. They learn to present an "I don't care" facade and to share the family viewpoint that all those within its boundaries are bad, even evil. The resulting unacceptable behavior of these children provokes social rejection and punishment, which further encourages self-loathing. Self-defeating behavior expresses their rage to an uncaring world.

Many of these families are embedded in a hostile community environment, and their functioning is affected by extreme poverty, racism, and a generalized sense of hopelessness regarding any improvement of circumstances. More often than not, there is a negative interaction between family and community, mirroring the negative relationship between individual and family. Such an environment makes great demands on family strengths and competence, with only the most resilient families and members able to thrive.

PRACTICAL USE AND RESEARCH

This approach to family assessment, based on general systems theory, was designed for training, research, and treatment. It has been quite useful in research (Beavers & Hampson, 1990; Hampson et al., 1990, 1991, 1994, 1999; Hampson & Beavers, 1996a, 1996b). It remains the basic tool of our training methodology, providing a practical, easily understood way for students to grasp a systemic perspective. Currently, we use the observational measures primarily for teaching; we use it for research only when we can obtain the necessary funds and personnel for such more intensive family evaluations. For our general work with clients, we rely more and more on the SFI (the simple pencil-and-paper test), because it has been shown to be well correlated with the observational measures in clinic samples. We have found that this is more sensitive to modest changes in family functioning and is, therefore, quite useful in determining movement in treatment. This self-report instrument and its scoring methodology are provided in Appendix 20.1.

Because the Family Studies Center works with inner-city families (primarily through Head Start Greater Dallas, Inc. and the Dallas Independent School System Special Education children and their families), we use the SFI as both a screening device whenever possible, and as a way to determine the effectiveness of intervention (Hampson & Beavers, 1996a). Inner-city families of our acquaintance are often suspicious of television cameras and one-way mirrors, and the SFI is a more easily accepted method of obtaining needed information about these families.

With increasing use of the instrument, our database is continuing to grow. Many researchers around the country and abroad contact us for permission to use the SFI. We gladly grant it and frequently receive the results of their studies, adding to our overall information regarding use of the SFI with families around the world. This instrument has been translated into nine languages and is used, by last count, in 15 countries. We have found that there is a widespread need for quick and useful evaluations of family functioning.

Recent studies in the United States that utilize the SFI include Diamond and Liddle (1996), Duff (1996), Johnson (2001), Knudson-Martin (2000), and Krawetz et al. (2001). Researchers and clinicians in many other countries are invested in the Beavers systems model, and utilize the SFI and/or the observational methodology. These countries include Canada (Laporte, Marcoux, & Guttman, 2001), Ireland (Carr, 2000; Drumm,

Carr, & Fitzgerald, 2000), Finland (Räiha, Lehtonen, Huhtala, Saleva, & Korvenranta, 1999; Räiha, Lehtonen, & Korvenranta, 1995), Norway (Haugland & Havik, 1998; Dundas, 1994), Sweden (Sundelin & Hansson, 1999), Denmark and Sweden (Wallin, Roijen, & Hansson, 1996), and Germany (Steininger & Frank, 1999).

Our more recent research has followed two major themes, both related to attempts to assist families through family or couple counseling. One rationale for the continued development of the assessment scales is the clinical utility for therapists and researchers to measure change globally and to help with intervention planning. Our book (1990) presented clinically based suggestions for therapists to use with certain types of families. Our more recent studies have confirmed that certain groupings of families fare better with certain forms of intervention and types of therapist relationships. The "normal" families at midrange levels and above, with less serious disturbance, tend to do quite well in therapy, as if they need more of a mentor or "coach" than a regulator. Below-average families in the clinical range are more disturbed and require more structure in therapy.

One set of research studies came from a cumulative 16-year experience with families and student therapists at our Dallas clinic. Families came from all walks of life, referred by schools, physicians, and others. Therapy was provided for all who came in, and many of the cases were completely subsidized. Given the research orientation of the institute, before the first session, all clients completed self-report forms at the initial session and were videotaped during the discussion task ("Discuss together what you would like to see changed in your family"). Both the therapist and teams of trained raters observed the family's interaction, then rated its competence and style using the updated Beavers Interactional Scales. At the third session, therapists completed a self-rating dealing with the degree of disclosure ("openness"), power differential, and partnership with that particular family/couple. All measures were scheduled to be repeated at the sixth session and again at termination.

The most salient and consistent finding across the families (Hampson & Beavers, 1996a, 1996b) and couples (Hampson et al., 1999) was the relationship between family competence at the outset and the gains made in therapy. With very few exceptions, the more competent systems fared best in treatment. There were strong associations between therapist-rated goal attainment, pre–post observational gains, and family-perceived goal attainment and the observational competence rating at the outset. A large portion of the "more competent" subjects were midrange families.

The number of therapy sessions was also related to outcome. As a general rule, those families that attended more sessions made greater gains. When families attending only one session were removed from the data, the overall improvement rate was 86.6%.

Many of the demographic and structural aspects of families, including ethnicity, single- versus two-parent families, gender of therapist, and structural types of families (foster, adoptive, step, multigenerational), were unrelated to therapy outcome. One demographic factor was consistent in predicting outcome in therapy: Larger families had worse treatment results than smaller families.

Functional qualities were much stronger predictors of therapy outcome. Different functional qualities of families are directly related to outcome with respect to the nature of the communication, emotional tone, coherence, and power differential in the therapy room. We have long asserted that families with different levels of competence and different styles need different qualities and relationships with their therapists. Families in dire need of clarity and coherence need someone who can structure, clarify, and direct, whereas such qualities might even be counterproductive in a midrange CP family (Beavers & Hampson, 1990).

To evaluate the impact of therapeutic relationship and style on outcome in family therapy, we studied a subset of 175 families from the larger sample of 434. These were families who came to at least three sessions and provided sufficient data about the therapeutic relationship and operating style. They were classified in terms of their initial competence and style: adequate families (15), midrange CP (38), midrange mixed (17), borderline CP (51), borderline CF (37), dysfunctional CP (9), and dysfunctional CF (8). There was a direct linear relationship between competence and outcome (Hampson & Beavers, 1996b).

For adequate families, the most advantageous therapeutic environment is one of collaboration, in which the therapist can be open and direct, with moderate to low levels of power difference. Midrange CP families, like adequate families, fared best with therapists who offered high levels of openness and low power differential. Those midrange CP families that made fewer gains had therapists with significantly lower levels of openness. Midrange mixed families who made greater gains in therapy had moderate levels of openness and partnership from their therapists, as well as a moderate amount of power differential.

Borderline CP families who attained the highest levels of goal attainment had therapists with significantly higher levels of partnership and openness, and significantly lower levels of power differential. This latter finding was a surprise to us, because our clinical experience has suggested that many of these control-oriented, rigid systems require a strong, directive therapist. However, the data suggest that these borderline CP families do better with higher levels of openness and partnership, and moderate levels of power differential.

Borderline CF families had less of a relationship between length of therapy and outcome. Of all the groups so far, they had the highest dropout rate, and there were no significant differences between high and low goal attainment groups on any of the therapist variables. At least a moderate degree of partnership appeared necessary for families to return, and for some gains to be made.

Dysfunctional CP families, so lacking in coherence and appropriate boundaries, apparently need a therapist who is a director. Although the overall goal attainment was relatively low on an absolute scale, families that did better in this group had therapists who employed a significantly higher power differential and significantly lower levels of openness and partnership. Therapists with stronger leadership and control strategies tended to do better with these chaotic families. Hence, the therapist qualities matched the emotional tone of these families. Once coherence is developed, the therapist can then begin modeling warmth and negotiation skills.

Finally, severely dysfunctional CF families showed a stronger relationship between number of sessions and outcome. Therapists who can get these families to return have accomplished a major task. Those families that fared better in treatment (although this group had the absolute lowest levels of goal attainment) had therapists with higher power differential, lower levels of openness, and significantly lower levels of partnership. The absolute differences between these therapist variables were fairly substantial, but the sample size (8 total) was small. Unfortunately, not too many of these families made it as far as three therapy sessions.

Overall, these data suggest that more competent families fare better in therapy and respond to therapists who join them, disclose strategy, and maintain more egalitarian partnerships. This mirrors the classic description of the "therapy alliance" (Greenberg & Pinsof, 1986). More dysfunctional families need more direction and few reasons why a certain strategy is suggested. Family style also makes a difference, with CP families in general responding to a more traditional therapist stance (warm, genuine, words as curative). CF families, whose style is more externalizing, and for whom words are typically ineffective for communication or change, typically require therapists who can structure and coordinate actions, with clear boundaries, because closeness is threatening to family members.

In a study of couples' progress in couple/marital therapy, we found the same main predictors (Hampson et al., 1999). The more competent the partners at the outset, and the more competent they believed themselves to be at the outset, the greater their gains in therapy. Also, number of children in the family was a significant predictor of outcome; couples with no or few children fared better in therapy than those with more children. From this observation, we found an additional variable predicting success in treatment: Childless couples versus those who had children at home. Childless couples fared significantly better in couple therapy. When a couple seeks help for that dyadic relationship, it helps if they can focus on their relationships, without child-rearing responsibilities.

Furthermore, whether or not this was the first or a later marriage for the couple also made a difference, but not as a single main effect (Hampson et al., 1999). This was also affected by whether or not there were children at home. Interestingly, the group that fared best in therapy was remarried couples with no children, followed by first-married couples with no children, then first-married couples with children. Remarried couples with children fared the worst in couple therapy; these more complicated family structures may need more time and guidance to work through issues of discipline and mixed emotional patterns.

In combination, these studies provide information related to normal family functioning. First, in helping families improve their functioning toward the healthy range, therapists can be assisted by tailoring strategies that depend on the family's competence and style. They can also be alerted to certain challenges and risk factors in treatment by using a relatively brief and inexpensive assessment procedure, with the observational scales, the SFI, or both. Second, we continue to search for more effective, practical, and low-cost ways to assist individuals and families. The conceptual framework and the instruments developed and described here guide our work.

REFERENCES

Anthony, E. J. (1969). The mutative impact on family life of serious mental and physical illness in a patient. *Canadian Psychiatric Association Journal, 14*(5): 433–453.

Beavers, J. A., Hampson, R. B., Hulgus, Y. F., & Beavers, W. R. (1986). Coping in families with a retarded child. *Family Process, 25,* 365–378.

Beavers, W. R. (1977). *Psychotherapy and growth.* New York: Brunner/Mazel.

Beavers, W. R. (1982). Health, midrange, and severely dysfunctional families. In F. Walsh (Ed.), *Normal family processes* (1st ed., pp. 45–66). New York: Guilford Press.

Beavers, W. R. (1985). *Successful marriage: A family systems approach to martial therapy.* New York: Norton.

Beavers, W. R., Blumberg, S., Timken, K. R., & Weiner, M. D. (1965). Communication patterns of mothers of schizophrenics. *Family Process, 4,* 95–104.

Beavers, W. R., & Hampson, R. B. (1990). *Successful families: Assessment and intervention.* New York: Norton.

Beavers, W. R., & Hampson, R. B. (2000). The Beavers Systems Model of family functioning. *Journal of Family Therapy, 22,* 128–143.

Beavers, W. R., Hampson, R. B., & Hulgus, Y. F. (1985). The Beavers Systems approach to family assessment. *Family Process, 24,* 398–405.

Beavers, W. R., Hampson, R. B., & Hulgus, Y. F. (1990). *Manual: Beavers Systems Model of Family Assessment.* Dallas: Southwest Family Institute.

Beavers, W. R., & Voeller, M. N. (1983). Family models: Comparing the Olson circumplex model with the Beavers systems model. *Family Process, 22,* 85–98.

Carr, A. (2000). Empirical approaches to family assessment. *Journal of Family Therapy, Vol. 22*(2): 121–127.

Diamond, G., & Liddle, H. A. (1996). Resolving a therapeutic impasse between parents and adolescents in multidimensional family therapy. *Journal of Consulting and Clinical Psychology, 64*(3), 481–488.

Drumm, M., Carr, A., & Fitzgerald, M. (2000). The Beavers, McMaster and Circumplex clinical rating scales: A study of their sensitivity, specificity and discriminant validity. *Journal of Family Therapy, 22*, 225–238.

Duff, S. E. (1996). A study of the effects of group family play on family relations. *International Journal of Play Therapy, 5*(2), 81–93.

Dundas, I. (1994). The Family Adaptability and Cohesion Scale III in a Norwegian sample. *Family Process, 33*(2), 191–202.

Erikson, E. H. (1963). *Childhood and society.* New York: Norton.

Greenberg, L. S., & Pinsof, W. M. (Eds.). (1986). *The psychotherapeutic process: A research handbook.* New York: Guilford Press.

Hampson, R. B., & Beavers, W. R. (1988). Comparing males' and females' perspectives through family self-report. *Psychiatry, 50*, 24–30.

Hampson, R. B., & Beavers, W. R. (1996a). Family therapy and outcome: Relationships between therapist and family styles. *Contemporary Family Therapy, 18*, 345–370.

Hampson, R. B., & Beavers, W. R. (1996b). Measuring family therapy outcome in a clinical setting. *Family Process, 35*, 347–360.

Hampson, R. B., Beavers, W. R., & Hulgus, Y. F. (1988). Comparing the Beavers and Circumplex models of family functioning. *Family Process, 27*, 85–92.

Hampson, R. B., Beavers, W. R., & Hulgus, Y. F. (1989). Insiders' and outsiders' views of family: The assessment of family competence and style. *Journal of Family Psychology, 3*, 118–136.

Hampson, R. B., Beavers, W. R., & Hulgus, Y. F. (1990). Cross-ethnic family differences: Interactional assessment of white, black, and Mexican-American families. *Journal of Marital and Family Therapy, 16*, 307–319.

Hampson, R. B., Hulgus, Y. F., & Beavers, W. R. (1991). Comparisons of self-report measures of the Beavers Systems Model and Olson's Circumplex Model. *Journal of Family Psychology, 4*(3), 326–340.

Hampson, R. B., Hyman, T. L., & Beavers, W. R. (1994). Age of recall effects on family-of-origin ratings. *Journal of Marital and Family Therapy, 20*(1), 61–67.

Hampson, R. B., & Pierce, J. A. (1993). *Within-family patterns of self-report ratings.* Unpublished manuscript, Southern Methodist University, Dallas, TX.

Hampson, R. B., Prince, C. C., & Beavers, W. R. (1999). Martial therapy: Qualities of couples who fare better or worse in treatment. *Journal of Marital and Family Therapy, 25*, 411–424.

Haugland, B. S. M., & Havik, O. E. (1998). Correlates of family competence in families with Paternal alcohol abuse. *Psychological Reports, 83*, 867–880.

Johnson, P. (2001). Dimensions of functioning in alcoholic and nonalcoholic families. *Journal of Mental Health Counseling, 23*(2), 127–136.

Kelsey-Smith, M., & Beavers, W. R. (1981). Family assessment: Centripetal and centrifugal family systems. *American Journal of Family Therapy, 9*, 3–21.

Knudson-Martin, C. (2000). Gender, family competence, and psychological symptoms. *Journal of Marital and Family Therapy, 26*(3), 317–328.

Korzybski, A. (1933). *Science and sanity.* Lancaster, PA: International Non-Aristotelian Library.

Krawetz, P., Fleisher, W., Pillay, N., Staley, D., Arnett, J., & Maher, J. (2001). Family functioning in subjects with pseudoseizures and epilepsy. *Journal of Nervous and Mental Disease, 189*(1), 38–43.

Laporte, L., Marcoux, V., & Guttman, H. A. (2001). Caracteristiques des familles de femmes presentant un trouble d'anerexie mentale restrictie compares a celles de familles temoins: A comparison of the characteristics of families of women with restricting anorexia nervosa and a control group. *Encephale,* *27*(2), 109–119.

Lewis, J. M., Beavers, W. R., Gossett, J. T., & Phillips, V. A. (1976). *No single thread: Psychological health in family systems.* New York: Brunner/Mazel.

Räiha, H., Lehtonen, L., Huhtala, V., Saleva, K., & Korvenranta, H. (1999). Excessively crying infant in the family. *European Child and Adolescent Psychiatry, 8*(2): 646–650.

Räiha, H., Lehtonen, L., & Korvenranta, H. (1995). Family context of infantile colic. *Infant Mental Health Journal, 16*(3), 206–217.

Reiss, D., with Neiderhiser, J. M., Hetherington, E. M., & Plomin, R. (2000). *Deciphering genetic and social influences on adolescent development: The relationship code.* Cambridge, MA: Harvard University Press.

Steininger, C., & Frank, R. (1999). Interactional processes in families of children with internalizing and externalizing disorders [Abstract]. *European Child and Adolescent Psychiatry, 8*(2), 209.

Stierlin, H. (1972). *Separating parents and adolescents.* New York: Quadrangle Press.

Sundelin, J., & Hansson, K. (1999). Intensive family therapy: A way to change family functioning in multi-problem families. *Journal of Family Therapy, 21,* 419–432.

von Bertalanffy, L. (1969). General systems theory—an overview. In W. Gray, F. J. Duhl, & N. D. Rizzo (Eds.), *General systems theory and psychiatry* (pp. 33–46). Boston: Little, Brown.

Wallin, U., Roijen, S., & Hansson, K. (1996). Too close or too separate: Family function in families with an anorexia nervosa patient in two Nordic countries. *Journal of Family Therapy, 18*(4), 397–414.

APPENDIX 20.1
SELF-REPORT FAMILY INVENTORY

NAME _____ DATE _____

FILE # _____ CHECK ONE: ___ FATHER ___ MOTHER ___ SON ___ DAUGHTER AGE ___

SELF-REPORT FAMILY INVENTORY: VERSION II

For each question, mark the answer that best fits how you see your family now. If you feel that your answer is between two of the labeled numbers (the odd numbers), then choose the even number that is between them.

		YES: Fits our family very well		SOME: Fits our family some		NO: Does not fit our family
1.	Family members pay attention to each other's feelings.	1	2	3	4	5
2.	Our family would rather do things together than with other people.	1	2	3	4	5
3.	We all have a say in family plans.	1	2	3	4	5
4.	The grownups in this family understand and agree on family decisions.	1	2	3	4	5
5.	Grownups in the family compete and fight with each other.	1	2	3	4	5
6.	There is closeness in my family but each person is allowed to be special and different.	1	2	3	4	5
7.	We accept each other's friends.	1	2	3	4	5
8.	There is confusion in our family because there is no leader.	1	2	3	4	5
9.	Our family members touch and hug each other.	1	2	3	4	5
10.	Family members put each other down.	1	2	3	4	5
11.	We speak our minds, no matter what.	1	2	3	4	5
12.	In our home, we feel loved.	1	2	3	4	5
13.	Even when we feel close, our family is embarrassed to admit it.	1	2	3	4	5

		YES: Fits our family very well		SOME: Fits our family some		NO: Does not fit our family
14.	We argue a lot and never solve problems.	1	2	3	4	5
15.	Our happiest times are at home.	1	2	3	4	5
16.	The grownups in this family are strong leaders.	1	2	3	4	5
17.	The future looks good to our family.	1	2	3	4	5
18.	We usually blame one person in our family when things aren't going right.	1	2	3	4	5
19.	Family members go their own way most of the time.	1	2	3	4	5
20.	Our family is proud of being close.	1	2	3	4	5
21.	Our family is good at solving problems together.	1	2	3	4	5
22.	Family members easily express warmth and caring towards each other.	1	2	3	4	5
23.	It's okay to fight and yell in our family.	1	2	3	4	5
24.	One of the adults in this family has a favorite child.	1	2	3	4	5
25.	When things go wrong we blame each other.	1	2	3	4	5
26.	We say what we think and feel.	1	2	3	4	5
27.	Our family members would rather do things with other people than together.	1	2	3	4	5
28.	Family members pay attention to each other and listen to what is said.	1	2	3	4	5

	YES: Fits our family very well		SOME: Fits our family some		NO: Does not fit our family
29. We worry about hurting each other's feelings.	1	2	3	4	5
30. The mood in my family is usually sad and blue.	1	2	3	4	5
31. We argue a lot.	1	2	3	4	5
32. One person controls and leads our family.	1	2	3	4	5
33. My family is happy most of the time.	1	2	3	4	5
34. Each person takes responsibility for his/her behavior.	1	2	3	4	5

35. On a scale of 1 to 5, I would rate my family as:

1	2	3	4	5
My family functions very well together			My family does not function well together at all. We really need help.	

36. On a scale of 1 to 5, I would rate the independence in my family as:

1	2	3	4	5
(No one is independent. There are no open arguments. Family members rely on each other for satisfaction rather than on outsiders.)		(Sometimes independent. There are some disagreements. Family members find satisfaction both within and outside of the family.)		(Family members usually go their own way. Disagreements are open. Family members look outside of the family for satisfaction.)

SELF-REPORT FAMILY INVENTORY SCORE SHEET

For each numbered item, fill in the score from the SFI. For items <BOLDED>, reverse the score and enter the reversed score on the score sheet.

HEALTH/COMPETENCE	COHESION	CONFLICT	LEADERSHIP	EXPRESSIVENESS
2 _____	2 _____	<5> _____	<8> _____	1 _____
3 _____	15 _____	6 _____	16 _____	9 _____
4 _____	<19> _____	7 _____	32 _____	<13> _____
6 _____	<27> _____	<8> _____		20 _____
12 _____	36 _____	<10> _____		20 _____
15 _____		<14> _____	SUM: _____	
16 _____		<16> _____		
17 _____	SUM: _____	<24> _____		SUM: _____
<18> _____		<25> _____		
<19> _____		<30> _____		
20 _____		<31> _____		
21 _____		34 _____		
<24> _____				
<25> _____				
<27> _____		SUM: _____		
28 _____				
33 _____				
35 _____				
36 _____				

SUM: _____

For interpretation, plot the SFI scores on the diagram.
1. Family Competence: Plot the Observation Competence Score Equivalent (CCSE) on the horizontal axis.
2. Family Style: Plot the SFI Scale Average on the vertical axis.

H/C	CCSE	COHESION	SFI SCALE	CONFLICT	LEAD	EXPRESS
95	10	25	5	60	15	25
90				57		24
86	9		4.5	54		23
81				51		21
76	8	20	4	48	12	20
71				45		19
67	7		3.5	42		18
62				39		16
57	6	15	3	36	9	15
52				33		14
48	5		2.5	30		13
43				27		11
38	4	10	2	24	6	10
33				21		9
29	3		1.5	18		8
24				15		6
19	2	5	1	12	3	6

CHAPTER 21

THE McMASTER MODEL
A View of Healthy Family Functioning

Nathan B. Epstein
Christine E. Ryan
Duane S. Bishop
Ivan W. Miller
Gabor I. Keitner

In this chapter, we discuss our view of healthy family functioning, the findings from our research, and the research of other investigators that relates to normal families. We describe the McMaster Model of Family Functioning (MMFF) from many points of view, including significant historical issues in its development and elaboration, the definition of the model, and its concepts. As an example, we describe one family according to the MMFF and discuss the variations that can occur within a normal range.

HEALTH AND NORMALITY

To attempt to arrive at a definition of a healthy or normal family may seem to be—or indeed may actually be—a fool's errand. It is exceedingly difficult to describe a healthy or normal individual. When we attempt to describe a normal family, the variables to consider multiply by quantum leaps. Those of us who conceptualize the family as a system of interacting individuals being acted upon and in turn acting on a number of other systems at obvious levels, such as surrounding subculture, culture, economic domain, and biological substrates of the individuals concerned, are often tempted to avoid this particular exercise. Nevertheless, the demands of systematic empirical research of the family are such that a series of benchmarks of family functioning must be developed. Thus, the markers of something approaching what is meant by "normal" and/or "healthy" are of greatest importance.

Normality is an ill-defined concept. It often seems to mean "not displaying any particular problems" (see Walsh, Chapter 1, this volume). For instance, when we conducted a computer search on the normal family, "normal" was not a category; we had to specify "not reconstituted," "not alcoholic," and so forth. When defined in this exclusionary way, "normal" is not a very useful concept. A normal family is described as not having a number of features, but there is no positive statement about what a normal family actually is.

Another common approach has been to equate "normal" with the statistical average. Measurements are taken on some sample, and the average score is taken to be the normal score for the population. If the sample is representative of the total population, then something is known of the distribution of the characteristic being measured in the whole population. But, for example, if the characteristic is the frequency with which husbands and wives discuss financial problems, and the average is once a week, it does not tell us much that is of use about families. For one thing, the current life situation of the family may influence the amount of discussion that is required. For another thing, if it could be assumed that other families were in similar life situations, can we think that families discussing finances once a week are functioning better than those discussing finances more or less often?

We argue that a clinically useful concept is "health." A healthy family is neither necessarily average nor merely lacking in negative characteristics. Rather, it has described, positive features. The MMFF contains a description of such a set of features.

McMaster Model of Family Functioning

The MMFF does not cover all aspects of family functioning. It focuses on the dimensions of functioning that are seen as having the most impact on the emotional and physical health or problems of family members. Within each dimension, we have defined concepts as ranging from "most ineffective" to "most effective." We hypothesize that "most ineffective" functioning in any of these dimensions can contribute to clinical presentation, whereas, "most effective" functioning in all dimensions supports optimal physical and emotional health.

The MMFF has evolved over more than 40 years. The initial study in the evolution of the model was conducted in the late 1950s at McGill University in Montreal, Canada, and was reported in *The Silent Majority* (Westley & Epstein, 1969). (This research is discussed in more detail later in this chapter.) The next stage in the development, described in the *Family Categories Schema* (Epstein, Sigal, & Rakoff, 1962), occurred in the early 1960s, also at McGill. From the late 1960s through the 1970s, work on the model took place at McMaster University, near Toronto. The model in its current form was first described by Epstein, Bishop, and Levin (1978). Since 1978, work on the model has taken place at Brown University in Providence, Rhode Island.

Useful ideas from the family literature, as well as from clinical, teaching, and research experience, have been incorporated into the model, which has been continually refined and reformulated. Aspects of family functioning were conceptualized and then tested in clinical work, research, and teaching. Problems arising in applying the model became the basis for reformulations. The result is a pragmatic model containing ideas that have proved useful in treating patients, teaching therapists, and conducting research. Ideas that have not been helpful in treatment, teaching, or research have been discarded or modified.

The model has been used extensively in a variety of psychiatric and family practice clinics (Epstein & Westley, 1959; Guttman, Spector, Sigal, Epstein, & Rakoff, 1972; Guttman, Spector, Sigal, Rakoff, & Epstein, 1971; Postner, Guttman, Sigal, Epstein, & Rakoff, 1971; Rakoff, Sigal, Spector, & Guttman, 1967; Sigal, Rakoff, & Epstein, 1967; Westley & Epstein, 1960) and by therapists who treated families as a part of a large family therapy outcome study (Guttman et al., 1971; Santa-Barbara et al., 1975; Woodward et al., 1974, 1975; Woodward, Santa-Barbara, Levin, Epstein, & Streiner, 1977). The framework has also been used in a number of family therapy training programs and was found to be readily teachable (Bishop & Epstein, 1979).

The model is based on a systems approach that refers to a group of individual units acting as one. The family is seen as an open system consisting of subsystems (individual, marital dyad) and relating to other, larger systems (extended family, schools, industry, religions). The unique aspect of the dynamic family group cannot be simply reduced to the characteristics of the individuals or interactions between pairs of members. Rather, there are explicit and implicit rules, plus action by members, that govern and monitor each other's behavior (Epstein & Bishop, 1973).

The crucial assumptions of systems theory that underlie our model can be summarized as follows:

1. The parts of the family are interrelated.
2. One part of the family cannot be understood in isolation from the rest of the system.
3. Family functioning cannot be fully understood by simply understanding each of the parts.
4. A family's structure and organization are important factors determining the behavior of family members.
5. Transactional patterns of the family system are among the most important variables that shape the behavior of family members.

In addition to the systems approach, we describe how a healthy, or, in our view, a normal family, should look on each of the dimensions. Often, such a description involves a value judgment. For instance, we would say that family members ought to be able to show sadness at appropriate times and to the degree called for by the situation. The judgment of appropriateness with respect to sadness is not clear-cut and varies among cultures. We take the position that knowledge of the culture to which a family belongs is necessary to understand a family, and the judgments of health or normality are relative to the culture of the family. We comment more on values later.

We assume that a primary function of today's family unit is to provide a setting for the development and maintenance of family members on social, psychological, and biological levels (Epstein, Levin, & Bishop, 1976). In the course of fulfilling this function, families will have to deal with a variety of issues and problems or tasks, which we group into three areas: the Basic Task Area, the Developmental Task Area, and the Hazardous Task Area.

The Basic Task Area, the most fundamental of the three, involves instrumental issues. For example, families must deal with the problems of providing food, money, transportation, and shelter.

The Developmental Task Area encompasses those family issues that arise as a result of development over time. These developments are often conceptualized as a sequence of stages. On the individual level, these include crises of infancy, childhood, adolescence, and middle and old age. On the family level, these might be the beginning of a marriage, the first pregnancy, or the last child leaving home. A number of authors have referred to developmental concepts and family functioning (Carter & McGoldrick, 1998; Hadley, Jacobs, Milliones, Caplan, & Spitz, 1974; Solomon, 1973).

The Hazardous Task Area involves handling crises that arise as a result of illness, accident, loss of income, job change, and so forth. There is also a substantial literature dealing with these topics (Hill, 1965; Langsley & Kaplan, 1968; Parad & Caplan, 1965).

We have found that families unable to deal effectively with these three tasks areas are most likely to develop clinically significant problems and/or chronic maladaptive functioning in one or more areas of family functioning.

Dimensions of Family Functioning

To understand how a family meets and addresses the tasks areas, as well as the structure, organization, and transactional patterns of the family, we focus on the following six dimensions: *problem solving, communication, roles, affective responsiveness, affective involvement,* and *behavior control.* These are outlined in Table 21.1. As stated by Epstein and Bishop (1981):

TABLE 21.1. Summary of Dimension Concepts in the McMaster Model of Family Functioning

Problem solving

Two types of problems:
    Instrumental and affective
Seven stages to the problem-solving process:
    1. Identification of the problem
    2. Communication of the problem to the appropriate person(s)
    3. Development of action alternatives
    4. Decision on one alternative
    5. Action
    6. Monitoring the action
    7. Evaluation of success
Postulated:
- Most effective when both instrumental and affective problems are solved.
- Most effective when all seven stages are carried out.
- Least effective when families cannot identify problem (stop before step 1).

Communication

Instrumental and affective areas
Two independent dimensions:
    1. Clear and direct
    2. Clear and indirect
    3. Masked and direct
    4. Masked and indirect
Postulated:
- Most effective when able to communicate well in both instrumental and affective areas.
- Most effective when clear and direct.
- Least effective when masked and indirect.

Roles

Two types of repetitive tasks:
    Necessary and other
Two areas of family functions:
    Instrumental and affective
Necessary family function groupings:
    1. Instrumental
      a. Provision of resources
    2. Affective
      a. Nurturance and support
      b. Adult sexual gratification
    3. Mixed
      a. Life skills development
      b. Systems maintenance and management
Role functioning is assessed by considering how the family allocates responsibilities and handles accountability for them.
Postulated:
- Most effective when all necessary family functions have clear allocation to appropriate individual(s) and accountability is built in.
- Least effective when few necessary family role functions are not addressed and/or allocation and accountability are not maintained.

(*continued*)

TABLE 21.1. *Continued*

Affective responsiveness

Two groupings:
  Welfare emotions (e.g., love, joy, concern) and emergency emotions (e.g., sadness, fear, anger)
Postulated:
  • Most effective when a full range of responses is appropriate in amount and quality to stimulus.
  • Least effective when range is very narrow (one or two affects only) and/or amount and quality is distorted, given the context.

Affective involvement

A range of involvement with six styles identified:
  1. Absence of involvement
  2. Involvement devoid of feelings
  3. Narcissistic involvement
  4. Empathic involvement
  5. Overinvolvement
  6. Symbiotic involvement
Postulated:
  • Most effective with empathic involvement
  • Least effective with symbiotic involvement and absence of involvement

Behavior control

Applies to three situations:
  1. Dangerous situations
  2. Meeting and expressing psychobiological needs and drives (eating, drinking, sleeping, eliminating, sex, and aggression)
  3. Interpersonal socializing behavior inside and outside the family
Standard and latitude of "acceptable behavior" determined by four styles:
  1. Rigid
  2. Flexible
  3. *Laissez-faire* (i.e., no standards)
  4. Chaotic (random implementation of styles 1–3)
Postulated:
  • Most effective: flexible behavior control
  • Least effective: chaotic behavior control

The McMaster model does not focus on any one dimension as the foundation for conceptualizing family behavior. We argue that many dimensions need to be assessed for a fuller understanding of such a complex entity as the family. Although we attempt to clearly define and delineate the dimensions, we recognize the potential overlap and/or possible interaction that may occur between them. (p. 448)

To date, our research has found no single dimension that predicts good or poor family functioning; nor have we found a ceiling or threshhold effect that adequately explains family patterns of healthy or unhealthy functioning. In the following section, we briefly discuss and define each dimension, and describe one family with very effective family functioning relative to that dimension. The Sampson family consists of a father, mother, and two sons, ages 3 and 4. We also provide commentary on what we consider the range of healthy or normal functioning for each dimension. A more detailed discussion of the model is presented elsewhere (Epstein & Bishop, 1981; Epstein et al., 1978).

Problem Solving

Definition

The term "family problem solving" refers to a family's ability to resolve problems to a level that maintains effective family functioning. Although not all family issues are problematic, those issues or problems that threaten the integrity of the family (or the emotional or physical health of its members) should be addressed and resolved. Prior to Epstein's early studies (Westley & Epstein, 1969), ineffective families were assumed to have more problems than more effectively functioning families. Surprisingly, studies showed that this was not the case; all families encounter more or less the same range of difficulties. Differences did occur, however, in the ways families addressed the problems. Families that functioned effectively solved their problems, whereas ineffectively functioning families dealt only partially, if at all, with their problems.

Family problems can be divided into two types: *instrumental* and *affective*. Instrumental problems relate to issues that are basic in nature, such as provision of money, food, clothing, housing, transportation, and so forth. Affective problems relate to issues of emotion or feeling, such as anger or depression. Families whose functioning is disrupted by instrumental problems rarely deal effectively with affective problems. However, families whose functioning is disrupted by affective problems may deal adequately with instrumental problems.

In the McMaster model, effective problem solving can be conceptualized as a sequence of seven steps:

1. Identifying the problem.
2. Communicating with appropriate people about the problem.
3. Developing a set of possible alternative solutions.
4. Deciding on one of the alternatives.
5. Carrying out the action required by the alternative.
6. Monitoring to ensure that the action is carried out.
7. Evaluating the effectiveness of the problem-solving process.

Effective families solve most problems efficiently and easily. Therefore, at times, it can be difficult to elicit information about the problem-solving steps that they have gone through. In families that have difficulties solving problems, it is usually easier to analyze their stepwise attempts at solving problems.

Families range along a dimension of problem-solving ability. Most effective families have few, if any, unresolved problems. Problems that exist are relatively new and are dealt with effectively. When a new problem situation occurs, the family approaches the problem systematically. As family functioning becomes less effective, family problem-solving behavior becomes less systematic, and fewer problem-solving steps are accomplished.

Clinical Description

The Sampsons cannot identify any major unresolved problems. A visit by the maternal grandmother, however, led to some difficulties with the children. They describe one son as cuddly, whereas the other is more active and independent. The independent one, who did not receive as much attention from his grandmother, became jealous and acted up when she visited. When his grandmother then scolded him, his behavior became more problematic. Mrs. Sampson first identified this problem and then discussed it with her husband. At the earliest reasonable opportunity, they discussed it with the grandmother. This was done in such a way that she was able to support them in maintaining discipline; at the same time, they helped her to relate more appropriately with each boy. The couple was flexible and made reasonable allowances for the grandmother, because she had come from a great distance and was only with them for a brief time.

They described another problem with the older son. He would not follow the rules they had laid down regarding where he could and could not play. Initially, they tried a number of disciplinary measures. Then, the mother realized that this was not working, and they reverted to a previously effective pattern of using rewards. Returning to a previously adaptive approach quickly led to positive results.

This family can discuss all problems in an open and clear way and also identify both the instrumental and the affective components of each problem. They communicate about problems at the earliest possible time, process alternatives quickly, make a decision, and begin to act. They make sure their actions are carried out, and they can describe their review of previously effective and ineffective methods.

Variations within Normal

Not all normal families demonstrate problem solving that is as effective as that just described. The Sampsons represent the positive extreme of healthy functioning. We conceptualize that a normal family can have some minor unresolved problems. However, such problems will not be of a degree or duration that creates major disruption in the family. Our example dealt with a child acting out during a grandmother's visit. The issue(s) confronting a family might be more serious. Job loss, terminal illness, or a family move may be disturbing to family members, but they may not be a problem for the family. A healthy functioning family will carry through with the steps listed earlier, including discussing the issues, communicating with one another, and deciding on appropriate action. Thus, the process of solving the problem is more important than its content.

A normal family can also be a little slower than the Sampsons to identify problems, to communicate with each other, and to act. Despite less efficiency, however, it will still manage to resolve most problems. It will resolve all instrumental problems; affective problems may present a little more difficulty. We also find that only the most effective families actually evaluate the problem-solving process.

Communication

Definition

We define "communication" as the exchange of verbal information within a family. Although all behavior can be seen as a form of communication, we focus on verbal communication because it is manifest and measurable. When looking at patterns of communication, one can examine an individual's style or, alternatively, the overall family style of communication. The MMFF focuses on the *family's* pattern of communication; we have found that using a limited definition of communication is more useful for both the therapist and the family members.

Communication is also subdivided into instrumental and affective areas, with the same ramifications for each, as was discussed for the problem solving dimension. In addition, two other aspects of communication are also assessed. Is the communication clear or masked, and is it direct or indirect? The clear versus masked continuum focuses on whether the content of the message is clearly stated or camouflaged, muddied, or vague. The direct versus indirect continuum focuses on whether messages go to the appropriate individuals or tend to be deflected to other people. Family members may be indirect in their communication by talking to one family member about another in front of that person(s) and/or assuming a message meant for another is directed at them. In other words, both the sender and receiver are involved in the family's communication patterns.

The clear versus masked and the direct versus indirect continua are independent; we can therefore identify four styles of communication. The following situation provides an example of each: Joan is late for a meeting with Bill. When she arrives, the following statements might be made:

1. *Clear and direct.* Bill says to Joan: "I'm upset that you're late, but let's get on with the meeting."

2. *Clear and indirect.* Bill says to someone else who is present: "I'm upset with Joan because she's late."
3. *Masked and direct.* Bill says to Joan: "Are you okay? You don't look well."
4. *Masked and indirect.* Bill says to someone else who is present: "People who come late are a pain."

Although we focus primarily on verbal communication, we pay attention to nonverbal behavior, especially when it contradicts the verbal information exchange. Contradictory nonverbal behavior contributes to masking and may also reflect indirectness of communication.

At the healthy end of the dimension, the family communicates in a clear and direct manner in both the instrumental and the affective areas. As we move toward the less effective end of the dimension, communication becomes less clear and less direct.

Clinical Description

The Sampson family is clear and direct in all their patterns of communication. There is no sense of hesitation or holding back, no talking around the issues. In addition, family members always direct their comments to the person for whom they are intended. Their talking is efficient and effective. This is equally true of the children, who were open and straightforward with their parents and the interviewer.

Variations within Normal

Toward the lower end of the normal functioning range, communication about conflictual issues may not be clear and direct. There can be some brief occasions of hesitations or beating around the bush (masking); trouble clearly hearing each other (masking and/or indirectness); or not clearly stating a personal point of view (indirectness). Clinicians learn through training and experience that there are many forms of expression and no "right" way of responding. Despite the variations (including cultural) in how family members express themselves, the therapist is able to discern whether communication within the family is effective.

Role Functioning

Definition

"Family roles" are defined as the repetitive patterns of behavior by which family members fulfill family functions. There are some functions that all families have to deal with repeatedly in order to maintain an effective and healthy system. We identify five such necessary family functions that are the basis for necessary family roles. Each of these areas subsumes a number of tasks and functions:

1. *Provision of resources.* This area includes those tasks and functions associated with providing money, food, clothing, and shelter.
2. *Nurturance and support.* This involves the provision of comfort, warmth, reassurance, and support for family members.
3. *Adult sexual gratification.* Both husbands and wives (or partners) personally find satisfaction within the sexual relationship and also feel that they can satisfy each other sexually. Affective issues are therefore prominent. A mutually desirable level of sexual activity is important. It has been our experience, however, that in some instances, both partners may express satisfaction with little or no activity.
4. *Personal development.* This includes those tasks and functions necessary to support family members in developing skills for personal achievement. Included are tasks related to the physical, emotional, educational, and social development of the children, and those relating to the career, avocational, and social development of the adults.
5. *Maintenance and management of the family system.* This area includes a variety of functions that involve techniques and actions required to maintain standards.
   a. Decision-making functions include leadership, major decision making, and questions of final decisions when there is no agreement. In general, these functions should reside at the parental level and within the immediate (or nuclear) family.
   b. Boundary and membership functions include issues and tasks concerned with extended family, friends, neighbors, boarders, family size, and dealings with any external institutions and agencies.
   c. Implementation and adherence of behavior control functions include disciplining children and maintaining standards and rules for the adult family members.
   d. Household finance functions include tasks such as monthly bills and managing household money.
   e. Health-related functions include caregiving, setting up and keeping medical appointments, identifying appropriate health problems, and maintaining compliance with health prescriptions.

Two additional and integral aspects of role functioning include *role allocation* and *role accountability*.

1. Role allocation is concerned with the family's pattern in assigning roles and includes a number of issues. Does the person assigned a task or

function have the power and skill necessary to carry it out? Is the task age-appropriate? Is the assignment done clearly and explicitly? Can reassignment take place easily? Are tasks distributed and allocated to the satisfaction of family members?

2. Role accountability looks at the procedures in the family for making sure that functions are fulfilled. This includes the presence of a sense of responsibility in family members and the existence of monitoring and corrective mechanisms.

At the healthy end of this dimension, all necessary family functions are fulfilled. Allocation is reasonable and does not overburden one or more members. Accountability is clear.

Clinical Description

The Sampsons are very clear regarding who carries out each of a variety of family tasks. They discuss each member's jobs, are comfortable with them, and do not feel overburdened. They share tasks in many areas but are also clear about their separate areas of responsibility. For example, the wife may prepare meals, whereas the husband is responsible for food shopping and cleanup.

The task of getting up with the children on weekend mornings is split, with one parent taking Saturday, the other Sunday. Their mutual involvement in dealing with the children was repeatedly demonstrated during the course of the interview, and the children showed no preference for one parent or the other.

The couple is satisfied with their financial resources but would prefer working fewer hours. They are quite clear about their roles in handling budgeting and financial organization. They set priorities and handle their finances so that they maximize their resources. The children clearly go to both parents for nurturance and support as appropriate, and the parents obtain their main support from each other.

Both partners are satisfied with their sexual functioning. They can discuss this in an open and straightforward manner and indicate their enjoyment in being personally satisfied, and in satisfying each other. In the course of their relationship, the wife has increasingly become more active in initiating sexual activity. They can handle issues such as one partner saying "no" to sex with tact and sensitivity, and without either of them having a sense of being rebuffed.

The wife is actively involved in decisions regarding the husband's career and his pursuit of avocational interests. He is aware of her need to be active outside the home, and he organizes his schedule to support this. She worked full time early in their marriage, and plans on returning to work, albeit part-time, when the children begin school. The husband and wife fully discussed their options, career/job choices, and long-range plans before making these decisions. The wife enjoys her active role with the children, yet also looks forward to reentering the workforce. They are always able to come to an agreement on major decisions.

In all of this role functioning, this family is amazingly clear in its member's ability to discuss the allocation of roles; in doing so, they play to individual strengths and interests. They keep track of whether the jobs allocated to each other are carried out. When one does not carry out a task, the other will either fill in or point out the problem.

Variations within Normal

Functioning less highly effectively than the Sampsons would still fall appropriately within the normal range. In our society, normally functioning families generally do not have difficulties with provision of resources except when circumstances are out of their control (e.g., times of economic recession, labor action). Families may be poor and have difficulties at some times in providing for food, clothing, or shelter. Financial difficulties can also lead to stress and occasional conflicts or arguments. But being poor does not in itself mean the family is not functioning effectively.

Nurturance and support are provided although it may not always be immediately available. Caring for an ill relative might add to the family's burden and put strain on the family's functioning—but it might not. This would be true for a family that is poor or one that is wealthy. One might argue that a poor family might have more strains and stresses to contend with than a wealthy family. A poor family may be able to handle family problems because it has effective family functioning, whereas a family with poor functioning is unable to deal with problems, despite its apparent advantages.

The couple may have minor dissatisfaction with the sexual relationship. Similarly, slight deficiencies in personal development and systems management and maintenance may also occur.

In general, these deviations from effective role functioning do not lead to persistent conflict. In some normal families, roles can be effectively handled even though most functions are carried out by one individual. In the most effective families, there is role sharing, which allows the family to deal with changes from the usual pattern (e.g., those caused by illness). Within the normal range of families, individuals carry out role functions willingly and possess (or learn) the required skills and abilities. Whether one person or several family members carry out the role functions, no individual is overburdened. Also, normally functioning families may not always maintain complete accountability, and there may be occasions when some tasks are delayed or not carried out. But, again, these situations do not lead to persistent conflict.

Affective Responsiveness

Definition

In this dimension, we examine the family's potential range of affective responses both qualitatively and quantitatively. We define "affective responsiveness" as the ability to respond to a given stimulus with an appropriate quality and quantity of feelings, and are concerned with two aspects of the quality of affective responses. First, do family members demonstrate an ability to respond with the full spectrum of feelings experienced in human emotional life? Second, is the emotion experienced at times consistent with the stimulus and/or situational context?

The quantitative aspect focuses on the degree of affective response along a continuum from absence of response through reasonable or expected responsiveness to overresponsiveness. Whereas the dimension considers the overall pattern of the family's responses to affective stimuli, it focuses more than any other on the capacity of individual members to respond emotionally, and not on their actual behavior.

In the clinical interview, therapists specifically ask each family member about his or her ability to feel certain emotions and to provide examples of how he or she personally experiences them (e.g., tenderness, anger). It is important to remember that this dimension does not assess the ways in which family members convey their feelings (an aspect of affective communication), but whether or not they have the capacity to feel the emotion.

We distinguish between two categories of affect: *welfare emotions* and *emergency emotions*. Welfare emotions consist of affection, warmth, tenderness, support, love, consolation, happiness, and joy. Emergency emotions consist of responses such as anger, fear, sadness, disappointment, and depression.

At the healthy end of the dimension, we conceive of a family that possesses the capability to express a full range of emotions. In most situations, members experience the appropriate emotion, and when an emotion is experienced, it is of reasonable intensity and duration. Although there is no single way to experience an emotion, a trained therapist will use the family's input during the clinical interview to determine the depth and breadth of family members' emotions. Obviously, cultural variability must also be considered in evaluating the affective responsiveness of families.

Clinical Description

All members of the Sampson family display a wide range of affect that is appropriate and in keeping with the situation. They have suffered no major losses in their extended family but can describe periods of sadness and loss in other circumstances. They respond with appropriate anger and disappointment to situations. Each family member has a good sense of humor and is able to be affectionate and caring. They not only describe how, earlier, the husband was more responsive across the range of emotions than the wife, but also how he has helped her become more responsive. As noted in the section on communication, they express all feelings in a clear and direct manner.

Variations within Normal

Even at a fairly healthy level on this dimension, families may contain a member who does not have the capacity to experience a particular affect. This dimension is not concerned with the variation that individual members may show in the timing of their emotional response. Rather, it concerns whether or not the member is capable of the response. For example, a family member may not be able to *experience* empathy, not that he or she is slow to feel empathy, or that empathy may be difficult for them to express. This distinction is important for the clinician to understand, so that it does not lead to frustration in family therapy on the part of the therapist and the other family members. A useful analogy might be the attempt to train someone to see colors when he or she is color blind.

Family members may occasionally respond with inappropriate affect and/or experience occasional episodes of under- or overresponding. However, the inappropriateness is temporary and is not disruptive.

Affective Involvement

Definition

"Affective involvement" is the extent to which the family shows interest in and values the particular activities and interests of individual family members. The focus is on the amount of interest the family demonstrates, as well as the manner in which the family members show interest and investment in one another. There is a range of styles, from a total lack of involvement at one end of the continuum to extreme involvement at the other. We identify six types of involvement as follows:

1. *Lack of involvement:* no interest or investment in one another.
2. *Involvement devoid of feelings:* some interest and/or investment in one another. This interest is primarily intellectual in nature.
3. *Narcissistic involvement:* interest in others only to the degree that their behavior reflects on the self.
4. *Empathic involvement:* interest and/or investment in one another for the sake of the others.
5. *Overinvolvement:* excessive interest and/or investment in one another.

6. *Symbiotic involvement:* an extreme and pathological investment in others that is seen only in very disturbed relationships. In such families, there is marked difficulty in differentiating one person from another.

We consider empathic involvement optimal for health. As families move in either direction away from empathic involvement, family functioning becomes less effective in this area.

Clinical Description

In the Sampson family, all members show an active interest in each other. The children respond appropriately for their age. The parents take an active interest in what is important to each other, even though their interests vary in several areas. They can respond to what is going on with each other without overidentifying or personalizing.

Variations within Normal

The Sampsons function very effectively on this dimension. However, some variation can occur within the healthy range. There may be instances of narcissistic interest of some members in others or occasional episodes of overinvolvement. However, these patterns are focused on a single individual and/or are not consistent.

Behavior Control

Definition

This dimension is defined as the pattern a family adopts for handling behavior in three areas: physically dangerous situations; situations that involve meeting and expressing psychobiological needs and drives; and situations involving interpersonal socializing behavior, both between family members and with people outside the family.

We are interested in the standards or rules the family sets in these areas and in the latitude it allows relative to the standard. We describe four styles of behavior control based on variations of the standard and latitude:

1. *Rigid behavior control:* Standards are narrow and specific for the culture, and there is minimal negotiation or variation across situations.
2. *Flexible behavior control:* Standards are reasonable, and there is opportunity for negotiation and change, depending on the context.
3. Laissez-faire *behavior control:* At the extreme, no standards are held, and total latitude is allowed, regardless of the context.

4. *Chaotic behavior control:* There is unpredictable and random shifting among styles 1–3, so that family members do not know what standards apply at any one time or how much negotiation is possible.

We view flexible behavior control as the most effective and chaotic behavior control as the least effective style.

Clinical Description

Mr. and Mrs. Sampson are very clear about rules of behavior. Their basic stance is to allow considerable exploration and activity by the children, and they tolerate a higher level of activity and noise than would many couples. However, they are very clear about what behavior is unacceptable, and they intervene consistently when such behavior occurs.

They support each other in this regard. They handle the children in a mutually supportive and consistent fashion. They make allowances when the situation calls for it (e.g., a visit by the grandmother), but they still maintain consistent patterns within that framework. They demonstrate superior techniques for handling the children's behavior. For example, during the interview, when one child got up to leave the room, he was politely told to stay and to close the door. When he persisted, he was told again, in a clear and slightly more forceful way. He complied and was immediately told, "Thank you, that's very good." On another occasion, when one boy was making quite a bit of noise, the father said, "Please yell more quietly." The child immediately spoke in a quieter voice.

This couple was considering becoming foster parents for a disturbed child. They could indicate with considerable insight the problems they felt they would face in this role. They knew that taking a disturbed child into the family setting would require a difficult shift in their standards of behavior and control. Although they had standards for their own children, they realized that tighter standards might initially be required when the disturbed child came to stay with them.

Variations within Normal

Within the range of normal functioning, there can be a number of variations on the above-mentioned example of very effective functioning. The family may be clear about the rules of behavior in general, while being indecisive, unclear, or lacking in agreement in one or two relatively minor areas (e.g., the parents may disagree about minor aspects of table manners, but the family members are aware of the general range). Such inconsistency should not, however, be a source of major conflict. Normally functioning families also may not use the most effective techniques and may therefore require more time to establish control.

It should be noted that this dimension also applies to the parents in the family. In normally functioning families, parents are able to describe what they expect from their partners, and what their partners expect of them. When one partner does not meet the other's expectations, they address the problem.

RESEARCH ON NORMAL FAMILIES

In our original study, *The Silent Majority* (Westley & Epstein, 1969), we sought to determine how the emotional health of individuals relates to the overall structure and functioning of their families. Since the publication of this study, extensive changes have occurred in our society with respect to values, views on marriage and divorce, and family composition. These changes have not only affected family life but they have also radically changed the methods of examining and evaluating families in many areas. The largest value shifts are those arising from changes related to the position of women in society and especially their role in today's family and the economy. These changes have had enormous effect on spousal and parent–child relationships, and they raise important questions about the fundamental makeup of a family household. The multiple varieties of family structure and organization that are common today were not even imagined when the initial study was conducted.

Despite all the changes that have taken place in families, we believe that two of the basic findings from the original study are still applicable, albeit with some clarification, as explained below.

First, we believe that the organizational, structural, and transactional pattern variables are more powerful in determining the behavior of family members than are intrapsychic variables. This statement refers to the relative power of the variables only and does not invalidate the contribution of intrapsychic factors to behavior.

Second, the most important finding of the *Silent Majority* study was that the emotional health of the children is closely related to the emotional relationship between their parents. When these relationships were warm and supportive, so that the husband and wife felt loved, admired, and encouraged to act in ways that they themselves admired, the children were happy and healthy. Couples who were emotionally close, met each other's needs, and encouraged positive self-images in each other were good parents. This positive relationship between husband and wife did not depend on their being emotionally healthy themselves as individuals, though, obviously, this was most beneficial. In some cases, one or both parents were emotionally disturbed, but they still managed to develop a good marital relationship. When this occurred, the children were emotionally healthy. It was as if the positive marital relationship had insulated the children and prevented contagion from the parent's psychopathology.

In our ongoing clinical and research work, we continue to be impressed by the importance of a loving and supportive relationship between parents. However, because of the societal changes noted earlier, we very often see families in which the adults are stepparents, cohabiting adults, single parents with or without a live-in partner, same-sex partners, and so on. Whether two parents, two adults, or a single parent head the family, we believe that the key factor in the family's functioning is the emotional climate maintained in the family system. The combination of strong support, genuine concern, and loving care, along with an absence of destructive comments or chronic hostility in the adult relationship, provides a foundation able to withstand strain from within or outside the family group that protects the ongoing interrelationships and development of family members. Single parents can establish a healthy functioning family by maintaining a supportive environment and developing a system of dealing with dissonance that is satisfactory to all family members. Finally, for any family with children, establishment and maintenance of appropriate adult–child boundaries are critical.

Over the years, a number of researchers using the MMFF have investigated different aspects of normal families. A few of the early studies that continue to hold our interest follow.

The Parent–Therapist Study

If we believe that disturbed family functioning leads to disturbed behavior in children, then a corollary is that superior family functioning should ameliorate or minimize it. Based on this assumption, colleagues in our research group tested the hypothesis that placing disturbed children in very effectively functioning families could have a remedial influence (Levin, Rubenstein, & Streiner, 1976; Rubenstein, Armentrout, Levin, & Herald, 1978). Their project, The Parent–Therapist Program: An Innovative Approach to Treating Emotionally Disturbed Children, compared the relative effectiveness of placing emotionally disturbed children in superior-functioning families with placing them in residential child-treatment centers. The families involved were interviewed and assessed with instruments we developed that measure family functioning according to the MMFF. Superior-functioning families were quite identifiable. This supported our view that the model could be applied to and discriminate among families with widely varying levels of functioning.

It was found that the families were as effective as the institutions in improving the functioning of the children. This finding supports the assumption that the behavior of individuals is strongly influenced by the structure and organization in the family of which they are a part.

The original design of the study called for the children to be placed in three different settings: in institutions, in families that were part of a collaborative network of parent–therapist families, and with individual parent–therapist families not tied into a network. It was quickly discovered that the last group could not deal with the assigned children. Even such highly effective families had limits to the stress they could handle. Less effective, but still healthy, families are probably even less able to handle such stresses. Presumably, they too can cope more effectively if they are part of a social network for support. These findings shed light on the popularity and apparent effectiveness of self-help groups—a phenomenon that has arisen in an explosive fashion in the past few decades to help people cope with a very wide range of human problems.

As a final comment on the parent–therapist project, it is interesting to note that none of the children treated were incorporated to the level of complete family membership. This supports our belief that aberrant behavior in an individual is not tolerated by a healthy family, and that healthy, well-functioning families deal clearly and effectively with boundary and membership issues.

The London Study

In 1979, Byles conducted a study of 30 families in which at least one child was being seen at a family medicine clinic for nonpsychiatric problems in London, Ontario, Canada. Although these families were not seeking help for psychiatric problems, there is no evidence that they were functioning extremely well according to our model; however, they can probably be considered "normal" in the average sense. Using the Problem Solving dimension of an early version of the Family Assessment Device (FAD), Byles found that some of these families had ineffective problem-solving techniques and a fairly high incidence of problems (Byles, 1979). The families that had the most trouble with the process of problem solving had the most areas of difficulty, consistent with the findings in *The Silent Majority*.

Another interesting finding was that families in which the oldest child was an adolescent had the most difficulties with problem solving. We have found that families with adolescent children experience more stress than families with children of other ages. These findings clearly highlight statements of most family researchers to the effect that families vary according to developmental stage and, therefore, all stages of family development must be studied (see Walsh, Chapter 1; Olson & Gorall, Chapter 19; McGoldrick & Carter, Chapter 14, this volume).

The Ontario Child Health Study

A series of reports came out of the Ontario Child Health Study (OCHS), a large community survey of 1,869 families set up, in part, to obtain estimates of the prevalence of emotional and behavioral disorders in children. Byles and his colleagues reported on the reliability and validity of the General Functioning (GF) scale of the FAD (Byles, Byrne, Boyle, & Offord, 1988). They were interested in learning "how the family unit works together on essential tasks. That is the essence of functioning" (p. 103). Study conclusions supported the construct validity of the GF scale as a measure of family functioning and as a useful assessment of overall family functioning when values of specific dimensions are not needed. Indeed, the GF scale was the best predictor of a psychiatric diagnosis in a child and correlated well with other issues such as alcoholism, marital separation, and violence. Finally, Byles et al. confirmed the approaches developed in the MMFF to assess family functioning with respect to healthy as well as pathological functioning.

The Retirement Study

In this project, our own research group studied the effect of family functioning, couple health, and retirement on the morale of 178 couples in their 60s (Bishop, Epstein, Baldwin, & Miller, 1988). The sample studied was a subset of Providence, Rhode Island, households selected originally by the Population Research Laboratory at Brown University in 1969, for a study of health and mobility (Speare & Kobrin, 1980). The proportion that reported optimal and less than optimal family functioning in the FAD were 63.5% and 36.5% for husbands and 67.0% and 33.0% for wives, respectively. Although perceptions about the effectiveness of their family functioning were similar across several dimensions, predictors of morale differed between men and women.

Health was the major predictive factor for the psychological well-being for husbands, whereas family functioning was more predictive of psychological well being for wives. Retirement status was not a significant factor for either husbands or wives. Such findings of differences in individual family members often recur in research on family functioning.

The Psychometric Study

Our group investigated the psychometric properties of the McMaster FAD using data obtained from large clinical, nonclinical, and medical samples (Kabacoff, Miller, Bishop, Epstein, & Keitner, 1990). Scale reliabilities were generally favorable, and the hypothesized structure of the FAD was supported. As an answer to previous criticism that the FAD was not developed through factor-analytic methods, this study reported "over 90% of FAD items loaded on factors hypothesized by the McMaster model" (p. 438). Based on this study, as well as other reports, the authors affirmed our earlier finding that the FAD provides a reliable and valid assessment of a wide range of families and confirms the constructs of the model (Miller, Epstein, Bishop, & Keitner, 1985).

We have stated explicitly in previous publications that there is overlap among some FAD scales. In fact, the GF scale was developed to correlate with other FAD dimensions (Epstein, Baldwin, & Bishop, 1983). Our rationale for this is, in part, that dimensions of family functioning are not likely to be totally independent of each other. Effective functioning in one area may facilitate or impede functioning in another area. For example, healthy family functioning in the area of problem solving may be useful in resolving some issues related to behavior control or role allocation. Likewise, difficulties that families may have with communication may exacerbate affective involvement or problem solving.

A more recent questioning of the factor-analytic structure of the FAD (Ridenour, Daley, & Reich, 1999, 2000) led our group to reassert the clinical underpinnings and family constructs of the MMFF (Miller, Ryan, Keitner, Bishop, & Epstein, 2000a, 2000c). Dimensions developed for the FAD are not purely self-report scale dimensions. Rather, they represent constructs used in a comprehensive model of family functioning that includes clinical interviews, family assessments, and family therapy (Miller, Ryan, Keitner, Bishop, & Epstein, 2000b).

The Quebec Group

A very productive research group led by Maziade and Thivierge at the University of Laval in Quebec City has used the MMFF and the McMaster Clinical Rating Scale (MCRS) in several investigations that focused on child psychiatric epidemiology.

Some of their findings included (1) the Behavior Control dimension was found to interact with the child's temperament in predicting middle-childhood clinical disorders (Maziade et al., 1985) but not academic achievement (Maziade et al., 1986); and (2) communication was shown to interact with extreme infant temperament to predict IQ in preschool years (Maziade, Cote, Boutin, Bernier, & Thivierge, 1987).

In another study (Maziade, Bernier, Thivierge, & Cote, 1987), the authors report:

> In an epidemiological framework, that is, when used in samples of the general population, the two MMFF dimensions under study [Behavior Control and Communication (our addition)] displayed a satisfactory level of interactor reliability. This suggests that trained investigators can deliver a satisfactory agreement when basing their rating on the process as well as on the content of the family interview. In addition, our data from this normal, nonclinical sample to some degree confirm that what the scale defines as a normal level of functioning (ratings of 4–5), corresponds to the functioning of a majority of nonclinical families in the population. The present data also bring into focus an important empirical quality that such an assessment device of family functioning must present: independence of SES [socioeconomic status]. (pp. 529–530)

RECENT DEVELOPMENTS

Our group continues to use the MMFF in both clinical work and in teaching, training, and research programs. Psychometric instruments developed from and based on the MMFF include the FAD (Epstein, Baldwin, & Bishop, 1983), the MCRS (Epstein, Baldwin, & Bishop, 1982; Miller et al., 1994), and the McMaster Structured Interview of Family Functioning (McSiff; Bishop, Epstein, Keitner, Miller, & Zlotnick, 1987).

The FAD, the oldest and most widely used of our instruments, was developed to assess a family's functioning from an internal, subjective perspective. In addition to computer-generated scoring programs, we are now able to offer the FAD in 16 languages: Afrikaans, Chinese, Croatian, Danish, Dutch, English, French, Greek, Hebrew, Hungarian, Italian, Japanese, Portuguese, Russian, Spanish, Swedish. In the process of being translated are Korean, Norwegian, and Thai versions of the FAD. Translation of the FAD was not a goal when the instrument was first developed. However, many clinicians and researchers from around the world have expressed an interest in using the FAD and have often worked with our research team to ensure an accurate translation.

The MCRS, a clinician-conducted interview, is used to provide an external rating of a family's functioning. The ability to follow the guidelines of the MCRS presupposes a thorough knowledge of the MMFF and the skills needed to conduct a family interview. We developed the McSiff in order to help trainees and paraprofessionals learn the model and obtain the information necessary to make an accurate assessment of the family. The McSiff systematically takes the interviewer and family members through a series of questions exploring each of the dimensions that make up the model.

Used for clinical, teaching, and research purposes, we recently revised the instrument, in part, to reflect changes in the composition of families; that is, we originally had structured the interview so that there were three forms of the McSiff, each geared to a specific family type (nuclear, married with no children, or the single-parent family). The new version does not specify any type of family composition but leads the interviewer through the assessment by a series of instructions and "skip-out" statements (Bishop et al., 2000).

Although we have used these instruments to help us assess family functioning in a variety of populations, most of our clinical and research focus centers on families in which one member has a psychiatric illness (e.g., severe depressive disorder, bipolar illness). Other studies examine the relationship between family functioning and caregiving for patients with a medical illness (e.g., stroke, Alzheimer's disease). In our studies, we have combined use of the research assessment tools with the clinical treatment approach based on the MMFF, that is, the Problem-Centered Systems Therapy of the Family (PCSTF, Epstein & Bishop, 1981). Over the past decade, we have also developed a telephone intervention (Family Intervention: Telephone Tracking, FITT) to assist families and caregivers through the period of transition required after a stroke (Bishop et al., 1998). This intervention is based on the MMFF and the PCSTF but uses telephone contacts with both patient and caregiver. Preliminary data suggest that use of this intervention decreases health care utilization while improving quality of life. It has recently been modified for use in studies involving populations diagnosed with HIV and Alzheimer's disease.

In addition, we have recently developed a research protocol that focuses on assisting family members in dealing with a newly diagnosed severe medical/surgical illness (e.g., prostate cancer). Members of our group have also begun to use our model and research tools as part of a community outreach program (1) for children and families at risk for depression, and (2) for parents who wish to gain insight into and/or improve their parenting skills.

We are currently in the process of bringing together—in one comprehensive volume—the clinical, teaching, and research efforts that have distinguished the McMaster approach to the evaluation and treatment of families (Ryan, Epstein, Keitner, Bishop, & Miller, in press). In addition to our own work based on the MMFF, we have accumulated over 150 references on studies that use various parts of the model covering a variety of topics—from family functioning in families with a member who has sustained a traumatic brain injury, to the functioning of families with adopted /foster care children, to adjustment and/or cross-cultural comparisons of family functioning across different ethnic groups.

This brief summary of the MMFF, as well as the synopsis of research findings, are indicators of the vitality of the McMaster approach and the variety of family studies being generated by the theoretical issues developed from the model. We continue to be gratified by the interest in our work and the McMaster approach, and are impressed by the enormous amount of family research being done today, with or without the use of our model. In the end, all these studies serve to throw further light on the functioning of healthy as well as pathological families.

REFERENCES

Bishop, D. S., & Epstein, N. B. (1979, July). *Research on teaching methods.* Paper presented at the International Forum for Trainers and Family Therapists, Tavinstock Clinic, London.

Bishop, D. S., Epstein, N. B., Baldwin, L. M., & Miller, I. W. (1988). Older couples: The effect of health, retirement, and family functioning on morale. *Family Systems Medicine, 6*(2), 238–247.

Bishop, D. S., Epstein, N. B., Keitner, G. I., Miller, I. W., & Zlotnick, C. (1987). *McMaster Structured Interview of Family Functioning (McSiff).* Providence, RI: Brown University Family Research Program.

Bishop, D. S., Epstein, N. B., Keitner, G. I., Miller, I. W., & Zlotnick, C., & Ryan, C. E. (2000). *McMaster Structured Interview of Family Functioning (McSiff).* Providence, RI: Brown University Family Research Program.

Bishop, D. S., Evans, R. L., Miller, I. W., Epstein, N. B., Keitner, G. I., Ryan, C. E., Weinter, D., & Johnson, B. (1998). *Family Intervention: Telephone Tracking: A treatment manual for acute stroke patients.* Unpublished manuscript, Brown University Family Research Program, Providence, RI.

Byles, J. (1979). *Study of families being seen at a family medicine clinic for nonpsyciatric problems.* Unpublished manuscript, McMaster University, Ontario, Canada.

Byles, J., Byrne, C., Boyle, M., & Offord, D. (1988). Ontario child health study: Reliability and validity of the general functioning subscale of the McMaster Family Assessment Device. *Family Process, 27,* 97–104.

Carter, E., & McGoldrick, M. (Eds.). (1998). *The expanded family life cycle.* Boston: Allyn & Bacon.

Epstein, N. B., Baldwin, L. M., & Bishop, D. S. (1982). *The McMaster Clinical Rating Scale (MCRS).* Providence, RI: Brown University Family Research Program.

Epstein, N. B., Baldwin, L. M., & Bishop, D. S. (1983). The McMaster Family Assessment Device. *Journal of Marital and Family Therapy, 9*(2), 171–180.

Epstein, N. B., & Bishop, D. S. (1973). State of the art—1973. *Canadian Psychiatric Association Journal, 18,* 175–183.

Epstein, N. B., & Bishop, D. S. (1981). Problem centered systems therapy of the family. In A. S. Gurman & D. P. Kniskern (Eds.), *Handbook of family therapy.* New York: Brunner/Mazel.

Epstein, N. B., Bishop, D. S., & Levin, S. (1978). The McMaster model of family functioning. *Journal of Marriage and Family Counseling, 4,* 19–31.

Epstein, N. B., Levin, S., & Bishop, D. S. (1976). The family as a social unit. *Canadian Family Physician, 22,* 1411–1413.

Epstein, N. B., Sigal, J. J., & Rakoff, V. (1962). *Family categories schema.* Unpublished manuscript, Jewish General Hospital, Department of Psychiatry, Montreal, Quebec, Canada.

Epstein, N. B., & Westley, W. A. (1959). Patterns of intra-familial communication. In *Psychiatric Research Reports 11* (pp. 1–9). Washington, DC: American Psychiatric Association.

Guttman, H. A., Spector, R. M., Sigal, J. J., Epstein, N. B., & Rakoff, V. (1972). Coding of affective expression in conjoint family therapy. *American Journal of Psychotherapy, 26,* 185–194.

Guttman, H. A., Spector, R. M., Sigal, J. J., Rakoff, V., & Epstein, N. B. (1971). Reliability of coding affective communication in family therapy sessions: Problems of measurement and interpretation. *Journal of Consulting and Clinical Psychology, 37,* 397–402.

Hadley, T. R., Jacob, T., Milliones, J., Caplan, J., & Spitz, D. (1974). The relationship between family developmental crisis and the appearance of symptoms in a family member. *Family Process, 13,* 207–214.

Hill, R. (1965). Generic features of families under stress. In H. N. Parad (Ed.), *Crisis intervention: Selected readings* (pp. 32–52). New York: Family Services Association of America.

Kabacoff, R. I., Miller, I. W., Bishop, D. S., Epstein, N. B., & Keitner, G. I. (1990). A psychometric study of the McMaster Family Assessment Device in psychiatric, medical, and nonclinical examples. *Journal of Family Psychology, 3*(4), 431–439.

Langsley, D. G., & Kaplan, D. M. (1968). *The treatment of families in crisis.* New York: Grune & Stratton.

Levin, S., Rubenstein, J., & Streiner, D. L. (1976). The parent–therapist program: An innovative approach to treating emotionally disturbed children. *Hospital and Community Psychiatry, 27,* 407–410.

Maziade, M., Bernier, H., Thivierge, J., & Cote, R. (1987). The relationship between family functioning and demographic characteristics in an epidemiological study. *Canadian Journal of Psychiatry, 32*(7), 526–533.

Maziade, M., Caperaa, P., Boudreault, M., Thivierge, J., Cote, R., & Boutin, P. (1986). The effect of temperament on longitudinal academic achievement in primary school. *Journal of the American Academy of Child Psychiatry, 25,* 692–696.

Maziade, M., Caperaa, P., Laplante, B., Boudreault, M., Thivierge, J., Cote, R., & Boutin, P. (1985). Value of difficult temperament among 7-year-olds in the general population for predicting psychiatric diagnosis at age 12. *American Journal of Psychiatry, 142,* 943–946.

Maziade, M., Cote, R., Boutin, P., Bernier, H., & Thivierge, J. (1987). Temperament and intellectual development: A longitudinal study from infancy to four years. *American Journal of Psychiatry, 144,* 144–150.

Miller, I. W., Epstein, N. B., Bishop, D. S., & Keitner, G. I. (1985). The McMaster Family Assessment Device: Reliability and validity. *Journal of Marital and Family Therapy, 11*(4), 345–356.

Miller, I. W., Kabacoff R. I., Epstein, N. B., Bishop, D. S., Keitner, G. I., Baldwin, L. M., & van der Spuy, H. I. J. (1994). The development of a clinical rating scale for the McMaster Model of Family Functioning. *Family Process, 33,* 53–69.

Miller, I. W., Ryan, C. E., Keitner, G. I., Bishop, D. S., & Epstein, N. B. (2000a). Commentary on "Factor Analyses of the Family Assessment Device by Ridenour, Daley, & Reich." *Family Process, 39,* 141–144.

Miller, I. W., Ryan, C. E., Keitner, G. I., Bishop, D. S., & Epstein, N. B. (2000b). The McMaster Approach to Families: Theory, assessment, treatment, research. *Journal of Family Therapy, 22*(2), 168–189.

Miller, I. W., Ryan, C. E., Keitner, G. I., Bishop, D. S., & Epstein, N. B. (2000c). Why fix what isn't broken?: A rejoinder to Ridenour, Daley, and Reich. *Family Process, 39,* 381–384.

Parad, H. J., & Caplan, G. (1965). A framework for studying families in crisis. In H. J. Parad (Ed.), *Crisis intervention: Selected readings* (pp. 53–72). New York: Family Service Association of America.

Postner, R. S., Guttman, H. A., Sigal, J. J., Epstein, N. B., & Rakoff, V. (1971). Process and outcome in conjoint family therapy. *Family Process, 10,* 451–473.

Rakoff, V., Sigal, J. J., Spector, R., & Guttman, H. A. (1967). *Communications in families.* Unpublished report on investigation, aided by grants from Foundations Fund for research in Psychiatry, Laidlaw Foundation.

Ridenour, T. A., Daley, J. G., & Reich W. (1999). Factor analyses of the Family Assessment Device. *Family Process, 38,* 497–510.

Ridenour, T. A., Daley, J. G., & Reich W. (2000). Further evidence that the Family Assessment Device should be reorganized: Response to Miller and colleagues. *Family Process, 39,* 375–380.

Rubenstein, J., Armentrout, J., Levin, S., & Herald, D. (1978). The parent–therapist program: Alternative care for emotionally disturbed children. *American Journal of Orthopsychiatry, 48,* 654–662.

Ryan, C. E., Epstein, N. B., Keitner, G. I., Bishop, D. S., & Miller, I. W. (in press) *McMaster model of family functioning: A comprehensive method for evaluation and treatment of families.* Philadelphia: Brunner/Mazel.

Santa-Barbara, J., Woodward, C. A., Levin, S., Steiner, D. Goodman, J., & Epstein, N. B. (1975, September). *The relationship between therapists' characteristics and outcome variables in family therapy.* Paper presented at the Canadian Psychiatric Association, Banff, Alberta.

Sigal, J. J., Rakoff, V., & Epstein, N. B. (1967). Indicators of therapeutic outcome in conjoint family therapy. *Family Process, 6*(2), 215–226.

Solomon, M. A. (1973). A developmental, conceptual premise for family therapy. *Family Process, 12,* 179–188.

Speare, A., & Kobrin, F. (1980, August). *Biases in panel studies of migration.* Paper presented at the American Statistical Association, Houston, TX.

Westley, W. A., & Epstein, N. B. (1960). Report on the psychosocial organization of the family and mental health. In D. Willner (Ed.), *Decisions, values, and groups* (Vol. 1, pp. 278–303). New York: Pergamon Press.

Westley, W. A., & Epstein, N. B. (1969). *The silent majority.* San Francisco: Jossey-Bass.

Woodward, C. A., Santa-Barbara, J., Levin, S., Epstein, N. B., & Streiner, D. (1977). *The McMaster family therapy outcome study: III. Client and treatment characteristics significantly contributing to clinical outcomes.* Paper presented at the 54th annual meeting of the American Orthopsychiatric Association, New York.

Woodward, C. A., Santa-Barbara, J., Levin, S., Goodman, J., Streiner, D., & Epstein, N. B. (1975, June). *Client and therapist characteristics related to family therapy outcome: Closure and follow-up evaluation.* Paper presented at the Society for Psychotherapy Research, Boston.

Woodward, C. A., Santa-Barbara, J., Levin, S., Goodman, J., Streiner, D., Muzzin, L., & Epstein, N. B. (1974). *Outcome research in family therapy: On the growing edginess of family therapists.* Paper presented at the Nathan W. Ackerman Memorial Conference, Margarita Island, Venezuela.

CHAPTER 22

UNRAVELING THE COMPLEXITY OF GENETIC AND ENVIRONMENTAL INFLUENCES ON FAMILY RELATIONSHIPS

Hilary Towers
Erica Spotts
David Reiss

Findings from the past decade of quantitative genetic research suggest that genes and environment frequently operate on individual behaviors, and on family relationships, in an interactive and nonlinear fashion (Collins, Maccoby, Steinberg, Hetherington, & Bornstein, 2000; Turkheimer, 2000). Since the publication of the second edition of *Normal Family Processes,* the field has made significant strides in the effort to begin to peel apart the layers of human behavioral complexity. The discovery that genetic factors account for a significant portion of variation in virtually every human behavior was an essential first step in addressing the broad issue of behavioral complexity. Twin, family, and adoption studies have confirmed moderate to substantial genetic influence on such widely varying conditions as schizophrenia, neurotic disorders, and autism (see review by McGuffin, Owen, O'Donovan, Thapar, & Gottesman, 1994), as well as social responsibility (Neiderhiser, Reiss, & Hetherington, 1996), cognition (Plomin & DeFries, 1999), and optimism (Plomin et al., 1992).

Likewise, the more recent discovery of genetic contributions to family *relationships,* such as parenting (Deater-Deckard, 2000; Dunn & Plomin,

1986; Elkins, McGue, & Iacono, 1997) and sibling relationships (Rende, Slomkowski, Stocker, Fulker, & Plomin, 1992), made an important contribution to our understanding of the complicated interplay between genes and family environment. Such findings confirm, again, the complexity of human behavior, namely, that most behaviors occur within the context of reciprocal, long-term relationships, which are themselves a representation of a very intricate pattern of interactions between people, formed over time. So, when a mother treats her adolescent harshly, and that adolescent displays unruly or "rowdy" behavior, we have learned that this association may reflect more than the psychological impact of the mother and the child on one another. Numerous alternatives now exist to account for such an association: Perhaps the adolescent's genetic propensity toward externalizing behavior plays a large role in evoking maternal negativity; perhaps these genetic tendencies toward impulsive behavior are ones the child shares with one or both biological parents, a phenomenon called passive gene–environment (GE) correlation. Alternatively, perhaps the heritable traits that impact the parent–child relationship most are those of the child, a phenomenon called evocative/active GE correlation.

Although the concept of GE correlation isn't a new one (see Chapter 5 by Bussell and Reiss entitled "Genetic Influences on Family Processes," in the second edition of this book), most genetically informed studies of parenting have been unable to isolate the *nature* of the GE correlation (e.g., evocative or passive) likely to be operating in parent–child associations. Consequently, we have been unsure about *whose* genes are really more important to the relationships of interest. In other words, are the behaviors of children associated with those of their biological parents only because of their 50% genetic similarity to one another? Or is it possible that children's own, heritable traits actually *shape* the behaviors of their parents toward them? The answer to this question has implications for many disciplines, both basic and clinical in orientation, since it speaks to the issue of the mechanisms underlying major family subsystems (in this case, the parent–child relationship). If heritable behaviors of the child evoke parental negativity, for instance, clinical efforts might be directed toward intervening more at the parent level. As we clarify in our discussion of GE interaction, there is accumulating evidence that favorable environmental conditions (e.g., in the home) can dramatically alter—or even eliminate—the impact of the same genetic factors that can cause psychopathology in unfavorable environments. In this sense, findings of genetic influence on family subsystems do not imply a hopeless scenario for families in distress. Neither does knowledge of genetic influence on behaviors imply that the home, or one's rearing environment, is not important. As we shall see, family environment, both of the "shared" and "nonshared" variety, plays an important and distinct role in human development.

The ability to distinguish between types of GE correlation in parent–child relationships is just one example of how the field of quantitative genetics has made significant gains in the effort to clarify the mechanisms underlying genetic and environmental influences on family relationships. Other equally important examples include identification of GE interactions, isolation of specific sources of sibling-specific environmental variation in behavior, and a focus on the potential for shared environment to moderate these sibling-specific associations. The purpose of this chapter is to provide an overview of some of the conceptual and methodological advances that have occurred within the field over the past decade. Information relevant to the study of family systems and processes is covered, with a particular focus on the following areas: (1) sensitivity of the family environment to variation in genotype (GE correlation), (2) sensitivity of genotype to the environment (GE interaction), (3) sibling-specific (or "nonshared") environments, and (4) the role of environmental factors shared by family members in shaping family relationships. Prior to a more detailed discussion of recent findings, we provide a brief definition and description of each conceptual area.

INTRODUCTION TO FOUR KEY QUANTITATIVE GENETIC CONCEPTS

Gene–Environment Correlation

GE correlation refers broadly to the estimated association between a person's environment (and the people in it) and that person's genetically influenced behaviors, and may be partitioned into three types (see Scarr & McCartney, 1983, for an in-depth description). Briefly, *passive* GE correlation refers to a correlation between a measure of the environment (e.g., parenting) and a genotype (e.g., that of a child), which is due to the 50% genetic-relatedness of the two. For example, a father may pass on to his child those genes that contribute to his own depression. A passive GE correlation could explain genetic influences on parent–child negativity in this example, because the depression genes shared by the father and the child also contribute to making the relationship strained and negative in tone. The two alternative types of GE correlation, *evocative* and *active*, represent the possibility that children's genetically influenced characteristics play an important role in shaping their own environments. Evocative GE correlation refers to the reaction of others (who *need not* be genetically related) to someone based on some genetically influenced trait of that person. For example, a husband may be overly critical toward a wife who is genetically predisposed to being gloomy and depressed. Or an adoptive mother may respond negatively to the difficult temperament of a newly adopted child. Active GE correlation refers to an individual's seeking out a particular environment based upon a genetically influenced characteristic. For example, Manke, McGuire, Reiss, Hetherington, and Plomin (1995) found that there are strong genetic influences on the quality of an adolescent's peer group. This suggest that heritable features of adolescents shape their choice of peer groups.

In the past couple of years, there has been an increase in the number of quantitative genetic studies that examine GE correlation directly. Such studies rely mainly on information regarding the characteristics of children adopted away at birth, their adoptive parents, and at least one biological parent. These adoption designs are ideal tools for assessing evocative GE correlation, because information on the psychiatric, biological, and criminal histories of the biological parent serves as a proxy for the adopted child's genetic characteristics. The adoptive parents constitute an environment entirely "disentangled" from the child's genes (because the adoptive parents share none of their segregating genes, or genes that cause human variation, with their adopted child). Finding an association between the heritable behaviors of an adopted child (e.g., the psychiatric or criminal characteristics of the biological parent) and the parenting of that child by his or her adoptive parents, then, suggests the presence of an evocative GE correlation. In the subsequent section on GE correlation, we examine recent findings of GE correlation with regard to parent–child relationships, in addition to anticipating the findings of an adult twin study designed to assess GE correlation between husbands and wives.

Gene–Environment Interaction

We can think of GE interaction as the "flip side" of GE correlation, although both can (and likely do) operate simultaneously to influence human behavior. GE interaction occurs when the environment has an impact on the degree to which genetic influences are expressed. Genetic influences may occur in some circumstances and not others. For example, one study of GE interaction in the development of antisocial behavior found that adolescent adoptees at genetic risk for becoming antisocial (indicted by the presence of an impulsive disorder in at least one birth parent) were much more likely to do so when placed into adoptive homes in which the environment was characterized by "adverse" factors, including a depressed adoptive mother or marital discord between the adoptive parents (Cadoret, Cain, & Crowe, 1983). Such a finding suggests that the compounded effect of genes and environment may outweigh the single, main effect of each, at least for certain behaviors. As we will see, the most current studies of GE interaction confirm the potential for one's family environment to alter the realization of his or her genetic blueprints.

Associations between Sibling-Specific Environments: "Nonshared Associations"

"Nonshared environment" refers to the repeated finding that children who are raised in the same family are often quite different from one another because of environmental influences on their respective behaviors. In fact, siblings from the same household are frequently just as *different* from one another, for reasons due to their environments, as they are *similar* to one another for genetic reasons, with both sources of influence ac-

counting for approximately half of the variation in a variety of human behaviors (see review by Plomin, Chipuer, & Neiderhiser, 1994). Such nonshared environmental influences may include different peer groups or
friendships, different parenting, different experiences of trauma, different work environments, and different romantic partners or spouses. However, as we shall see, the difficulty has been in finding evidence of the substantial and systematic impact of any of these variables on sibling
differences. Nonshared environment remains a "hot topic" in the field of
quantitative genetic research, because it has been shown to be important
to a wide array of behaviors across the entire lifespan, yet its *systematic* causes remain elusive (Turkheimer & Waldron, 2000). In a subsequent section
on nonshared environment, we examine recent efforts to identify sources
of nonshared environmental influence on behaviors, including some preliminary analyses of nonshared associations using an adult-based twin
study we are conducting. We then discuss some of the recent speculation
about why it has been so difficult to find large, systematic effects of variables that cause within-family differences.

Shared Family Environment

There remains broad agreement today within the field of quantitative genetics that "the general family environment is not a very important determinant of variations in children's outcomes" (Bussell & Reiss, 1993, p.
161). This conclusion is based on the quantitative genetic finding that
when young siblings are similar with respect to constructs such as IQ
(Scarr & Weinberg, 1983) and personality (Loehlin, Willerman, & Horn,
1987), it is usually for *genetic* reasons, and not because of "shared" influences within their environment, such as common parenting, common
friends, or family socioeconomic scale level. Although it is true that shared
environmental influences appear to account for less variation in many
human behaviors than nonshared ones (new, preliminary twin data provide exceptions to this "rule," as described in the next section), some researchers are beginning to reexamine the relevance of shared environment within the context of more sophisticated models of influence
(McHale & Pawletko, 1992; Turkheimer, Haley, Waldron, D'Onofrio, &
Gottesman, submitted). For example, it has been suggested that factors
traditionally conceptualized as working exclusively "between families" may
moderate nonshared environmental factors. The basis for such proposals
is described in a following section on shared environment.

CONCEPTUAL AND METHODOLOGICAL ADVANCES

Gene–Environment Correlation

Evidence for the association between one's genotype and characteristics of
his or her social environment has been accumulating over the past several

years (Deater-Deckard, 2000; Ge et al., 1996; O'Connor, Deater-Deckard, Fulker, Rutter, & Plomin, 1998; van Os, Park, & Jones, 2001), although such studies continue to be relatively rare. The reason these studies are relevant to research concerned with family process is that most theories linking child adjustment to family "environment," including parenting behaviors, have presumed that these associations were caused by environmental mechanisms (e.g., Patterson, 1982), due, primarily, to the reliance of these theories on data collected using designs that provide no information on genetic influences. Most often, any observed correlations between the two have been interpreted as evidence of socialization. Although such research has made an invaluable contribution to our knowledge of the importance of parent–child relationships to children's functioning, what we know now from twin studies suggests that the influence of children's genetic factors on their own behavior is roughly equal to that of their family environment. More importantly, these same genetic factors have been shown to correlate with behaviors exhibited by family members toward the child, which may indicate the role of children's heritable characteristics in shaping their own family environment.

For example, a cross-sectional examination of adopted adolescents and their families found that the association between parenting and negative adolescent outcome could be explained by evocative GE correlation (Ge et al., 1996). Results from this study indicate that the same genes that contribute to antisocial behavior in adolescents also seem to evoke specific parenting practices in their adoptive parents. In other words, it was the children's genes that accounted for the association between parenting, on the one hand, and child outcome, on the other. A separate, more recent adoption study confirmed the presence of a GE correlation mechanism for the same parent–child relationship construct, only employing a longitudinal design (O'Connor et al., 1998). O'Connor and colleagues found that 7- to 12-year-olds who were at genetic risk for becoming antisocial, a risk assessed by measuring antisocial behavior in their biological parents, were more likely to evoke negative parenting from their adoptive parents than were those adopted children not at genetic risk. Such a finding confirms that we are capable of predicting problematic relationships between adopted children and their adoptive parents from knowledge of the presence of psychopathology in their birth parents. Interestingly, the same study found that a range of the adopted children's *internalizing* behaviors, although significantly heritable and associated with parenting, did *not* account for negative parenting patterns of their adoptive parents. In most instances, it seems that the more salient heritable characteristics of children, such as externalizing or aggression, are those most likely to evoke reaction from parents (although we discuss an exception to this pattern below).

The GE correlation mechanism observed in these two studies (Ge et al., 1996; O'Connor et al., 1998) is thought to account for at least some of the genetic influence often observed on certain measures traditionally considered to be environmental, such as negative parenting. The process is likely reciprocal and compounds itself with time, such that a child's externalizing behavior is only intensified by the negative parenting it evoked, causing a further increase in parental negativity, and so on. In fact, a recent publication was the first to make this parent–child reciprocity, or "mutuality," the explicit focus of genetic analysis (Deater-Deckard & O'Connor, 2000). The study was also unique in its findings of GE correlation between *positive* child and parent behaviors. Three aspects of mother–child dyadic mutuality, including cooperation, emotional reciprocity, and responsiveness, were assessed in two separate, genetically informed samples of young children. Results of genetic analyses of these relationship constructs showed both substantial genetic and nonshared environmental influences on all three aspects of mother–child mutuality. In other words, within each family, the two siblings' mutual relationships with their mothers were both similar to and different from (i.e., relationship-specific) one another. When they were similar, it was due to the impact of some aspect of the children's genetically influenced behavior on the mother's parenting, and not to the children's similar rearing experiences, or shared environment. This inference was based on the finding that siblings who were most genetically similar to one another (e.g., identical twins) had more similar, mutual relationships with their mothers than did siblings who were less genetically similar (e.g., fraternal twins). These results suggest the potential for evocative GE correlation mechanisms to play a role in the interactions between children as young as 3 years old and their parents.

Findings such as these are consistent with earlier work that confirms children and adolescents are not merely passive recipients of parenting efforts, but instead often actively elicit and affect parents' behaviors through the children's own heritable traits (Lytton, 1980; Scarr & McCartney, 1983). But what about the potential for GE correlation to occur within family relationships other than those between parents and children? Such instances will have implications for the workings of normal family processes to the extent that they impact the various subsystems that characterize families (e.g., the marriage relationship). Although research examining GE correlation within family subsystems has been concerned primarily with parent–child associations, there have been reports of GE correlation among other family subsystems, including sibling (Plomin, Reiss, Hetherington, & Howe, 1994; Stocker & Dunn, 1994) and marital (Block, Block, & Gjerde, 1986) relationships. However, such publications, to date, have focused on circumstances surrounding the *child* for whom genetic and environmental data have been collected. The following description of preliminary findings from an adult-based twin study provides one example of current efforts to identify and describe GE correlation patterns in *adult* family subsystems.

The Twin Mothers (TM) sample consists of 326 adult monozygotic (MZ) and dizygotic (DZ) twin pairs of women with at least one adolescent child, and their spouses or live-in partners of a minimum of 5 years. One primary goal of the TM project (Reiss et al., 2001) has been to identify genetic and environmental underpinnings of the husband–wife family subsystem. Because the focus of assessment in the TM sample is the adult twin women's genes, one form of GE correlation in this context refers to the role of the women's heritable characteristics in eliciting, and potentially constraining, relationships with their husbands. Much like the finding of child genetic influence on the association between child behaviors and parenting (discussed earlier), this type of mechanism would be indicated by a finding of wives' genetic influence on the association between a characteristic of the husband and of the wife.

For example, there is a strong correlation in the TM data between a husband's and a wife's perceptions of their overall marital satisfaction. Interestingly, both wife and *husband* reports show moderate genetic influence on the extent to which they view the marriage as satisfactory. The finding of genetic influence on the husband's perceptions in this sample is particularly fascinating, because it indicates that the effect of the wife's genes is not just on her perceptions of the marriage. The wife's genes also influence her husband's perceptions. This is because any observed genetic influence on behaviors in the TM sample can only reflect that influence emanating from the *wives* (we have no genetic data on the husbands). The wives' genetic characteristics are somehow associated with their husbands' perceptions of marital satisfaction. While it is possible that this association merely reflects assortative mating (i.e., a wife seeks out a husband compatible with her heritable characteristics), it may also be true that the husband is *responding* to some heritable trait of the wife, and that this response leads him to feel a certain way about the marriage. Only further study of the mechanisms underlying both the husband's and wife's perceptions of the marital subsystem will shed light on this important distinction.

To date, there appear to be no other published studies of GE correlation among adult family subsystems such as marriage and adult sibling relationships. Although the detection of mechanisms underlying the parent–child relationship is an important first step, the mental health of individual family members—and of children in particular—is known to be closely related to other relationships that exist within the family, like marriage (Harold, Fincham, Osborne, & Conger, 1997; Stocker & Youngblade, 1999) and sibling relationships—both in childhood (Volling & Belsky, 1992) and adulthood (Stocker, Lanthier, & Furman, 1997). In accordance with a true systems approach to family research, future quantitative genetic studies should begin to search for the mechanisms responsible for creating and maintaining GE correlations among all of the various subsystems of the family.

Gene–Environment Interaction

In animal studies, researchers can assign one genetic strain to two contra-dicting environments and do the same for a second genetic strain, known as "cross-fostering." In fact, some of the most useful information we have obtained concerning the potential relevance of the early rearing environ-ment to gene expression has come from rearing experiments using non-human mammals (Suomi, 2000). Most Old World monkeys (e.g., rhesus) and chimps share approximately 90–95% and 99%, respectively, of their genes with human beings. This means that while the analog isn't perfect, animal models of the mechanisms underlying biological/gene–behavioral links constitute an indispensable part of human studies—including re-search aimed at illuminating family processes.

Take, for example, the problem of childhood aggression—not infre-quently the focus of family therapy intervention. A series of animal studies shows biological evidence of strong associations between the serotonergic functioning and highly aggressive behavior of a group of preadolescent rhesus monkeys (Champoux, Higley, & Suomi, 1997; Mehlman et al., 1994). The studies found that low levels of a particular serotonin metabo-lite (5-HIAA) in the cerebrospinal fluid (CSF) of these monkeys are highly predictive of certain patterns of extremely aggressive and often deadly be-haviors, including life-threatening tree-to-tree leaps, attacks on dominant members of one's troop, and interactions with peers and nongroup mem-bers characterized by damage to vital tissues (Mehlman et al., 1994). Fur-thermore, it appears that individual differences in rhesus monkey levels of 5-HIAA are genetically influenced (Higley et al., 1993). These findings are particularly interesting in light of recent work suggesting that an identical biological mechanism may account for acts of aggression in *human* chil-dren and adults. Human studies have found evidence for a link between 5-HIAA concentrations and numerous forms of aggression, including ani-mal torture by children (Kruesi, 1989), children's disruptive behavioral disorders (Kruesi et al., 1990), adult male convicts (Linnoila et al., 1983), successful suicides (Mann, Arango, & Underwood, 1990), and men with personality disorders who score high on scales of aggression (Brown, Lin-noila, & Goodwin, 1990), to name a few.

Even more provocative are findings from a prospective study con-ducted with rhesus monkeys demonstrating a moderating effect of *early rearing environment* on this well-documented association between one's ge-netic propensity toward low CSF 5-HIAA levels and one's aggressive be-haviors (Bennett et al., 1998). It seems that whether monkeys develop a relationship *with their mother* is a critical factor in determining the expres-sion of their genetic risk toward aggression. For instance, the study found an association between a "polymorphism," or variation in DNA associated with specific behaviors, and negative behavioral outcomes for the mon-keys. Specifically, having a short version of a transporter gene implicated in serotonergic activity was associated with depressed serotonergic functioning and increased alcohol consumption for those monkeys reared by their *peers*. Alternatively, being raised by one's mother seemed to serve as a "buffer" to these negative effects among monkeys with the same short version of the gene, who showed reduced risk for excessive alcohol consumption and high social dominance. These findings provide more evidence of the role of the early environment in the biological and genetic processes involved in *human* functioning than is commonly acknowledged.

Although animal experiments are certainly better suited to assess specific GE interactions, numerous studies have demonstrated the usefulness of adoption designs for uncovering GE interactions among humans, focusing on psychiatric illnesses ranging from depression and alcoholism (Cadoret, 1995; Cadoret et al., 1996) to schizophrenia (Tienari et al., 1994; Tsuang, Stone, & Faraone, 2001) and antisocial personality disorder (Bohman, 1996). The basic premise of most of these studies is that children adopted at a young age into a new "environment," or home, come with genetic characteristics (usually indexed via the psychiatric status of their biological parent). If the environment is capable of either constraining or modifying their genetic tendencies, then we would expect to find that the developmental trajectories of individuals with the same genetic propensities (e.g., toward antisocial behavior) *differ* as a function of whether they are placed into a supportive or a disruptive adoptive home.

For example, Bohman (1996) found that male children with a genetic propensity toward criminality (as indexed by criminal behavior of a biological parent) who experienced unstable preadoptive (e.g., multiple temporary placements) or adverse adoptive conditions (e.g., low socioeconomic status) evidenced much higher rates of petty criminality than did those children with the same genetic risk placed into stable adoptive conditions. Similarly, schizophrenic symptoms (e.g., thought disorder) appear among children at genetic risk for schizophrenia who are raised in a home with a schizophrenic parent (Kinney et al., 1997), and full-blown schizophrenia is present among those adopted into homes with multiple problems (Tienari et al., 1994). Remarkably, there is an *absence* of these symptoms among adoptees who have a genetic liability toward schizophrenia but were adopted into well-adjusted families.

These results confirm a recent statement by Suomi, in reference to his study of GE interaction in monkeys: "It is hard to imagine that the situation would be any less complex for humans" (2000, p. 253). Indeed, this area of human research is in its infancy. Still, what we have observed thus far makes at least one point very clear: Having a genetic propensity toward a particular behavior—good or bad—is not a "recipe" for expression of that behavior. Knowledge of an individual's genotype (a not-too-distant prospect), combined with early intervention at the level of the family environment, may well prove to be the critical combination for preventing serious psychopathology.

The Search for Nonshared Environmental Associations

The topic of nonshared environmental variation in behavior, or within-family differences, has been of primary interest to quantitative geneticists for some time. This interest is derived from one simple fact: Across a very wide range of individual characteristics and behaviors, children raised in the same home are more often *different* from one another than they are similar (Reiss et al., 1994). Most importantly, these behavioral differences are the product of some aspect of the children's environment—and not to differences in their genes. How do we know this to be the case? Just as genetic influences on behaviors are inferred from comparisons of different sibling types, so can these nonshared environmental outcomes be detected through similar comparisons. For example, identical twins are 100% genetically identical. This means that when members of an identical twin pair exhibit different behaviors, these differences cannot be due to genetic differences: They must be the result of differential effects of factors within each twin's respective *environment*. As we shall see, this unique opportunity to separate the effects of genes and environment on behavior has made identical twins very popular among behavioral geneticists.

Prior to a review of some of the more recent efforts to identify nonshared environmental associations, a brief discussion of an important distinction is necessary. While it is clear that within-family differences are substantial for most behaviors, until recently, the *sources* of these differences have remained "anonymous"; that is, quantitative genetic analyses of individual behaviors at one time point (i.e., univariate, cross-sectional analyses) can only tell us that siblings are different because of factors in their environments. An example using the MZ twin methodology (cited earlier) clarifies this point. If the adjustment behavior of interest is depression, and we find there are substantial differences in levels of depression *within MZ twin pairs,* then a nonshared environmental influence on depression is indicated. However, we still don't know what factors are causing, or contributing to, these behavioral differences. It is only fairly recently that people have begun to assess the causes of within-family differences by examining nonshared environmental associations between proposed environmental factors (e.g., peer relations) and adjustment (e.g., depression). In the simplest form of these bivariate analyses, MZ differences for an environmental factor may be correlated with MZ twin differences for an adjustment factor, with the purpose of revealing the relationship between the two, which represents "pure," noshared environmental association. In the past decade or so, this effort to uncover nonshared environmental associations has become widespread (see review in Turkheimer & Waldron, 2000). The following section provides a brief overview of the major findings produced by recent studies searching for causes of within-family environmental differences.

The second edition of *Normal Family Processes* (Bussell & Reiss, 1993) referred to the Nonshared Environment in Adolescent Development (NEAD) project (Reiss et al., 1994), an effort only recently undertaken at the time of publication. NEAD's goal was to clarify environmental sources of sibling differences. Since then, all the major findings from this project have been reviewed in book form (Reiss, Neiderhiser, Hetherington, & Plomin, 2000). It is notable that the title of one particular section on genetic and environmental associations between family relationships and adolescent adjustment speaks directly to the current topic: the silence of the nonshared family environment. Seven different indices of adolescent adjustment were assessed in NEAD, including depressive symptoms, antisocial behavior, cognitive agency, sociability, social responsibility, autonomy, and global self-worth. Negative, positive, and controlling aspects of parents' behaviors toward their adolescents, in addition to positive and negative aspects of the siblings' relationships with one another, were assessed using multiple reporters, including parents, children, and observers.

Despite the presence of nonshared environmental influence on both adolescent adjustment and parenting at specific time points (sibling relationships were due almost entirely to shared environment), there was virtually no systematic impact of differential parenting practices on sibling differences in adjustment across the interval of early to late adolescence. This conclusion was based on (among results of other, more complex analyses) the observation that MZ twin differences in adolescent adjustment were not substantially associated with differences in the way their parents treated them. It had been expected that the factors contributing to differential parenting would also contribute to, or at least correlate with, factors influencing differential sibling adjustment. Findings from the NEAD project suggested otherwise: Differential sibling adjustment in adolescence is apparently the result of factors in the environment other than differential parenting. For example, recent quantitative genetic studies have turned their focus toward the impact of extrafamilial influences, such as peers (Iervolino et al., 2002; Manke et al., 1995).

The MZ twin difference method is ideal in its relative simplicity and its stringency, because reduced sample sizes and the general tendency for MZ twins to be *more* rather than less similar to one another than DZ twins decreases the likelihood of finding significant associations. Yet very few quantitative genetic analyses have employed the use of MZ differences. Of those that have, the reported associations have almost exclusively relied on self-reports of both the environment, which are often retrospective, and current psychological adjustment (Baker & Daniels, 1990; Bouchard & McGue, 1990). While this doesn't diminish the importance of their findings, exclusive reliance on within-reporter difference correlations (i.e., correlations between two measures reported by the same informant) is subject to the same criticism that applies to standard, two-variable correlations, namely, that the correlations are more likely to represent rater bias of some sort than are more objective, across-reporter correlations.

However, one very recent MZ difference analysis of nonshared environmental influences on the socioemotional development of preschool children provides evidence for at least moderate and, in some cases, substantial nonshared environmental family associations using parent, interviewer, and observer ratings (Deater-Deckard et al., 2001). In this study, across-rater MZ difference correlations between interviewer reports of parental harshness, for example, and parent reports of the children's problem behaviors, emotionality, and prosocial behavior were .36, .38, and −.27, respectively. Cross-rater MZ difference correlations were also significant between (1) parental positivity and child positivity, (2) parental positivity and child problem behavior (a negative association), (3) parental negative control and child prosocial behavior (a negative association), and (4) parental harsh discipline and child responsiveness (a negative association). These findings can be interpreted as evidence that the differential parental treatment of very young siblings living in the same family *matters*—and it matters *apart from any genetic traits of the child.* For example, when a parent is harsh toward one child and less harsh to the other, the child receiving the harsh discipline is more likely to have behavior problems, be more emotionally labile, and be less prosocial than the sibling.

Of course, one alternative explanation (not directly testable with cross-sectional data) is that differences in the children's behaviors elicit differences in the parents, or that the relationship is reciprocal. As an interesting and related aside, preliminary analysis of parent–child data from the TM sample (described earlier) shows several substantial cross-rater MZ difference correlations between the differential parenting patterns of adult twin women and characteristics of their adolescent children. Although directionality cannot be confirmed in this cross-sectional sample either, such findings in an *adult-based* sample imply that differences in the children are contributing to differences in (or nonshared variation in) parenting behaviors of the mothers, because the mothers' genes and environment are the focus of assessment.

Regardless of the direction of effect, the associations reported by Deater-Deckard and colleagues (2001) are remarkable for at least two reasons. First, within-family differences for at least certain traits have been shown to increase over time—and to be less easily detected in early childhood, when parents are more likely to treat their children similarly (McCartney, Harris, & Bernieri, 1990; Scarr & Weinberg, 1983). Finding associations between differential parenting, a family environment variable, and childhood behaviors with a sample of 3½-year-old children is notable and has implications for clinical intervention efforts that are discussed later in the chapter. Second, the fact that these associations exist across three different rater "perspectives" lends credence to the validity of the associations: They cannot be attributed entirely to the bias of a single reporter. Third, unlike univariate analyses of nonshared environment, analyses of multivariable associations minimize the amount of measurement error in the estimate of nonshared environment.

In light of this apparent success, one may ask, why all the excitement over nonshared environment? Again, the issue is an inability to isolate *systematic* sources of within-family differences in behavior, which are so prevalent. In other words, when single studies have succeeded in specifying sources of sibling differences, there has been a general failure to replicate these findings across samples. A recent meta-analysis of the effect produced by candidate sources of nonshared environment on behavior found the average effect size of studies *using genetically informed designs* to be roughly 2% (Turkheimer & Waldron, 2000). Revelations of this kind have stirred discussion about the definition of nonshared environment itself (Maccoby, 2000; Rowe, Woulbroun, & Gulley, 1994), and some researchers have begun to examine directly the issue of *how* nonshared environment may operate by examining the interplay between shared and nonshared environmental events (Jenkins, Rasbash, & O'Connor, 2001; McHale & Pawletko, 1992; Turkheimer et al., submitted). At the crux of the issue for those who question the traditional approach to searching for nonshared environmental influence on behavior is the issue of whether attention should be focused only on environmental events, factors, or people unique to each sibling—or whether environmental events (e g , family socioeconomic status) that are *shared* among siblings might also impact the extent of differences between them. This leads us to our discussion of a reconceptualization of shared environment.

Shared Environment: Revisited

Where there has been failure among quantitative genetic studies to replicate most nonshared environmental associations, there has certainly been success in replicating a separate but related phenomenon: the relative lack of importance of shared family environment in causing *across*-family similarities in most behaviors. Shared environmental influence is indicated in behavioral genetic research by a finding of sibling similarity in behavior across all sibling types—regardless of the siblings' genetic similarity. For example, if adopted-together siblings, who share 0% of their segregating genes, are very similar in behavior, this indicates that factors in the siblings' common environment are making them similar. For example, one might expect that marital discord would have a relatively similar impact on children living in the same household. Were this the case, we would expect an association between marital distress in the home and the extent to which *multiple* siblings within the same family are well adjusted. In the case of a shared environmental effect, we would not expect marital satisfaction to have a differential impact on within-family sibling adjustment. As it happens, the importance of factors we might assume to be experienced as "shared" by immediate family members—parental socioeconomic status, parental education (because parents are often similar to one another with regard to level of education), marital discord, and family size—doesn't appear to have the shared effect on family members we would predict (Plomin & Bergeman, 1991). These factors don't cause family members to be similar to one another in their behaviors. But might they cause at least some family members to be *different* from each another?

Several very recent sets of analyses, each coming from separate labs, suggest that this seeming contradiction is not only a possibility but also an often untested (and thus undetected) reality. The National Longitudinal Survey of Children and Youth (NLSCY) is a design that includes some 3,860 families from various Canadian provinces, each family with two to four children, 4–11 years old. A recent investigation of the role of child- and family-level effects on differential parenting patterns within this sample showed that differential parenting (the prototypical nonshared environmental variable) was itself a function of, or moderated by, shared environmental factors (Jenkins et al., 2001). For example, the study found that differential parental positivity (more praise directed toward one child than the other, activities enjoyed more often between parent and one child over the other, etc.) was *more frequent* in homes characterized by low socioeconomic status, high marital dissatisfaction, and larger family size. In addition, the study found differential parental negativity to be highest among single-parent families and families in which marital dissatisfaction was great.

Findings from another study using data from a genetically informative sample, the National Perinatal Collaborative Study, also examined the effects of socioeconomic status (a shared environmental factor) on genetic and environmental variation in child IQ (Turkheimer et al., submitted). The study showed that at low levels of family socioeconomic status, the amount of variation in child IQ due to nonshared environment was large. In other words, siblings in families of low socioeconomic status were more likely to *differ* in their IQ levels than were siblings from high socioeconomic status households. Among families in which financial stress was absent (i.e., high socioeconomic status), sibling IQ differences caused by the environment seemed to dissipate. Findings such as these suggest that we may have created a false dichotomy, of sorts, in our conclusions about the relative influence of shared and nonshared environment on behavior. Just as most behaviors are influenced by both nature (genes) and nurture (environment), so it may prove to be the case that many of our behaviors are influenced by both *types* of environment, shared and nonshared, only in ways more complicated than previously thought.

Let us take as one final example of this concept an analysis of peers as nonshared environmental influences on child and adolescent behaviors

(Rowe et al., 1994). Peers are commonly described in the quantitative genetic literature as a potential source of nonshared influence on child and adolescent adjustment, because it is generally assumed that siblings within the same family associate with *different* peers. However, a simple analysis of frequencies using data from the Arizona Sibling study, a survey of siblings ranging from 10 to 16 years in age, showed that the siblings' frequency of contact with friends that were classified as "mutual" to both siblings within a pair was actually quite high. In other words, 47.4% of brother pairs, 34.5% of sister pairs, and 24.8% of mixed-gender sibling pairs reported contact with mutual friends. Because these findings came as somewhat of a surprise to the researchers, it was suggested that variables such as the amount of time spent with mutual friends, or the number of mutual friends, should be assessed as potential *moderators* of nonshared associations between peer networks and adolescent adjustment. In other words, the impact of a mutual friend (seemingly shared, but effectively nonshared) on a sibling's adjustment may depend on the amount of time the friend and the sibling spend together. Perhaps the point to be gleaned from each of these studies is that (at least sometimes) it may be the intricacies of an experience, and the nature of the relationship under study, that matter—and not simply whether the experience is shared or nonshared within a sibling pair.

CONCLUSIONS

We have discussed examples of recent advances in our understanding of four different quantitative genetic concepts, each of which is highly relevant to our understanding of how families function. In the first two sections, we described two mechanisms that may account for a major part of the interaction between genetic and social processes that occurs both between and within the various family subsystems. In the latter two sections, we focused on *specific* environmental mechanisms that most likely act as supplements to, or in conjunction with, GE correlation and interactions. Thus, the question remains: How might we account for these related but distinct mechanisms in terms of a comprehensive developmental theory of family process? The short answer is that much more longitudinal research is needed to confirm the sequence and timing of genetic and environmental interplay among different family members.

However, behavioral genetic findings from various studies of parent–child relationships—both studies of GE correlation and interaction, and studies of specific environmental influence—do lend support to a nonadditive, reciprocal theory of family adjustment, in contrast to a one-way, additive model of influence (Deater-Deckard et al., 2001; Deater-Deckard & O'Connor, 2000; O'Connor et al., 1998; Reiss et al., 2000). Findings from the few longitudinal studies conducted to date suggest the potential for a "family relations–effects" model (Reiss et al., 2000), by which a genetically influenced child behavior sparks a reaction (either negative or positive) from a parent. The parental response in turn serves to reinforce the initial child behavior, and so on. According to this model, a family subsystem (e.g., parent–child) is capable of *mediating* the genetic influence so often observed on adolescent adjustment behaviors. Research showing the ability of 3-year-olds to evoke positive responses within a mother–child interaction (Deater-Deckard & O'Connor, 2000), in addition to evidence for strong genetic influence on temperament in infancy (Braungart, Plomin, DeFries, & Fulker, 1992), illustrates what may be considered the basis for such a developmental trajectory.

If these early, heritable behaviors do indeed turn out to be genetic precursors to subsequent adjustment of the child, then what is left to be demonstrated is the mediating role of parenting on that later adjustment construct. Longitudinal analyses from the NEAD project provide some indirect support for this part of the family relations equation, since there is some evidence that genetic influence on family processes (like parenting) in early adolescence often *precedes* changes in child adjustment from early to late adolescence (Reiss et al., 2000). Researchers used genetic analyses to gain insight into whether such a sequence might be operating between different family processes (parent and sibling variables) and adolescent adjustment constructs. In a majority of cases, the findings supported such a model of effect. For example, a negative association was found between maternal and paternal positivity (both shown to be influenced by an unidentified, genetically influenced behavior of the child) in early adolescence and the child's antisocial behavior in later adolescence. It is interesting to speculate about what may be going on here: Perhaps the parents are responding to some positive heritable characteristic of the child that exists alongside the more "testy" behavior. Whatever the mechanism, the implications for early intervention are clear: The parental response to the child in early adolescence appears to have the effect of *protecting* the child from a pathway to "full-blown" antisocial characteristics.

So we see that the family relations–effects model accommodates behavioral genetic evidence of child genetic effects on family environment, but the model must also account for the large body of psychosocial evidence that family influence on child and adolescent adjustment is substantial (e.g., Conger & Elder, 1994; Kochanska, 1997; Patterson & Bank, 1989). While the longitudinal NEAD findings give us some clues about the *order* of GE interplay, analyses of GE interaction and specific shared and nonshared environmental influences on behaviors are critical for isolating the effects of environment on family processes. Recall the MZ difference analysis that suggested a strong impact of differential parenting on childhood adjustment, *independent* of child genetic effects (Deater-Deckard et al., 2001). It is noteworthy that some of the same differential parent–child relationships observed in this study were also observed in a separate MZ difference study of parenting and adolescent adjustment (Pike, Reiss, Hetherington, & Plomin, 1996). Results such as these, in combination with findings from studies showing that family environment may actually *moderate* both genetic propensities and nonshared environment, are evidence that family environment does matter. On a related note, it is important to remember that part of the influence that parents have on their children may well be grounded in heritable behaviors of the *parents* (Neiderhiser et al., submitted), which may or may not be shared with a given child, because parents and children share only 50% of their genes. Parent-based genetic designs, in which the parents are the twins or siblings of interest, are needed to reveal the extent of such influence.

We are really only beginning to understand the complexities of GE operations within the family. As the enigma surrounding the issue of nonshared environment illustrates well, the "trick" in linking specific influences to family process constructs has been to do so *consistently* across samples. Based on the general lack of consistency of findings from studies of nonshared environmental associations, some researchers in the field have concluded that the reason we cannot isolate *systematic* sources of within-family differences is because these sources are themselves *unsystematic* shared and nonshared environmental experiences that will likely remain undetected by our research designs (Turkheimer, 2000). This hypothesis may well prove unable to be rejected. Undoubtedly, there is so much about human nature that escapes even our most sophisticated methodology: The distinction between "real" behaviors and people's subjective perceptions of behavior patterns (the latter is generally what psychologists have to work with) testifies to this challenge. As noted by Turkheimer, this "chaotic psychological reality" may frustrate psychologists searching to explain what is predictable about human behavior. However, it is ultimately the *unpredictable* part of human behavior and interaction that makes us rational beings with free will.

This being said, the three goals of human developmental psychology are the description, explanation, and optimization of behavior (Baltes, Reese, & Lipsitt, 1980). Part of meeting these goals necessarily entails a thorough assessment of those factors that shape development over the entire lifespan. For example, behavioral genetic evidence to date suggests entirely different mechanisms underlying the link between *children's* own adjustment patterns and behaviors of their parents toward them, and that between *parents'* relationships with their spouse and their child. In the former, genetic factors emanating from the child appear to be important. In the latter, those factors in the environment that make siblings different from one another (perhaps the children and spouses themselves) are most important in determining the quality of adult marriages and parent–child relationships (Spotts et al., submitted; Towers et al., in preparation).

So far, our study of nonshared environmental associations (with the exception of unpublished data from the TM project) has been limited almost exclusively to analyses of children and adolescents. As has already been noted, it has been observed that within-family differences in at least certain characteristics increase with age (McCartney et al., 1990). This makes intuitive sense, because siblings, after they leave home, often go their separate ways—rent their own place, get a job, get married, and so on. Once this happens, a whole host of new people and experiences in the siblings' respective environments may be influential in terms of their behaviors. It seems at least a viable possibility that primary sources of non-shared environmental influence on behavior are to be found in adulthood. As mentioned earlier, analyses from TM project indicate that the majority of the covariation in reports of marital satisfaction by middle-age, adult women and their husbands is due to some aspect of the nonshared environment of the twin women (Spotts et al., submitted). Future research might address the role of *husbands'* genetic and environmental histories in shaping the marital relationship.

Finally, our success in quantifying the relative impact of GE factors (and their mutual interplay) on human behavior has profound implications for therapeutic intervention. For example, the purpose of many types of therapy is often to produce changes in individuals' social environments. How much more effective these therapies may be when based on the knowledge that a particular psychosocial intervention has the potential to alter the mechanisms of genetic expression for a particular trait. Such knowledge may, in fact, enable clinicians to target an intervention toward "knocking out" the *evocative* effects of extreme problem behaviors in young children, which are a function of the heritability of these behaviors. For example, intervention research has demonstrated the potential for altering behavioral responses of mothers toward their infants with difficult temperaments (van den Boom, 1994). The intent is not only to change mothers' behaviors or thought processes but also to eliminate the *evocative association* between the infants' irritable behaviors and their mothers' corresponding expressions of hostility. The combination of an adoption design and a preventive intervention study would make possible an assessment of whether therapy has actually disrupted the pattern of negative maternal response to children's heritable behaviors. Awareness of the different genetic mechanisms underlying both individual traits and relationships will also help to inform clinicians as to why certain forms of intervention are effective in treating some problems but not others. The task before us is to begin to expand our search for the genetic and environmental determinants of individual behaviors to include the interactive GE bridges between various subsystems of the family.

REFERENCES

Baker, L. A., & Daniels, D. (1990). Nonshared environmental influences and personality differences in adult twins. *Journal of Personality and Social Psychology, 58*(1), 103–110.

Baltes, P. B., Reese, H. W., & Lipsitt, L. P. (1980). Life-span developmental psychology. *Annual Review of Psychology, 31,* 65–110.

Bennett, A. J., Lesch, K. P., Heils, A., Long, J., Lorenz, J., Shoaf, S. E., Champoux, M., Suomi, S. J., Linnoila, M., & Higley, J. D. (1998). Serotonin transporter gene variation, strain, and early rearing environment affect CSF 5-HIAA concentrations in rhesus monkeys (*Macaca mulatta*). *American Journal of Primatology, 45,* 168–169.

Block, J. H., Block, J., & Gjerde, P. F. (1986). The personality of children prior to divorce: A prospective study. *Child Development, 57,* 827–840.

Bohman, M. (1996). Predispositions to criminality: Swedish adoption studies in retrospect. In G. R. Bock & J. A. Goode (Eds.), *Genetics of criminal and antisocial behavior: Ciba Foundation Symposium 194* (pp. 99–114). Chichester, UK: Wiley.

Bouchard, T. J., & McGue, M. (1990). Genetic and rearing environmental influences on adult personality: An analysis of adopted twins reared apart. *Journal of Personality, 58*(1), 263–292.

Braungart, J. M., Plomin, R., DeFries, J. C., & Fulker, D. W. (1992). Genetic influence on tester-rated infant temperament as assessed by Bayley's Infant Behavior Record: Nonadoptive and adoptive siblings and twins. *Developmental Psychology, 28*(1), 40–47.

Brown, G. L., Linnoila, M., & Goodwin, F. K. (1990). Clinical assessment of human aggression and impulsivity in relation to biochemical measures. In H. M. Van Praag, R. Plutchik, & A. Apter (Eds.), *Violence and suicidality: Perspectives in clinical and psychobiological research* (pp. 184–217). New York: Brunner/Mazel.

Bussell, D. A., & Reiss, D. (1993). Genetic influences on family process: The emergence of a new framework for family research. In F. Walsh (Ed.), *Normal family processes* (2nd ed., pp. 161–181). New York: Guilford Press.

Cadoret, R. J. (1995). Familial transmission of psychiatric disorders associated with alcoholism. In H. Begleiter (Ed.), *Alcohol and alcoholism* (pp. 70–81). New York: Oxford University Press.

Cadoret, R. J., Cain, C. A., & Crowe, R. R. (1983). Evidence for gene–environment interaction in the development of adolescent antisocial behavior. *Behavior Genetics, 13*(3), 301–310.

Cadoret, R. J., Winokur, G., Langbehn, D., Troughton, E., Yates, W. R., & Stewart, M. A. (1996). Depression spectrum disease: I. The role of gene–environment interaction. *American Journal of Psychiatry, 153*(7), 892–899.

Champoux, M., Higley, J. D., & Suomi, S. J. (1997). Behavioral and physiological characteristics of Indian and Chinese-Indian hybrid rhesus macaque infants. *Developmental Psychobiology, 31,* 49–63.

Collins, W. A., Maccoby, E. E., Steinberg, L., Hetherington, E. M., & Bornstein, M. H. (2000). Contemporary research on parenting: The case for nature and nurture. *American Psychologist, 55,* 218–232.

Conger, R. D., & Elder, G. H. (1994). *Families in troubled times: Adapting to change in rural America.* Hawthorn, NY: Aldine.

Deater-Deckard, K. (2000). Parenting and child behavioral adjustment in early childhood: A quantitative genetic approach to studying family processes. *Child Development, 71*(2), 468–484.

Deater-Deckard, K., & O'Connor, T. G. (2000). Parent–child mutuality in early childhood: Two behavioral genetic studies. *Developmental Psychology, 36*(5), 561–570.

Deater-Deckard, K., Pike, A., Petrill, S. A., Cutting, A. L., Hughes, C., & O'Connor, T. G. (2001). Nonshared environmental processes in socio-emotional development: An observational study of identical twin differences in the preschool period. *Developmental Science, 4*(2), F1–F6.

Dunn, J., & Plomin, R. (1986). Determinants of maternal behavior towards three-year-old siblings. *British Journal of Developmental Psychology, 4,* 127–137.

Elkins, I. J., McGue, M., & Iacono, W. G. (1997). Genetic and environmental influences on parent–son relationships: Evidence for increasing genetic influence during adolescence. *Developmental Psychology, 33*(2), 351–363.

Ge, X., Conger, R. D., Cadoret, R. J., Neiderhiser, J. M., Yates, W., Troughton, E., & Stewart, M. A. (1996). The developmental interface between nature and nurture: A mutual influence model of child antisocial behavior and parent behaviors. *Developmental Psychology, 32*(4), 574–589.

Harold, G. T., Fincham, F. D., Osborne, L. N., & Conger, R. D. (1997). Mom and Dad are at it again: Adolescent perceptions of marital conflict and adolescent psychological distress. *Developmental Psychology, 33,* 333–350.

Higley, J. D., Thompson, W. T., Champoux, M., Goldman, D., Hasert, M. F., Kraemer, G. W., Scanlan, J. M., Suomi, S. J., & Linnoila, M. (1993). Paternal and maternal genetic and environmental contributions to CSF monoamine metabolites in rhesus monkeys (*Macaca mulatta*). *Archives of General Psychiatry, 50,* 615–623.

Iervolino, A. C., Pike, A., Manke, B., Reiss, D., Hetherington, E. M., & Plomin, R. (2002). Genetic and environmental influences in adolescent peer socialization: Evidence from two genetically sensitive designs. *Child Development, 73,* 162–174.

Jenkins, J. M., Rasbash, J., & O'Connor, T. (2001, April). *Understanding the sources of differential parenting: The role of child and family level effects.* Paper presented at the biennial meeting of the Society for Research in Child Development, Minneapolis, MN.

Kinney, D. K., Holzman, P. S., Jacobsen, B., Jansson, L., Faber, B., Hildebrand, W., Kasell, E., & Zimbalist, M. E. (1997). Thought disorder in schizophrenic and control adopters and their relatives. *Archives of General Psychiatry, 54,* 475–479.

Kochanska, G. (1997). Mutually responsive orientation between mothers and their young children: Implications for early socialization. *Child Development, 68,* 908–923.

Kruesi, M. J. (1989). Cruelty to animals and CSF 5-HIAA. *Psychiatry Research, 28,* 115–116.

Kruesi, M. J., Rapoport, J. L., Hamburder, S., Hibbs, E., Potter, W. Z., Lenane, M., & Brown, G. L. (1990). Cerebrospinal fluid monoamine metabolites, aggression, and impulsivity in disruptive behavior disorders of children and adolescents. *Archives of General Psychiatry, 47,* 419–426.

Linnoila, M., Virkkunen, M., Scheinin, M., Nuutila, A., Rimon, R., & Goodwin, F. K. (1983). Low cerebrospinal fluid 5-hydroxindoleacetic acid concentration differentiates impulsive from nonimpulsive violent behavior. *Life Sciences, 33,* 2609–2614.

Loehlin, J. C., Willerman, L., & Horn, J. M. (1987). Personality resemblance in adoptive families: A 10-year follow-up. *Journal of Personality and Social Psychology, 53,* 961–969.

Lytton, H. (1980). *Parent–child interaction: The socialization process observed in twin and single families.* New York: Plenum Press.

Maccoby, E. E. (2000). Parenting and its effects on children: On reading and misreading behavior genetics. *Annual Review of Psychology, 51,* 1–27.

Manke, B., McGuire, S., Reiss, D., Hetherington, E. M., & Plomin, R. (1995). Genetic contributions to adolescents' extrafamilial social interactions: Teachers, best friends, and peers. *Social Development, 4,* 238–256.

Mann, J. J., Arango, V., & Underwood, M. E. (1990). Serotonin and suicidal behavior. *Annals of the New York Academy of Science, 600,* 476–485.

McCartney, K., Harris, M. J., & Bernieri, F. (1990). Growing up and growing apart: A developmental meta-analysis of twin studies. *Psychological Bulletin, 107*(2), 226–237.

McGuffin, P., Owen, M. J., O'Donovan, M. C., Thapar, A., & Gottesman, I. I. (1994). *Seminars in psychiatric genetics.* London: Gaskell Press.

McHale, S., & Pawletko, T. M. (1992). Differential treatment of siblings in two family contexts. *Child Development, 63*(1), 68–81.

Mehlman, P. T., Higley, J. D., Faucher, I., Lilly, A. A., Taub, D. M., Vickers, J. H., Suomi, S. J., & Linnoila, M. (1994). Low cerebrospinal fluid 5-hydroxindoleacetic acid concentrations are correlated with severe aggression and reduced impulse control in free-ranging primates. *American Journal of Psychiatry, 151,* 1485–1491.

Neiderhiser, J., Reiss, D., & Hetherington, E. M. (1996). Genetically informed designs for distinguishing developmental pathways during adolescence: Responsible and antisocial behavior. *Development and Psychopathology, 8,* 779–791.

Neiderhiser, J. M., Reiss, D., Pedersen, N., Cederblad, M., Hansson, K., Lichtenstein, P., Neiderhiser, J., & Elthammer, O. (submitted). Genetic and environmental influences on mothering of adolescents: A comparison of two samples.

O'Connor, T. G., Deater-Deckard, K., Fulker, D., Rutter, M., & Plomin, R. (1998). Genotype–environment correlations in late childhood and early adolescence: Antisocial behavioral problems and coercive parenting. *Developmental Psychology, 34*(5), 970–981.

Patterson, G. (1982). *Coercive family process: A social learning approach.* Eugene, OR: Castalia.

Patterson, G. R., & Bank, C. L. (1989). Some amplifying mechanisms for pathologic processes in families. In M. R. Gunnar & E. Thelen (Eds.), *Systems and development: The Minnesota Symposia on Child Psychology* (Vol. 22, pp. 167–209). Hillsdale, NJ: Erlbaum.

Pike A., Reiss, D., Hetherington, E. M., & Plomin, R. (1996). Using MZ differences in the search for nonshared environmental effects. *Journal of Child Psychology and Psychiatry, 37*(6), 695–704.

Plomin, R., & Bergeman, C. S. (1991). The nature of nurture: Genetic influence on "environmental" measures. *Behavioral and Brain Sciences, 14*(3), 373–427.

Plomin, R., Chipuer, H. M., & Neiderhiser, J. M. (1994). Behavioral genetic evidence for the importance of nonshared environment. In E. M. Hetherington, D. Reiss, & R. Plomin, (Eds.), *Separate social worlds of siblings: The impact of nonshared environment on development* (pp. 1–31). Hillsdale, NJ: Erlbaum.

Plomin, R., & DeFries, J. C. (1999). The genetics of cognitive abilities and disabilities. In S. J. Ceci & W. M. Williams (Eds.), *The nature–nurture debate: The essential readings: Essential readings in developmental psychology* (pp. 177–195). Malden, MA: Blackwell.

Plomin, R., Reiss, D., Hetherington, E. M., & Howe, G. W. (1994). Nature and nurture: Genetic contributions to measures of the family environment. *Developmental Psychology, 30*(1), 32–43.

Plomin, R., Scheier, M. F., Bergeman, C. S., Pedersen, N. L., Nessleroade, J. R., & McClearn, G. E. (1992). Optimism, pessimism and mental health: A twin/adoption analysis. *Personality and Individual Differences, 13*(8), 921–930.

Reiss, D, Neiderhiser, J. M., Hetherington, E. M., & Plomin, R. (2000). *The relationship code: Deciphering genetic and social influences on adolescent development.* Cambridge, MA: Harvard University Press.

Reiss, D., Pedersen, N., Cederblad, M., Hansson, K., Lichtenstein, P., Neiderhiser, J., & Elthammer, O. (2001). Genetic probes of three theories of maternal adjustment: Universal questions posed to a Swedish sample. *Family Process, 40*(3), 247–259.

Reiss, D., Plomin, R., Hetherington, E. M., Howe, G. W., Rovine, M., Tryon, A., & Hagan, M. S. (1994). The separate worlds of teenage siblings: An introduction to the study of the nonshared environment and adolescent development. In E. M. Hetherington, D. Reiss, & R. Plomin (Eds.), *Separate social worlds of siblings: The impact of nonshared environment on development* (pp. 63–109). Hillsdale, NJ: Erlbaum.

Rende, R. D., Slomkowski, C. L., Stocker, C., Fulker, D. W., & Plomin, R. (1992). Genetic and environmental influences on maternal and sibling interaction in middle childhood: A sibling adoption study. *Developmental Psychology, 28,* 484–490.

Rowe, D. C., Woulbroun, J., & Gulley, B. L. (1994). Peers and friends as nonshared environmental influences. In E. M. Hetherington, D. Reiss, & R. Plomin (Eds.), *Separate social worlds of siblings: The impact of nonshared environment on development.* Hillsdale, NJ: Erlbaum.

Scarr, S., & McCartney, K. (1983). How people make their own environments: A theory of genotype–environment effects. *Child Development, 54,* 424–435.

Scarr, S., & Weinberg, R. A. (1983). The Minnesota Adoption Studies: Genetic differences and malleability. *Child Development, 54,* 260–267.

Spotts, E. L., Neiderhiser, J. M., Towers, H., Hansson, K., Lichtenstein, P., Cederblad, M., Pedersen, N. L., Elthammar, & Reiss, D. (submitted). Genetic and environmental influences on marital relationships. *Journal of Family Psychology.*

Stocker, C., & Dunn, J. (1994). Sibling relationships in childhood and adolescence. In J. C. DeFries, R. Plomin, & D. W. Fulker (Eds.), *Nature and nurture during middle childhood* (pp. 214–232). Oxford, UK, Cambridge, MA: Blackwell.

Stocker, C. M., Lanthier, R. P., & Furman, W. (1997). Sibling relationships in early adulthood. *Journal of Family Psychology, 11*(2), 210–221.

Stocker, C. M., & Youngblade, L. (1999). Marital conflict and parental hostility: Links with children's sibling and peer relationships. *Journal of Family Psychology, 13*(4), 598–609.

Suomi, S. (2000). A biobehavioral perspective on developmental psychopathology: Excessive aggression and serotonergic dysfunction in monkeys. In A. J. Sameroff, M. Lewis, & S. M. Miller (Eds.), *Handbook of developmental psychopathology* (2nd ed., pp. 237–256). New York: Kluwer Academic/Plenum Press.

Tienari, P., Wynne, L. C., Moring, J., Lahti, I., Naarala, M., Sorri, A., Wahlberg, K. E., Saarento, O., Seitma, M., Kaleva, M., & Lasky, K. (1994). The Finnish adoptive family study of schizophrenia: Implications for family research. *British Journal of Psychiatry, 23*(Suppl. 164), 20–26.

Towers, H., Spotts, E. L., Neiderhiser, J. M., Hansson, K., Lichtenstein, P., Cederblad, M., Pedersen, N. L., Elthammar, O. & Reiss, D. (in preparation). Children as a source of nonshared environmental variation in mothers' parenting.

Tsuang, M. T., Stone, W. S., & Faraone, S. V. (2001). Genes, environment and schizophrenia. *British Journal of Psychiatry, 178*(Suppl. 40), S18–S24.

Turkheimer, E. (2000). Three laws of behavior genetics and what they mean. *Current Directions in Psychological Science, 9*(5), 160–164.

Turkheimer, E., Haley, A., Waldron, M., D'Onofrio, B., & Gottesman, I. I. (submitted). Socioeconomic status modifies heritability of IQ in young children. *Psychological Science.*

Turkheimer, E., & Waldron, M. (2000). Nonshared environment: A theoretical, methodological, and quantitative review. *Psychological Bulletin, 126*(1), 78–108.

van den Boom, D. C. (1994). The influence of temperament and mothering on attachment and exploration: An experimental manipulation of sensitive responsiveness among lower-class mothers with irritable infants. *Child Development, 65*(5), 1457–1477.

van Os, J., Park, S. B. G., & Jones, P. B. (2001). Neuroticism, life events and mental health: Evidence for person–environment correlation. *British Journal of Psychiatry, 178*(Suppl. 40), S72–S77.

Volling, B. L., & Belsky, J. (1992). The contributions of mother–child and father–child relationships to the quality of sibling interaction: A longitudinal study. *Child Development, 63*, 1209–1222.

PART VI

Social Policy Perspectives: Social Constructions of Family Health

CHAPTER 23

FAMILY POLICY

Dilemmas, Controversies, and Opportunities

Ann Hartman

To embark on an examination of family policy is to be cast adrift in a sea of conflicting and strongly held moral and value positions. It is understandable that this should be the case. Public policy consists of often strongly contested values and preferences translated into law and program through the political process. It has enormous power to reward and punish, to encourage and prohibit, to shape behavior and exert control. When this power and intimate, private, human relationships meet, the impact can be enormous. It is at that intersection that family policy comes into being, implicitly, if not explicitly.

It would seem that the controversy around family policy has become increasingly intense in the last decade. Although both political parties embraced "the family" in the 1992 and 1996 elections, by 2000, there was almost complete silence on the subject. It is possible that by then, political pundits advised that issues around the family were so controversial, and positions on the right and the left were so inconsistent and conflicting, that taking almost any specific stance on the family was a no-win proposition.

Family policy is controversial because imbedded in it are a number of value and ideological issues that sharply divide America. These issues have locked Americans into intense, even at times violent struggles, and have undermined the rather naive notion that flourished two decades ago: that the government could simply pass laws and develop programs to "support families." The issues are expressed in the following questions:

1. How is the family to be defined? Are some family forms to be pre-ferred or privileged over other family forms?
2. What is the nature of the family–state relationship? To what extent is "family business" the business of the state?
3. To what extent is the government responsible for the welfare of the people?

These are not easy questions, and they lead one to think that perhaps Joseph Barbaro (1979) was right when he took a strong and lonely posi-tion against family policy over 20 years ago. In the midst of the enthusiastic acceptance of the idea that social policies should be focused on the family, he took the position that policies specifically directed at the family are anathema in a free society. He was not only concerned that many people whose life arrangements fell outside of the desired definition of the family would be excluded and discriminated against but also that policies could be used to proscribe and control behavior in this very private part of human life. These concerns, as demonstrated in the following pages, were well founded. Support grows for the use of family policy to shape behavior and define family life.

In this chapter, I attempt to navigate the stormy sea of controversy surrounding family policy. But first, it may be useful to try to define family policy, a task that has been revisited time and time again by policy experts. Then, some of the major subtexts of family policy are explored. Finally, I discuss a few major areas of family policy and examine value conflicts and underlying agendas.

WHAT IS FAMILY POLICY?

Clearly, most laws and programs enacted by federal, state, and local gov-ernments have impact on families, whether these enactments and actions focus on economic, military, agricultural, medical, or social matters. All areas of government action have some direct or indirect effect on social well-being, social structures, and quality of life. Does this mean that all pol-icy is family policy? If we took that position, we would be overwhelmed by the complexities of our enormous bureaucracy and lose the family. Per-haps Kahn and Kamerman's (1978) old distinction is still the most useful. They clearly separate explicit policies designed to achieve specific goals re-garding families from those policies not intended to affect families but that nonetheless have consequences for families. There has been growing awareness of the indirect influence of government policy on family life. The Family Impact Seminars were developed in the 1970s to focus on the effect of public policy on families, and both Presidents Reagan and Clin-ton, through executive order, required that family impact assessments be performed on any federal initiative. These actions attempted to encourage "a family perspective" in policymaking. In this chapter, however, I limit our focus to those policies specifically related to family life, to "family business." These enactment's and programs may emanate from federal, state, or local governments, and from executive, legislative, or judicial bodies, although my focus here is primarily but not exclusively on federal policy.

DEFINING THE FAMILY

One of the most potentially oppressive prerogatives is the ability to define others, to establish the nature of reality, to characterize identities, and to identify desirable statuses, which include some and exclude others. One such prerogative, that of defining the American family, constitutes a major subtext in family policy.

The State has had a monopoly on defining the family, encoding various values and beliefs in enactments and procedures at every level of government. Perhaps the most common and one of the broadest descriptions is that used by the Bureau of the Census, which defines the family as two or more people living together and connected by blood, marriage, or adoption. Clearly, even this fairly broad definition excludes many families. This is not a minor or purely semantic issue. The word "family" appears over 2,000 times in the United States Code, as well as in the various states' codes. For example, "family" appears over 2,000 times in the New York Code, and over 4,000 times in the California Code. In any family policy, those who are defined as family are included in entitlements and services. Others that fall outside the definition are not only marginalized and ineligible for entitlements but also their relationships are disqualified.

Not only are some family arrangements recognized and others ignored but also even within the accepted definitions of family and kinship, some relationships are preferred or privileged over others. An amazing example of this is the Supreme Court's unaccountable decision that permitted illegitimate as well as legitimate children to recover inheritance for the wrongful death of their mother (*Levy v. Louisiana,* 1968) but permitted states to limit the out-of-wedlock children's right to inherit from their father (*Lalli v. Lalli,* 1978)! Adoption law and policy provide another example. Laws in most states privilege the relationship through adoption over the biological relationship, closing adoption records and making it illegal to give either adoptees or birth parents identifying information.

Exclusionary and privileged definitions of the family, however, are being challenged. Adoptees and birth parents are pressing for open adoption records and slowly, state by state, they are having some success. Gay and lesbian advocates have assumed major leadership in the struggle to expand the definition of the family with both success and failure as local, state, and federal lawmakers have responded to this issue and as cases challenging the marginalized status of gay and lesbian families are being heard in courts throughout the nation. In 1989, in a groundbreaking opinion, New York State's highest court found that a longtime partner of a man who had died could retain the lease on a rent-controlled apartment they had shared—a right that had been limited to cohabiting family members. The court, in this historic decision, cited the lived experience of the people involved, stating that the government's proper definition of the family should not "rest on fictitious legal distinctions or genetic history, but instead *should find its foundation in the reality of family life*" (*Braschi v. Stahl Associates*, 1989; emphasis added).

Since that time, other concrete steps have been taken that recognize gay and lesbian families. Registration of domestic partnership has become available in many communities; the provision of health insurance and other spousal benefits to same-sex partners has been widely instituted by companies, municipalities, and educational institutions. Courts have taken action in a variety of cases concerning employee benefits, coparent adoption, bereavement leave, visitation rights, and so on. All of these cases turn around the key issue, the definition of the family, asking whether same-sex domestic partners have the same rights as married heterosexual partners. The response to this question varies from state to state, court to court, and case to case.

The most dramatic example of the struggle over family definition has been the failed effort in Hawaii to legalize marriage between same-sex partners. In 1996, it looked as if same-sex marriage might become law in Hawaii. This so panicked members of the U.S. Congress that they rushed to pass a major and clearly unconstitutional piece of "family policy" legislation, the Defense of Marriage Act. Subsequently signed into law by "gay-friendly" President Clinton, this legislation not only defined marriage as a union between one man and one woman and denied Social Security benefits to same-sex couples, but it also stipulated that no state was required to recognize a same-sex marriage performed in another state.

The State of Vermont's passage of a Civil Union Law was another major step in broadening the definition of the family. Under this statute, those who commit to a civil union have many of the same rights, privileges, and responsibilities as do married couples. Initially, there was considerable backlash as "Take Back Vermont" signs appeared in charming, white clapboard villages. In time, however, frightened Vermonters discovered that nothing catastrophic happened, and the signs began to disappear. Although the effort to legalize same-sex marriage failed, the effort changed the boundaries of the possible. Whereas 10 years ago the idea of civil union would have been shocking, today it seems to many like a rather modest request!

Despite the fact that there has been some rather remarkable movement toward expansion of the definition of the family, a powerful backlash is growing apace. A proposed 28th Amendment to the Constitution was announced on July 2001, by a group of conservative scholars and religious leaders. This amendment would not only limit marriage to a bond between a man and a woman, but it would also deny "legal incidents" of marriage to anyone else. This means that local or state statutes allowing unmarried partners of either sex to share health plans, leases, pensions, hospital visits, or adoption of each other's children would be nullified. Although the advocates for this amendment have set a 10-year goal for the success of their campaign, the effort to institute this kind of discrimination should alarm all Americans, because gays and lesbians are canaries in the coal mine when it comes to civil rights (Goldstein, 2001).

The backlash is evident in more immediate ways, as will be obvious throughout this chapter. At this point, the major thrust in family policy is not toward the acceptance and support of diverse families but toward the development of policies that privilege a particular model of the nuclear family and seek to shape behavior by punishing those who live differently (see Walsh, Chapter 1, this volume).

THE BOUNDARY BETWEEN
THE STATE AND THE FAMILY

The second subtext of family policy discourse concerns the extent to which, and under what circumstances, the State shall enter family life. The family–State relationship is clearly crucial to family policy, and an examination of the transactions at the boundary between the family and the State, and the nature of the State's excursions across that boundary, explicates that relationship.

These boundary definitions and decisions are again value-based. Several cherished American beliefs give direction to the State regarding family relationship. Paramount is the view, a clarion call of patriarchy, that "a man's home is his castle." This powerful metaphor defines the family as surrounded by impenetrable walls and stipulates that within the walls of the family, man is king.

Slowly, over the years, the State has put limits on family inviolability, particularly in regard to the protection of children. The State may, and does, enter and even dismember a family on behalf of abused or neglected children. It has been less ready to intervene in the marital relationship. For example, the landmark decision that strengthened the boundary between the family and the State, *Griswold v. Connecticut* (1965), protected couples' privacy and began to protect reproductive rights by establishing that it is unconstitutional for a state to make the possession or use of contraceptives by married couples a criminal offense.

The State has also been slow to intervene in the marital relationship to protect abused and battered wives, although finally, in 1994, with the passage of the Violence Against Women Act, it increased money for services to abused women and established a national domestic violence hotline. People on both the right and the left hold inconsistent views on the State's intrusion into family life. Those on the right favor intruding into family life through the prohibition of abortion and the sharp curtailment of reproductive rights. They also favor prayer in the schools, whereby the State intrudes in the family's socialization role. On the other hand, they oppose sex education in the schools as a usurpation of family authority and have generally taken a position against State intervention to protect women from their husband's violence. Those on the left take equally inconsistent positions, favoring reproductive rights and the separation of religion and the State, but supporting the entry of the State into the family for the protection of women and sex education in the schools.

THE MARRIAGE MOVEMENT

The current push to promote marriage through use of the power of the State is a dramatic intrusion across the family–State boundary. Although political conservatives have been generally opposed to the expansion of the State's role in family life, alarm over divorce and the high proportion of single-parent–headed families in our nation has led to the growing "marriage movement." Marriage has become touted as the solution to poverty, delinquency, and substance abuse. The Heritage Foundation urged President Bush to set up an office of marriage to create a "marriage-friendly" bureaucracy.

How ready are the Congress or the states to move aggressively in this direction? Although the Welfare Reform Act of 1996 allowed states to use welfare funds to encourage marriage, only four states made use of this opportunity. Recently, however, there has been more effort to develop policies to encourage marriage, particularly for people on welfare, as will be explored later.

The "marriage movement" is not just directed at the poor. Three states have passed covenant marriage laws that bar divorce except under extreme circumstances, and require premarital and predivorce counseling and a waiting period of up to 2½ years should a couple wish to divorce on a "no-fault" basis. For the most part, the idea of covenant marriage, supported primarily by evangelical Christian groups, has not been enthusiastically received. Several states have considered this legislation and rejected it, and in states where covenant marriage is available, very few couples have made this choice.

States are also getting into "divorce prevention." Oklahoma is using $10 million of its Temporary Assistance to Needy Families (TANF) grant to develop community-based marriage-strengthening programs in cooperation with religious leaders and to train people to teach marriage skills courses (Peterson, 2000). Arizona has published a free "Healthy Marriage Handbook" and is offering a voluntary program of workshops to teach effective communication and conflict resolution. Utah and Wisconsin have also initiated TANF-financed marriage-strengthening programs. These programs have been controversial, with critics questioning the State's intrusion into this very personal area and expressing concern about the weakening boundary between church and State. Some also feel that the TANF money should be exclusively devoted to welfare for people in poverty.

The marriage movement, however, although slow in being translated into public policy, has been very successful in capturing the media and influencing discourse about families, blaming "family breakdown" for all of our social ills and publishing research, some of which is highly suspect, that predicts dire outcomes from divorce and for children raised in any way other than a family headed by a married heterosexual couple (Wallerstein, Blakeslee, & Lewis, 2001). A recent longitudinal study has challenged these negative accounts (Hetherington & Kelly, 2002).

Finally, in terms of the state's intrusions into family life, I must add that autonomy and privacy are clearly tied to class. A long tradition in the United States makes it not only permissible but desirable for the State to enter a family's life, if that family requires financial aid. It was believed that such aid should be contingent and structured in such a way as to manipulate the family's behavior and to "rehabilitate." In the 1960s, personal services were separated from income maintenance in an attempt to end the practice of using money to manipulate welfare recipients' behavior. We have now moved in the opposite direction, announcing in the Welfare Reform Act that a primary purpose of financial assistance is to alter the recipient's behavior.

FAMILY–STATE COLLABORATION IN CARING

A third central value position that underlies family policy discussions and legislative decisions concerns the nature of the shared responsibility between the State and the family. The State intervenes in the family not only for order and control but also to meet social need. Robert Moroney, who has studied family–State relationships in England and the United States, writes that "the structure of the welfare state has been shaped by a number of beliefs concerning the responsibilities that families are expected to carry for the care of the socially dependent and a set of conditions under which this responsibility is to be shared or taken over by society"(1980, p. 1).

In the past 25 years, we have witnessed a major shift in the pattern of sharing between the State and the family. Deinstitutionalization in health and mental health care, and permanency planning and family preservation in child welfare programs have all been efforts to meet the needs of dependent populations in the "least restrictive environment," and the family has tended to be considered the most favorable and least restrictive environment. These trends in service provision, strongly supported by progressives and most health care and social welfare professionals, have shifted the care of dependent populations to the family. It was promised that this change would be accompanied by supports for the family and extensive community- and home-based services to help families take on this addition responsibility. Unfortunately, deinstitutionalization was quickly followed by a sharp move to the right, with major cuts in a variety of services for the family and a change in the economic situation, which now often requires that two paid workers maintain a family. Women, who have traditionally provided care, are now in the workplace and suffering considerable conflict over their jobs, their caretaking responsibilities, and their families. What began as a progressive movement toward deinstitutionalization and family-centered services has too often become the State's withdrawal from the task of caring for the dependent, so that the family and the caretakers in the family, usually women, have to do more with less. The extent to which the current political climate is cold toward the support of the family is seen in the struggle even to get a minimum family leave act passed. The continuing shift of State responsibility to the family is dramatically demonstrated in "welfare reform," to which we now turn.

ECONOMIC SECURITY

Economic security is the bedrock upon which all family policy rests. In fact, some believe that if true economic security were guaranteed to all Americans through a strong economy, nondiscriminatory employment practices, education and job training, a universal nonstigmatizing income support plan, and a national health plan, then little other family policy would be required, because individuals and families in all their different forms could meet their needs through the purchase of resources and services. However, currently policymakers are moving away from the universal provision of economic security. Americans have been very reluctant to establish the kind of universal, nonstigmatized family support available in most advanced industrialized nations. Again, we see the powerful operation of deeply held values shaping social policy. American culture has never been fully liberated from the Puritan views of its founders. We see in modern language in our welfare policy the Puritan conviction that poverty is a great affliction and sin is its cause, that all work is sanctified, and that charity is the cause, not the cure, of poverty. These convictions, often unspoken, have found their most complete expression in the Welfare Reform Act of 1996.

What, then, is the current economic situation for American families? America has been going through two revolutions that have wrought major changes in the economic life of the nation. First, there has been major revolution in our economic system. The move to a postindustrial global economy produced an extraordinary economic boom but did not bring economic security to most American families. The result of the boom has been the widening of the gap between the very rich and the rest of the population. Most of the enormous wealth accumulated in the 1990s went to the very rich. "Forty percent of the total real income between 1983 and 1998 went to the top 1 percent of income recipients, 42 percent went to the next 19 percent and 12 percent accrued to the to the bottom 80 percent"(Stille, 2001, p. 1). The income of working families remained relatively static. Most American families have fought the downward drift by becoming two-worker families. Most single parents must struggle to survive on one paycheck. The one exception to this income depletion has been at the lower end of the spectrum, as the tightening of the labor market and the increase in the minimum wage has led to some improvement in the wages of the lowest paid workers.

The pressures faced by American families are enormous. The cost of medical care, day care for children while their parents work, and decent housing stretches most families. The cost of a college education, the surest predictor of income in the complex technological labor market, has escalated. Many families are without medical insurance or are covered only marginally. Job security is a thing of the past. Labor unions that once offered workers protection are considerably weakened. Large firms have shown a profit by drastically downsizing, without regard for seniority or company loyalty. Unemployment insurance offers a buffer in the face of unstable employment, but this resource is limited in terms of both amount and length of time available. In the meantime, Americans are encouraged to spend for the sake of our consumer-driven economy, and many do, accumulating enormous debt. With the slowing of the economy, the repayment of consumer debt will become more and more difficult.

The second revolution that has occurred over the past two decades has been the steady dismantling of the social and economic support programs so laboriously constructed since the passage of the social welfare legislation in the Roosevelt administration. This trend was most dramatically demonstrated in the abolishment of Aid to Families with Dependent Children and the passage of "welfare reform," with its clear and very specific repudiation of the principle of "entitlement," its abandonment of the commitment that every American is *entitled* to economic support if in need. The "safety net" is gone, and the responsibility for the welfare of the citizenry has been shifted to the states.

WELFARE REFORM

In the Welfare Reform Bill, the extent to which social and family policy expresses value positions is clearly demonstrated. The introductory section of the bill includes "findings," "facts" that state the ideological basis of the legislation, echoing the convictions of those in the marriage movement. The first three "findings" set the tone:

1. Marriage is the foundation of a successful society.
2. Marriage is an essential institution in a successful society, which promotes the interests of children.
3. Promotion of responsible fatherhood and motherhood is integral to successful child rearing and the well-being of children (Zuckerman, 2000).

The Personal Responsibility and Work Opportunity Reconciliation Act (PRWORA), which became law in 1996, had three major objectives. First, it was primarily designed to cut benefits and spending on low-income programs. For example, it sharply limited legal immigrants' and disabled children's access to public benefits and reduced the Food Stamp Program.

Second, not only did the bill eliminate the federal entitlements, but it also did not require the states to provide any financial aid. It gave the states unprecedented discretion over the design and administration of welfare monies and froze the size of the block grants to 1994 or 1995 allocations, ending open-ended federal funding.

Third, the federal agenda was clearly and specifically to change peoples' behavior and to use federal money, funneled through the states for an experiment in social engineering to change the supposed "culture of welfare." These objectives were to be met through the program at the heart of PROWRA, TANF, the replacement for AFDC. In section 401 of the bill (H.R. 3734), the purposes are clearly stated.

(a) IN GENERAL—The purpose of this part is to increase the flexibility of the states in operating a program designed to
  (1) provide assistance to needy families so that children may be cared for in their own homes or in the homes of relatives;
  (2) end the dependence of needy parents on government benefits by promoting job preparation, work, and marriage;
  (3) prevent and reduce the incidence of out-of-wedlock pregnancies and establish annual numerical goals for preventing and reducing the incidence of these pregnancies; and
  (4) encourage the formation and maintenance of two parent families. (H.R. 3734: Personal Responsibility and Work Opportunity Reconciliation Act of 1996)

The state plans, although they may vary a great deal, must conform in certain ways to achieve the stated goals. First, states must require that parents and caretakers receiving assistance engage in work or work-related activities within 2 years or less. Second, they must develop a plan and take action to reduce out-of-wedlock pregnancies. States that are successful in reducing such pregnancies receive a bonus of $20–25 million. Third, the states must conduct a program designed to reach law enforcement officials, educators, and relevant counseling services to provide education and training in the area of statutory rape, so that teenage pregnancy-prevention programs may be expanded in scope to include men. Finally, no family shall receive assistance for more than 5 years in total.

President Clinton and the Democratic leadership were opposed to some of the more draconian rulings in the act, and over the next few years, some adjustments were made.

What Has Been the Impact of Welfare Reform?

Congress must revisit TANF in 2002 for reauthorization, and discussions have been heated about what should be done. It is almost impossible to know what the impact of welfare reform has been, because the unprecedented boom of the 1990s came into being at the same time. Furthermore, each state has developed different plans, and to evaluate the programs nationwide is an impossibility. There are, however, some certainties. Since the passage of the bill, there has been a marked decrease in welfare rolls and in expenditures for welfare. When the law passed, 4.4 million families were receiving assistance. By the end of 1999, that number had been cut to 2.4 million. The percentage of poor single mothers who received welfare benefits in the paid workforce grew from 39% in 1994 to 57% in 1999. It is clear that two of the objectives of the bill have been achieved. People have left welfare and entered the paid labor force. The question is, was this welfare reform or the booming economy? All those who extol the virtues of the bill deny that it is the economy, whereas its critics take the opposite position.

People have been encouraged or forced off welfare and into work. Most states adopted the federal limit of 5 years for receipt of benefits, although 20 states adopted shorter time limits. In two-thirds of the states, assistance could be cut off for noncompliance with the work requirements. In most states, the opportunity for training and education was sharply restricted, and most people who left welfare entered low-skill and poorly paid jobs. Most states extended some supports to families after they entered the workforce. Reports are now being made available on how those who left welfare have fared. Most are earning at or slightly above minimum wage in intermittent employment, and although they may have more cash income, their expenses are higher (transportation, child care, etc.) and they have often lost food stamps and other benefits. The legislation seems to have moved people in poverty on welfare to become members of the working poor (Loprest, 1999, 2001). And, we must remember, this was during of time of economic boom. As the economy slows, we will perhaps have a better test of welfare reform. A recent study released by the Economic Policy Institute reports that the areas in which most of those who left welfare obtained jobs—retail trade, restaurants, personnel supply, and hotels and other lodging—have been hardest hit by the recent slowdown. Furthermore, those who left welfare for work are often the last hired and thus the first fired (Boushey, 2001). There is grave concern about what will happen to these unemployed ex-welfare recipients when they attempt to return for public assistance. As the 5-year limit for any kind of assistance approaches, there are still over 2 million families on welfare. Are they simply to be cut off?

TANF has been less successful in achieving its goal of changing the "culture of welfare." The "illegitimacy bonus" offered to states that have been the most successful in reducing rates of births to unmarried parents has been awarded to states with miniscule reductions. For example, Michigan received $25 million for a reduction of .009% from 1996 to 1999. Alabama was rewarded with a .249% reduction. The only credible change was in the District of Columbia, where out-of-wedlock births were reduced by 3.976% (Solot & Miller, 2002).

The effort to encourage or support marriage has also been minimal, with only four states shifting TANF funds to marriage programs. However, with the change in the Administration, the idea that marriage is the solution to poverty has been more enthusiastically accepted, and there is a strong push to make marriage incentives a requirement in the reauthorization of TANF. West Virginia is already offering an additional $100 per month assistance to recipients who will marry. The Health and Human Services Assistant Secretary for Family Support has advocated preferential treatment of married couples in the allocation of benefits. In the 2003 budget proposal sent to Congress, President Bush shifts $100 million of the funds for the "illegitimacy bonus" to pay for experimental programs aimed at getting single parents to marry (Graves, 2002).

To Reform Welfare Reform

The reauthorization of welfare reform is an excellent opportunity to reform welfare reform, although in the current political climate, it seems unlikely that a progressive bill will be enacted. What would truly reformed welfare reform look like? First, concerning the move from welfare to work, almost all agree that this is an important and useful policy position, at least for women with school-age children. Work not only provides economic support but also social contact, social place, and a sense of being a part of this very work-centered culture. Almost all of those who left welfare have stated that they would not want to go back on welfare even if they could. They prefer to work. However, as reported earlier, many of the jobs are low-skill, low-paid jobs. If we are serious about moving people permanently into the workforce, training and education must be made available. Without an upgrading of skills, former welfare recipients will continue to labor for little pay in insecure and often deadening jobs, with little opportunity for advancement. Second, other family supports must be strengthened to make work viable: Health care, paid family medical leave, and day care are essential.

There appears to be voter support for the reform of welfare reform and for addressing inequality. In a review of a number of polls, it appeared that although Americans were divided on the causes of poverty, they agreed that work should be the cornerstone of antipoverty efforts. However, they also felt that individual effort is not enough to erase economic insecurity and supported policies that would enable work and supplement earnings. Ninety percent said that society should do whatever is necessary to make sure that everyone has equal opportunities. Americans believe in work, but fairness is also a very cherished value (New Opportunities: Overview and Summary, 2001). Although there seems to be public support for reforming the welfare system, it seems unlikely in the current political and economic climate that the 2002 reauthorization will include progressive change.

WORK AND THE FAMILY

Women entering the paid workforce have created a major social revolution that has totally changed American families' participation in the workforce. In the United States, 99% of women will work for pay at some time in their lives (Facts about Working Women, n.d.). In 2000, in only 29.2% of married couples with children under 18 was the father employed and the mother at home. In 64.2% of these families, both parents were in the workforce. The proportion of all married couples, with or without minor children, in which only the husband worked was 19.2%. The employment rate for unmarried mothers with children under 18 was 78.9%, an increase of 11.6% since 1994, whereas the rate for married mothers was unchanged. This may well be the impact of the welfare to work policies. Of particular interest are mothers with very young children. Labor force participation for unmarried mothers with children under 1 year old was 58%, an increase of 13% since 1994. The overall rate of mothers in the workforce with infants has declined from 59 to 55% in the past 2 years. The decline has occurred among mothers who are white, married, and living with their husbands, age 30 or more, and have completed at least 1 year of college. (U.S. Bureau of Labor Statistics, 2001)

Women go out to work for two reasons, the first being economic necessity. Because the real value of wages has deteriorated over the last two decades, it frequently takes two incomes to maintain a family. Second, many women want to go to work to acquire and use knowledge and skills, to be participating actors in the world outside the home, to earn an income that decreases their dependency on others, and to establish a social place and a network of friends and colleagues.

This major change in American family life has significant implications for family policy. However, neither governmental policy nor employers have kept abreast of this major revolution or made the adjustments required by such a fundamental change in our socioeconomic system. Employers and governmental bodies, for the most part, continue to operate as if only fathers are at work, and mothers are at home providing full-time care to children, elders, and other dependent family members (Levitan & Gallo, 1990). This is causing considerable strain for the working people caught between the demands of family and job. And not only do workers and their families suffer, but employers are also faced with high rates of absenteeism and turnover, and with worried and distracted employees unable to function at an optimal level. Some firms have learned how expensive chronic work–family conflict is for their operation and have become more sensitive to family needs, establishing some positive initiatives to reduce this conflict, such as information and referral services, employee assistance programs, family leave guarantees, child care, and elder care support. However, there are reports that even when these supports are available, there is subtle pressure not to take advantage of them.

The recommendation that a married couple with children work only a total of 60 hours out of the home has been enthusiastically adopted by several groups concerned about the state of the American family and the welfare of children (Combined 60-Hour Workweek, 2001). The problem with such a recommendation is that the split would in all likelihood be 40 hours for the man and 20 for the woman. This is already a solution for many families, because many women are working part-time. This often, however, condemns women to low-paying jobs, poor benefits, and ineligibility for advancement (Kim, 2000).

In recent decades, benefit packages, including employer-provided and government-managed provisions, have become an increasingly important part of compensation, until they now represent 30% of worker's actual pay. For the most part, they continue to be based on the family of former times—the father in the workplace, the mother at home with children. This means that such benefits tend to be inadequate or redundant and to disadvantage many (Wiatrowski, 1990). For example, if both marital partners are working in situations that include family health benefits as part of compensation, either their coverage is unnecessarily duplicated or one of them elects not to be covered by his or her employer and receives less real compensation than his or her fellow employees. Furthermore, if a limited definition of the family is used in the distribution of benefits, families that fall outside the definition face discrimination and also receive less compensation.

Some employers, responding to the growing diversity in family forms and work lives, are offering cafeteria-style benefit plans that allot to workers a certain amount of money for benefits and allow them to choose among a number of options to create individualized packages that meet their families' needs.

Although some firms are becoming more responsive to families, it is likely that a restructuring of the world of work to become supportive to families will have to come through some sort of governmental intervention—through mandatory regulations or the use of tax breaks, an old and very effective federal strategy to manipulate companies' behavior. Currently, there is little optimism that such changes will take place, until we have a major shift in governmental philosophy or American business and industry learn what most other modern industrialized countries have known for a long time: that secure, unstressed, and supported workers are productive workers.

A minimalist but nonetheless important venture into the regulation of business and industry with the aim supporting the family, the Family and Medical Leave Act, finally became law early in the Clinton Administration, after having been vetoed by President Bush. This act gives workers up to 12 weeks of unpaid, job-protected leave for a serious illness, birth, adoption of a child, or serious illness of a parent or spouse. The measure exempts companies with fewer than 50 workers and also the 10% of the workers in the highest salary range. Family leave benefits are not available to unmarried domestic partners, children not related by birth or adoption, or for the care of ill and aging fictive kin.

The next step in the very halting effort to support families in the workplace is to expand the coverage of the Family and Medical Leave Act and to pay workers on leave. One plan is to make workers on leave eligible for unemployment insurance. The fact that there was such resistance to the minimal initial bill does not make the passage of paid leave very likely.

Other initiatives that could begin to reduce the gap between the world of work and the family are job sharing, flex time, and facilitation of part-time employment rather than penalizing part-time workers in relation to benefits and promotion, pay equity, support for elder care, and child care and family-centered employee assistance programs. Also important is career support that allows women to interrupt their careers to have a family without being penalized. Tax breaks for firms that would institute family-sensitive policies and programs would encourage business and industry to move in this direction and to learn that they, as well as their workers and their families, benefit from such changes. Finally, unpaid work in the home continues to be unrecognized economically in the benefit and Social Security structure. Although clearly an option that has gathered little support, those who are concerned about the economic situation of women have proposed tax credits for homemakers (Schroeder, 1989).

CHILD CARE POLICY

As women have entered the workforce, policies and programs concerning child care have become increasingly important. Value issues, political positions, and economic and welfare reform issues all converge around child care. In part, the question seems to be this: Should women go to work or should they stay home and take care of their children? The answer to this question depends not only on values and political positions but also on the social class and economic situation of the mother involved.

First, what is the federal government's policy concerning child care at this time? There are two different approaches to child care support: One, for the middle class, is a subsidy for child care expenses through Dependent Care Tax Credit; the other is for low-income families, through direct subsidy from federal block grants administered by the states.

In 1996, PRWORA not only changed welfare but also radically altered federal child care policy. First, the separate child care funding streams were consolidated into a single Child Care and Development Block Grant, which includes child care for low-income and welfare families, Head Start, and the 21st Century Learning Centers that grant federal assistance to help schools provide recreational and learning-based activities in a safe place for children after the end of the regular school day.

The amount of money available to the states for child care was expanded through both increasing child care funds and allowing states to transfer TANF funds to child care. In the new law, the states were no longer required to provide child care assistance to families on or transitioning off welfare, and finally, the states were given almost complete discretion over every aspect of providing child care to low-income families. For example, the states determine the eligibility requirements for child care assistance and determine parent's copayment responsibilities. Standards of care are primarily left up to the states, with few requirements remaining in the federal policy (Greenberg, 1998).What has been the result for families and children as a result of this reorganization and these new initiatives?

First, as expected, it depends on where a family lives; the situation varies tremendously from state to state. For example, a study by the General Accounting Office found that in the first year of the program, one state's expenditures went up 62%, whereas in another, expenditures rose only 2%. Eligibility also varies a great deal. Although the government allows states to provide child care assistance to families with annual incomes up to 85% of the state's median income, only four states do so (New Investments in Childcare Needed, 2002). In half of the states, families with annual incomes above $25,000 are ineligible. A number of states are cutting off assistance to families that may be above the poverty line but clearly cannot afford child care. Furthermore, states differ in regard to their demand for copayments, with 40 of the states demanding copayment from families with incomes below the poverty line (Childcare Basics, 2001).

There is considerable difference among states in terms of the standards required of day care providers, the rates the states are willing to pay, and the going salary for day care workers, one predictor of quality of care. In most states, there are few or no training requirements for staff, and with high rates of turnover resulting in part from low pay, on-the-job experience cannot compensate for lack of training.

Finally, with the pressures faced by the states to get women off the welfare rolls and into the workforce, the effort is to get as many children into child care as feasible, for as little expenditure as possible. This means that rates paid to providers are often kept at a minimum and the level of parent copayments is raised.

What, then, is actually happening to low-income families in need of child care? In spite of increased funding, quality, affordable child care continues to be unavailable for most low-income families. In 2000, only 1.5 million of the 9.9 million eligible children were receiving subsidized care (Childcare Basics, 2001). This is not only because of limited resources and unaffordability, but also TANF and other low-income families are often unaware that they are eligible. Child advocates have been working to disseminate information about eligibility. There are also long waiting lists in many states, and preference is given to families on welfare or at risk of becoming financially dependent. Therefore, many families among the working poor must patch together informal child care or spend a large percentage of their limited income for care.

Furthermore, studies indicate that the quality of most care centers ranges from mediocre to poor; many are actually a threat to children's health and development (Childcare Basics, 2001). Afterschool programs are extremely limited, and a Bureau of the Census study found that 7 million children are home alone and unsupervised after school (Childcare Basics, 2001).

The Politics of Child Care

Ambivalence, confusion, and controversy shape child care policy in the United States. First, there is confusion about its purpose. Is its purpose to provide quality developmental care for children or to get mothers off welfare and into the workforce? There are two answers to this in our child care system. The goals of Head Start are clear: to prepare children from low-income families to enter school through a developmental program including education, nutrition, and health care. Head Start is not a program of child care for working parents; the schedules are neither flexible nor extensive enough to meet those needs. There have been arrangements between some Head Start programs and other community resources to offer a program that would cover a parent's working hours, but this is not the usual pattern. On the other hand, the goal of the child care program does not appear to be the provision of a developmental or enriching experience for children but rather to enable their parents to get off welfare and into the workforce. This leads to the question: How is it that some low-income children receive developmental care while others are placed in often-mediocre or even dangerous caretaking situations? Many political issues surface in the child care debate. What should the state's role be in providing services? Should expenditures for social programs be reduced or expanded? Should women be supported in their efforts to join the workforce? Should poor women with very young children be forced to go to work?

As reauthorization of TANF approaches, the progressive agenda is expressed in H.R. 3113, The TANF Re-Authorization Act of 2001, introduced by 31 cosponsors as a reform of welfare reform. In the area of child care, it includes increased funding for child care, the reinstatement of guaranteed child care for TANF recipients, and the continuation of child care for 2 years after a recipient leaves TANF, if income is lower than 250% of the poverty level. The bill also includes protection against sanctions for noncompliance with the work requirements arising from lack of appropriate child care. Finally, for parents on TANF, full-time care for a child under the age of 6 or disabled will be countable as work. In other words, poor women may be supported to remain home to care for preschool-age children (TANF Reauthorization Act of 2001 H.R. 3113 Summary, 2001). It is unlikely that this bill will receive extensive support, but it does provide a position from which to negotiate.

The position of the ultraconservatives and religious right on child care can be found in the publications of the Family Research Council, the Heritage Foundation, and such groups as Concerned Women for America. These organizations take a strong position against any support to help working-class and middle-income women move into the workforce. They particularly target the Dependent Tax Care Credit, which is called a part of the "war against the family." Brian Robertson (2001) of the Family Research Council states that child care tax relief shifted the tax burden to single-income families "who were not only funding a program for which they received no direct benefit but also in effect, funding their own destruction" (p. 1). He claims that most women would choose to stay home and care for their children if they could afford it, and that the increased tax burden has "driven women out of the home to earn." The answer he proposes is tax relief for all families with preschool children. This, of course, would be a "family allowance" that would benefit only those families with good earnings. Families that have little taxable income would receive little or no help. The extent to which the voices from the far right will influence the current Congress and Administration will depend on whether they consider support from the right essential to their maintenance of control of the legislature and the White House.

The recent history of the parties' differences on child care may provide some guidance for the future. The Clinton Administration focused considerable attention on child care and development. These were keen interests of Mrs. Clinton, who became the major villain in the eyes of the child care conservatives. Two White House Conferences were held in the second term, one on child care and one on development. The Clinton agenda was to "help working families pay for childcare, build the supply of good after school programs, improve the safety and quality of care and promote early learning" (Childcare: The Unfinished Agenda and Accomplishments, 1998).

When the Human Services Reauthorization Act was signed in October 1998, Head Start was reaffirmed and funding was increased, although not doubled as the President had wished. Some funds were appropriated for afterschool programs, and money was secured to help start improvement of quality of care. Other key elements of this child care initiative were blocked by the Congress, including increased funding for child care, expansion of child care tax credits to include more families, and the institution of tax breaks for businesses that offer child care assistance to workers.

The Republican-controlled Congress that enthusiastically supported welfare reform and getting poor women out of the home and into the workforce has been less interested in supplying funds to support these efforts and provide quality day care. It has also been reluctant to extend child care tax credit to more families. It would appear, at least for the right wing of the Republican Party, that poor women should go to work, and that in families with more financial resources, mothers should stay home. As discussed in the previous section, a trend in this direction can be identified; the number of working unmarried mothers with infants has risen sharply, whereas more middle-class women with infants are staying home.

HEALTH CARE POLICY

Another crucial family policy issue concerns the delivery of health care to families. Our health care system has been trapped by our inability as a nation to come to terms with the major metapolicy issue in health care delivery. Americans have been unable to "discuss and decide whether basic health care is a social good that is intrinsically related to individual liberty, independence, and equal opportunity and, therefore, a collective obligation or a private good to be left as an individual responsibility" (Shapiro, 1991, p. 6). We are clear on the belief that people have a right to life, at least when no exotic intervention is required to maintain it, but not clear about whether they have a right to health.

Our health care system had been shaped by the changing policy positions of national leadership concerning the collective obligation to provide care. Until the Reagan presidency, the federal government had moved steadily toward assuming more and more responsibility for the health of the nation, particularly for the most vulnerable populations. Medicare, Medicaid, and maternal and child health programs developed and flourished. Hopes were high for some sort of national health plan, and in the 1970s, such plans were brought to the Congress, although none survived.

During the Reagan–Bush administrations, there was a steady reduction in the federal government's involvement in and expenditure on health care. Programs were widely and deeply cut, and the responsibility for financing care steadily shifted to the patient, the family, and to localities. Cost-containment measures and managed care were vigorously instituted. Limited hospital stays shifted the burden of care to families at the same time that the programs that might support families in providing care were reduced or eliminated.

Our national health care policy supported the drift toward privatization and an increasingly market-driven health care system. This Social Darwinian view of the distribution of health care services leads quite dramatically to the survival, not necessarily of the fittest, but of those with the greatest power and command of resources, and the most extensive and generous insurance coverage. The combination of privatization and competition has led to the development of for-profit medical facilities that can cream off the well-insured, high-fee patients, leaving the voluntary hospital, and particularly the public city and county hospitals, to care for those without resources and often the sickest. This competition and neglect has promoted a two- or three-track health care system based on ability to pay.

This raises the controversial issue of the rationing of health care. Many vociferously oppose rationing on moral and ethical grounds, but we are rationing health care now, on the basis of the ability to pay. Somehow we must face the fact that a heroic effort to forestall death in extreme situations "reduces resources available for other forms of life saving and life enhancing measures" (Fischer, cited in Silverman, 1992, p. 151).

The Clintons, with enthusiasm and surprising naivete, took on health care reform in the first year of the President's term with disastrous results. Undoubtedly, they tried to do too much too fast and underestimated the enormous power of the forces organized to maintain control over the vast amounts of money and resources that go into health care every year. Unfortunately, this move may well have made it more difficult to achieve less extensive reforms. In the ensuing 8 years, third-party payers have gained even more power and control, and managed care, usually controlled by insurance companies, often means that the bottom line is dictating medical decisions. Millions of Americans continue to be without insurance, and millions who are insured have little or no choice as to who provides them with care. Interestingly, the specter of loss of choice was used to defeat government insurance plans.

Medicaid and S-CHIP (State Children's Health Insurance Plan) continue to provide states with health-care funds for low-income families. Again, just as with TANF, states have considerable discretion as to how these funds are administered, and each state's plan is unique. Although it is generally assumed that Medicaid provides a safety net for low-income families in terms of health care needs, the fact is that many families in need are ineligible. For example, in more than half the states, a parent in a three-person family, working full time at minimum wage, is considered to have "too much income" to be eligible for Medicaid (Millions of Americans Are Falling through the Health Care Safety Net, 2001).

The Politics of Health Care Delivery

The availability of health care continues to be of great concern to the American public and a very controversial and crucial political matter. One major issue up for discussion concerns ways to empower and protect patients in the increasingly elaborate, bureaucratized, and impersonal health care system. Patients, often having lost the ability to chose their physician and increasingly directed by managed care, have become more and more disempowered, and efforts in Congress to pass a Patient's Bill of Rights, or managed care reform, continue to bog down. In the summer of 2001, a Democratic bill was passed in the Senate and a Republican bill in the House. The bills are quite similar and considerably watered down compared to the one introduced by Democratic leadership and defeated during the Clinton administration. A compromise, however, has not been worked out. One contentious issue revolves around the nature and extent of employers', insurers', and HMOs' liability. There is considerable difference of opinion about patients' or families' right to sue. The Senate bill gives the patient greater possibilities for redress than does the House bill. Furthermore, the Republican bill would override state bills that go beyond the federal allowances in granting protections and redress, whereas the Democratic bill does not, an interesting reversal of Republicans' usual "state's rights" position (Athey, 2002). At issue here is "the right to good health care" and the extent to which the government should intervene to protect the citizenry from the vicissitudes of the marketplace. In the case of medical care, the power differential between the patient and all the actors in the health care industry sharply limits patients' ability to chose, to obtain all the services they need, to leave a service with which they are unhappy, or to seek redress for poor service. The far right, siding with the powerful insurance industry, takes the position that the government is incapable of regulating quality or access to health care, and that government intervention would lead to greater costs, lower quality, and ever-increasing numbers of uninsured persons (Gavora, 1997).

A second approach to the problem of patient disempowerment in the health care system has been to institute the requirement for public disclosure of performance information about health care institutions and providers. Those who favor this approach feel that such requirements would make the system more accountable and give patients and their families more knowledge upon which to base their health care decisions. They also feel it would motivate health care providers to increase self-regulation. Those opposed are concerned about the potential for undermining trust in the professions, restricting access to high-risk procedures, and focusing too much attention on selected performance areas. In this, the Information Age, there is more pressure for disclosure, because people are well aware that knowledge is an essential ingredient of power.

Another current issue is the growing numbers of families losing health care coverage. By November 2001, over 900,000 workers who lost their jobs as unemployment escalated also became uninsured. Discussions are rife concerning how to deal with this growing problem. The Democrats favor government subsidization of the Consolidated Omnibus Budget

Reconciliation Act (COBRA) that keeps health insurance connected with employment. Currently, four out of five people who lose their jobs do not purchase COBRA, which typically costs over $7000 a year for family coverage. The Bush plan, on the other hand, favors the use of individual tax relief for medical insurance costs, and in the long run favors individual responsibility for the maintenance of health insurance rather than employer-based coverage. The tax relief would be limited to premiums for individually purchased coverage. As with any plan that relies on tax breaks, this favors only those with taxable incomes.

The issue of Medicaid coverage continues to surface. Whereas there has been an effort to increase funds and extend eligibility for Medicaid, the Bush Medicaid Policy, Health Insurance Flexibility and Accountability, although giving states the freedom to expand coverage, limits spending of federal funds to the current levels. Again, as we are faced with "guns or butter" choices; in the current atmosphere, it is unlikely that any real improvement in health care coverage will be forthcoming.

Finally, there is continuing concern but a deadlock over legislation dealing with medications for the elderly. As the cost of drugs continues to escalate, many elderly must choose between adequate food and their needed medications. Congress continues to be unable to agree on a way to assume some of this overwhelming burden. Now that the budget surplus has vanished in tax cuts, war expenditures, and a recession, and with a Republican Administration and control of the House, the hope that we may somehow resolve this or other health care delivery problems recedes.

REPRODUCTIVE RIGHTS AND ASSISTED REPRODUCTION

The birth, in 1978, of Louise Brown, the first product of *in vitro* fertilization, and the subsequent rapid development of assisted reproductive technology (ART) have raised major policy questions and demand new ways to think about conception, parenthood, and the family. Currently, the conflict around abortion continues, and questions emerging from ART have far exceeded the nation's ability to formulate consistent policy relating to the ethical, legal, and rights issues involved. Imbedded in reproductive rights and policy controversy are conflicting convictions about when life begins, the fetus's right to life versus the mother's right to control her own body, and parental rights versus the birth mother's right to privacy. ART raises further questions, for example, concerning the establishment of parental identity, the ownership of *in vitro* embryos, and what should happen to unused embryos.

These questions revolve, in part, around the nature of the boundaries between the family and the State. The trend to limit the states' interference in the intimate lives of people began with the Supreme Court decision in 1965 in the case of *Griswold v. Connecticut.* This was followed, in

1973, by *Roe v. Wade,* which made it unconstitutional to prohibit a woman from terminating a pregnancy in the first trimester. Both of these decisions were based on the Bill of Rights and the Fourteenth Amendment, which support the right to privacy of individuals in personal matters.

It must be remembered that such a position guarantees noninterference but not self-determination. Social supports and resources are required for true self-determination. *Roe v. Wade* really won women the right to be left alone. Subsequent legislation has reinforced this. For example in *Harris v. McRae* (1980), the Supreme Court upheld the right of Congress and state legislatures to refuse to pay for abortions for poor women, and in *Rust v. Sullivan* (1991) the Court upheld the right of the government even to refuse support for abortion counseling, information, or referral. This famous gag rule prohibits staff (with the exception of physicians) of medical facilities that receive federal funds from any discussion of abortion.

The current situation means that those with information, access, and resources may achieve reproductive choice. It has become a privilege of the economically secure and enormously burdensome or unattainable for those with limited resources. Not only those with limited resources but also teenagers face constraints in their attempts to terminate a pregnancy. In many states, minors are required to obtain parental consent. The Supreme court has ruled that such laws must include a judicial bypass, that is, that the Court may give permission without parental notification.

Roe v. Wade, a highly controversial decision, demonstrates that social policy enactments can lead but cannot get too far from the sentiments of large groups of American people without generating backlash and consistent efforts to undermine the position. Across the nation, states are passing laws and policies that constrain and limit access to abortion. Furthermore, support has been withdrawn from other means of supporting reproductive self-determination. Funds have been cut for all aspects of family planning and research on contraception. The most recent test of the Supreme Court's position of abortion declared Nebraska's attempt to ban "partial birth abortion" unconstitutional by the slim margin of one vote. A new appointment to the Supreme Court could lead to a reversal of *Roe v. Wade* and drastically limit reproductive choice.

The new issues resulting from ART are many and complex, and courts and legislatures across the country are struggling with them. It is essential that there be clarity about these new technologies. Approximately 75,000 babies are born through ART annually, 60,000 from donor insemination and 1,500 through the use of *in vitro* fertilization. One thousand births are occurring through gestational parenthood each year and the number is growing (Shapiro, Shapiro, & Paret, 2001). The major issue involved is the determination of parenthood. If a child were the product of an embryo from a male and a female donor, carried by a "gestational mother" (formerly called the surrogate mother) and raised by social or "intentional" parents, five people would have some kind of parental relationship to the child. The separation of fertilization from sexual intimacy, and even from the person who will bear the child, raises a number of complicated issues. Policy around parental determination is in the hands of the states and thus differs in different locations.

The National Conference of Commissioners on Uniform State Laws has developed and recommended passage of the Uniform Parentage Act. The major part of the act concerns definitions of and procedures for determining paternity. The financial obligations entailed in paternity may well explain this emphasis, although throughout the ages, issues of determining paternity have been vital and are certainly one reason for the control of women in cultures historically and today.

The law takes up the position of the male or female donor, making it very clear that genetic donors are not the child's legal parents and have neither the rights nor the responsibilities of parenthood. They can make no claim, nor can they be sued for support. As this position becomes accepted in the various states, the clarity has eased some of the anxiety of donors and birth parents, because it offers protection from interference. It is interesting to note that, according to the law, the husband of a wife so inseminated is only the father if he has given his consent. Furthermore, in the case of a single mother, the law makes it clear that the child has no legally recognized father.

The other, even more difficult issue concerns the parentage of a child born of a gestational mother (or surrogate mother). The highly publicized, painful, and bitter struggles that have arisen between gestational and intentional or even genetic mothers have led to efforts to develop policy. At this point, gestational motherhood is dominated by the use of contractual agreements, but there is considerable disagreement about whether this is the correct approach (Capron & Radin, 1994). As of December 2000, 11 states honored such agreements; 6 states voided them, among them New York. Many states have not acted as yet. The model parentage law takes the position that because people will continue this practice, it is important to bring some sort of order out of the chaos, and recommends that contracts should be used. The law outlines the process and the required content for the contractual agreements, including a home study similar to that done in adoption and to ensure reasonable compensation for the gestational mother.

The model law does not deal with many of the other issues raised by ART. For example, the struggle over the ownership and disposition of frozen embryos, highly publicized when a divorcing couple fought over possession, raises complex issues. Also, ART raises to a new level the question of when human life begins. Does it really begin *in vitro,* in the petri dish? The current administration's position sharply limiting the use of discarded embryos for stem cell research implies that it does. This stance has enormous implications for reproductive rights. What then should happen to unneeded embryos? Should they be kept indefinitely? Should they be destroyed? Should they be adopted? The advances in technology have raised questions in family policy that we could not have imagined a short time ago.

FINAL COMMENTS

I would like to conclude this brief journey through the controversial world of family policy with a few comments.

First, family policy is a matter of values that divide the nation. Controversy about the family is on the front lines of the "cultural wars." At this point, it is unlikely that those in power will follow the wisdom of the New York judge who wrote that the definition of the family should find its foundation in the reality of family life (*Braschi v. Stahl,* 1989). Instead, the growing trend seems to be use of family policy to reward certain kinds of families, and disqualify and punish those who do not fit the required definitions—in a sense to deny or attempt to change that reality.

Second, family policy is deeply political. It is about power—the power to make laws, the power to distribute the resources of this wealthy nation. It is also about power in the sense that issues about the family are very much on the agendas of both political parties and an enormous number of advocacy and pressure groups, lobbyists, and "think tanks."

Third, in the current political climate, there appears to be a growing danger that the power of the State will be increasingly used to shape the private lives of the people. The boundaries between private life and the government are being threatened. It is hoped that another treasured American value, individualism, will serve as a bulwark against this threat.

Fourth, it is clear that strong government intervention is needed to protect people against the vicissitudes of capitalism and of the marketplace. As the individual and the family become increasingly disempowered in the face of the global economy and the enormous governmental, economic, and medical bureaucracies, only a strong federal government can provide a framework for protection. However, the extent to which those very systems influence the government through campaign financing, power brokering, and well-supported lobbying leaves one questioning whether such protection can be made available.

Finally, and sadly, it would appear that this nation has abandoned the ethic of care, although the human response to the crisis of September 11, 2001, seemed to belie this. This trend has been increasingly apparent since the end of the Johnson administration and even the administrations of Presidents Carter and Clinton, both of whom embraced the caretaking role of government, were unable to reverse it. As we become deeply involved in the morass of an undefined and at this moment, undeclared, and endless "war," and see our nation's resources being consumed in this war, it seems unlikely that the state will resume its caretaking role.

This trend, however, is reversible. Most Americans believe in fairness and justice, and want to live in a fair and just society. Furthermore, as the income gap becomes more and more evident, and as more people find themselves unable to maintain an adequate lifestyle, pressures will build for change. Family scholars and practitioners must not succumb to hopelessness and helplessness. In times such as these, it is even more important to speak out and take action in the public arena. People with knowledge about and experience with families must bear witness, inform public discourse, counter backlash, reframe debates, and influence public policy in a way that recognizes and respects the broad diversity of families, and responds to their needs in our changing world.

REFERENCES

Athey, J. (n.d.). The patient's bill of rights: Where it will land, nobody knows. Excerpts from *Benefits and Compensation Law Alert.* Retrieved January 28, 2002, from *http://www.hyhero.com/benefits/patients.shtml*

Barbaro, F. (1979). The case against family policy. *Social Work, 24,* 455–457.

Boushey, H. (2001). *Last hired, first fired: Job losses plague former TANF recipients.* Economic Policy Institute Issue Brief No. 171. Retrieved December 22, 2001, from *http://www.epinet. org/Issuebriefs/ib171. html*

Braschi v. Stahl. New York Court of Appeals, July 6, 1989, No. 108. (1989).

Capron, A. M., & Radin, M. (1994). Choosing family law over contract law as a paradigm for surrogate motherhood. In T. Beauchamp & L. Waters (Eds.), *Contemporary issues in bioethics* (4th ed., pp. 258–269). Belmont, CA: Wadsworth.

Childcare basics. (2001, April). Children's Defense Fund. Retrieved December 22, 2001, from *http://www.childrensdefense.org/cc_facts.htm*

Combined 60-hour work week. (2001). *Religion, Culture and Family Project.* Retrieved July 11, 2001, from *Family-Project@uchicago.edu*

Comments on TANF reauthorization. (2001, November 30). Center on budget and policy and priorities. Retrieved January 22, 2002, from *http://www.cbpp.org/11-30-01wel.htm*

Facts about working women. (n.d.). AFL–CIO fact sheet. Retrieved on January 2, 2002 from *http://www.aflcio.org/women/wwfacts.htm*

Gavora, C. L. (1997, November 21). *Congress and consumers beware: The Patient's Bill of Rights is a bill of goods.* Retrieved from the Heritage Foundation December 23, 2001: *http://www.heritage.org/library/catagories/health/fyl164.html*

Goldstein, R. (2001, July 25–31). By amending the Constitution, the right hopes to ban what it can't stop. *The Village Voice,* retrieved August 17, 2001, from *http://www.vil;lagevoice.com/issues/0130/goldstein.php*

Graves, B. (2002,February 5). Bush proposes marriage as a way out of welfare. From *The Oregonian,* retrieved February 6, 2002, from the Council on Contemporary Families: *ccf@listserv.uh.edu*

Greenberg, M. H. (1998). *Childcare policy two years later.* Retrieved on January 17, 2002 from the Center for Law and Social Policy: *http://www.clasp.org/pubs/childcare/childcarepolicyarticle.mhg.htm*

Griswold v. Connecticut. 381 U. S. 479, 486. (1965).

Harris v. McRae. 448 U. S. 297. (1980).

Hetherington, E. M., & Kelly, J. (2002). *For better or for worse: Divorce reconsidered.* New York: Norton.

Kahn, A., & Kamerman, S. (1978). Families and the idea of family policy. In S. B. Kamerman & A. Kahn (Eds.), *Family policy: Government and families in fourteen countries* (pp. 1–16). New York: Columbia University Press.

Kim, M. (2000). Women paid low wages: Who they are and where they work. *Monthly Labor Review, 23*(9), 26–30.

Lalli v. Lalli. 439 U. S. 259. (1978).

Levitan, S., & Gallo, F. (1990). Work and family: The impact of legislation. *Monthly Labor Review, 113,* 34–40.

Levy v. Louisiana. 391 U. S. 68. (1968).

Loprest, P. (1999). How families that left welfare are doing: A national picture. B1 in Series, *New federalism: National survey of American families.* Retrieved from Urban Institute, May 8, 2001: *http://www.newfederalism.urban.org/html/series_b/ anf_b1.html*

Loprest, P. (2001). How families that left welfare are doing? A comparison of early and recent welfare leavers. B36 in Series, *Nee Federalism: National Survey of American Families.* Retrieved May 8, 2001, from *http://www.newfederalism.urban.org/ html/series_b/b36/b36.html*

Moroney, R. (1980). *Families, social services and social policy: The issue of shared responsibility.* Rockville, MD: National Institute of Mental Health.

New investments in childcare needed. (2002). Children's Defense Fund. Retrieved December 22, 2001, from *http://www.childrensdefensefund.org/ cc_basics.htm.*

New opportunities: Overview and summary. (2001). Demos. Retrieved January 26, 2002, from *http://demos_USA.org/pubs/poreport/default.asp?page=pobs/poreport/summary.htm.*

Ortiz, E. T., & Bassoff, B. (1987). Military taps: Emerging military family service roles for social workers. *Employee assistance quarterly, 2*(3), 55–66.

Personal Responsibility and Work Opportunity Reconciliation Act of 1996 (H. R. 3734). Retrieved May 8, 2001, from *http://thomas.loc.gov/cg-bin/query/ D?c104:1:./temp/~c10400LgXrF:e29376:*

Peterson, K. S. (2000, March 23). Oklahoma weds welfare funds to marriage. *USA Today,* National Center for Policy Analysis. Retrieved January 20, 2002, from *http://www.ncpa.org/pd/social/pdo323ooa.html*

Robertson, B. C. (2001, January–February). The politics of childcare: Why daycare subsidies do not help parents or kids. *Family Policy, 14*(1). Retrieved January 2, 2002, from *http://www.frc.org/get/fpo/aa.cfm*

Roe v. Wade. 410 U. S. 113, 153. (1973).

Rust v. Sullivan 500 U. S. 114L. ed. 2nd 233, 111. SCT. (1991).

Schroeder, P. (1989, November). Towards a national family policy. *American Psychologist,* pp. 1410–1413.

Shapiro, H. (1991). Princeton University, Princeton, NJ. Unpublished manuscript.

Shapiro, V., Shapiro, J., & Paret, I. (2001). *Complex adoption and assisted reproductive technologies: A developmental approach to clinical practice.* New York: Guilford Press.

Silverman, E. (1992). Hospital bioethics: A beginning knowledge base for the neonatal social worker. *Social Work, 37*(2), 150–154.

Solot, D., & Miller, M. L. (2002). *Let them eat wedding rings: The role of marriage promotion in welfare reform.* Boston: Alternatives to Marriage Project.

Stille, A. (December 15, 2001). Grounded by an income gap. *The New York Times,* retrieved December 29, 2001, from *http://NYTimes.com/2001*

TANF Reauthorization Act of 2001 (H. R. 3113) Summary. (2001). NOW Legal Defense and Education Fund. Retrieved January 21, 2002, from *http://www.now/def.org/html/issues/wel/tanf_summary.htm*

U.S. Bureau of Labor Statistics. (October 10, 2001). *Labor force participation for mothers with infants declines for the first time.* U.S. Bureau of the Census, U.S. Department of Commerce News, retrieved December 15, 2001, from *http://www.census.gov/press-release/www/2001/cb01–170.html*

Wallerstein, J., Blakeslee, S., & Jewis, J. (2001). *Unexpected legacy of divorce: The 25 year landmark study.* New York: Hyperion Press.

Wiatrowsjki, W. J. (1990). Family related benefits in the workplace. *Monthly Labor Review, 113,* 28–33.

Zuckerman, D. (2000, Winter). Welfare reform in America: A clash of politics and research. *Journal of Social Issues,* pp. 578–599.

INDEX

Index

Health problems (*see* Chronic illness)
Health professionals, family interactions, 483–485
Healthy family
  Beavers Systems Model, 556–563
  characteristics, 556–563
  definition, 6, 7
  limits to, 563
  McMaster Model, 581–607
  sociocultural factor, 6, 7
Help-seeking, family beliefs, 479
Heterosexism
  and religion, 349–351
  and same-sex families, 177, 185
  therapy challenge, 48
Hierarchical issues, family therapy, 32
Hispanics (*see also* Latinos)
  cultural diversity, 16, 17
  gender differences in earnings, 312
  religious preferences, 347
  U.S. census, 246, 247
Historical era effects, 377
Home office workers, 71, 72
Homophobia, 177, 185, 190, 191
Homosexuality (*see* Same-sex families)
Hope, and resilience, 408
Housework
  dual-earner families, 79, 80, 310
    myths, 310
  family connection opportunities in, 84
  gender norms, 305, 308–310
  racial and ethnic differences, 79
  women's perceptions, 80
Humor, in successful marriages, 505
Husbands (*see also* Fathers)
  parenthood transition response, 436, 510, 511
  and power needs, divorce predictor, 502
  retirement adjustment, 601

Ideal family, definition, 6, 7
Identity development
  adolescents, 390
  adoptees, 220, 221
  cultural context, 240, 241
  theoretical models, 382, 383
  transitions, 426
"Illegitimacy bonus," 646
Immigrant families, 280–300
  children, 288–290
  cultural clashes, 237, 238
  "double consciousness" in, 291
  extended families, 286–288
  generational conflicts, 288, 289
  life-cycle transitions, 296, 297
  loss experience, 282–284, 296, 297
  resilience, 285, 286
  rituals, 291–295
  sense of coherence, 285, 286
In vitro fertilization, 657

Income disparities
  married couples, 67
  single-parent families, 123
  socioeconomic classes, 18, 642, 643
Indirect communication, 589, 590
Individualism, "Western" view, 240
Individuation, adoptees, 220, 221
Infant irritability effects, 440
Infertility, and adoption, 212
"Insiders' perspective," 530, 550, 551–554
  (*see also* Self-report scales)
Instrumental problems, 587–589
Interfaith marriage
  complications, 342, 343
  rates and attitudes, 351
Intergenerational relations/conflicts
  contemporary trends, 18, 19
  immigrants, 288, 289
  and parenthood transition, 432, 433
Intermarriage, and cultural patterns, 249
Internalizing behavior
  centripetal families, 553, 565
  in children's school adaptation, 444–446
  family process predictors, 444–446
  parenting interplay, adoption studies, 613
International adoption, 211, 224–226
Intimacy, optimal families, 559, 560
"Invisibility factor," 262
"The invulnerable child," 400
Iranians, family therapy issues, 255, 256
Irish, family therapy issues, 253–255
Italians, family therapy issues, 252–255

Jewish culture, and family therapy, 253–255
Jewish faith
  beliefs, 348, 352
  and interfaith marriage, 343, 351
  and marriage, 343
Job stress (*see* Work stress)
Joint custody, effect on children, 109

Kinship network
  African Americans, 268, 276
  resilience factor, 412
Kosovar Family Professional Educational Collaborative, 418, 419

Lalli v. Lalli, 637
Latinos (*see also* Hispanics)
  collectivist orientation, 289
  definition of, 245
  dual-earner families, 66
  intergenerational relations, 289
Leadership, flexibility levels, 519
Learned optimism, 408
"Least restrictive environment" policy, 641, 642
Legal rights, stepparents, 165